# DICTIONARY OF HEALTH SERVICES MANAGEMENT

Thomas Timmreck, Ph.D.
Editor

NATIONAL HEALTH PUBLISHING
OWINGS MILLS, MD.

# DICTIONARY
# OF
# HEALTH SERVICES
# MANAGEMENT

NATIONAL HEALTH PUBLISHING
ALLIED WITH NATIONAL LAW PUBLISHING
99 PAINTERS MILLS ROAD
OWINGS MILLS, MARYLAND 21117
(301) 363 6400



ISBN—0-932500-11-0

# A

**abandon**
1. To leave or give up entirely, completely and finally. 2. To relinquish one's rights.

**abandonee**
1. The one who is abandoned. 2. The abandoned party. 3. The party to whom a right is abandoned or relinquished by another.

**abandonment**
1. The entire giving up of one's rights, property, or obligations with no intent of reclaiming them. 2. When a person leaves another person having an injury or illness that is considered an emergency without another person taking over and providing care. A patient in an acute care setting can be abandoned if a health care provider quits caring for a patient before they have found a new health care provider to provide care. 3. Children are abandoned if they are deserted and if the intent is permanent.

**abandonor**
The one who does the abandoning.

**ab ante**
1. Prior. 2. Before. 3. To happen or occur in advance.

**ab antiquo**
1. Since olden times. 2. Old rules or ideas. 3. Things that have been that way.

**abatable nuisance**
A nuisance that is easily abated or stopped, or can be permanently enjoined without causing irreparable economic loss.

**abate**
1. To decrease. 2. To put an end to. 3. To diminish. 4. To destroy or end. 5. To lessen or reduce. 6. Stop.

**abduction**
1. Criminally or illegally taking away another person. This could be of concern in health care when this person is under the care of another. 2. Kidnapping.

**aberration**
1. Deviation from normal. 2. Mental illness.

**abet**
1. To encourage. 2. To aid or incite. 3. To order, help or assist a person to commit an illicit act.

**abettor (abetter)**
One who abets.

**abeyance**
1. Temporary inactivity. 2. Supervision of personal property. When there is no one to whom it can be given it is in abeyance until a proper owner appears. 3. To be held in suspension.

**ab inconvenienti (Lat.)**
1. The literal meaning is "From inconvenience". 2. An argument founded upon the hardship of the case and the inconvenience or disastrous consequences which would follow a different course of reasoning.

**ab initio (Lat.)**
1. From its initiation. 2. From its inception. 3. Since the beginning or completely from the beginning.

**abnormal**
1. Deviating from the usual, average or normal. 2. Out of the ordinary.

**abortion**
1. The act of bringing forth or destroying a human fetus before it is capable of maintaining life. 2. Termination of a pregnancy before the fetus has attained viability, i.e. become capable of independent extra-uterine life. Viability is usually defined in terms of the duration of pregnancy, weight of the fetus, and/or, occasionally, the length of the fetus. Viability is usually attained at 28 weeks of gestation, with a fetal weight of approximately 1000 g. This definition is based on the observation that infants below this weight have little chance of survival, while the mortality of infants above 1000 g. declines rapidly. Different types of abortions are distinguished: early—less than twelve completed weeks of gestation; late—more than twelve weeks; induced—caused by deliberate action undertaken with the intention of terminating pregnancy; spontaneous—all abortions other than induced ones. See also stillbirth.

**above cited**
A phrase for "cited or stated earlier in this record".

**abrogate**
1. To repeal. 2. To annul. 3. To abolish. 4. To destroy. 5. To cancel, such as a law.

**abscond**
1. To hide. 2. To leave a jurisdiction in order to avoid legal process. 3. To flee after a wrongdoing. 4. To covertly leave the jurisdiction of a court. 5. To hide in order to avoid legal process.

**absolute right**
A right given to a person which allows uncontrolled dominion over the subject, person or item at all times and for all purposes.

**absque (Lat.)**
Without.

**abstention doctrine**
A doctrine that allows a Federal court to refuse to decide a case, even if it has the power to. A policy of the Federal courts giving a court discretion to decline to exercise its jurisdiction to hear a case.

**abstinence**
Refraining from use of alcohol, drugs, food, sex, etc.

**abstract**
1. A summary. 2. A short overview of a subject with the substance of the document presented. 3. In pharmacy, a drug in two parts, where one part of the abstract is compounded with milk sugar. Abstracts differ from extracts, as abstracts are double strength.

**abstracting**
1. The process of forming a summary. 2. Isolating or separating out of a particular aspect of an object.

**abstraction**
1. The ability to do generalized thinking, form ideas or sort out information. 2. In law, it is the fraudulent taking of money or items of worth.

**abstract of record**
1. A short complete history of a case as found in a record. 2. An abbreviated overview of all the proceedings of a case complete enough to show that questions presented for review by an appellate court have been properly reserved.

**abulia**
1. Lack of ability to make decisions. 2. A lack of will.

**abuse**
1. To use improperly, i.e. abuse of drugs. 2. Sexual molestation of a child or regularly harming a child. 3. To mistreat. 4. To verbally insult another person. 5. To over tax. 6. Misuse of a privilege. 7. Wrongful practice. 8. Improper or excessive use of program benefits, resources or services by either providers or consumers. Abuse can occur, intentionally or unintentionally, when services are used which are excessive or unnecessary; which are not the appropriate treatment for the patient's condition; when cheaper treatment would be as effective; or when billing or charging does not conform to requirements. It should be distinguished from fraud, in which deliberate deceit is used by providers or consumers to obtain payment for services which were not actually delivered or received, or to claim program eligibility. Abuse is not necessarily either intentional or illegal. See also drug dependence.

**abuse of discretion**
Poor, unreasonable or unsound decisions made by an administrator or person in a position of authority.

**abut**
To touch on to, to border, to join up to.

**acarophobia**
The fear of small objects such as spiders and needles.

**acatalepsia**
Lack of ability to comprehend and reason.

**acceleration**
1. To move faster. 2. To shorten the time for performance on a contract. 3. To cause to come sooner.

**acceptability**
1. The acceptability of health care services is a measure of consumer satisfaction with the services they receive, the manner in which the services are delivered, the ease with which services are obtained, and their confidence in the providers of the services. 2. An individual's (or group's) overall assessment of medical care available to him. The individual appraises such things as the cost, quality, results, and convenience of care, and provider attitudes in determining the acceptability of health services provided. See also accessibility and availability.

**acceptance**
1. In contract law it is to agree to be bound by the precise terms of an offer, thereby creating a binding contract. 2. Agreeing to become bound by the terms of a contract. 3. Willingness to pay a negotiable instrument.

**accessibility**
1. Accessibility to health care services refers to the degree to which the system inhibits or facilitates the ability of an individual to gain entry and to receive services. Thus, accessibility includes geographic, architectural, transportation, social, time and financial considerations. 2. A characteristic of a health care system. 3. An individual's (or group's) ability to obtain medical care. Access has geographic, financial, social, ethnic and psychic components and is thus very difficult to define and measure operationally. Many government health programs have as their goal to improve access to care for specific groups or equity of access in the whole population. Access is also a function of the availability of health services, and their acceptability. In practice access, availability and acceptability, which collectively describe health system characteristics, determine the choice and types of health care people use and are very hard to differentiate. See availability, acceptability.

**accessibility of services/facilities**
The ease with which area residents can gain access to the existing health facilities and avail themselves of the services being provided therein. Barriers that impede access to health services and facilities may include factors such as architecture, geography, economics, language, etc. See accessibility.

**accessory**
1. Anything that is joined to, incident to, or part of another thing. 2. Contribution to; aiding. 3. Helping a person commit an illicit act. 4. One who helps a person commit an illegal act.

**accident**
1. An unexpected, unplanned event which may involve injury. 2. An event or occurrence which was unforeseen and unintended. 3. Something done unintentionally. 4. A mishap which lacked intent.

**accidental bodily harm**
In insurance, it is injury to the body of an insured person as a result of an accident.

**accidental death benefit**
Same as double indemnity. See these words.

**accidental injury**
A definite impairment of function or traumatic injury to a body structure resulting from an unexpected outside force or object, occurring without foresight or expectation at an identifiable time and place. Not to be confused with medical emergency.

**accident and health insurance**
1. Insurance which provides benefits which are payable in case of disease, accidental injury, or accidental death. 2. A contract wherein the insurer, in consideration of premiums paid, agrees to pay the insured medical and hospital benefits in case of disease or accidental injury.

**accident prone**
A tendency for a person to have accidents with underlying psychological implications.

**accommodation**
The progress or change of a person's cognitive processes to sufficiently matured level enabling the solving of problems that could not be solved previously.

**accomplice**
One who with intent participates with another in the commission or attempted commission of an illicit act.

**account**
In finance it is a segment of the ledger in which gains and losses are accumulated for separate assets, liabilities, equities, revenues, and expenses. The title of an account is called a chart of accounts.

**accountability**
1. Being held responsible. 2. Responsible for and answering for the expenditure of money and the commitment of resources based on gains or results achieved. Having stewardship over money and other resources, with evaluation of acceptable use judged in relation to the reaching of specified goals.

**accountable**
1. Responsible, liable, explainable. 2. To furnish a justification or detailed explanation of financial activities or responsibilities. 3. To furnish substantial reasons or convincing explanations. Accountability entails an obligation to periodically disclose in adequate detail and consistent form to all directly and indirectly responsible or properly interested parties the

purposes, principles, procedures, relationships, results, incomes, and expenditures involved in any activity, enterprise or assignment so that they can be evaluated by the interested parties. The concept is important in health planning and regulation programs (such as health systems agencies) which should be accountable to the public and those they affect for their actions.

**accounting system**
All of the records, ledgers, and procedures used in recording, retrieving, and reporting financial information, position and operations.

**accounts payable**
1. The money that is owed to others. 2. Liabilities on open account, owed by the facility to other persons or companies for goods furnished and services provided.

**accounts receivable**
1. The money owed to you or your organization, institution or facility. 2. Open account of amounts owed to your company by outside persons or businesses for goods furnished and services provided by your organization.

**accounts receivable turnover**
The net amount of money or billings for a period of time, divided by the average balance of net accounts receivable. The formula is used to determine the effectiveness of collection policies.

**accredit**
The act of officially recognizing or approving something such as a health professional or an institution.

**accreditation**
1. The process by which an agency or organization evaluates and recognizes a program of study or an institution as meeting certain predetermined standards. The recognition is called accreditation. Similar assessment of individuals is called certification. Standards are usually defined in terms of: physical plant, governing body, administration, medical and other staff, and scope and organization of services. Accreditation is usually given by a private organization created for the purpose of assuring the public of quality. (Such as the Joint Commission on Accreditation of Hospitals.) Accreditation standards are not always available to the public. In some situations governments recognize accreditation in lieu of, accept it as the basis of, or require it as a condition of licensure. Public or private payment programs often require accreditation as a condition of payment for covered services. Accreditation may either be permanent once obtained or for a specified period of time. Unlike a license, accreditation is not a condition of lawful practice but is intended as an indication of high quality practice, although where payment is effectively conditioned on accreditation it may have the same effect.

**Accreditation Association For Ambulatory Health Care (AAAHC)**
A non-profit organization extablished to improve the quality of care rendered by ambulatory care organizations. The AAAHC develops

uniform standards for ambulatory health care organizations, provides consultants and educational services. It also conducts voluntary peer on-site reviews and inspections of ambulatory health care facilities.

**accredited**

1. To be officially authorized or vouched for. 2. The verification of having high quality and standards of service. 3. When applied to any program of education, it means a program accredited by a recognized body or bodies, or by a State agency, approved for such purpose by the Commissioner of Education. When applied to a hospital, school, college, or university (or a unit thereof) it means a hospital, school, college, or university (or a unit thereof) which is accredited by a recognized body or bodies, or by a State agency, approved for such purpose by the Commissioner of Education, except that a program, or a hospital, school, college, or university (or unit thereof) which is not, at the time of the application, eligible for accreditation by such a recognized body or bodies or State agency, shall be deemed accredited in the following cases if the Commissioner of Education finds, after consultation with the appropriate accreditation body or bodies, that there is reasonable assurance that the program, or the hospital, school, college, or university (or unit thereof), will meet the accreditation standards of such body or bodies.

**Accredited Record Technician (ART)**

A person knowledgeable, trained, and skilled in medical record keeping systems and procedures who has completed an accredited educational program and has satisfactorily passed a national accreditation examination. Passing the examination entitles an individual to use the initials ART after his or her name as proof of their qualifications as a thoroughly trained specialist in the assembling, analyzing, abstracting and maintenance of the medical record. ARTs will often be responsible for supervising many of the medical record department's day-to-day functions. Records are reviewed for completeness and accuracy by the ART, who also indexes and classifies all diagnoses and operations performed during the patient's hospitalization. This information is retrieved and prepared for hospital statistics, reports on diseases for public health authorities, special studies for the medical staff such as quality of care reviews, and in response to authorized inquiries for insurance or legal purposes. Also see Medical Records Administrator, Registered Records Administrator, RRA.

**accrual**

A method of accounting used to show expenses and income over a period of time, whether cash has changed hands during that period or not. The process of gaining something. See accrue.

**accrual basis of accounting**

An accounting method that identifies money within the period in which goods or services are provided for a fee. It identifies expenses within the time period in which goods, services, or resources were consumed for a fee. Money is credited to the time period in which it is earned, regardless of when payments are received, and expenses are charged in the time period in which they occurred and are incurred, regardless of when cash is disbursed to pay the expenses.

**accrue**
To gain, accumulate or happen. To come into fact or to come into existence. A "cause of action" can come into existence as a law when filed as a legal claim. The length of time allowed for a legal action to accrue is often determined by statutes of limitation. See accrual.

**accumulated depreciation**
The account showing the total depreciation recorded for an asset or capital item since the time it was acquired. Older and less used terms are allowance for depreciation or reserve for depreciation.

**accumulation**
In insurance it is an increase in the amount of benefits provided by some policies, as a reward to the insured for continuous renewal.

**accusation**
1. A charge formally made in court stating that a person is guilty of committing a crime. 2. Any charge brought against a person or corporation. 3. An indictment or information.

**accusatory instruments**
The official documents that charge a person with a crime.

**accused**
1. The defendant in a criminal case. 2. One whom an accusation is made against.

**achluphobia**
Fear of the dark.

**acid**
Slang for lysergic acid diethylamide (LSD).

**acid test ratio**
The sum total of cash, saleable securities, and current receivables divided by current liabilities. Also referred to as the quick asset ratio or liquidity ratio; used in determining liquidity of a business or corporation.

**A computer system sometimes used in larger hospitals or by Medicare insurance companies, in which both numeric and alphabetic data are processed in the form of electrical pulses. Both the information to be processed and the instructions to process it are stored in the memory cells of the computer. Work is performed with a minimum of human effort. Large electronic-computer systems are mostly self-directing.**

**acquiescence**
1. A silent agreement. 2. To know about an act, behavior, or occurrence and remaining silent about it, as it may be for your betterment.

**acquisition charge**
A financial charge assessed against the holder of a loan for paying off a loan early.

**acquisition cost**
The immediate cost of selling, underwriting, and issuing a new insurance policy, including clerical costs, agents' commissions, advertising, and medical inspection fees. Also refers to the cost paid by a pharmacist or other retailer to a manufacturer or wholesaler for a supply of drugs.

**acquit**
1. To set free. 2. To be judicially discharged from an accusation.

**acquittal**
1. A formal legal judgement of a person's innocence. 2. To be released from a commitment or obligation.

**acrophobia**
Fear of high places.

**act**
1. Any behavior, occurrence or action taken that may have legal consequences. 2. A law formally passed by a legislative body.

**act in pais**
A judicial act not a matter of record and performed out of court.

**actio (Lat.)**
1. An action. 2. A right. 3. Any legal proceedings that are necessarily taken in order to enforce a right. 4. A lawsuit.

**actio damni injuria (Lat.)**
An action for damages.

**actio ex delicto (Lat.)**
An action arising from a tort.

**action**
1. A judicial remedy. 2. To enforce a right. 3. To punish an offender. 4. A lawsuit. 5. Behaviors or acts that are done. 6. The filing of a claim or answering to a charge.

**Activity Director**
One who directs recreational activities in long term health care settings. See Recreational Therapist and recreational therapy.

**activity services**
According to JCAH for psychiatric, alcoholism and drug abuse facilities accreditation purposes, these are structured activities designed to develop an individual's creative, physical, and social skills through participation in recreational, art, dance, drama, social and other activities.

**act of commission**
1. An intentional act which is harmful or injurious. 2. Intentionally doing a criminal act.

**act of omission**
1. Failing to take necessary precautions so as to insure another person is not harmed. 2. Being negligent. 3. The lack of action when action is required to benefit another person.

**actual charge**
The amount a physician or other practitioner actually bills a patient for a particular medical service or procedure. The actual charge may differ from the customary, prevailing, and/or reasonable charges under Medicare and other insurance programs. See also fractionation.

**actual damage**
See damages, actual.

**actuary**
In insurance, a person trained in statistics, accounting, and mathematics who determines policy rates, reserves, and dividends by deciding what assumptions should be made with respect to each of the risk factors involved (such as the frequency of occurrence of the peril, the average benefit that will be payable, the rate of investment earnings, if any, expenses, and persistency rates), and who endeavors to secure as valid statistics as possible on which to base his assumptions.

**actus (Lat.)**
An act.

**acute**
1. Short term, short stay. 2. Sharp or severe. 3. Any severe condition or disease that has a sudden onset and short course (opposed to chronic.).

**acute brain syndrome**
A reversible form of organic brain disease which results from acute diseases, pulmonary dysfunction, cardiac insufficiency, long term high temperature, malnutrition, alcoholism, trauma or other factors. Diagnosis of this syndrome is difficult. Symptomatology includes: fluctuations in mood and mental capacity, confusion, easy distractibility and possible hyperactivity. Early diagnosis and treatment are essential for recovery.

**acute care**
Short term health care.

**acute care hospital**
A short term care hospital with an average length of stay of less than 30 days. See hospital, general, average length of stay, hospital, acute care.

**acute disease**
A disease which is characterized by a single episode of a fairly short duration from which the patient returns to his normal or previous state and level of activity. While acute diseases are frequently distinguished from chronic diseases, there is no standard definition or distinction. It is worth noting that an acute episode of a chronic disease (an episode of diabetic coma in a patient with diabetes) is often treated as an acute disease.

**ad (Lat.)**
At; by; for; to.

**adaptation**
1. Coping behavior. 2. The ability to handle the demands of the environment by means of a combination of autoplastic maneuvers involving a change in the self and alloplastic maneuvers involving alteration of the external environment with the end result being successful adaptation or adjustment. "Maladjustment" refers to unsuccessful adaptation.

**adapted physical education**
See corrective therapist.

**adaptive mechanism**
See mental mechanisms.

**ad curiam (Lat.)**
To court.

**ad curiam vocare (Lat.)**
To summon to court.

**ad damnum (Lat.)**
To the damage. That part of a pleading that states the money loss or damages claimed by the plaintiffs.

**addict**
A person who has a habit of use, such as drugs, and who can no longer exercise self-control over that use.

**addicting drug**
Any drug that produces both withdrawal symptoms and tolerance.

**addiction**
Habitual use of a drug, of which the deprivation causes symptoms of distress and a driving impulse to take the drug again. See drug addiction, abuse, and dependence.

**additives**
Any of a wide range of chemical substances added to foods or other products in low percentages, to stabilize certain end products.

**additur (Lat.)**
It is increased. 1. An increase in the amount of damages awarded by the court, which usually is over the amount awarded by jury. 2. On a motion for a new trial, a plaintiff is denied the new trial on the condition that the defendant pay damages larger than those already awarded in a judgement, where a court believes the award to be too low.

**ademption**
1. A revocation of a legacy. 2. A gift left in a will but given before death. 3. To credit a decedent's estate for gifts to an heir or devisee already given before death.

**adequate and well-controlled studies**
Investigations that must be conducted by a new drug sponsor to demonstrate that a new drug is effective. As amended in 1962, the Federal Food, Drug, and Cosmetic Act requires that drug sponsors provide substantial evidence of effectiveness. Thus, this gives this term a special definition: "evidence consisting of adequate and well-controlled investigations, including clinical investigations, by experts qualified by scientific training and experience to evaluate the effectiveness of the drug involved, on the basis of which it could fairly and responsibly be concluded by such experts that the drug will have the effect it purports or is represented to have under the conditions of use prescribed, recommended, or suggested in the labeling thereof" (section 505(d) of the Act). FDA regulations further delineate the types of studies which must be conducted to satisfy this requirement, and permit waiver in certain cases. The study protocol must minimize bias and must assure comparability between test and control groups. Generally, four types of control are recognized: comparing treated and untreated patients, comparing results of new drug use with a placebo, comparing results of new drug use with results from a regimen of therapy known to be effective, and comparing results of new drug use with experience that is historically derived. The statute and regulations do not explicitly require that safety of a new drug be established by adequate and well-controlled studies; nor do they set forth explicit criteria for safety testing.

**adhesion contract**
A contract in printed standard form, submitted on a take-it-or-leave-it basis. Adhesion contracts are common in situations where one party's bargaining position is substantially weaker than the others. A court may refuse to enforce a contract of adhesion.

**ad hoc (Lat.)**
For one special purpose, such as an ad hoc committee which is a committee that meets only one or two times for a special purpose and the committee ends once this special purpose has been met.

**ad hominem (Lat.)**
To the person. A personal attack on another person rather than arguing against his position.

**ad idem (Lat.)**
Proving the same point.

**ad infinitum (Lat.)**
Without limit; infinity.

**adjective law**
The rules governing legal procedure and practice. This is distinguished from substantive law, which determines rights and duties.

**adjourn**
1. To let out or dismiss. 2. To postpone.

**adjudicate**
1. To judge. 2. To evaluate or assess. 3. To finally decide.

**adjudication**
1. Judgement or evaluation. 2. The formal process of giving, declaring or recording a judgement. 3. The act of declaring a person bankrupt by a court. 4. In health insurance this is the process of reviewing claims to determine the services eligible for reimbursement.

**adjunct**
Additional. Added upon. United with.

**adjunct disability**
In the Veterans Administration health care program, a nonservice-connected disability associated with or held to be aggravating; a service-connected disability.

**adjunction**
A permanent addition or attachment; for example: a wing added to a hospital.

**adjunctive radiotherapy physics services**
Those treatments necessary to conduct radiation therapy for optimal patient care, performed in consultation with a qualified radiological physicist (e.g., patient dosimetry, design and construction of beam shaping devices).

**adjuration**
1. Swearing under a solemn oath. 2. Swearing under the penalty of a curse or commitment to a deity.

**adjusted death rate**
See case severity.

**adjusted rate of return**
The rate of return of money on a long-term project, as determined by adjusting the cash flow of the project for the time value of money. Also called discounted rate of return.

**adjuster**
1. A person employed by an insurance company who assesses, adjusts or determines the dollar amount of a claim or debt. A health insurance adjuster determines and settles medical care claims.

**adjusting entry**
Any new entry made at the end of an accounting period to show a record of an accounting action that was not recorded during the regular accounting period or process.

**adjustment**
1. In psychology the way a person relates to society and himself. 2. In insurance the settling of the amount the insured is entitled to receive under his policy.

**ad litem (Lat.)**
For the suit; to meet the needs of a lawsuit; for purposes of litigation.

**administer**
1. To take charge of and manage. 2. To take charge of business or an organization. 3. To conduct or manage something.

**administration**
1. To take charge of the management or running of a public service, a health care organization, or part of a governmental health agency. 2. The guidance of an undertaking toward the achievement of its purpose. Administration and management are so similar and irregularly distinguished that they may be considered synonymous, although they have been distinguished by applying administration to public activities and management to private, or by describing one as concerned with the execution of that policy once formulated. See also planning, goals and objectives. See Health Service Administration.

**administrative**
According to JCAH for psychiatric, alcoholism and drug abuse facilities accreditation purposes, this is related to the fiscal and general management of a facility rather than to the direct provision of services to patients.

**administrative agency**
A branch of the government created to carry out laws and policies. For example: the public health department is a local health administrative agency and the Health Systems Agency is a regional or state governmental administrative agency.

**administrative board**
A body of people set up by an agency or hospital to hold hearings or determine policy. See governing body.

**administrative decision**
A decision rendered by a commission established by legislation, such as OSHA, SSA, or FDA.

**administrative discretion**
Decisions made by administrative officials that are not covered by a policy, law or rule, and which depend on professional judgement. Upon judicial review of an administrative decision, there is an area of such professional judgment which the court will not disturb in the absence of abuse of discretion.

**administrative law**
1. Laws made for the adequate management of an administrative agency. 2. Regulations created by administrative agencies. 3. Branch of law dealing with government power and determining the manner of its activity.

**administrative remedy**
An administrative agency providing an internal solution to a problem related to the agency's jurisdiction rather than going to court or before considering litigation. Generally administrative remedies must be exhausted before seeking relief from the judicial system.

**administrative services**

1. Those services provided to assure adequate management of medical care resources as well as adequate management of the patient care environment.

**administrator, (Medicare)**

The governing body appoints a qualified administrator who is responsible for the overall management of the facility, enforces the rules and regulations relative to the level of health care and safety of patients, and to the protection of their personal and property rights, and plans, organizes, and directs those responsibilities delegated to him by the governing body. Through meetings and periodic reports, the administrator maintains ongoing liaison among the governing body, medical and nursing staffs, and other professional supervisory staff of the facility, and studies and acts upon recommendations made by the utilization review and other committees. In the absence of the administrator, an employee is authorized, in writing, to act on his behalf.

**administrator-clinic**

The chief officer responsible for the management of a medical group's administrative activities except for doing the physician's duties of patient care. The administrator is trained in management and business and reports to the Board of Directors, usually comprised of the physicians who own the medical group practice.

**administrator of skilled nursing facility**

A person who: (1) is licensed as required by State law; or (2) if the State does not have a Medicaid program, has no licensure requirement, he or she must be a high school graduate (or equivalent), has completed courses in administration or management approved by the appropriate State agency, and has three years of supervisory management experience in a skilled nursing facility or related health program; or (3) if the administrator of a hospital in which there is a hospital-based distinct-part skilled nursing facility, in a State that does not license skilled nursing facility administrators, meets the legal federal requirements. See qualified administrator.

**admissibility (of evidence)**

1. The worthiness of evidence. 2. Evidence that meets the legal rules of evidence and that is allowed to be considered by a jury.

**admissible evidence**

Evidence that may be properly received by a court for consideration in a case.

**admission**

1. The act of admitting. 2. Allowing one to enter. 3. Assertion of a fact. 4. A voluntary statement admitting that a fact or set of events is true or happened which become a part of the record. 5. If a party admits a fact the opposing party does not have to prove it. 6. The formal acceptance by a hospital or other inpatient health care facility of a patient who is to be provided with room, board, and continuous nursing service in an area of the hospital or facility where patients generally stay at least overnight.

**admission by adoption**
In evidence, a statement made in the presence of the defendant which is of such a character and is made under such circumstances as to require a denial if untrue.

**admission certification**
A form of medical care review in which an assessment is made of the medical necessity of a patient's admission to a hospital or other inpatient institution. Admission certification seeks to assure that patients requiring hospital level of care, and only such patients, are admitted to the hospital without unnecessary delay and with proper planning of the hospital stay. Lengths of stay appropriate for the patient's admitting diagnosis are usually assigned and certified, and payment by any program requiring certification for the assigned stay is assured. Certification can be done before (preadmission) or shortly after (concurrent) admission.

**admission notice**
Communication from a hospital, skilled nursing facility or other institution to health insurance companies to determine a patient's eligibility and benefits.

**admission of evidence**
1. A court allowing evidence to be considered. 2. A judge allowing a jury to consider evidence.

**admissions**
Number of patients accepted and admitted into a hospital for inpatient service in certain periods of time. Births are not counted as admissions.

**admissions office**
This department is also referred to as admitting, admitting department or office, which arranges and schedules paper work for patients for admission, keeps a waiting list, and a list of empty beds. The admissions office may assign rooms and beds, and collect initial data and nonmedical information about the patient and his family for the patient's record before being taken to his room. Other units of concern of the hospital are identified when the patient is admitted.

**admitted assets**
Assets of an insurance company recognized by a State regulatory body or other examining body in determining the company's financial condition.

**admitting physician**
The physician responsible for admission of a patient to a hospital or other inpatient health facility. The physician remains responsible for the care of the patient once admitted (see private patient). If in an indigent care facility such as a county hospital in a city, then the housestaff usually becomes responsible. Some facilities have all admitting decisions made by a single physician (typically a rotating responsibility) called an admitting physician.

**admitting privileges**
See staff privileges.

**admonition**
1. An oral reprimand given by a judge instead of giving the convicted person a jail sentence or another type of punishment. 2. Advice or caution from a judge to a jury.

**admonitory tort**
1. An intentional tort. 2. A case in which a mild punishment is given to the wrongdoer as this is viewed to be more important than compensating the injured party.

**adolescence**
The period of life that begins with the onset of secondary sex characteristics and ending with somatic growth or maturation. Between ages 11 and 21.

**adolescent medicine**
A relatively new medical specialty that focuses its practice on general medicine for the patient of the adolescent age group (11-21 years).

**adopt**
1. To put a law into effect. 2. To establish the legal relationship of parent and child between parties not naturally so related.

**ad respondendum (Lat.)**
For the purpose of answering.

**adult**
1. Of legal age. 2. A person over the age of majority as set by state law. 3. The age when full rights are to begin. 4. Refers to older patients or the special care or services offered to older persons such as adult day care centers.

**adulteration**
1. The production of a quality product with an item of lesser quality than the original genuine product. 2. Mixing inferior products or harmful materials in with quality ones, to increase volume, gain money, lower costs, etc. In health care the adulteration of drugs is always a legal concern.

**adultery**
A common grounds for divorce, adultery is sexual intercourse between a married person and any other person who is not the legal husband or wife.

**advance appropriation**
In the Federal budget, an appropriation provided by the Congress one or more years in advance of the fiscal year in which the budget authority becomes available for obligation. Advance appropriations allow State and local governments, and others sufficient time to develop plans with assurance of future Federal funding. An advance appropriation is sometimes mistakenly referred to as forward funding, which involves an agency in obligating funds in the current year for outlay to programs that are to operate in subsequent fiscal years.

**adversary**
The opposing party in a suit, writ or action; the opponent in litigation.

**adversary proceeding**
A trial court or a hearing where contesting parties present opposing views.

**adversary system**
A system in American law. The judge serves as a decision maker between opposing parties.

**adverse interest**
Having needs and wishes which oppose the interests of a party with whom you work or are associated with.

**adverse selection**
Disproportionate insurance of risks who are poorer or more prone to suffer loss or make claims than the average risk. It may result from the tendency for poorer risks or less desirable insureds (sick people) to seek or continue insurance to a greater extent than do better risks (healthy people), or from a tendency for the insured to take advantage of favorable options in insurance contracts. Favorable, as compared to adverse, selection, when intentional, is called skimming.

**adverse witness**
A witness showing opposition through prejudice, thus open to leading questions and cross-examination by the side that requested the witness appear.

**advisory group (board)**
1. A committee of persons who serve as an advice-giving body, yet are unlike a board of governors or board of directors. The advisory board has no authority or power over the organization that established it. 2. For PSRO programs purposes, it is an organization required under Section 1162(e) of Public Law 92-603 to advise and assist a Statewide Professional Standards Review Council, or a PSRO in a state without a Statewide Council, in carrying out PSRO program objectives. An advisory group is an ongoing, formal mechanism whereby health care practitioners other than physicians and representatives of hospitals and other health care facilities participate in the Professional Standards Review Organization program.

**advocate**
1. A person who pleads for another person or an organization. 2. A person who defends or pleads a "cause" of another.

**aero-**
Prefix meaning air.

**aerobe**
Microorganisms that require oxygen for growth.

**aerosols**
Liquid droplets or solid particles sprayed as a mist in air, that are fine enough to remain afloat or dispersed in the air for a period of time.

**affect**
Emotions. This is opposed to the cognitive or intellectual domain. These are the inner feelings and the external reaction to feelings.

**affect, blunted**
A disturbance of emotions that shows dullness in ones feelings. It can be observed in schizophrenia.

**affective**
Founded in, pertaining to or arising from feelings, emotions, or certain mental states.

**affective disorders**
Emotional problems marked by personality changes, alterations in mood, lack of self-esteem and psychological confusion. Reactive depression and mania are frequent affective disorders observed.

**affective interaction**
Interpersonal transactions that are emotionally charged.

**affiant**
One who makes and signs an affidavit.

**affidavit**
1. Any voluntarily sworn statement or declaration of fact that is done in writing with the person swearing that the facts are true. 2. A declaration written or sworn to, under oath before an official permitted by law to administer such an oath.

**affiliated hospital**
One which is affiliated in some degree with another health program, usually a medical school. Some definitions in fact limit the term to mean hospitals with close or extensive affiliations with medical school, nursing schools, and schools of allied health.

**affiliated hospital (or affiliated outpatient facility)**
An affiliated hospital is a hospital or outpatient facility which is not owned by, but is affiliated with, a school of medicine, allied health, nursing, health administration, osteopathy, or dentistry, which meets eligibility conditions.

**affiliation**
An agreement (usually formal) between two or more otherwise independent programs or individuals which defines how they will relate to each other. Affiliation agreements may specify: procedures for referring or transferring patients from one facility to another; joint faculty and/or medical staff appointments; teaching relationships; sharing of records or services; or provision of consultation between programs. See also affiliated hospital.

**affinity**
Related to by marriage; a husband is related to his wife's sister by affinity.

**affirmative action**
A legal requirement that governmentally related organizations take affirmative steps to avoid discrimination in hiring and promotion.

**affirmative defense**
A defendant's answer that is more than a denial of facts to a complaint. It provides new facts and arguments that could cause the defendant to win even if the complaint is true.

**affirmative relief**
Relief or compensation granted a defendant which is apart from any claim made against him by the plaintiff.

**a force (Lat.)**
Of necessity.

**aforesaid**
Said previously or already mentioned.

**a fortiori (Lat.)**
A good possibility; having a strong reason to believe. For a greater reason.

**aftercare**
1. After hospitalization. In counseling, in psychiatry, physical therapy, occupational therapy, this is a continuing program of rehabilitation to continually help the effects of therapy and the patient to adjust to his new environment and the community's work setting. It also refers to home health care provided after discharge from a hospital or nursing home where a patient is still in need of some skilled health care. 2. According to JCAH for psychiatric, alcoholism and drug abuse facilities accreditation purposes this is services that are provided to a patient after discharge and that support and increase the gains made during treatment. See home health care.

**age adjusted death rate**
See case severity, age specific death rate, crude death rate.

**aged**
One with an advanced age. Some authorities or programs classify anyone over 65 years of age as aged. There is no known time when a person becomes old. Aged can become a comparative definition.

**age dependency ratio**
A demographic measure. A ratio that is used to assess changing age composition in a population. It is based on an aggregation of those that are too young or to old to provide their own financial or social well-being. The age-dependency ratio is used to determine how many dependents every 100 working members of a group must support. Using simple statistics to reflect age distributions, this ratio can be calculated for various populations. Thus, it is possible to compare those that are age dependent among diverse societies.

**age distribution**
A descriptive statistical measure used to determine the proportional age mix in a population.

**ageism**
The image of and attitudes toward an individual simply because he or she is old. The extent to which the public in general perceives the elderly. The negative or positive perception a society has of the aged population.

**age limits**
Stipulated minimum and maximum ages, below and above which a health insurance company will not accept applications and may not renew policies.

**agency**
A relationship whereby one person represents or acts on behalf of another, under and by the other person's authority.

**age norms**
Guidelines used to determine age-appropriate behavior within a given set of expected roles. Age norms provide a guide to acceptable behavior but do not supply detailed stipulations or exceptions for each and every possible case.

**agent**
1. A person who represents or acts on behalf of another, with that person's implied or expressed permission and authority i.e. a nurse in carrying out health care under the directions of a physician is his agent. 2. In insurance it is an insurance company representative licensed by the state who solicits, negotiates, or effects contracts of insurance, and services the policyholder for the insurer.

**age of majority**
Legal age. It can be 18 to 21 years of age depending on the state. Over the age of minority. The age at which a person receives legal adult rights and obligations.

**age specific birth rate**
The number of live births in a selected age group per 1,000, 10,000, or 100,000 in that same age group.

**age specific death rate**
The number of deaths reported in a selected age group per 1,000 or 10,000 or 100,000 population in that same age group.

**aggravation**
1. Increasing the severity of a crime. 2. Actions that make the seriousness of a crime worse.

**aggregate indemnity**
The maximum dollar amount payable for any disability, period of disability, or covered under an insurance policy, also called "policy limits."

**aggression**
1. Forceful behavior that could be verbal or a physical act. 2. The reaction of rage, anger and hostility. 3. Any forceful physical, verbal or nonverbal symbolic act. 4. As referred to in assertiveness training, it is directly standing up for personal rights and expressing thoughts, feelings and beliefs in a forceful, hostile, dishonest, inappropriate way which violates the rights of the other person. Obtaining one's desires is insured by humiliating, degrading, belittling, or overpowering other people so that they become weaker and less able to defend their needs and rights. This is a negative, inappropriate approach and is not being assertive.

**aggressive collection**
Using a variety of methods to collect a debt, such as attachment, garnishment, etc.

**aggressive drive**
Destructive impulses aimed at others or at oneself. In psychiatry it may be known as the death instinct.

**aggrieved party**
The party that has been injured, harmed or has had personal or property rights violated by another party.

**aging accounts receivable**
A method of reviewing and classifying accounts receivable. Time elapsed since the receivable came due or the time that has passed since the last payment was made. This process is used for the purpose of evaluating credit and long overdue bill collection policies. This process may also be used in estimating the amount of difficult to collect or uncollectible accounts receivable as of a given date.

**agitation**
Anxiety associated with severe restlessness.

**agoraphobia**
Fear of open places.

**agraphia**
Being unable to write.

**agreement**
1. Having unity in an opinion. 2. In contract law it is the "meeting of the minds". Two or more parties having equal sentiment to enter into a contract. 3. To form a valid contract.

**agreement number**
See identification number.

**agromania**
An unhealthy interest in living alone or in seclusion.

**AHA**
American Hospital Association. See these words.

**AHCCCS**
Arizona Health Care Cost Containment System. See these words.

**AHEC**
Area Health Education Center. See these words.

**AHPA**
America Health Planning Association. See these words.

**aichmophobia**
Fear of pointed objects. This is usually a fear that it will be used on someone else.

**aid and abet**
To know and intentionally help or encourage another to commit a crime.

**aide**
A worker found in hospitals and nursing homes who helps with the non-nursing chores such as changing patients clothes, changing the diapers of incontinent elderly patients, showering patients, changing beds, etc. Most of these workers are usually females and require no specific educational level or credential.

**aider**
A procedure, where once a verdict had been reached and those facts upon which the verdict is based are presumed to have been proven to be true.

**Aid to Families with Dependent Children (AFDC)**
A federal program created to provide medical aid to families with dependent children. Any child under age 21 is eligible.

**Aid to the Blind (AB)**
A federally created program that provides financial assistance to states to assist them in providing medical aid to the blind.

**Aid to the Permanently and Totally Disabled (APTD)**
A federal program used to provide medical care to the permanently and totally disabled who are medically indigent.

**ailurophobia**
Fear of cats.

**A.I.P.**
Annual Implementation Plan. See these words.

**air quality control region**
A geographical region where two or more communities share a common air pollution problem. Designated by the Secretary of Health and Human Services, these regions are required to set and enforce air quality standards.

**alarm reaction**
The initial and basic reaction of the human body to a stressor. See Stress.

**alcohol and drug abuse specialist**
These personnel work with patients and their families on problems of alcohol and drug abuse or dependence. Among their more important functions are encouraging patient self-analysis and personality development, and the provision of emotional support and behavioral guidance, especially for institutionalized patients. They usually function as members of health teams which include physicians, psychologists, and social workers.

**Alcohol Drug Abuse and Mental Health Administration**
A division of the U.S. Public Health Service. This Agency brought together 3 other government health agencies: 1) Drug Abuse and Mental Health, 2) National Institutes on Alcohol Abuse and Alcoholism, 3) National Institutes of Health.

**Alcoholic and Narcotic Addict Rehabilitation Amendment**
A public law passed in 1968 that provides additional provisions to the Community Mental Health Centers Act. This amendment provided for funds for construction of community mental health facilities as well as employment of medical personnel to provide treatment to addicts. Financing for special training programs was also provided.

**alcoholic psychoses**
Mental illness from alcoholism including organic brain damage. See also Delirium tremens, Korsakoff's psychosis, Hallucinosis.

**Alcoholics Anonymous (AA)**
A rehabilitation organization for alcoholics formed in 1935.

**alcoholism**
Physical and psychological dependence on or addiction to alcohol. A chronic disorder manifested by repeated drinking of alcoholic beverages in excess of the dietary and social uses and norms of the community and to an extent that interferes with the drinker's health, or his social or economic functioning. The definition of alcoholism in both theory and practice is highly variable: sometimes requiring only excessive drinking or interference with the drinker's functioning rather than both; sometimes requiring, in addition to the above, physical signs of drug dependence, or being recognized as present without either. There are many, variable systems for separating different types of alcoholism and grading its severity. See also drug abuse.

**aleatory contract**
An agreement or contract which is contingent upon an uncertain future event.

**alexia**
The inability to grasp the meaning of written words and sentences.

**-algia**
suffix meaning, pain.

**algophobia**
Fear of pain.

**alienable**
1. That which can be sold. 2. That which can be transferred. 3. Subject to removal.

**alienate**
1. To estrange. 2. To transfer, convey, or dispose of property to another.

**alienation**
1. A psychological term for feelings of detachment from society or even oneself. 2. Avoidance of emotional experience, to estrange oneself.

**alienation clause**
A part of an insurance policy that voids or ends policy if what is being insured is sold or otherwise transferred.

**alienation of affection**
Withdrawing of love, companionship, or affection of another person. A defunct law in many states.

**alienist**
A psychiatrist or psychologist who provides expert opinion about mental illness or sanity.

**alignment**
The positioning of bone structures or body parts that facilitates effective body function.

**allay**
To subdue or reduce in intensity; to make quiet, calm, or reduce fear.

**allegation**
1. Something alleged, asserted, stated or charged. 2. A statement in the pleading that provides the facts that one side expects to prove. 3. the first plea by the plaintiff in a case.

**allege**
To declare without proof; to assert; charge or make an allegation.

**allergy-immunology technician**
These individuals are trained to prepare and administer the materials prescribed by a physician, who usually specializes in allergy-immunology, to desensitize individuals to various environmental and food allergens.

**all fours**
Two cases are on "all fours" if they are alike in a legal manner; so factually similar that the rationale of one case with equal logic is equal to another.

**allied health educator**
This person teaches in an allied health specialty in which he/she was trained so to prepare students in the same discipline. The term "allied health educator" is typically not specific to one occupation, but prepares educators in their various allied health disciplines.

**allied health personnel**

**allied health personnel**
Specially trained and licensed (when necessary) health workers
Allied health personnel means individuals with training and responsibilities for (A) supporting, complementing, or supplementing other than physicians, dentists, podiatrists and osteopaths. The term has no constant or agreed upon detailed meaning: sometimes being the professional functions of physicians, dentists, and other health used synonymously with para-medical personnel; sometimes meaning professionals in the delivery of health care to patients, or (B) assisting environmental engineers and other personnel in environmental all health workers who perform tasks which must otherwise be performed by a physician; and sometimes referring to health workers health control and preventive medicine activities. who do not usually engage in independent practice. In a legal sense a nurse is considered allied health personnel as the nurse is an agent to the physician and has to work under his orders as he is the principal in this working relationship.

**Allied Health Professions Personnel Training Act (1966)**
A federal law passed to establish programs for construction of training facilities for training allied health care providers such as nurses, medical technologists, dental hygienists. Student loans, grants and scholarships were also provided. Loans for physicians and dentists who practice in rural areas were cancelled.

**allocated benefit provision**
A provision in an insurance policy under which payment for certain benefits (such as miscellaneous hospital and medical services like X-rays, dressings and drugs) will be made at a rate for each specified (scheduled) in the provision. Usually there is also a maximum that will be paid for all such expenses. An allocated benefit is one which is subject to such a provision. In an unallocated benefit provision no specification is given of how much will be paid for each type of service although the provision sets a maximum payable for all the listed services.

**allocation**
1. The setting up of an allotment or shares. 2 To have set apart for a specified purpose.

**allocation basis**
A systematic method of assigning indirect costs to two or more cost areas. This is useful in determining full costs for preparation of billing rates.

**allocution**
A formality of the court whereby a defendant is asked whether he has anything to say in his behalf toward stopping his sentencing.

**allograph**
1. A legal paper that is written or signed by one person for another party who is not a part of the agreement. 2. A signature by proxy.

**allopathic physician**
Usually used in contrast to osteopathic and homeopathic; a physician practicing a philosophy of medicine which views the role of the physician as an active interventionist who attempts to counteract the effect of a disease by using treatments, surgical or medical, which produce effects opposite to those of the disease. A homeopathic physician, on the other hand, generally uses a drug therapy which reinforces the body's natural self-healing process. Almost all physicians in the United States would be considered allopathic. See homeopathy

**alloplasty**
Adapting to stress by trying to change the environment.

**allowable charge**
A generic term referring to the maximum fee that a third party will use in reimbursing a provider for a given service. An allowable charge may not be the same as either a reasonable, customary or prevailing charge as the terms are used under the Medicare program.

**allowable costs**
Items or elements of an institution's costs which are reimbursable under a payment formula. Both Medicare and Medicaid reimburse hospitals on the basis of certain costs, but do not allow reimbursement for all cost. Allowable costs may exclude, for example, uncovered services, luxury accommodations, costs which are not reasonable, expenditures which are unnecessary in the efficient delivery of health services to persons covered under the program in question (it would not be allowable to reimburse costs under Medicare involved in provding services to newborn infants), or depreciation on a capital expenditure which was disapproved by a health planning agency. See also section 223 and 1122.

**ALOS Average length of stay in the hospital**
See average length of stay, also case severity, length of stay.

**alteration**
1. Making something different from what it was before. 2. A change or modification.

**alter ego (Lat.)**
1. Other self. 2. When individual shareholders act through a corporation for personal rather than corporate purposes, they can be held personally liable for the consequenses of the acts as the corporation was their alter ego.

**alternate delivery system (ADS)**
New methods of delivering health care (such as Health Maintenance Organizations) which emphasize preventive care, cost containment, new methods of payment or other innovations.

**alternating role**
A mental illness pattern characterized by the periodic switching from one type of behavior to another.

**alternative birthing center**
Can be independent facilities or facilities adjoining a hospital. Strives to provide a home-like atmosphere emphasizing the cheerful and comfortable. Nurse-midwives, under supervision of an obstetrician, may deliver the baby. Unexpected complications of mother or child can be dealt with in an adjacent high-risk suite or hospital.

**alternative pleading**
1. Declaring facts that exist separately but cannot exist at the same time in the same pleading. 2. A pleading in common law where separate facts are difficult to determine and it is unclear which set of facts a person is intended to rely upon as the basis for recovery. "When a plaintiff pleads his case in the alternative, one version of which is good and the other not, his petition will, on demurrer, be treated as pleading no more than the latter, since it will be construed most strongly against him." 93 S.E. 2d. 3, 5. See election of remedies.

**alternative relief**
In a pleading, a plaintiff asks for relief in ways that might be contradictory, i.e. asking for either the return of a borrowed oxygen tank or for the payment of its value.

**alternatives to long-term institutional care**
The whole range of health, nutritional, housing and social services designed to keep persons, particularly the aged, disabled and retarded, out of institutions like skilled nursing facilities which provide care on a long-term basis. The goal is to provide the range of services necessary to allow the person to continue to function in the home environment. Alternatives to institutional care include day-care centers, foster homes or homemaker services, home health agencies and meals-on-wheels.

**alzheimer's disease**
A disease of progressive mental deterioration; usually considered a presenile dementia.

**AMA**
American Medical Association.

**ambiguity**
Being ambiguous.

**ambiguous**
1. Uncertainty in meaning. 2. When a statement can be understood in two or more meanings. 3. Uncertain or obscure possibility that a document can have two or more meanings or can be interpreted in more than one way.

**ambit**
1. Limits or scope of something. 2. A boundary line, limit or border.

**ambivalence**
Strong or overwhelming simultaneous contrasting attitudes, beliefs, ideas, feelings, and drives toward an object, person, or goal.

**ambulance**

A vehicle especially designed to carry and transport sick, injured or wounded persons at high speed to a health care facility for advanced treatment. Advanced emergency care and resuscitation measures can be performed in the vehicle, as it is equipped with two-way radios, oxygen systems, suction devices, litters, blood pressure devices, stethoscopes and other medical and safety equipment. Five types of equipment are needed: basic, safety, access, emergency care and communication. The vehicle must have emergency vehicle markings and large flashing lights. Most ambulances are now of the van-type automobile. Helicopters and airplanes are also commonly used as ambulances.

**ambulance chaser**

1. A lawyer who follows ambulances to automobile accidents to try to get the legal business that could come from some negligent act. 2. Slang for any attorney who solicits legal business.

**ambulance emergency medical technician**

Responds to medical emergency calls, provides first aid, and transports the injured to medical facilities. Qualified to administer only basic life support services, such as artificial resuscitation.

**ambulant**

Able to walk or move about.

**ambulation**

Walking or getting about in an upright position, unassisted by any walking device.

**ambulatory**

1. Movable; not fixed; changeable; revocable. 2. A patient who is not bedridden and is capable of walking. 3. able to walk or move about. 4. Capable or adapted to walking. 5. In law, something that can be changed or altered; not fixed.

**ambulatory care**

All types of health services which are provided on an outpatient basis, in contrast to services provided in the home or to persons who are inpatients. While many inpatients may be ambulatory, the term ambulatory care usually implies that the patient has come to a location other than his home to receive services and has departed the same day. See ambulatory setting, hospital-sponsored ambulatory care department.

**ambulatory service settings**

Residential care in which patients are able to move about unaided to receive health care services. Inpatient-patients must remain in a short term health care setting on a 24-hour basis, and usually require assistance. Outpatient-services which are available to patients on a walk-in appointment basis.

**ambulatory setting**

Outpatient or walk-in type Health Care Services that provide health care to patients who travel to the provider to receive services. An ambulatory setting has no provision for patients to stay overnight. See ambulatory care, hospital-sponsored ambulatory care department.

**ambulatory surgery**
Elective surgery provided to the patient on an out-patient, walk-in, same-day basis in an appropriately equipped and staffed health facility, with surgery conducted under general anesthesia with no overnight stay in the hospital required.

**ambulatory surgery center**
An outpatient same-day care health facility specializing in the simpler types of surgical treatment on an outpatient basis by a licensed physician, which do not require an overnight stay. A physician's office or the outpatient department of a hospital are not considered ambulatory surgery centers. An ambulatory surgery center is a separate free-standing, self-contained facility with all essential surgical equipment and personnel needed for quality surgery to be performed.

**ambulatoy automatism**
A form of automatism wherein a person unconsciously wanders about, performing involuntary acts.

**amenable**
Liable; responsible to answer.

**amend**
To change or revise, to improve, correct or review.

**amendment**
1. A change. 2. A revision. 3. The changing of a bill through legislation or changing a law that already has been passed.

**American Association of Health Care Facilities (AAHCF)**
Organized in 1949 by a group of concerned leaders in the nursing home field. These persons gathered together to discuss mutual goals and objectives of nursing homes. Today the membership of The American Association of Health Care Facilities consists of the proprietary and nonproprietary nursing home institutions.

**American College of Nursing Home Administrators (ACNHA)**
ACNHA was organized in 1962 as an individual membership professional society for long-term administrators. ACNHA assesses memberships through an advancement program, using experience, formal education, continuing education, professional activity, and civic/community activity as criteria for becoming a nominee, member, or fellow. The ACNHA's major goals and purposes are to: advance the quality of patient care in long term care institutions to the highest level possible, to promote the well being of the public and maintain the dignity of nursing home administration, and to establish standards of performance for nursing home administrators.

**American Dental Association**
The major professional organization for licensed practicing dentists. It has a board of trustees and a house of delegates who establish standards,

policies and accredits professional dental school internships, and residency programs. It published professional journals and provides information services and is involved in public health education, audiovisual service, research, statistics, etc.

**American Dietetic Association**
A professional organization responsible for establishing educational and supervised clinical experience requirements and standards of practice in the profession of dietetics.

**American Digest System**
A collection of all of the summaries of law cases ever reported in America. This includes: up to 1896: Century Digest. Also for every ten year period thereafter is Decennial Digest and General Digest. Case summaries presented are by subject by the Key Number System.

**American Group Practice Association (AGPA)**
Founded in 1949, AGPA represents private health care group practice practitioners in the United States. The Association is directed by a board of trustees selected from delegates representing the AGPA institutional members. Membership size varies with physician staffs, ranging from three to hundreds, with organization structures including partnerships, corporations, foundations and associations. Most groups are single or multispecialty. Affiliated with AGPA is the American Academy of Medical Directors which encourages educational and publications activities for physicians who serve as medical directors and/or have both management and health care provider responsibilities.

**American Health Care Association (AHCA)**
The nation's largest federation of licensed nursing homes and allied long term health care facilities. AHCA was founded in 1949 to promote high professional standards in long term health care delivery and quality care for patients and residents in safe surroundings at fair payment for services rendered. All AHCA members must be licensed by their state governments, as must the administrators who manage them. AHCA represents its members on issues before Congress, the Federal regulatory and executive authorities, and before the press and public at large. AHCA and its affiliated state associations work closely with individual members to achieve their objectives at all levels of government and public opinion. The American Health Care Association, formerly the American Nursing Home Association, consists of Skilled, Intermediate, and Residential Care Facilities, as well as Adult Day Care, Mental Health, and Child Care services. Membership includes both propietary (tax-paying) and non-proprietary (tax-exempt) facilities.

**American Health Planning Association**
It is one of the youngest major health associations in the United States, but its aims are the most ambitious, its potential the most exciting, and its breadths of concern the widest. With active participation from every affected sector of this society, the AHPA is designed to promote whatever changes are required to make health care services more responsive to local needs, more rational, more effective and more efficient. AHPA was founded in 1971.

**American Jurisprudence**
A legal encyclopedia, cited as Am. Jur. or Am. Jur. 2d (second series).

**American Law Reports**
Reprints of significant American cases usually followed by an annotation of similar cases dealing with the same legal principle cited as ALR, ALR 2d, ALR 3d or ALR 4th depending upon the edition.

**American Medical Association (AMA)**
The major physician association, founded in 1847. The AMA is a federation of subunits known as constituent medical societies. These medical societies are composed of local, county and city medical societies. The AMA is an educational, scientific, and information non-profit organization concerned with advancing medical knowledge and promoting high quality medical care by evaluating medical education, and examining health care delivery systems that will be responsive to the overall medical and health care needs of the public.

**American Nurses' Association**
The official national organization and spokesman for registered nurses. It was founded in 1896 and exists to improve the standards of nursing and to promote the general welfare of the professional nurses.

**American Nursing Home Association**
Changed to the American Health Care Association. See these words.

**American Public Health Association**
Founded in 1872, it is a non-governmental professional society representing all disciplines and specialties in public health. Together with the membership of its affiliated associations and regional branches, APHA is the largest public health association in the world, with a combined membership of over 55,000.

**American School Health Association**
A national professional organization concerned solely with the health of the school-age child. It promotes comprehensive school health programs for school health services, health education, and a healthful school environment. Founded in 1927, it establishes guidelines for Standards of Excellence and Competency for the school heath team including: health educators, school nurses, physicians, dentists, dental hygienists, and other health professionals. It also serves as a professional liaison for the various disciplines in the field of school health. It provides cooperation with local, state, and national organizations in behalf of all school health personnel.

**America Psychological Association**
Founded in 1892 and incorporated in 1925, is the major psychological organization in the United States. The purpose of the APA is to advance psychology as a science, as a profession, and as a means of promoting human welfare. It attempts to accomplish these objectives by holding annual meetings, publishing psychological journals, and working toward improved standards for psychological training and service.

**amicus curiae Lat.)**
1. Friend of the court. 2. One who is allowed to appear in court even though he has no standing as a party.

**amino acid**
One of a group of organic acids that are mostly made up of nitrogen. These are considered to be the building blocks of proteins.

**Am. Jur.**
American Jurisprudence, a legal encyclopedia.

**amnesty**
1. Deliberately overlooking an offense. 2. Removal by the government of penalties or guilt of a crime. 3. To grant a pardon.

**amortization**
1. Settling a debt. 2. The periodic payment of a debt that covers accrued interest and part of the principal. 3. The act or process of extinguishing a debt, usually by equal payments at regular intervals over a specific period of time.

**amortize**
1. To end, extinguish or to deaden. 2. To transfer or sell.

**amphetamine**
A drug that is a central nervous system stimulant.

**ampule**
A small, sealed glass flask or container used to preserve a sterile medication or drug solution, originally a French invention.

**ANA**
American Nurses' Association. See these words.

**anaerobe**
Any microorganism that can live and grow without the presence of oxygen.

**anal eroticism**
Pleasurable sensation of the anal region.

**analgesia**
When one feels little or no pain.

**analgesic**
Something that causes analgesia, usually a drug or ointment.

**anal incontinence**
The loss of the ability to voluntarily control bowel (fecal and gaseous) discharges.

**analog computer**
1. In medical records it is a computer that measures variables by physical analogies in continuous form. Other than use in hospitals it is used primarily in scientific research. 2. A computer operating on analog

data by performing physical processes on these data. This is contrasted with a digital computer.

**anal sex**
Sexual intercourse in the anus. See also sodomy.

**analysis**
1. The process of separating things into classes or parts. 2. To examine information or circumstances to determine their parts or elements. 3. In computerized medical records or billing it is used as an examination to distinguish the component parts of a record separately and in their relation to the whole. 4. In psychology or psychiatry this refers to psychoanalysis. See qualitative analysis, quantitative analysis, vector analysis.

**anamnesis**
In psychiatry it is the patient's medical history, particularly using the patient's ability to recall.

**anatomist**
An anatomist teaches medical, dental and allied health students about the human body's structure and function. As a researcher he/she may be involved in any aspect of biomedical research from problems at the molecular level to those concerned with the entire body. After college, 4 years of study at a medical school leading to a PHD or M.D. degree is required.

**ancillary**
1. Aiding. 2. Auxiliary. 3. A supportive role that helps a main function, effort or proceeding. 4. Supportive aid or service. 5. That which is subordinate to or is in support of. Such as ancillary services of a hospital are support services which help in the daily functioning of the health care facility. Such services include central supply, department of materials management, housekeeping, etc. See ancillary services.

**ancillary benefits**
Health or medical Insurance that pays for tests, treatments, therapies and procedures and other extra services provided or given to the patient.

**ancillary charges**
Those extra charges made to the patient for any unusual or special service, or diagnostic tests or treatments such as a C.T. scan, lab test, x-rays, etc.

**ancillary expenses**
See miscellaneous expenses.

**ancillary services**
Hospital, or other inpatient services other than room and board, and professional services. They may include X-ray, drug, laboratory or other services not separately itemized, but the specific content is quite variable. See also miscellaneous expenses.

**andro-**
Prefix meaning male.

**androgyny**
Having both female and male characteristics.

**anesthesia**
1. Absence of sensation, usually caused by a drug or gas. 2. Loss of sensation or feeling; an induced loss of the sense of pain.

**anesthesiologist, qualified**
According to JCAH for psychiatric, alcoholism and drug abuse facilities accreditation purposes, this is a doctor of medicine who practices the science of anesthesiology, which involves the administration of a drug or gas to cause a partial or complete loss of sensations, and who is fully licensed to practice medicine in the state in which he or she practices.

**anesthesiologist's assistant**
Performs diagnostic and therapeutic tasks under the supervision and direction of the anesthesiologist. Activities of the anesthesiologist's assistant may include care and proper usage of anesthesia equipment, monitoring of patients during anesthesia, and postanesthesia care.

**anesthesiology**
A clinical service provided in hospitals that utilizes this specialty of medicine to administer local and general anesthetics, usually in surgery. The department often includes anesthesiologists and /or nurse-anesthetists.

**anesthetist**
As used in JCAH accreditation, this is a generic term used to identify anesthesiologists, other physician anesthetists, or qualified nurse or dentist anesthetists.

**angiogram**
A diagnostic method used to visualize the veins and arteries by introducing a radioactive dye into the blood stream.

**anibiotic**
Any drug containing any quantity of any chemical substance produced by a microorganism which has the capacity, in dilute solution, to inhibit the growth of, or to destroy, bacteria and other microorganisms (or a chemically synthesized equivalent of such a substance). Antibiotics are used in the treatment of infectious diseases.

**anilingus**
Oral, anal, sexual, and sensual stimulation, legally considered a sexual deviant practice.

**animal technician**
An animal technician assists the veterinarian, biological or biomedical researcher, or other scientist in the care and management of animals. This technician is knowledgeable in basic principles of normal and abnormal life processes, and in routine laboratory and animal health care procedures.

**animus (Lat.)**
Intention.

**animus furandi (Lat.)**
Intention to steal.

**animus revertendi (Lat.)**
Intention to return (to a place).

**animus revocandi (Lat.)**
Intention to revoke.

**Annual Implementation Plan (AIP)**
1. A plan which the National Health Planning and Resources Development Act of 1974 (P.L. 93-641) requires health systems agencies to prepare or update annually, specifying, and describing how to implement, and giving priority to, short-term objectives which will achieve the long range goals of the agency, detailed in its health system plan. Section 1513 of the PHS Act describes the place of AIP's in the larger context of agency functioning. 2. A document presenting the decisions reached by a Health Systems Agency with regard to its short-range objectives and priorities and the tactical actions and resource changes that should occur in the next year, toward bringing about the long-term achievements set forth in the Health Systems Plan.

**annuity**
A regular periodic payment on a yearly basis. A fixed annual payment.

**annul**
To void; to end, to nullify ab initio.

**anomaly**
1. A marked deviation from normal; an abnormality. 2. When a structure or organ is malformed or has an irregular formation. (e.g. congenital anomalies are missing fingers or toes or heart defects.)

**anomie**
1. Without a sense of association with society, experiencing lack of social cohesion. 2. A person with no fixed values or moral standards.

**anorexia**
Lack or loss of appetite. Hunger is considered a physiological phenomenon, whereas appetite is considered psychological in origin. Anorexia can be stimulated by mental or thought processes or by environmental experience such as unattractive smells or food.

**anorexia nervosa**
A serious and life endangering emotional disorder concerned with the lack of appetite that is self-imposed and is characterized by fasting, dieting, over physical exercise, and self-starvation which can result physical, emotional, and mental problems and even death.

**answer**
1. To reply to. 2. A counterstatement of facts in a pleading. 3. A response to a complaint. 4. A formal reply in a lawsuit.

**antabuse**
A drug used in the treatment of alcoholics to discourage further use of alcohol.

**ante-**
Prefix meaning before.

**ante (Lat.)**
Before.

**antepartum care**
Includes usual prenatal services (e.g., initial and subsequent history, physical examination, recording of weight, blood pressure, fetal heart tones, routine chemical urinalyses, maternity counseling, etc.)

**anterior frame**
Frame on which the patient lies when in a prone position.

**antero- or anterio-**
Prefix meaning front.

**anti-**
Prefix meaning against.

**anti (Lat.)**
Against.

**antianxiety drug**
A drug used to reduce the symptoms of pathological anxiety without influencing cognitive or perceptual functioning. It is a minor tranquilizer and an anxiolytic drug.

**antibiotic certification**
An FDA program in which each batch of every antibiotic drug for human use is certified by FDA as possessing the necessary characteristics of identity, strength, quality, and purity to adequately insure safety and effectiveness in use. Before an antibiotic is eligible for certification, FDA must approve the drug as safe and effective under procedures that are substantially equivalent to those for approving new drugs. Similar procedures exist for batch certification insulin. Both antibiotic and insulin certification services are supported by user fees.

**antibody**
Any immunoglobulin which naturally combines with an antigen to fight off infection, pathogens, harmful bacteria, or toxins.

**anticipatory breach**
In contract law a breach prior to a duty to perform, indicating an intention not to perform.

**anticipatory grief**
Knowing in advance that the death will occur. This permits one to adjust without acute shock and emotional trauma due to the actual death. It is believed that previous knowledge of death lessens the emotional upset and stress of the loss of a loved one.

**anticipatory socialization**
Learning of and preparing for obligations, expectations and rights of a new role, prior to actually assuming it, thereby making adjustment much easier.

**antidepressant drug**
A drug used to treat pathological depression.

**antidiscrimination laws**
1. In insurance, this can be a State law which prohibits insurers from giving preferential terms or rates, not warranted by the rating of the risks involved. 2. In general use this term refers to equal and fair treatment or selection for jobs, school, positions, etc.

**antimanic drug**
A drug, such as lithium. This is used to reduce or alleviate the symptoms of mania.

**antiophobia**
Fear of floods.

**antipsychotic drug**
Any drug used to treat psychosis, particularly schizophrenia. It could be a major tranquilizer.

**antipyretic**
1. Tending to reduce or relieve fever. 2. A substance that reduces pain or fever. 3. A substance that is effective in treating burns.

**antiseptic**
1. Any agent that inhibits the growth of microorganisms. 2. A germicide. 3. Any substance that kills pathogens or living tissue.

**antisocial personality**
Inability to get along with members of society; having repeated conflict with individuals and groups.

**anti-substitution laws**
State laws that require the pharmacist to "dispense as written." The effect is to prohibit a pharmacist from substituting a different brand name drug for the one prescribed, or from substituting a generic equivalent drug in place of a drug prescribed by brand name, even if the drug that would be substituted is considered to be therapeutically equivalent to the drug prescribed and perhaps is less expensive. Drug reimbursement programs such as the Maximum Allowable Cost Program, which will limit reimbursement to the lowest cost at which a drug is generally available, will be more effective if they override anti-substitution laws.

**antitrust acts**
Statutes that protect commerce from unlawful business trusts and monopolies.

**anxiety**
The belief in an unreal danger or threat. Physiological changes that occur which can include increased heart rate, uneven breathing, trembling and

sweating. Physiological changes and uncomfortable emotional feelings of impending danger. An overwhelming feeling of being powerless. The inability to see that the threat is unreal. A prolonged feeling of tension and readiness to attack the threat.

**anxiety neurosis**
A mental state that is characterized by panic and anxious overconcern.

**A.P.A.**
American Psychiatric Association. American Psychological Association.

**apathy**
The lack of feeling, interest and emotional involvement.

**apgar scores**
Measurements taken soon after birth used to determine physical normality. The scores are based on color, respiratory effort, heart rate, reflex action, and muscle tone. Used routinely, to detect the effects of drugs taken by pregnant mothers.

**APHA**
American Public Health Association. See these words.

**aphasia**
1. Speech disorder due to organic brain damage or dysfunction. 2. A condition that manifests the loss of the ability to write or speak coherently and to understand written or spoken language.

**aphasia related to stroke**
Problems related to aphasia (loss of language) with the stroke patient is the inability to understand language or to use language. The following are three classes of aphasia in which aphasic patients are most commonly classified: 1) The expressive type of aphasia is observed in a patient when the inability to speak and write is predominant. 2) The receptive type of aphasia is observed in a patient when the inability to understand speech and writing is predominant. 3) The mixed type of aphasia is most frequently found among aphasic patients, for it is unusual to see a clearly defined aphasia.

**apizootic**
An epidemic among animals.

**apnea**
The cessation of breathing.

**a posteriori (Lat.)**
1. From the end result back to the cause. 2. An argument founded on fact or experimentation that demonstrates a cause. 3. From the result or effect to the cause. 4. A form of deductive reasoning which tries to show what facts come first.

**apparent defect**
A defect in a product that was not hidden and readily discoverable upon inspection, as opposed to a latent defect.

**appeal**
Application to a higher court to challenge a decision that is claimed as an error of a lower court.

**appearance**
1. To show up in court as a party to a lawsuit. 2. The formal showing up in court. 3. Being present in court.

**appellant**
1. The person who appeals a case to a higher court. 2. One who makes an appeal.

**appellate**
Pertaining to appeals.

**appellate court**
A higher court that hears appeals from lower courts.

**appellate jurisdiction**
The authority given to a higher court to hear cases of lower trial courts and has the power to make decisions about these cases without a retrial.

**appellee**
The party appealed against by the appellant in an appeal to a higher court.

**apperception**
Significance of and meaning one's own beliefs, experiences, knowledge, attitudes, thoughts, and emotions. See also Perception.

**applicant**
According to JCAH for psychiatric, alcoholism and drug abuse facilities accreditation purposes, this is an individual who has applied for admission to a program but who has not completed the intake process.

**application**
In health insurance this is a signed statement of facts requested by the insurance company on the basis of which the insurance company decides whether or not to issue a policy. This then becomes part of the health insurance contract if the policy is issued.

**appoint**
1. To fix by decree. 2. To constitute, or establish. 3. To designate. 4. To give a person a job, duty or responsibility. 5. Conferring power upon someone to carry out a responsibility.

**appointment scheduling**
The management task of allotting time and patient/physician meetings for the care of a patient.

**apportion**
1. To allot or portion out. 2. Dividing something according to a pre-determined plan. 3. To divide into fair shares.

**appose**
1. To put questions to. 2. To examine the clerk of records about his records.

**appraisal**
1. Estimating the value of something by a fair and impartial appraiser. 2. Unbiased estimation of the value of property.

**appraise**
To estimate the quality or value of something.

**appreciation**
A raise or increase in value or price.

**apprehension**
1. To take into custody. 2. Fear of an upcoming event.

**appropriate**
1. To assign a particular use. 2. To claim an exclusive right. 3. To acquire or take possession of something. 4. Suitable for a particular person, condition, occasion, or place; proper; fitting. A term commonly used in making policy, usually without specific indication of which aspects of the person or thing to which the term is applied are to be judged appropriate, or how and by what standard those aspects are to be judged. A good example occurs in P.L. 93-641, in section 1523(a)(6) which requires State health planning and development agencies to periodically review existing institutional health services and make public findings "respecting the appropriateness of such services." No indication is given in the law or legislative history of what the agencies are to find either appropriate or inappropriate (the costs or charges, necessity, quality, staffing, administration, or location of the services), or what methods and criteria are to be used.

**appropriateness of care**
For PSRO programs purposes, it is used to describe proper settings for delivery of medical care (e.g., acute care hospital when needed and long-term care facility only) when it is proper and required.

**appropriation**
1. In the Federal budget, it is an act of Congress that permits Federal agencies to incur obligations and to make payments out of the Treasury for specified purposes. An appropriation usually follows enactment of authorizing legislation. An appropriation is the most common form of budget authority, but in some cases the authorizing legislation provides the budget authority. Appropriations are categorized by their period of availability (one-year, multiple-year, no-year), the timing of Congressional action (current, permanent), and how the amount of the appropriation is determined (definite, indefinite). 2. A legislature's setting aside of money for a specific purpose for example: A Health Planning appropriation. 3. The taking of property by the government.

**approved**
According to JCAH for psychiatric, alcoholism and drug abuse facilities accreditation purposes, this means acceptable to the authority having jurisdiction.

**approved drugs and biologicals (Under Medicare)**
Such drugs and biologicals as are: (a) approved for inclusion in the United States Pharmacopoeia, National Formulary, or United States Homeopathic Pharmacopoeia; or (b) included (or approved for inclusion) in AMA Drug Evaluations or Accepted Dental Therapeutics, except for any drugs and biologicals unfavorably evaluated therein; or (c) not included (nor approved for inclusion) in the compendia listed in the above paragraphs of this definition, may be considered approved if such drugs: (1) were furnished to the patient during his prior hospitalization, and (2) were approved for use during a prior hospitalization by the hospital's pharmacy and drug therapeutics committee (or equivalent), and (3) are required for the continuing treatment of the patient in the facility. (In the case of Medicaid, drugs approved by the State Title XIX agency, are included).

**appurtenance**
1. That which is a part of something else. 2. An extra right. 3. Something annexed, attached to or belonging to a major thing, and which also passes with ownership.

**appurtenant**
Belonging to or added on to.

**a priori (Lat.)**
1. From the first, from the preceding. 2. Opposite of a posteriori. 3. Looking at cause-effect relationships. 4. Starting with cause going to the end result, a form of reasoning which tries to discover what facts came first and what followed one after another. 5. To reason or argue with the factual and historical knowledge that certain facts are true.

**aqueo-**
Prefix meaning water.

**arbiter**
1. One authorized to judge or decide; an adjudicator. 2. A person who decides a disagreement. 3. A person selected to decide a controversy with authority behind his decision.

**arbitrament**
The decision of an arbitrator.

**arbitrary**
1. Not controlled by a principle; capricious. 2. Any action taken or made without any supervision or any set of principles or policies used in decision making. 3. Left to the judgment of the court, not statutes.

**arbitration**
A method of settling controversies or disputes by enlisting the services of an unofficial third party to hear and consider arguments in order to

determine an equitable settlement. The settling or judgement of disputes between two parties by an arbiter or arbitrators has most often been associated with collective bargaining in labor disputes since the early 1940s. As of recent years, it has become common to have controversies of various natures reviewed for judgement by third parties with their decision being final and binding. One main purpose for arbitration is a screening mechanism which substitutes for the litigation process. Arbitration has been confused with mediation with the basic differences between these two being that the decision of arbitration is a binding decision which is often referred to as "award," whereas in mediation, a compromise is sought, in which a third party assists in reaching decisions. The concept of arbitration in recent years has been used in hearing malpractice suits prior to going to court. See malpractice screening panels.

**arbitration clause**
A clause in a contract compelling the parties of the contract to arbitrate differences and controversies that may arise from the contract.

**arbitrator**
An unbiased third party through which a controversy is decided: an arbiter.

**area health education center (AHEC)**
An organization or system of health, educational and service institutions whose policy and programs are frequently under the direction of a medical school or university health science center and whose prime goals are to improve the distribution, supply, quality, utilization, and efficiency of health personnel in relation to specific medically underserved areas. The primary objectives are to educate and train the health personnel specifically needed by that underserved community and to decentralize health manpower education, thereby increasing manpower supplies and providing a linkage between the health and educational institutions in scarcity areas. In practice, each AHEC has as its nucleus one or more public or nonprofit hospitals, some distance away from the medical school or university health science center, but whose educational efforts are under the effective guidance of such medical center. The development of AHECs were assisted by the old department of HEW.

**area of responsibility**
A major aspect of the role which encompasses an aggregate of related functions.

**area-wide agreement**
A single labor agreement made by one union which also makes the same agreement with many hospitals in the same geographical area.

**areawide comprehensive health planning agency (areawide A agency, or 314(b) agency)**
A former sub-state (usually multi-county) agency assisted under the old section 314(b) of the PHS Act, created by the Comprehensive Health Planning and Public Health Service Amendments of 1966 (P.L. 89-749), and charged with the preparation of regional or local plans for the

coordination and development of existing and new health services, facilities, and manpower. The agencies were authorized to review and comment upon proposals from hospitals and other institutions for development of programs and expansion of facilities, but had no significant powers of enforcement. Up to three quarters of the operating costs of the 314(b) agencies could be supported by Federal project grants. The balance of the costs were obtained from voluntary contributions from any source, including the health care providers affected by the agencies' plans. Under the provisions of the new health planning law, P.L. 93-641, existing 314(b) agencies have been replaced by health systems agencies which have expanded duties and powers.

**arguendo (Lat.)**
Accepting something as true for the sake of argument.

**argument**
1. Debate and discussion using facts, reasoning and legal documents to persuade a shift of opinion. 2. In-court presentation of facts and opinions to sway a decision.

**argumentative**
1. Stating reasons and facts with intent to prove something. 2. Stating conclusions and reasons.

**Arizona Health Care Cost Containment System (AHCCCS)**
Since Arizona is the only state to not adopt Medicaid, it has developed a proposed related program to meet state health care needs of the poor. A few differences the AHCCCS proposal has from Medicaid include: eligibility for services for indigents is determined by income and resources rather than participation in other public assistance programs; to establish a stabilized risk pool, services for high risk populations (65 and older) will continue to be provided by the counties; most care will be provided on a cost containment rather than fee for service basis; co-payment by all participants is required; will serve persons other than indigents in a cost-effective fashion with no federal financial participation sought for these persons; non-inclusion of references to family planning, home health care, transportation other than emergency ambulance, and nurse midwives; long-term care services will be provided by the counties in conformance with new legislation which promotes the use of less costly as well as less restrictive forms of care contrasted with the Medicaid promotion of the most restrictive and costly form of long-term care (skilled nursing care); the private enterprise system will be used to manage the system, contain costs and prevent fraud.

**arm board**
A special table-like device, attached to an operating table, to aid in giving injections.

**arraign**
1. To call a defendant before a court to hear charges, usually to enter a plea of guilty or not guilty. 2. To accuse or charge with faults.

**arrears (or arrearages)**
1. Something kept in reserves. 2. Money owed that is due or unpaid. 3. Unpaid debts.

**arrest**
1. To seize or take by power or force. 2. Legal apprehension of a person. 3. Taking a person into legal custody to answer for criminal charges. This may involve the use of force if necessary. 4. To end or stop a disease, condition or disorder or to stop it from getting worse.

**arrest of judgement**
1. The staying of a decision. 2. The temporary stopping of the court's judgement because of wrong proceedings.

**arrogation**
1. To claim something unwarrantedly. 2. Claiming or taking something in a manner that is over bearing or without having the right to.

**A R T**
Accredited Records Technician. See these words, also see Medical Record Technician.

**arteriogram**
A diagnostic method used to enable visualization of the arteries by introducing radioactive dye into the blood stream.

**arteriosclerosis**
A pathological condition in which the walls of the arteries become thick and hardened.

**article**
1. A part of a document. 2. A clause in a contract. 3. A distinct part of a document that has two or more parts. 4. In ecclesiastical law, to accuse. 5. A method of binding.

**articles**
1. The separate parts of an instrument, document, policy, etc. such as articles of agreement. 2. Parts of a formal document that make it a whole work.

**articles of incorporation**
A legal document used to create a corporation.

**art therapist**
The art therapist applies the principles and techniques of art to the rehabilitation of patients. These individuals work with mentally ill or mentally retarded patients and with temporarily or permanently disabled patients.

**Aschheim-Zondek test (AZT)**
A test used to test for pregnancy where a urine specimen from a female is injected into a female mouse.

**asepsis**
The absence of disease-producing pathogens and microorganisms.

**ASHA**
American Speech and Hearing Association. Also American School Health Association. See these words.

**ASPH**
Association of Schools of Public Health.

**asphyxia**
A condition resulting from the lack of oxygen being inspired into the body.

**aspiration**
1. The removal of fluids or gases from a cavity of the body by suction. 2. The act of inhaling.

**asportation**
1. Illicit removal of goods from where they are left. 2. Carrying away items illegally.

**assault**
1. An illegal threat of physical harm or an attempt to do harm. 2. Show of force or an action that could be taken to cause a person to feel in danger of physical attack or physical harm.

**assent**
1. To admit as true consent. 2. To approve an agreement. 3. Compliance.

**assertion**
See assertiveness.

**assertiveness**
Used in assertiveness training for managers, administrators, supervisors and women's groups. Assertion is taught. Being assertive is not being aggressive. Expression is made without dominating, humiliating, or degrading the other person. Assertion involves respect, not deference. The goal of assertion is communication and compromise. In compromises, neither person sacrifices basic integrity and both get some of their needs satisfied. See aggression and non-assertion.

**assertiveness training**
See assertiveness.

**assess**
1. To fix a sum against, such as a tax or fine. 2. To set an amount. 3. To place a value on something, usually for tax purposes.

**assessed valuation**
Determining the value of real estate for tax purposes that is usually less than present market value.

**assessment**
1. In insurance, a charge upon carriers to raise funds for a specific purpose such as meeting the administrative costs of a government required program (usually state government) or a special organization authorized by government, and provided for in law or regulation. Applied

to all carriers handling a specific line of coverage subject to regulation by the government in question and based upon a formula. 2. According to JCAH for psychiatric, alcoholism and drug abuse facilities accreditation purposes this is those procedures by which a program evaluates an individual's strengths, weaknesses, problems and needs.

**assets**
1. Anything a person owns that is of value. 2. Money and property owned by a person or an organization.

**asset turnover**
A ratio net sales to average assets representing the activity portion of the return on investment.

**assign**
1. To designate or appoint for a particular purpose or duty. 2. To transfer a contractual right to another. 3. An asset or belonging.

**assigned risk**
A special type of insurance, such as malpractice insurance, that insurance companies write only because it is required by law. A risk which underwriters do not care to insure (such as a person with hypertension seeking health insurance) but which, because of State law or otherwise, must be insured. Insuring assigned risks is usually handled through a group of insurers (such as all companies licensed to issue health insurance in the State) and individual assigned risks are assigned to the companies in turn or in proportion to their share of the State's total health insurance business. Assignment of risks is common in casualty insurance and less common in health insurance. As an approach to providing insurance to such risks, it can be contrasted with pooling of such risks (see insurance pool) in which the losses rather than the risks are distributed among the group of insurers.

**assignee**
The one to whom rights at law or whose property rights have been transferred for the benefit of others or oneself. An assignee may be designated by a court, specially appointed or named in a deed.

**assigner**
One who assigns.

**assignment**
1. In insurance and under medicare, an agreement is when a patient assigns to another party, usually a provider, the right to receive payment from a third-party for the service the patient has received. Assignment is used instead of a patient paying directly for the service and then receiving reimbursement from public or private insurance programs. In Medicare, if a physician accepts assignment from the patient, he must agree to accept the program payment as payment in full (except for specific coinsurance, copayment and deductible amounts required of the patient). Assignment, then, protects the patient against liability for charges which the Medicare program will not recognize as reasonable. 2. The transfer of property. 3. A claim or right to another person or a

second party. 4. The transfer of one's right to collect an amount payable under an insurance contract. Also known as Assignment of benefits. 5. A transfer of a right or a claim or property. Also see assign.

**assignment of benefits**
An agreement where the patient assigns any or all benefits to be paid to the health care provider by his health or medical insurance If a provider accepts assignment, he accepts the amount paid by the third party payer for that particular service. In most cases, the provider has the choice of accepting or rejecting assignment of benefits.

**assignment of error**
A declaration made by an appellant court against a trial court, setting forth the errors complained of to determine from the record the effect of the alleged errors.

**assignor**
One in law who assigns or transfers claims, property or rights under law.

**assimilation**
The process whereby a person is able to encounter and react to new situations by using the defense or adjustment mechanisms they already possess.

**Assisted Health Insurance Plan (AHIP)**
One of three parts of one of a proposed approach to national health insurance, the Comprehensive Health Insurance Plan. AHIP is designed to provide health insurance coverage for low income and high medical risk people. It would be available to anyone electing coverage, at a premium no greater than 150 percent of the average group premium for private health insurance in the State. Premiums and cost sharing would be indexed to income. AHIP would replace Medicaid and would be State administered under contract with fiscal intermediaries. The plan would be financed by premiums, and subsidized by State and Federal revenues under a matching formula.

**associate degree program**
A program which educates registered nurses or other allied health professionals in a junior college, the associate degree being given upon junior college graduation. The student's classroom and laboratory teaching is principally provided in the college and clinical teaching in an affiliated hospital. See also diploma school and baccalaureate degree program.

**associate degree school of nursing**
A department, division, or other administrative unit in a junior college, community college, college, or university which provides primarily or exclusively a two-year program of education in professional nursing and allied subjects leading to an associate degree in nursing or to an equivalent degree, but only if such program, or such unit, college, or university is accredited.

**association**
1. In psychology it is the relationship between ideas and feelings. 2. In research or epidemiology, the general name for a relationship between

two variables. Two related variables, such as age and the incidence of diabetes, are said to be 'associated.' Several different types of association are recognized: such as artifactual, causal, and chance. 3. A society or group of persons with common interests who create an organization for this common purpose, to transact business and activities pursuant to the members' mutual advantage. 4. Union of things.

**association group**
A group composed of members of a trade or business association, which purchases insurance under one master health insurance agreement.

**Association of Humanistic Psychology (AHP)**
An organization created for the development of the human sciences in ways which recognize one's distinctive human qualities and work toward fulfilling one's innate capacities as individuals and members of society. Established to link people together who have humanistic beliefs of people, to encourage others to treat all in a humanistic way and to demonstrate that being humanistic to others can be realized in the life and work of all people.

**Association of University Programs in Health Administration**
An international cooperative effort to improve health services delivery through education for administration. The university programs are a primary resource for improving administrative technology, which is fundamental to high quality and effective delivery of medical care. It is also fundamental to the appropriate allocation of scarce and expensive community health resources. Through graduate and undergraduate programs, community service, research and continuing education, the member universities are advancing administrative technology and preparing qualified administrative leadership for health services. The Association is a corporation organized in 1948 as a consortium of faculties, assisting the participating universities in achieving their individual and collective objectives. Its work is supported by a unique partnership of industry, health organizations, individuals, foundations, government and the universities.

**assuming insurance company**
See reinsurance.

**assumption of risk**
In some states, if you knowingly expose yourself, or your property, to certain dangers, you cannot collect damages if harm or damage occurs.

**assurance**
Synonymous with insurance.

**asthenic personality**
Lack of enthusiasm, lacks capacity for enjoyment, low tolerance for stress and tires easily.

**astigmatism**
An eye disorder caused by an imperfectly curved lens or cornea. Different surface curvatures will thus produce an unequal focal plane on

the surface of the retina so some parts of the object are in focus and others are not.

**astringent**
An agent or substance that causes contraction. It usually is applied topically.

**asyndesis**
A language disorder common in schizophrenia. The combining of unconnected ideas and images by a person suffering from schizophrenia.

**ataxia**
The lack of either physical or mental coordination. In neurology, it refers to loss of muscular coordination. In psychiatry, it refers to lack of coordination between feelings and thoughts; the disturbance is found in schizophrenia.

**athletic trainer**
An allied health care professional who treats, cares for and rehabilitates athletic injuries. They provide treatment and rehabilitation procedures as prescribed by the team physician. Trainers give first aid, tape injuries, supervise diets, and assist in purchasing and fitting athletic equipment. A 4 year bachelor's degree in athletic training is the minimum education. Graduate training is recommended and some physical therapists become athletic trainers. College graduates without an athletic training degree can qualify by completing additional undergraduate and graduate courses and a minimum of 900 hours of supervised clinical experience.

**atomic energy**
Energy released in nuclear reactions or when a neutron splits an atom's nucleus or when two nuclei are joined together under millions of degrees of heat; more correctly called nuclear energy.

**atomic power**
The production of thermal power in a nuclear reactor.

**at risk**
1. The state of being subject to some uncertain event occurring which connotes loss or difficulty. In the financial sense, this refers to an individual, organization (like an HMO) or insurance company assuming the chance of loss—through running the risk of having to provide or pay for more services than paid for through premiums or per capita payments. If payments are adjusted after the fact so that no loss can occur, then there is no risk. Losses incurred in one year may be made up by increases in premiums or per capita payments in the next year, so the "risk" is somewhat tempered. A firm which is at risk for losses also stands to gain from profits if costs are less than premiums collected. For a consumer being financially at risk usually means being without insurance or at risk for substantial out-of-pocket expenses. 2. A second use of the term relates to the special vulnerability of certain populations to certain diseases or conditions; ghetto children are at risk for lead poisoning or rat bite; workers in coal mines are at risk for black lung disease.

**attachment**
1. The taking of goods, persons, property or estates into custody. 2. A writ providing for the seizure of property or persons in order to bring them into custody of the court for the purpose of satisfying a judgement. A hospital may attach a patient's bank account or property to make sure that a person pays a debt that occurred from a lawsuit.

**attending physician**

**attending physician**
The physician legally responsible for the care given a patient
The physician legally in charge of and responsible for treatment in a hospital or other health program. Usually the private and health care provided to the patient. physician of a private patient is also responsible for the patient's outpatient care. The attending physician for a public patient is typically chosen by the hospital upon the patient's admission from among members of its medical staff, or is one of its teaching physicians. See physician, attending.

**attention**
Concentration; in psychology it is that aspect of consciousness that relates to the focusing on certain aspects of an experience.

**attention getting**
A mental mechanism used to satisfy or relieve inner tensions by acting out, being ill mannered, tattling, or doing other behaviors, either positive or negative, to get attention focused upon one's self.

**attest**
1. To swear to; certify or witness. 2. To put a person under oath. 3. To declare. 4. To bear witness to.

**attestation**
1. A testimony; an official declaration that supports fact or evidence. 2. The witnessing of the execution of a written document. 3. Signing as a witness.

**attest function**
The act of a noninvolved certified public accountant (CPA) auditing and reviewing the fairness of an organization's or health care facility's financial statements and then explaining the findings to those having a direct concern.

**attitude**
A constant belief, predisposition, or set of behaviors directed toward a person, situation, circumstance or object.

**attorneys lien**
The right of an attorney to hold money or property already in his hands to pay for attorney's fees.

**attractive nuisance**
If potentially dangerous property is maintained so that children might be attracted to it, then the property owner can be held liable if the children get hurt even if the children are at fault.

**atypical child**
A child with problematic personality development; often used with brain-damaged or autistic children.

**audi alteram partem (Lat.)**
To hear the other side. No man should be condemned without a chance to defend himself.

**audiological assessment**
According to JCAH for psychiatric, alcoholism and drug abuse facilities accreditation purposes, this is the audiological tests for delineating the site of auditory dysfunction, including such tests as pure tone air-conduction and bone-conduction threshold, speech reception thresholds, speech discrimination measurements, impedance measurements, and others.

**audiologist, qualified**
According to JCAH for psychiatric, alcoholism and drug abuse facilities accreditation purposes, this is an individual who is certified by the American Speech-Language-Hearing Association as clinically competent in the area of audiology, or an individual who has documented equivalent education, training, and/or experience.

**audiologists**
These health care providers specialize in diagnostic evaluation of hearing and conduct research related to hearing disorders. Using electroacoustic instrumentation, audiologists determine the range, nature, and degree of hearing function. They coordinate audiometric results with other diagnostic data, such as educational, medical, behavioral, and social information. They plan, direct, conduct, or participate in aural rehabilitation programs. These programs include such activities as hearing-aid selection and orientation, auditory training, speech reading, speech conservation, counseling, and guidance. The audiologist may also provide consultant services to educational, medical, and other professional groups, or teach audiology-related courses in educational institutions. See qualified audiologist.

**audiology**
The study, examination, appreciation and treatment of hearing defects, including the use of auditory substitutional devices (hearing aids) and other therapy. See also audiologist and speech pathologist.

**audiometric screening**
According to JCAH for psychiatric, alcoholism and drug abuse facilities accreditation purposes, this is a process that may include such tests as pure tone air-conduction thresholds, pure tone air-conduction suprathreshold screenings, impedance measurements, or observations of reactions to auditory stimuli.

**audio response unit**
In computers, it is a device that provides verbal replies to questions directed to the computer through a dial telephone input unit.

**audit**

1. An examination of an account of a financial status. 2. To check and examine. 3. A methodical approach to the examination and review of business records or medical records.

**audit, financial**

According to JCAH for psychiatric, alcoholism and drug abuse facilities accreditation purposes, this is an independent review by a public accountant certifying that a facility's financial reports reflect its financial status.

**auditor**

1. An official authorized to check the accounts of others. 2. One who examines financial accounts for accuracy.

**AUPHA**

Association of University Programs in Health Administration. See these words.

**authenticate**

As used in JCAH accreditation, this means to prove authorship, for example, by written signature, identifiable initials, or computer key. The use of rubber stamp signatures is acceptable only under the following conditions: 1) The individual whose signature the rubber stamp represents is the only one who has possession of the stamp and is the only one who uses it; and 2) The individual places in the administrative offices of the hospital a signed statement to the effect that he is the only one who has the stamp and is the only one who will use it. According to JCAH, when accrediting long term care facilities, the use of rubber stamp signatures is acceptable only if the physician whose signature is represented on the rubber stamp is the only one who has possession of the stamp and the only one who uses it, and if a signed statement is on file stating that he or she is the only one who has the stamp and is the only one who will use it.

**authentication**

According to JCAH for psychiatric, alcoholism and drug abuse facilities accreditation purposes, this is proof of authority and responsibility by written signature, identifiable initials, computer key, or other method. The use of a rubber stamp signature is acceptable only under the following conditions: the person whose signature the rubber stamp represents is the only one who has possession of the stamp and is the only one who uses it, and this person gives the chief executive officer a signed statement that he or she is the only one who has the stamp and is the only one who will use it.

**authority**

1. The power or right to command or administer. 2. Power to act. 3. An official declaration. 4. A precedent or decision of a court.

**authority having jurisdiction**

According to JCAH for psychiatric, alcoholism and drug abuse facilities accreditation purposes this is the organization, office, or individual responsible for approving a piece of equipment, an installation, or a procedure.

**authorization or authorizing legislation**
In the Federal budget, it is when legislation has been enacted by Congress which sets up or continues the legal operation of a Federal program or agency indefinitely or for a specific period of time, often it is for three years. Such legislation is a prerequisite for subsequent appropriations, or other kinds of budget authority to be contained in appropriation acts. It may limit the amount of budget authority to be provided subsequently or may authorize the appropriation of 'such sums as may be necessary.' In a few instances budget authority may be provided in the legislative authorization (see backdoor authority). The term also refers to annual dollar limits specified in authorizing legislation on amounts which may be appropriated for the authorized program.

**authorize**
1. To make legal. 2. To give authority or official power. 3. To give the authority to act. 4. To officially permit.

**auto-**
Prefix meaning self.

**autodidactic**
Any person who is an inner-directed self-starter, self-teacher who questions reality, instead searches for underlying meanings and new ways of organizing information about the world. Believed by some professionals to be a personality characteristic of many creative persons.

**autoerotism**
Sexual arousal of self. Often used interchangeably with the term masturbation.

**automated, multichannel tests**
The following list contains those pathology tests which can be and are frequently done as groups and combinations on automated multichannel equipment: albumin, bilirubin (direct), bilirubin (total), calcium, carbon dioxide content, chlorides, cholesterol, creatinine, globulin, glucose (sugar), lactic dehydrogenase, phosphatase (alkaline), phosphorus, potassium, protein (total), sodium, transaminase (glutamic oxalacetic SGOT), transaminase (glutamic pyruvic SGPT), urea nitrogen, uric acid.

**automation**
1. In medical records or the hospital business office it is a process in which work is done with a minimum of human effort, in which the process is largely self-regulating. 2. The investigation, design, development and application of health care or record processing methods of rendering processes automatic, self-moving, or self-controlling.

**automatism**
1. A mental state where the person unknowingly commits certain acts that he would not have consciously committed. 2. Behavior that lacks direction and is not controlled by conscious thought.

**automysophobia**
Fear of smelling bad or of being unclean.

**autonomic**
1. Self-controlling; capable of independent function. 2. An automatic, yet separate, function.

**autopsy**
Examination of the body after death (post mortem, therefore also called a 'post' or 'post mortem') to determine the cause of death. The autopsy rate (percentage of deaths receiving autopsies in a hospital) is sometimes considered a measure of the quality of a hospital. Consent for an autopsy, except where exception is made by law, is required from the dead person's survivors.

**autoptic evidence**
Evidence gained from the examination of a dead body in search for the cause of death.

**auxiliary**
Supplementary. Giving aid or support.

**availability**
A measure (in terms of type, volume and location) of the supply of health resources and services relative to the needs (or demands) of a given individual or community. Health care is available to an individual when he can obtain it at the time and place that he needs it, from appropriate personnel. Availability is a function of the distribution of appropriate resources and services, and the willingness of the provider to serve the particular patient in need. 2. The extent to which health care services are present in a specified geographic area. The mere presence or absence of a given service is the simplest measure of its availability. A better measure of availability is whether or not a particular service is present in the appropriate quantity. The extent to which health care resources (manpower, facilities, equipment) are present in an area is often used as a substitute measure of service availability. 3. A characteristic of a health care system. See also access and acceptability.

**availability of service/facilities**
The procedures the health care consumer has to follow in order to utilize existing health services. Refers to the existence of facilities and/or services on the basis of need regardless of the time at which the need occurs. See accessibility and availability.

**available bed days**
The average number of beds available in a health care facility that can be used for patient care. This is determined by taking the number of beds available times the number of days in a given time period. Thus, a 100-bed hospital would have 36,500 available bed days per year.

**aver**
1. To affirm; confirm. 2. To prove. 3. To declare. 4. To justify. 5. To formally allege.

**average cost**
The fixed costs plus variable total costs divided by the number of units of product produced or number of units of service rendered.

**Average Daily Census**
The total number of patients occupying a bed and receiving in-patient care on an average day (excluding newborns). This is determined by counting the number of patients in the hospital every day at midnight (midnight census).

**average deviation**
The average or mean of all differences between each observation in a series of numbers and the median of the series of the numbers.

**average length of stay (ALOS)**
Using days as a measure of time, it is the average amount of days in-patients in a health care facility stay in a given period of time. ALOS is determined by dividing the number of patient days by either the number of admissions or the number of discharges and deaths. See case severity, length of stay.

**averment**
1. An offer to prove what is alleged. 2. A statement of facts to justify or prove.

**aversion therapy**
A form of behavior therapy based on respondent conditioning. Stimuli related to undesirable behavior are paired with a painful or unpleasant occurrence, resulting in the elimination of the negative, undesirable behavior. For example, the feelings, looks, smell and taste of cigarettes are paired with nausea induced by over use so that the patient wants nothing more to do with cigarettes.

**aversive therapy**
A form of conditioning or behavior therapy where one is made to associate an unpleasant or painful experience with undesirable behavior in order to eliminate the undesirable behavior. See aversion therapy.

**aviation trip insurance**
A short-term policy protecting individuals as passengers of scheduled aircraft. It is generally obtained at airports.

**award**
1. A document containing the decision of arbitration. 2. To formally give to or to grant. 3. The decision of an arbitrator in a dispute is an award. 4. To determine or to judge; to grant.

**axiom**
Self-evident truth or an established principle.

**aypnia**
Insomnia; inability to sleep.

**AZT**
Aschheim-Zondek test. See these words.

# B

**backdoor authority**

In the Federal budget, legislative authority for the obligation of funds outside the normal appropriation process is sometimes called backdoor spending. The most common forms of backdoor authority are borrowing authority (authority to spend debt receipts) and contract authority. In other cases, (e.g., interest on the public debt) a permanent appropriation is provided that becomes available without any current action by the Congress. Entitlement authority is sometimes included as a form of backdoor authority, since the enactment of the basic benefit legislation may effectively mandate the subsequent enactment of the appropriations to pay the statutory benefits. Section 401 of the Congressional Budget and Impoundment Control Act of 1974 specifies certain limits on the use of backdoor authority. Examples of programs that have backdoor authority are the Environmental Protection Agency's construction grant program and the social security trust funds.

**back-up hospital**

A hospital that provides inpatient care and special services which cannot be gotten in a neighborhood health center. The back-up hospital is the health care facility affiliated with neighborhood health centers to provide lacking and needed services not otherwise available for adequate patient care or treatment.

**bactericide**

A bacteria-destroying substance.

**bacterio-**

Prefix meaning bacteria.

**bad debts**

The amount of income lost by a provider because of failure of patients to pay amounts owed. The impact of the loss of revenue from bad debts may be partially offset for proprietary institutions by the fact that income tax is not payable on income not received. They may also be recovered by increasing charges to paying patients by a proportional amount. Some cost-based reimbursement programs reimburse certain bad debts (see reasonable cost).

**bad faith**

1. Untrustworthy. 2. Dishonesty which may or may not involve fraud. The opposite of "good faith" implying a design to mislead another or do fraud. 3. To neglect or refuse to complete a contract or fulfill a duty; not done by an honest mistake but by an unrighteous motive.

**bail**
Money or property deposited with the court to obtain the release of an arrested person from jail until time of trial. This money, in the form of a bond, will become the property of the court if the person does not appear in court or at the proper time.

**bail bond**
A bond offered and deposited with the court as bail money that is put up by an arrested person or others such as a bail bond company. The deposit promises that the accused person will show up in court or lose the bond to the court.

**bailee**
One who receives money or property from another as bailment. The one who is loaned or entrusted with property or money that is part of a bailment.

**bailiff**
A deputy or court official who keeps order and peace in the courtroom. The officer of the court who is responsible for the prisoner, safety of the jury and keeping order during a trial.

**bailment**
1. Delivery of personal property or money to another person, who holds it in trust for temporary care, such as a loan which is returned when certain requirements are met. 2. Providing goods or money to the court to be held in exchange for the release of an arrested person. 3. Putting up bail for the release of an arrested or jailed person.

**bailor**
One who bails or delivers property, goods or money to another under a bailment contract.

**bait and switch**
Advertising a product or service at one price to get people to come and look at it with purchasing it in mind then trying to get them to buy a different item. This may be against the law if the original item is not the one made available or if it is not the actual one advertised.

**balance sheet**
A summary of the financial status of a company, hospital or health care facility at a given time. It usually provides an accounting of all assets and all liabilities of the institution.

**Balkan frame**
A frame attached lengthwise over a bed for the purpose of attaching splints, tractions, or providing a means of mobility to bedridden patients.

**bandage**
A special material used to wrap or bind an injury or a body part.

**banker's lien**
An interest in property or money owned by a banker as security to extinguish a debt. If proper legal steps were taken, a hospital or nursing home could use such a lien to secure a debt owed to the facility.

**bankrupt**

1. To be declared legally insolvent. Under the Federal Bankruptcy Act, a person may have all debts discharged once all property and money is turned over to a trustee to pay creditors proportionately. 2. A method by which an organization in financial trouble can be restructured by the court and have all property turned into cash to pay creditors. 3. To fail at a business and to be unable to pay debts, thus legally declaring so and giving up all property to the court for distribution to creditors.

**bar**

1. A system of law and courts. 2. An organized group of lawyers. 3. The practice of law in a particular court system. 4. The part of some courtrooms where prisoners stand. 5. To prevent, stop or put up a barrier or prohibition through legal objection. 6. Nullifying of a claim or action.

**bar act**

State law states what and how a lawyer may practice.

**Bar association**

A professional society or organization established so that lawyers may participate and share the benefits of membership in it. See association.

**barbiturate**

A highly addictive drug that depresses the central nervous system. This depressant is derived from barbituric acid. The drugs commonly used as hypnotics and for sedatives. Some more common barbiturates are phenobarbital and seconal.

**bar diagram**

A graph that is similar to a histogram except that the width of the bars have no significance.

**Bard-Parker forceps**

A special type of forceps commonly used to handle or transfer sterile supplies.

**bar examination**

The written exam that a law student must pass in order to practice law in the state administering it. Some states use the same exam so if it is passed in one state, he or she can practice in other states through reciprocity.

**bargain**

1. A contract or mutual agreement. 2. An agreement to buy, sell or exchange.

**bargaining agent**

1. A bargainer. 2. One who makes a bargain, contract or mutual agreement. 3. A union that has the sole right to represent all the employees of a health care facility or institution.

**bargaining unit**

Employees in a health care facility who are an in-house representative labor group for the purposes of being represented by a union.

**bariatric medicine**
The branch of medicine that treats obesity through anorectic drugs.

**barium**
A metallic element commonly introduced into the body in solution as a contrast medium for x-ray of the gastrointestinal tract.

**barium sulfate**
White powder used as a contrast medium which is given either orally or by enema for radiographic diagnostic procedures.

**barratry**
The practice of exciting, encouraging or stirring up lawsuits; a lawyer's attempt to create lawsuits for his or her own financial gain.

**barrier technique**
A medicine practice used to control, destroy, or limit the speed of pathogenic diseases or infections.

**barrio (Spanish)**
The district, ward or neighborhood in which most of the Mexican-Americans of a city live.

**basal metabolic rate**
The rate at which energy is expended by the body to maintain its functions at rest.

**base case**
See reference projection.

**baseline data**
Basic information and facts about a patient.

**base pay**
A starting, basic or beginning rate of pay for a job level; the fundamental pay excluding bonuses, overtime, etc.

**base year**
1. A 12 month period starting from the month and day of establishment, initiation or attachment. 2. The first year from which a program started. The foundation year; the year something was established or founded; the starting year.

**basic health services**
The minimum supply of health services which should be generally and uniformly available in order to assure adequate health status and protection of the population from disease, or to meet some other criteria or standards. Given that all possible services cannot be supplied to the entire population, little information exists as to what set of services constitutes appropriate minimum services and of how to assure its availability.

**baso-**
Prefix meaning base.

**bassinets**
Bassinets, incubators, and isolators maintained for use in a hospital nursing room for newborn babies.

**batch processing**
In data processing, it is when a number of similar input data items are grouped and processed for a single computer run using the same computer program.

**battered child syndrome**
Physical harm and damage to a child as a result of repeated beatings and abuse usually done by a parent.

**battery**
1. Any intentional, illegal, unwanted, unprovoked, beating, touching or any harmful physical contact to a person by an object or another person. 2. The act of beating, hitting or battering another person with the intent of beating them up or causing physical harm.

**bearer**
Any person holding, in possession of, or presenting a note or a negotiable instrument, such as a check.

**bed**
A bed in a hospital or other inpatient health facility. Hospitals, nursing homes and other health care facilities are measured by the number of beds they have. Many definitions require that the beds be maintained for continuous (24 hour) use by inpatients. Beds are often used as a measure of capacity (hospital sizes are compared by comparing their number of beds). Licenses and certificates-of-need may be granted for specific numbers or types of beds: e.g. surgical, pediatric, obstetric, or extended care. Facilities may have both licensed and unlicensed beds; and active and licensed but unused beds. Other qualifying adjectives are frequently used to categorize beds: e.g. available, occupied, pediatric, maternity, acute care or observation beds. To have more beds in health care facilities in an area or region than are needed is said to be over bedded.

**behavior**
Any act or response that has an observable and measurable specific frequency, duration, and purpose, conscious or unconscious in origin.

**behavioral diagnosis**
Determining the specific health behaviors that are likely to affect a person's health status or need.

**behavioral health**
A field of health care that uses patient education, health education and behavioral procedures to alleviate problems of health or illness, disease, conditions and disorders by changing self-defeating or self-destructive behaviors, i.e., smoking, and/or activating positive health behaviors that are lacking. Prevention, behavior change and health activation are the major focuses.

**behavioral medicine**
The use of behavioral procedures applied to problems of illness, disease, disorders, conditions, disabilities or behaviors contributing to these, with attention focused on behavior change, prevention, diagnosis, treatment, and rehabilitation, with a goal of optimum health.

**behavioral objective**
A statement or plan created to achieve a desired outcome that spells out in specific terms who is to do how much of what, and by when.

**behavioral psychotherapy**
A type of therapy that uses observable behavior, rather than focusing on thoughts and feelings. It aims at systematic improvement and the elimination of maladaptive behaviors. Various conditioning and learning theories are combined with a directive approach including techniques adapted from other systems of psychotherapy.

**behavior control**
Exercising influence over others by changing the environmental contingencies to achieve a goal or behavior change.

**behavior modification**
The application of operant conditioning principles to behavioral problems with the intent of changing behavior and managing behavior or health problems. Management of behavior is achieved by the control of reinforcers of the behavior. This behavior change modality has been utilized in changing both physical and mental disorders, i.e. smoking and obesity.

**behavior therapy**
A therapy designed to modify the client's behavior. Behavior therapy is derived from learning theories, and focuses on modifying observable and quantifiable behavior by means of manipulation of the environmental and behavioral variables thought to be functionally related to the behavior that is to be changed. Some of the approaches include operant conditioning, shaping, token economy and systematic desensitization.

**belief**
A confidence, opinion, judgement or expectation about the truth or knowledge of a case that is not all based on fact nor only on suspicion.

**bench**
1. The place where judges sit. 2. A court of law. 3. Judges collectively. 4. The seat of Justice.

**bench warrant**
An order issued directly by a judge or court to the police for the arrest of a person charged with contempt of court or a crime.

**Bender-Gestalt test**
A psychological test used to measure the ability to reproduce a set of geometric designs. It is useful for detecting perceptual and visuomotor co-ordination thus detecting brain damage.

**bene-**
Prefix, meaning well or good.

**benefice**
A benefit, a kindness, a favor, the doing of good acts.

**beneficiary**
1. A person designated in an insurance policy to receive a specified cash payment upon the policyholder's accidental or natural death or an injury or illness. 2. In the case of medical insurance, one who is eligible to receive, or is receiving, benefits from an insurance policy or health maintenance organization. Usually includes both people who have themselves contracted for benefits and their eligible dependents. See also subscriber and insured.

**benefit**
1. In insurance, a sum of money provided in an insurance policy payable for certain types of loss, or for covered services, under the terms of the policy. The benefits may be paid to the insured or on his behalf to others. 2. In prepayment programs like HMOs, benefits are the services the program will provide a member whenever, and to the extent needed. 3. The amount payable by the carrier toward the cost of various covered medical or dental services. 4. The medical or dental service or procedure covered by an insurance policy or program. 5. To have the advantage or privilege.

**benefit-cost analysis**
Evaluating the relationship between the benefits and costs of a particular project or activity. See cost benefit analysis.

**benefit package**
In insurance it is the specific services provided in the insurance program to persons enrolled in a particular health care plan. In labor and employment it is the set of benefits that offset and assist in the employees' income, such as health and life insurance paid by the company.

**benefit period**
The period of time for which payments for benefits covered by an insurance policy are available. The availability of certain benefits may be limited over a specified time period, for example by two well-baby visits during a one-year period. While the benefit period is usually defined by a set unit of time, such as a year, benefits may also be tied to a spell of illness. See Medicare benefits.

**benefits (proration)**
A method of dividing health insurance benefits into sub-units when multiple item coverage is provided.

**benefits, health**
Those outcomes or increases experienced in one's health status or quality of life that are related to health-care processes.

**benefit year**
In health insurance, a 365-day period (which may or may not be a calendar year) during which a certain benefit (such as major medical payments) are provided.

**benestressor**
Any occurrence, event, experience, life change, achievement, advancement, success or recognition that is beneficial or positive which causes stress to be experienced by a person, yet causes much less damage than distress or dystressors. See dystressor.

**benign**
Not malignant; a tumor that does not metastasize.

**bereavement**
1. Loss of a loved one by death. 2. The act or process of mourning over a loss or death.

**best evidence rule**
A legal rule whereby primary evidence of a fact, such as an original document can be introduced, presented, or explained, before a copy or facsimile can be introduced or before testimony can be given concerning the fact or document.

**bestiality**
Sexual deviation where a person engages in sexual activity with an animal. Sexual intercourse by a human with an animal. This is a crime in many states. See sodomy.

**beyond a reasonable doubt**
In criminal law this the amount or level of proof needed to convict a person of a crime.

**bi-**
Prefix meaning two.

**BIA**
Bureau of Indian Affairs.

**bias**
1. Pre-established or pre-acquired information or opinion that makes it difficult to be fair and impartial. 2. Preconceived opinion by a judge about persons that makes him or her inclined to lean to one side unfairly so to have a pre-assessed judgement.

**bid bond**
A bond taken out to provide surety for a bid on a contract.

**bigamy**
The crime of entering a second marriage while maintaining the first marriage. The crime of marrying two husbands or two wives at the same time.

**bilateral contract**
1. An agreement wherein both parties have participated equally in the negotiations. 2. A two-sided agreement.

**bilis (Spanish)**
1. Bile. 2. A disorder in the Mexican-American culture caused by anger and envy.

**bilk**
1. To deceive or defraud. 2. To get away without paying.

**bill**
1. A draft of a law presented to a legislature. 2. A written declaration, statement, or complaint, usually against someone who suffered by someone breaking the law. Used in both criminal and civil law. 3. A financial statement sent to a patient itemizing money owed. 4. A public notice.

**bill of costs**
An itemized statement of costs charged against the losing party in a legal action.

**bill of credit**
A written request that credit be given to the bearer based on the security of the one who wrote it.

**bill of exceptions**
A written statement of a party's objections to rulings, actions and instructions made by a judge during a trial, which statement forms the basis for an appeal.

**bill of exchange**
A written document, from one person to another, unconditionally ordering the receiver to pay a specific amount to a third person.

**bill of indictment**
A written document presented to a grand jury which states the accusations of a crime. If evidence shows this is factual, it is labeled a true bill.

**bill of lading**
1. A cargo list. 2. A document provided by a shipping company that lists all goods or property for transport. The terms of the shipping agreement can also be stated in this document. It also is used to acknowledge the receipt of the goods.

**bill of parcels**
A list of items purchased and the value of each listed on the invoice.

**bill of particulars**
A detailed written statement of charges or pleadings of a plaintiff or prosecutor given at the request of the defendant.

**Bill of Patient Rights**
Legal and ethical principles utilized by health care facilities to ensure that patients are treated in a manner that recognizes their dignity and human rights. The basic rights of patients are: The right to be furnished with information on diagnosis, treatment and prognosis; to participate in any and all decisions about their treatment and health care. The Bill allows for complaints to be registered and for corrective action to be made. See patients rights, patients bill of rights.

**bill of review**
A new lawsuit brought requesting that a court consider setting aside a prior decree.

**binary code**
The language of the computer based on a 2 digit numeric system, represented by two distinct characters, usually 1 and 0.

**binder**
1. A written memorandum in contract law stating the most important items agreed upon. 2. A temporary contract until a formal policy of title insurance can be drawn up. 3. In medicine, a type of abdominal bandage. 4. In law, a collection of cases or court decisions that are added to a book as they become available.

**binding arbitration**
When the outcome of arbitration is binding on both parties to the dispute.

**binding authority**
The previous decisions of appellate courts which must be considered and followed by a judge when deciding a case. See stare decisis.

**binding instruction**
Instructions to a jury which must be followed to arrive at a specified decision, on the basis of whether the jury concludes certain facts to be true or false.

**binding receipt**
A receipt given for a premium payment accompanying the application for insurance. This binds the company, if the policy is approved, to make the policy effective from the date of the receipt.

**binding review**
For PSRO programs purposes, it is a PSRO review for which determinations are final and affect payments by Title XVIII fiscal intermediaries and Title XIX state agencies.

**bind over**
1. A court order that an accused be held in custody pending a proceeding against him. He may then be permitted to post bond and be released. 2. To obligate an accused person to appear in court.

**bio-**
Prefix meaning life.

**bioavailability**

1. The extent and rate of absorption of a dose of a given drug, measured by the time-concentration curve for appearance of the administered drug in the blood. The concept is important in attempting to determine whether different brand name drugs, a generic name as opposed to a brand name drug, or, in some cases, different batches of the same brand name drug, will produce the same therapeutic effect. 2. The same drug made by two different manufacturers or different batches of the same drug made by the same manufacturer may demonstrate differing bioavailability. There is debate as to differences which are therapeutically significant. See also Maximum Allowable Cost Program, antisubstitution, and bioequivalence.

**bioequivalence**

1. Describes drug preparations which have the same bioavailability. Such drugs are chemically equivalent although chemically equivalent preparations are not always bioequivalent. Bioequivalence is a function of bioavailability and the terms are often used synonymously. 2. Chemically equivalent drugs which are bioequivalent have the same treatment effect although therapeutically equivalent preparations need not be either chemically or bioequivalent.

**biofeedback**

An anti-anxiety or body function control technique based on fundamental learning principles where the average person learns to make a certain response when he or she receives information or feedback as whether he or she has made a correct response, or that are moving he or she closer to the desired goal. Electronic monitoring is used to give the patient immediate and continual signals, readings (feedback) related to changes in bodily functions of which one is not normally aware of, such as brain waves, blood pressure, and heart rate. Through control of the mind, the patient strives to learn to control the function of various body parts, functions or organs.

**biologics**

1. Biological products or biologicals. 2. Any virus, therapeutic serum, toxin, antitoxin, or analogous product of plant or animal origin used in the prevention, diagnosis, or treatment of disease. 3. Biologics, vaccines and blood plasma products, are regulated by the Bureau of Biologics, a division of the Food and Drug Administration. They differ from drugs in that biologics are usually derived from living microorganisms and cannot be synthesized or readily standardized by chemical or physical means. They tend to be chemically less stable than drugs, their safety cannot be as easily assured and they are never as chemically pure as drugs.

**biology**

The science of life and living organisms.

**biomedical and consumer product safety**

Those measures taken to insure that drugs, cosmetics, therapeutic devices and all types of consumer products including cleaning fluids, pesticides and children's toys are safe and appropriate for their intended use, and are clearly labeled as to potential harm resulting from abuse or misuse.

**biomedical engineer**
The biomedical engineer utilizes engineering ideas and techniques in the development of new instruments, equipment, processes, and systems for the medical care of patients and the improvement of health systems.

**biomedical engineering technologist/technician**
Assembles, repairs, and adapts medical equipment to assist biomedical engineers, physicians, and scientists in the development and maintenance of medical equipment and systems for the delivery of health care. (Biomedical Equipment Technologist)

**biomedical research**
Research concerned with human and animal biology, and disease and its prevention, diagnosis and treatment. It contrasts with health services research which is concerned with behavioral science and organizational behavior in various aspects of health services.

**biometry**
The application of mathematics, statistics, research to biology; measuring the processes and functions related to living things.

**bionics**
The science of the creation and function of electronic and mechanical devices or systems that operate similarly or in the same way as body parts or living organs.

**biopsy**
The removal and examination of living tissue.

**biostatistician**
A person with advanced training in the application of mathematics and statistics to research related to health care, medicine and health planning. Usually this requires a Masters or PhD in biostatistics/statistics/math. See health statistician.

**biostatistics**
The application of mathematical statistics and techniques to research information related to medicine, biomedical science, health and social problems, public health, vital statistics and demography.

**birth control**
The intentional limiting of the number of children born. This is done through the control of sexual activity or by the use of contraceptives. See family planning.

**birthing room**
Comfortable homelike room in a hospital for labor and delivery. Women are not moved to a surgical-type suite for delivery. See alternative birthing center.

**birth rate**
1. The rate at which babies are born in a specific population. 2. A formula used to determine the birth rate which is a fraction, whose numerator is the total number of births in a population during a given period and whose denominator is the total number of person-years lived

by the population during that period. The latter is generally approximated by the size of the population at the mid-point of the period multiplied by the length of the period in years. The birth rate is usually stated per 1,000. Like other rates in which the population at the mid-point of the period is used as the denominator of the fraction, this is sometimes called the central birth rate. Where birth rate is used without qualification, the live birth rate is generally meant and only live births appear in the numerator. The total birth rate, based on live births and late fetal deaths, is sometimes calculated. Legitimate birth rates and illegitimate birth rates, with legitimate and illegitimate births respectively, are computed; and the illegitimacy ratio, the number or illegitimate births per 1,000 total births, is frequently used. See fertility rate. (See appendix I)

**birth rates**
See crude birth rate, age specific birth rates.

**bit-binary digit**
1. In computerized medical records it is a single character in a binary number. 2. Each of the eight intersections making up a computer cell. See Magnetic core.

**black letter law**
Legal principles that are universally accepted by most judges.

**black light**
Ultraviolet light radiation; causes pigmentation of the skin.

**black lung**
Common name for pneumoconiosis, a chronic severely debilitating lung disease caused by inhaling coal dust and principally found among coal miners. Certain medical benefits for the victims of the disease are available under title IV of the Federal Coal Mine Health and Safety Act of 1969 (P.L. 91-173), as amended by P.L. 92-303.

**blackmail**
1. Threats or danger used for extortion. 2. To extort money from a person by threats of exposing illicit activities that could destroy one's reputation or have a negative effect on a relationship. For this to be blackmail, and not just extortion, some state laws require it to be in writing.

**blanching**
The pressing of a patient's fingernail with your fingernail to determine if blood is circulating to it or if there is an impairment in circulation to a patient's limbs and fingers. The fingernail should become white looking when momentarily pressed and then quickly return to its normal pink color if circulation is normal. If it is not normal, it may stay white. This test is used to insure circulation to limbs and fingers when they are bound with bandages, casts, etc.

**blanket medical expense (coverage)**
A provision (usually included as an added feature of a policy primarily providing some other type of coverage, such as loss of income insurance)

which entitles the insured to collect, up to a maximum established in the policy, for all hospital and medical expenses incurred, without limitations on individual types of medical expenses.

**blanket overhead rate**
One method of determining overhead and dividing or apportioning it to projects, services or activities, using only one rate for the whole organization.

**blanket policy**
1. To cover everything by one policy. 2. A flexible insurance policy with broad coverage.

**blank indorsement**
Signing a draft or check, without specifying who can cash it.

**blind spot**
A term used in psychiatry indicating an area of a person's personality that he is totally unaware of. These areas of unawareness are often hidden by repression in order to avoid painful emotions.

**block**
In computerized medical records it is a set of things, such as words, characters, or digits handled as a unit. See Block Diagram Symbol.

**block diagram**
In computerized medical records it is a schematic chart, setting forth the detailed sequence of operations to be performed for handling a particular application. A tool used in computer programming.

**block diagram symbols**
In computerized medical or business records they are symbols used in a block diagram to represent the basic instructions prepared for a computer. The terms "block" and "symbol" are used interchangeably.

**blood bank**
Some hospitals maintain a blood bank services and others do not. This service provides a constant supply of blood and plasma, for use in the health care facility.

**blood bank technologist**
A medical technologist, working under the direction of a pathologist, physician, or laboratory director, prepares, collects, classifies, stores, and processes blood including the separated components of whole blood. He or she also does detection and identification of antibodies in patient and donor bloods, as well as selection and delivery of suitable blood for transfusion.

**blood pressure**
The pressure at which the heart pushes the blood as it pulsates through the arteries.

**Blue Cross**
An independent, not for profit membership health insurance corporation providing protection against the costs of hospital care, and in some

policies protection against the costs of surgical and professional care. (See Blue Cross Association and Blue Cross plan.)

**Blue Cross Association (BCA)**

The national nonprofit organization to which the 70 Blue Cross plans in the United States voluntarily belong. BCA administers programs of licensure and approval for Blue Cross plans, provides specific services related to the writing and administering of health care benefits across the country, and represents the Blue Cross plans in national affairs. Under contract with the Social Security Administration (SSA), BCA is intermediary in the Medicare program for 77 percent of the participating providers (90 percent of the participating hospitals, 50 percent of the participating skilled nursing facilities, and 76 percent of the participating home health agencies). See also Health Services, Inc. and Blue Shield Plan.

**Blue Cross plan**

A nonprofit, tax-exempt health service prepayment organization providing coverage for health care and related services. The individual plans should be distinguished from their national association, the Blue Cross Association. Historically, the plans were largely the creation of the hospital industry, and designed to provide hospitals with a stable source of revenues, although formal association between the Blue Cross and American Hospital Associations ended in 1972. A Blue Cross plan must be a nonprofit community service organization with a governing body with a membership including a majority of public representatives. Most plans are regulated by State insurance commissioners under special enabling legislation. Plans are exempt from Federal income taxes, and, in most States, from State taxes (both property and premium). Unlike most private insurance companies, the plans usually provide service rather than indemnity benefits, and often pay hospitals on the basis of reasonable costs rather than charges. There are 70 plans in the United States. See also Health Services, Inc. and Blue Shield Plan.

**Blue Shield**

An independent, not for profit membership health insurance association providing protection against the costs of physician services, surgery, and other items of medical care. Some policies also offer protection against the costs of hospital care. See also Blue Shield Plan.

**Blue Shield Plan**

A nonprofit, tax-exempt plan of a type originally established in 1939 which provides coverage of physician's services. The individual plans should be distinguished from the National Association of Blue Shield Plans. Blue Shield coverage is commonly sold in conjunction with Blue Cross coverage, although this is not always the case. The relationship between Blue Cross and Blue Shield plans has been a cooperative one; as the two organizations have a common board, one management, and are located in the same building. Blue Shield plans cover some 65 million Americans through their group and individual business. In addition, plan activities affect some 20 million persons through participation in various government programs, including Medicare (32 plans act as carriers under part B), Medicaid, and CHAMPUS. Most States have enacted special enabling legislation for the Blue plans. See also Medical Indemnity of America, Inc.

**BNDD**

Bureau of Narcotics and Dangerous Drugs. (Housed under the Department of Justice.)

**board certified**

Describes a physician or other health care professional who has passed an examination given by a medical specialty board and been certified by that board as a specialist in a specific area. The examination cannot be taken until the professional meets requirements set by the specialty board for board eligibility.

**board eligible**

Describes a physician or other health care professional who is eligible for specialty board examination (including those who may have failed the examination if they remain eligible). Each of the specialty boards have requirements which must be met before the examination for specialty board certification can be taken. Usually this includes graduation from an approved school, have approved training experience of specified type and length, and specified time in practice or on the job. The minimum time required after graduation from medical school to become board eligible is generally three to five years. Government and other types of health programs which define standards for specialists often accept board eligibility as equivalent to board certification, since the only difference is that the board certified professional has passed an examination.

**boarding homes**

Organized or informal facilities which provide room and board (to those desiring it, often the aged), and, sometimes, custodial care for a fee. The provision of medical supervision, social activities or counseling is not normally included as it is in a nursing home. They are not licensed as health facilities and usually are not subject to licensure at all.

**board of directors**

A group of people chosen to supervise the business activities, select key employees, and plan for the future development of the health care facility or enterprise. Members are usually elected to the board. Persons are usually elected because of their business ability and it is not essential that members of the board of directors hold stock in the health care business organization. The board of directors also have power to take such actions as are necessary or proper to conduct the business activities of the hospital or health care organization.

**Board of Directors, hospital**

A hospital governing board, which is called a Board of Directors, Board of Trustees, or Governing Board, is usually elected by a community, church, stockholders, etc., depending upon ownership and tax status (profit or not-for-profit). A typical board of 5 to 15 members meet monthly and is governed by bylaws and elects its own officers and chooses its own committees. The committees usually consist of the executive, finance, building, fund raising, etc. The board chooses and appoints, the administrator, physicians to the medical staff, and make major financial and administrative decisions beyond the usual day to day decisions delegated to the hospital administrator.

**board of governors**
See board of directors.

**Boards of Health**
A committee or board of citizens including one physician, selected and appointed by elected and governing officials such as mayor or county commissioners, to serve as an advisory and governing board to oversee administrative function of the public health department and the community's health.

**bodily heirs**
Lineal descendants.

**body contact-exploration maneuver**
A psychotherapy approach utilizing physical touching of others to gain awareness of feelings, sensations and emotions created and aroused by the experience. A technique used in encounter groups.

**body execution**
Official and legal authority to put a person in jail and deprive him or her of their freedom.

**body language**
The presentation of a person's thoughts and feelings by means of his or her bodily activity gestures, actions or posture.

**boilerplate**
1. A general standardized form for a document. 2. In a contract, it is the sections and paragraphs of general nature that do not deal with material specific to the contract.

**bona fide (Lat.)**
1. Genuine; without fraud. 2. In good faith. 3. Actual; real. 4. Honest; without deception.

**bond**
1. A written obligation with agreement to pay a specified amount of money upon certain conditions being met. 2. A written agreement to do or not do something with an amount paid as security or bail. 3. A document used to show proof of a debt. 4. A binding agreement.

**bonus**
One method of paying an incentive-type wage to an employee over normal salaries. This lump sum payment is for meritorious performance and is preferred to a dividend as it is not taxable, and can be a tax write-off for the organization.

**booking**
1. The recording of charges. 2. Facts written down by the police about an arrest. This includes identification and background information and other related facts.

**book of original entry**
A journal or record in which an accounting action is first recorded.

**book value**
1. Proven assets minus liabilities. 2. The value of any assets as recorded on a hospital or health care facility's accounting statement. 3. Net worth of the institution.

**borderline state (borderline psychosis)**
When symptoms of a mental disorder are so unclear that it is difficult to determine if the patient is psychotic or nonpsychotic.

**borrowed servant**
An employee temporarily under the control of another. An example is when a nurse employed by a health care facility is "borrowed" by a surgeon in the operating room. The temporary master of the borrowed servant will be held responsible for the act of the borrowed servant under the doctrine of "respondeat superior". See respondeat superior.

**boycott**
1. To ban use of a product, business or service. 2. To ban doing business with and attempting to stop others from trading with a company or business. 3. A primary boycott in labor law involves directly boycotting a union and the employer. A secondary boycott is banning the company from doing business with support companies.

**Bradford frame**
A rectangular frame (3 x 7 ft.) made from sturdy pipes which has two strips of movable canvas stretched across it and is used as a bed frame for patients with bone diseases (usually of the hip or spine) or is used for serious fractures. This frame allows immobilized patients to carry on bowel and urinary functions without moving or changing position.

**Bradley Training (Husband-coached childbirth)**
Developed over 30 years ago by Robert Bradley, an obstetrician. Oriented towards preparation before labor including doing what comes naturally, relaxing and breathing deeply. Encourages direct involvement of the expectant father.

**bradylalia**
Abnormally slow speech, common in depression.

**brainwashing**
1. A method of manipulating human thought and behavior against the will of those involved. 2. A systematic effort of indoctrinating persons to a way of believing and thinking.

**brain waves**
See EEG.

**Brandeis brief**

The Brandeis brief gathers and presents opinions from authorities in fields germane to the argument, but without a pertinent legal basis. Named for Louis D. Brandeis, [Muller v. Oregon 208 U.S. 412 (1908).]

**brand name**

The registered trademark given to a specific drug product by its manufacturer. Also known as a trade name. There are no official rules governing the selection of brand names. According to the Pharmaceutical Manufacturers Association, the objective is to coin a name which is "useful, dignified, easily remembered, and individual or proprietary." Drugs are primarily advertised to practitioners by brand name. When a physician prescribes by brand name, anti-substitution laws in most states forbid the pharmacist from substituting either a brand or generic name equivalent made by a different manufacturer, although either may be less expensive than the drug prescribed. However, some states have changed these laws to allow the use of a generic substitute.

**breach**

1. Failing to observe terms of an agreement. 2. The breaking of a law or the violation of a duty.

**breach of contract**

1. Failure to perform or fulfill any promise or contractual agreement. 2. Failing to carry out the terms of a contract by overlooking the legal ramifications of the promise to perform. 3. Violating by the omission of a legal duty or confidence. 4. Failure to perform on all or part of a contract, where there is no legal excuse for such failure.

**breach of promise**

1. Failing to keep one's word. 2. Breach of promise as in to not marry someone after a promise was made to do so. An outdated principle.

**breach of warranty**

The violation of any agreement or representation concerning the condition, content, or quality of a product, but with no fraudulent misrepresentation.

**break**

1. To stop by force. 2. To overwhelm. 3. To disperse or scatter. 4. Using force to illegally enter into a building or room. 5. To intrude; to enter by force. 6. To breach such as breaking in, breaking and entering.

**breakeven point**

The level where total monies equal total costs. The point where the income line meets the total cost.

**breaking bulk**

1. Illegally opening a bulk package and taking part of the contents or contaminating the contents. 2. An offense by a carrier in which part of the contents of a bulk package, box or bale in shipment are removed or converted.

**bribery**

1. The act of offering, giving, taking or receiving of rewards or things of value to influence a public official. 2. To receive a false judgement or an illegal performance.

**brief**

1. A written summary or brief statement. 2. A concise written statement prepared for a lawsuit explaining the case. A brief should contain a fact summary, law summary and shows how the law applies to the facts. 3. A summary of a published opinion.

**brief services**

See services, also levels of service.

**bring suit**

1. To seek out an attorney in order to start a lawsuit, by filing the proper papers with the court. 2. To present a lawsuit in a court of law.

**broker**

1. Any person who is paid to act as an agent to make bargains or enter into contracts. 2. One who deals in buying and selling money or notes.

**broker (insurance)**

1. One who writes insurance. 2. An insurance solicitor, licensed by the state, who does business with a variety of insurance companies and who represents the buyers of insurance rather than the companies, even though he or she is paid commissions by the companies.

**bronchogram**

An x-ray of the bronchial tree using an iodized oil dye introduced into the body as contrast medium.

**bronchoscope**

A specialized lighted instrument used to visually examine the bronchi of the lungs.

**bronchoscopy**

To visually examine the bronchi.

**brown lung**

New popular name for byssinosis; a chronic, disabling lung disease caused by chronic inhalation of cotton dust and prevalent among textile workers. Similar to, but not the same as, black lung. Federal benefits, like those available for miners disabled by black lung, are not available for people with brown lung.

**bruja (f.), brujo (m.) (Spanish)**

1. Witch, sorcerer, magician. 2. One with cursing and healing powers. 3. Brujo (male) also a conjurer, wizard and warlock.

**budget**

1. A detailed financial plan for carrying out Health Service or Hospital program activities in a specified period, usually a fiscal year. The budget typically accounts for all the program's proposed income, by source, and expenses, and by purposes such as salaries and capital costs, for the year.

Expenses are sometimes related to the program's goals and objectives. 2. Money provided for a particular purpose. 3. A plan or schedule of expenses. 4. An estimate of money needed over a certain time period.

**budget authority (BA)**
In the federal budget, authority provided by law to enter into obligations which will result in immediate or future outlays of government funds, except that it does not include the authority to insure or guarantee the repayment of indebtedness incurred by another person or government. The basic forms of budget authority are: appropriations, contract authority, and borrowing authority. Budget authority is classified by the timing of Congressional action (current or permanent) or by the manner of determining the amount available (definite or indefinite).

**budget variance**
The difference between actual costs incurred and the budget that has been adjusted to the real activity level.

**bulk sales acts**
A statute enacted to prevent the secret bulk sale of a business, merchandise or stock of a business. By these statutes a business must list items to be sold and give creditors notice of intent to sell. This helps prevent the defrauding of creditors.

**bulk transfer**
In the Uniform Commercial Code, a bulk transfer is considered an unusual way of doing business or maintaining inventories. Rules are made against "bulk sales," "bulk mortgages," or "bulk transfers" to protect creditors from being cheated.

**burden of proceeding**
To be required to present evidence on a certain question in a lawsuit, even before the other party is obligated to.

**burden of proof**
1. A requirement of proving an assertion or a disputed fact. 2. The legal principle used to determine which party has to prove the facts. 3. Burden is placed on a certain party to come forth with evidence and proof.

**bureaucracy**
1. A large organization or an administrative agency that has a hierarchy or chain of command type organizational structure. 2. An organization with well defined or specialized positions and responsibilities; inflexible rules and procedures. The delegation of authority is usually downward, utilizing all levels.

**Bureau of Biologics**
A subdivision of the U.S. Food and Drug Administration in charge of the control of biological material used in the control and prevention of disease such as serums, vaccines, antitoxins, antibiotics, toxins, blood plasma, etc.

**Bureau of Drugs**
A subdivision of the U.S. Food and Drug Administration in charge of the regulation of drugs. See Kefauver-Harris Amendment.

**Bureau of Health Facilities Financing, Compliance, and Conversion**
Shortened to the Bureau of Health Facilities.

**Bureau of Health Insurance (BHI)**
An agency within the Social Security Administration (SSA) which administers the Medicare program. Actual operation of the program is carried out through arrangements with intermediaries and carriers, who operate under contract with BHI/SSA and receive all policy guidance from the Bureau.

**Bureau of Health Manpower**
See Bureau of Health Professions.

**Bureau of Health Professions**
The Bureau of Health Professions is a component of the Health Resources Administration, Public Health Service, U.S. Department of Health and Human Services. The Bureau supports development of the human resources needed to staff the U.S. health care system. It is concerned with health professions education, credentialing of health care personnel, and analysis of data to project needs for health professions personnel. On March 18, 1980, the name of the Bureau of Health Manpower was changed to Bureau of Health Professions.

**Bureau of Quality Assurance (BQA)**
A federal level governmental agency within the Health Resources Administration which administers the Professional Standards Review Organization program.

**burned-out anergic schizophrenic**
A chronic form of schizophrenia. Symptoms include apathy and withdrawal with minimal psychotic symptoms but with persistent schizophrenic thought processes.

**burn unit**
A hospital special care unit providing intensive care to burn patients. See special care unit.

**business insurance**
An insurance policy which provides benefits principally to a business (like a hospital) rather than to an individual. It is issued to indemnify a business for the loss of services of a key employee or partner who becomes disabled.

**business interruption insurance**
A special form of insurance providing continual income to cover payroll or loss of business income due to interruption of business activity due to injury, loss, fire or other peril.

**business judgement rule**
If the executives of a corporation, such as a hospital, make honest, wise, and careful decisions and stay within their powers, the courts will not

interfere with the functions of the organization even if the results are not always good.

**business office**

This department is responsible for handling, compiling, and sending out patient's bills. It also collects money from the patient insurance companies, governmental bodies, and other types of third party payers. The director of the business office insures that financial records are properly maintained, budgets prepared, and cost analysis reports are kept and completed and that payrolls are efficiently handled.

**business record exception**

This principle provides for an exception to the "hearsay, exclusion rule." Thus, original, routine records used in transacting business could be used as evidence in a trial. This could include medical and hospital business records.

**business trust**

A company such as a hospital established as a trust that is similar to a corporation.

**buy in**

The business arrangement used to purchase or acquire an interest in a medical group practice. This is possible only if the group is a corporation, or partnership or is made into one of these legal structures.

**by-laws**

1. Subordinate laws created by groups or corporations for policy and control of the membership. 2. A secondary law, rules, or policies adopted by an organization. 3. According to Medicare, the governing body, in accordance with legal requirements, creates and adopts effective patient care policies, administrative policies and bylaws that are used in the governing and operation of the facility. Such policies and bylaws are in writing, dated, and made available to all members of the governing body which ensures that they are operational, reviewed, and revised as necessary. 3. According to JCAH for psychiatric, alcoholism and drug abuse facilities accreditation purposes, this is the laws, rules, or regulations adopted for the government of the facility. Also used for the laws, rules, or regulations of the professional staff.

[illegible] ... organization [illegible] are not [illegible].

**business office**

The department [illegible] responsible for handling, collecting, and sending out patient bills. It also collects money from the patient, insurance companies, government agencies, and others [illegible] for the patient. The director of the business office makes sure that [illegible] property [illegible], [illegible] prepared, and [illegible] kept and completed [illegible] records are [illegible].

**business record exception**

This principle [illegible] an exception to the hearsay exclusion [illegible] original [illegible] record is used [illegible] the business could be used as evidence in a legal [illegible] hospital [illegible] records.

**business trust**

A company such as a [illegible] trust, [illegible] similar to a corporation.

**bylaws**

The business activities of [illegible] corporation [illegible] medical group practice. [illegible] provide [illegible] [illegible] or [illegible] [illegible] [illegible] bylaws.

**bylaws**

Subordinate laws [illegible] corporation [illegible] control [illegible]. A [illegible] law [illegible] adopted by an organization [illegible] according to Medicare [illegible] in accordance with legal requirements [illegible] patient care [illegible] administrative [illegible] and bylaws [illegible] the governance and operation of the facility. [illegible] written [illegible] and [illegible] of the [illegible] rules [illegible] review [illegible] necessary [illegible] bylaws [illegible] above [illegible] regulations adopted [illegible] the [illegible] of the facility [illegible] rules [illegible] professional [illegible].

# C

**C.A.**
1. Court of Appeals. 2. Abbreviation for chronological age.

**cabinet**
A group of department heads or group of people that advise the President or state governors.

**cacodemonomania**
When a person believes he is possessed by a devil or evil spirit.

**C.A.H.E.A.**
Committee on Allied Health Education and Accreditation. See these words.

**calendar year**
January 1 through December 31 of any given year.

**California relative value studies (CRVS)**
Procedure coding manual (numbering system) used by physicians to evaluate difficulty of procedures used in patient care and/or payments. See relative value schedule and procedure coding manual.

**calorie**
A unit of heat; the amount of heat energy required to raise the temperature of 1 gram of water 1 degree centigrade.

**calumny**
Slander; false accusation of a crime.

**cancel**
1. To void or draw a line across. 2. To make invalid; annul. 3. To end, abolish; to do away with; to stop.

**cancellation**
Under the Uniform Commercial Code, cancellation is the recission of a contract on the basis of the other party's breach of the contract.

**Candy stripers**
Teenage volunteer workers in health care facilities. See volunteer services.

**cannabis**
Marijuana; a euphoria causing drug from the Indian hemp plant, cannabis sativa. See marijuana.

**canon**
Any law, rule or principle, in general, often related to a church such as the Catholic canon.

**canon law**
1. Laws governing a church, especially where the religion is the society's laws. 2. English church laws or laws related to religion.

**canons of construction**
Principles used to guide the legal interpretation or construction of written documents.

**canons of ethics**
1. A form of ethics used until 1969 when the Code of Professional Responsibility, which delineates the ethical standards of the legal profession, was put into practice.

**canons of judicial ethics**
Older rules of conduct for judges which are being replaced by the Code of Judicial Conduct.

**capacity**
1. Legal power to act; legal qualification or ability. 2. Legal right to do something once majority is reached.

**CAPER**
Computer Assisted Pathology Encoding and Reporting System. A computerized medical reporting system written into the MUMPS system (see MUMPS), which serves as a comprehensive pathology information-management system for hospitals. Presently in use at Massachusetts General Hospital. It automatically labels each transaction with a patient number, consolidates information on different specimens from the same patient taken at different times, and provides immediate access to each specimen's analysis status. It is also used in research and for teaching.

**capias (Lat.)**
You take. A document from a judge or court commanding the police to arrest or take a person into custody.

**capital**
1. Fixed or durable non-labor inputs or factors used in the production of goods and services, the value of such factors, or money specifically available for their acquisition or development. This includes, for example, the buildings, beds, and equipment used in the provision of hospital services. Capital goods are usually thought of as permanent and durable (in cases of doubt, those lasting over a year) and should be distinguished from such things as supplies. Refers also to investment in self (human capital, for example, where presentive care is purchased because of the positive effect such care may have on one's ability to sustain future earning capacity). See also capital depreciation and working capital. 2. First in importance, principal, head; chief; major. 3. Money or wealth.

**capital asset**
Depreciable property such as equipment or buildings which is not held for sale in the regular course of business.

**capital cost**
The financial requirements invested in the development of a new activity. These costs do not include any costs of operations, but instead, include all costs incurred prior to the operation of the activity.

**capital depreciation**
The decline in value of capital assets (assets of a permanent or fixed nature, goods and plant) over time with use. The rate and amount of depreciation is calculated by a variety of different methods (e.g., straight line, sum of the digits, declining balance) which often give quite different results. Reimbursement of health services usually includes an amount intended to be equivalent to the capital depreciation experienced by the provider of the services in conjuction with their provision. See also debt service, section 1122 and funded.

**capital expenditure review (CER)**
Review of proposed capital expenditures of hospitals and/or other health facilities to determine the need for, and appropriateness of, the proposed expenditures. The review is done by a designated regulatory agency such as a State health planning and development agency and has a sanction attached which prevents (see certificate-of-need) or discourages (see "section 1122") unneeded expenditures.

**capital expenditures**
1. In health planning this means an expenditure on health care equipment or facilities which exceeds the expenditure minimum (which usually is $150,000) or which substantially changes the services of a facility. This determination is usually based on the previous 12 month period. 2. The purchase of capital assets.

**capital gains tax**
A tax placed on the profit made from selling stocks, property, or capital assets. Federal income tax on capital gains is at a lower rate than on regular earned income.

**capital losses**
Losses realized from sale of capital assets.

**capital offenses**
Crimes punishable by death. Very serious crimes such as murder or treason are the most common capital offenses.

**capital stock**
1. Stock issued by a corporation. 2. The assets or property of a corporation. 3. The value given to a corporation.

**capitation**
A method of payment for health services in which an individual or institutional provider is paid a fixed, per capita amount for each person served without regard to the actual number or nature of services provided to each person. Capitation is characteristic of health maintenance organizations but unusual for physicians (see fee-for-service). Also, a method of Federal support of health professional schools authorized by the Comprehensive Health Manpower Training Act of

1971, P.L. 92-157, and the Nurse Training Act of 1971, P.L. 92-158 (section 770 and 810 of the PHS Act), in which each eligible school receives a fixed capitation payment from the Federal government for each student enrolled, called a capitation grant.

**capitation tax**
A tax on each person or head (individual) at a fixed rate; referred to as a "head tax."

**capricious**
Willful, wanton, and deliberate; purposefully allowed or done in an irrational manner.

**captain of the ship**
In the operating room, the physician/surgeon is considered by law to be totally responsible and has to have authority over all activities and personnel much as the "captain of the ship." In a real sense, surgery could not be conducted smoothly under any other organization structure. *McConnel vs. Willians,* 361 PA. 355, 65 A2d 243 (1949), it is stated "...he is in the same charge of those who are present and assisting him as is the *captain of a ship* over all on board." The Captain of the Ship Doctrine is when the person in charge makes all the decisions and is ultimately responsible for all those under his supervision. See respondeat superior.

**carbohydrate (CHO)**
An energy producing nutrient that is the largest single item consumed by man aside from water. It is a nutrient composed of carbon, hydrogen, and oxygen, common foods that are CHO are starches and sugars. CHO is found most in foods that are of plant origin, such as potatoes, rice and grain products. A major animal source is milk. The chemical symbol is $(CH_20)_n$.

**carbonless paper**
A paper product employing colorless chemicals placed on the backs of paper in order to produce duplicate copies rather than carbon paper. It is used to reproduce something on subsequent sheets in a set.

**carcino-**
Prefix meaning cancer.

**cardiac arrest**
The sudden and unexpected cessation of effective heart functioning. See heart attack, heart failure, myocardial infarction.

**cardiac monitor**
A specialized graph or oscilloscope which measures and records the heart's function.

**cardio-**
Prefix meaning heart.

**cardiology technician**

Performs diagnostic cardiac testing under the supervision of a physician. Tests are non-invasive in nature, and may include electrocardiography, vector cardiography, stress-testing, and echo-cardiography.

**cardiopulmonary technician**

Performs a wide range of tests related to the functions of the heart-lung system. Diagnostic tests may be invasive or non-invasive. Assists in cardiac catheterization and cardiac resuscitation. Also assists in the treatment and rehabilitation of heart-lung patients, including their post-operative care and out-patient testing.

**cardiovascular perfusionist**

Perfusionists operate the heart/lung machine needed for complete or partial cardiopulmonary (heart-lung) bypass during the time that surgery is performed to repair defects of the heart of large blood vessels. The machine is also used in cases of respiratory failure. Specialized experience combined with advanced knowledge of anatomy, pathology, physiology, pharmacology, biochemistry, hematology, cardiology, and surgery are needed to recognize and deal with problems associated with the equipment, surgery, or patient's condition. They must know the limitations of every piece of equipment used and be able to keep it working properly during every moment of surgery. This requires an understanding of what the surgeon is doing, since the need for changes in any part of the procedure must be recognized, often on a split-second basis, and carried out in consulation with the physician. Other duties which perfusionists may be required to perform include using the heart/lung machine to give anesthetics and other drugs on prescription and to control body temperature of the patient. Perfusionists are employed by hospitals, surgeons, or professional health corporations. They always work in a hospital setting, regardless of who employs them. They often work more than 40 hours per week, depending on the operating schedule, and they are on call for emergencies, which frequently occur. This term covers cardiopulmonary technicians, cardiorespiratory technicians, cardiovascular technicians, and circulation technologists. Although the names may vary slightly, all perform the same general functions, including performing a wide range of tests related to the functions and therapeutic care of the heart-lung machinery for extracorporeal circulation, assist in cardiac catheterization and cardiac resuscitation, and assist in the postoperative monitoring, care, and treatment of heart-lung patients.

**care**

1. Safekeeping, protection, or custody; watchful regard. 2. attention or heed; to look after. In any health care situation, a person must act with "reasonable care."

**care, ambulatory**

See ambulatory care.

**care, emergency**
Care for patients with severe, life-threatening, or potentially disabling conditions that require intervention within minutes or hours. See emergency care.

**care, primary**
Medical care delivery which emphasizes first contact care and assumes ongoing responsibility for the patient in total health maintenance and therapy of illness. It is comprehensive in the sense that it takes reponsibility for the overall coordination of the care of the patient's health problems, be they biological, or social.

**care, secondary**
Services provided by medical specialists who generally do not have first contact with patients (e.g., cardiologist, urologists, dermatologists). In the United States, however, there has been a trend toward self-referral by patients themselves for these services, rather than referral by primary care providers.

**care team**
Under Medicare for home health care, it is the physician, pertinent members of the agency staff, the patient, and members of the family who assist in the health care of the patient.

**care, tertiary**
The more complex services and the more narrowly defined care practices, much more specialized than primary care and includes both ambulatory and inpatient care services. Most are inpatient care, such as open heart surgery and other advanced and high technological services and care.

**carnal knowledge**
Sexual intercourse.

**carrier**
1. An insurance company that "carries" the insurance. Often referred to as insurer, underwriter, or administrative agent. 2. A commercial health insurer, a government agency, or a Blue Cross or Blue Shield plan which underwrites or administers programs that pay for health services. Under the Medicare Part B (Supplemental Medical Insurance) Program and the Federal Employees Health Benefits Program, "carriers" are agencies and organizations with which the program contracts for administration of various functions, including payment of claims. See also intermediary and third party. 3. In public health, it is a person who is not ill but who carries a disease and may or may not show the symptoms of the disease, but can transmit it to others. 4. An organization employed to transport persons or property for hire, as in *common carrier.*

**carriers (disease)**
Any persons or animals that harbor a specific infectious agent without any discernible clinical evidence of the disease, but who can also be reservoirs or sources of infection. There can be "healthy carriers" who lack any clinical manifestations of the disease or there can be "incubatory" or "convalescent" carriers, in which the carrier state is in

the incubation stage of a disease. A carrier state may be short, temporary or chronic. Some diseases known to produce carriers are typhoid, diphtheria, cholera and scarlet fever.

**carrier's lien**
The legal right to retain or hold items or property until all bills and costs have been paid. This is usually a practice carried out by transport companies or shipping companies.

**carry back**
A tax law that allows the use of losses in the prior year on the current tax report in order to reduce taxes. Also referred to as carry over.

**carryback and carryforward**
In tax law it is the provision in which a loss may be carried back to three previous years, and forward to five succeeding years as an offset to operating income in each of those three and five years.

**carry over**
See carry back.

**cartel**
An association or monopoly of companies doing the same type or a similar kind of business. Often a cartel is used to fix prices and control stocks.

**case**
1. A lawsuit; a dispute set for trial in a court. 2. Convincing evidence or grounds for a cause of action. 3. An appellate decision.

**casebook**
Published books of written judicial opinion and the facts of cases. These books are mostly used in teaching law.

**case-control study**
A study in which groups of individuals are selected because they do (the cases) or do not (the controls) have the disease whose cause and other attributes are being studied; the groups are then compared with respect to their past, existing, or future characteristics judged likely to be relevant to the disease to see which of the characteristics differ, and how, in the cases as compared to the controls.

**case fatality ratio**
The numbers of deaths from a specific disease in a certain period of time per 100 episodes of the disease that occurred in the same time period. A ratio instead of rate is figured because the deaths could be the results of episodes that started at an earlier time.

**case history**
Information gathered on an individual, usually used in the practice of psychology, psychiatry, and medicine.

**case-in-chief**
The main or chief evidence acquired for and presented by one party of a lawsuit, this does not include evidence presented in opposition on the other party's side of the case.

**case incurred**
In health insurance, claims which originated, and for which the insurance is liable, during a given period.

**Case Law**
Law based on judicial decisions which set precedents for future cases; recorded judicial decisions; law based on judges' opinions on lawsuits.

**case method or case study system**
A teaching method used in some aspects of law school and the teaching of law by studying of cases (judicial opinions).

**case-mix**
The diagnosis-specific makeup of a health program's workload. Case-mix directly influences the length of stays in, and intensity, cost and scope of the services provided by a hospital or other health program.

**case of first impression**
See impression, case of first.

**case severity**
It has been found that one of the best measures of case severity is ALOS (average length of stay in the hospital). The longer the average length of stay, the greater the average severity of illness. (Average length of stay can also be affected by other factors such as the demand for hospital beds. The higher the occupancy rate the shorter the average length of stay.) Following this logic, ALOS is adjusted to take out differences in pressure for beds by use of the following equation: A* = (00) Occupancy-corrected ALOS, where A* is the average length of stay corrected for differences in pressure for beds. Then the hospital's death rate is adjusted for differences in case severity by use of the following equation using severity-adjusted death rate (SADR): SADR = 100 DR. - 0.94 (A* - A*), where SADR is severity adjusted death rate (the final quality of medical care measure); A*, the mean average length of stay corrected for occupancy differences for all the hospitals.

**cases treated**
The number of patients cared for by a health program during a year. Inpatient discharges and outpatient visits can be combined into an aggregate weighted index of hospital output.

**cash basis accounting**
An accounting method used to determine income based on that which is received and what expenses are deductible for the year in which they are paid. This is distinguished from accrual basis accounting.

**cash surrender value**
The cash value of an insurance policy if surrendered to the insurance company that wrote the policy.

**cassette**
1. In radiography, it is a light proof box containing x-ray film used to take the x-ray. The box contains special screens that fluoresce under the x-rays and causes the image to appear on the film. 2. A small case containing film, magnetic tape or video tape.

**cast**
A mixture of plaster of Paris or gypsum and water and stockinette which is placed around an injured or broken bone or body part to immobilize the injured parts.

**casualty**
Any injury caused by an accident; an inevitable accident; accident or injury without design.

**casuistry**
A technique for solving case of right and wrong based on principles of ethics; subtle but evasive reasoning used to determine right from wrong or questions of duty.

**cata-**
Prefix meaning down.

**cataract**
A lens of the eye which is no longer transparent. Its development is associated with the loss of blood supply to the lens with advanced age and with abnormally high exposures to ultraviolet light. The cataract may be abnormally hard or abnormally soft when compared to a normal lens.

**catastrophe policy**
See major medical policy.

**catastrophic anxiety**
The anxiety associated with organic brain syndromes in that a patient is aware of his condition and can do nothing about it or cannot accept it, which in turn causes overwhelming anxiety.

**catastrophic health insurance**
Health insurance which provides protection against the high cost of treating severe or lengthy illnesses or disabilities. Generally such policies cover all or a specificed percentage of medical expenses above an amount that is a deductible or is the responsibility of the insured or the responsibility of another insurance policy up to a maximum limit of liability. Generally there is no maximum amount of coverage under these plans; however, many include some coinsurance. See also major medical.

**catastrophic illness**
Any illness that causes costs and expenses in very large amounts. Any sickness in which hospital and other inpatient costs exceed a certain percentage of annual net income, or the amount of such income in excess of public assistance levels, whichever sum is smaller.

**catastrophic insurance**
Insurance against catastrophic illness. Also referred to as major medical insurance. See catastrophic health insurance.

**catatonia**

A mental state characterized by muscular rigidity and immobility. It is associated with the schizophrenic form of psychosis.

**catchment area**

A geographic area defined and served by a health program or institution such as a hospital or community mental health center. Delineated on the basis of such factors as population distribution, natural geographic boundaries, and transportation accessibility. Should be contrasted with service, medical market, or medical trade area. All residents of the area needing the services of the program are usually eligible for them, although eligibility may also depend on additional criteria (age or income). Residents of the area may or may not be limited to obtaining services from the program, be known to, or enrolled in the program. The program may or may not be limited to providing services to residents of the area or under any obligation to know of, register, or have the capacity to serve all residents of the area. Used in mental health care to identify a geographical area for which a mental health services facility includes or has responsibility for. See community psychiatry.

**categorical assistance**

Government financial assistance programs that have requirements other than financial need, such as medicare which is determined by age.

categorically needy

Persons who are both members of certain categories of groups eligible to receive public assistance, and economically needy. As used in Medicaid, this means a person who is aged, blind, disabled, or a member of a family with children under 18 (or 21, if in school) where one parent is absent, incapacitated or unemployed and, in addition, meets specified income and resources requirements which vary by State. In general, categorically needy individuals are persons receiving cash assistance under the AFDC or SSI programs. A State must cover all recipients of AFDC payments under Medicaid; however, it is provided certain options (based, in large measure, on its coverage levels under the old Federal/State welfare programs) in determining the extent of coverage for persons receiving Federal SSI and/or State supplementary SSI payments. In addition, a State may cover additional specified groups, such as foster children, as categorically needy. A State may restrict its Medicaid coverage to this group or may cover additional persons who meet the categorical requirements as medically needy.

**categorically related**

In the Medicaid program, the requirements (other than income and resources) which an individual must meet in order to be eligible for Medicaid benefits; also individuals who meet these requirements. Specifically , any individual eligible for Medicaid must fall into one of the four main categories of people who are eligible for welfare cash payments. He must be "aged", "blind", or "disabled" (as defined under the Supplemental Security Income Program, title XVI of the Social Security Act) or a member of a family with dependent children where one parent is absent, incapacitated, or unemployed (as defined under the Aid to Families with Dependent Children Program, title IV of the Social

Security Act). After the determination is made that an individual is categorically related, then income and resources tests are applied to determine if the individual is poor enough to be eligible for assistance (categorically needy). As a result of this requirement, single persons and childless couples who are not aged, blind, or disabled and male headed families in States which do not cover such groups under their AFDC programs cannot receive Medicaid coverage no matter how poor they are.

**categorical program**
Originally, a health program which concerned itself with research, education, control and/or treatment of only one or a few specific diseases. Now more generally used for a program concerned with only part, instead of all, of the population or health system. Even more generally used by the present administration to refer to any existing program which it feels the Federal government should cease to support.

**catharsis**
The healthful and therapeutic release of self talk and thoughts through talking them out of the conscious state of mind and is often accompanied by the appropriate emotional reaction. Thoughts are released into awareness from the repressed area of the unconscious.

**catheter**
1. A plastic or rubber tube that is inserted into the bladder to allow the urine to flow out. 2. Any tube used to allow passage into a structure for the purpose of injecting or withdrawing fluids.

**catheterization**
Having a tube inserted into the urinary tract to allow the passage of urine. Catheterization can be done to other areas of the body such as cardiac catheterization.

**catheterize**
To insert a catheter into a hollow of the body, usually the urinary tract, to allow urine to pass from the bladder via a plastic tube.

**cathexis**
Conscious or unconscious attachment of emotions and significant thought to an idea or object.

**cathode-ray-tube (CRT)**
Used in medical records, an electronic vacuum tube containing a screen on which output data of a computer can be displayed in graphic form or by character representation. It depicts letters and numbers similar to the way images are projected on the tube of a television set.

**CAT scanner**
See CT scanner, also computerized axial tomography.

**causa (Lat.)**
Cause. Purpose; motive; reason.

**causa mortis (Lat.)**
In thinking about the cause of death or an approaching death.

**cause**
1. An action in court. 2. Legal procedures by which a party gains its claim, lawsuit or case. 3. That which produces an effect. 4. Motive or reason enough; grounds for a case; producing an effect. 5. Something that, if prevented, removed or eliminated, will prevent the occurrence of the event in question, and/or, if permitted, introduced or maintained, will be followed by the event in question. A necessary cause is a cause that must exist if a given event is to occur, but may not itself result in the event. A sufficient cause is one which is inevitably followed by a given event or the existence of a given thing.

**cause fatality rate**
The number of deaths from a certain disease or specific cause per 1,000 or 10,000 reported cases of the same diseases, conditions, or disorder.

**cause of action**
Enough evidence and facts to support a lawsuit.

**cause specific death rate**
The number of deaths from a specific disease or cause in a period of time, usually a year, per 1,000, 10,000 or 100,000 population and is estimated in the middle of the year.

**caveat (Lat.)**
Warning. A notice filed with the proper legal authorities ordering a named party to cease activities until the issue is heard in court.

**caveat emptor (Lat.)**
Let the buyer beware. A term that suggests that the buyer is responsible to determine if goods that are bought are good or work properly.

**caveat venditor (Lat.)**
Let the seller beware. A term that suggests that the seller is responsible for deficiencies in goods or products sold.

**C.C.A.**
Circuit Court of Appeals.

**cease and desist**
A legal order to discontinue, stop and to do no more; a directive to quit. An order from an administrative agency that is similar to an injunction.

**cede**
To assign. To yield; to admit; to grant. To give up or surrender. To resign.

**ceding insurance company**
See reinsurance.

**cell**
1. A storage unit in a computer. 2. In biology, the structural and functional unit of an organism consisting of protoplasm, a nucleus and a cell wall.

**censor**
1. To review, examine, eliminate or stop. To put under censorship. 2. One who conducts censorship.

**censorship**
1. To censor; the act of censoring. 2. Denial of freedom of speech or freedom of the press, however not all censorship necessarily means a violation of the First Amendment.

**census**
See Average Daily Census.

**Center for Disease Control (CDC)**
Organization within the department of Health and Human Services serving as a focal point for disease control and public health activities. The Center provides facilities and services for the investigation, prevention and control of diseases; supports quarantine and other activities to prevent the introduction of communicable diseases from foreign countries; conducts research into the epidemiology, laboratory diagnosis, prevention and treatment of infectious and other controllable diseases at the community level; provides grants for work on venereal disease, immunization against infectious diseases, and disease control programs; and sets standards for laboratories. Activities focus on the improvement of the health care system through emphasis on prevention, health education, and investigations, surveillance and control operations, including training of State and local health workers in specific control techniques or methodologies, rather than through direct treatment.

**Center For Research in Ambulatory Health Care Administration (CRAHCA)**
The research organization of the Medical Group Management Association. It is a charitable, scientific and educational organization, devoted to the development of programs and services that contribute to the professional competence and personal growth in ambulatory health care and in clinic administrators. The Center is funded through grants and contracts from private foundations, governmental agencies and the private sector.

**centigrade (Celsius)**
A metric system temperature scale in which temperature goes from zero to 100 with zero degrees equaling freezing or 32 degrees Fahrenheit.

**central city**
The older part of a city, often having old apartment buildings, hotels and houses with low rent, thus attracting low income, poor and deprived persons. This in turn creates many special public health and health care delivery problems.

**central medical supply**
See central supply.

**central processing unit (CPU)**
In a hospital business office or in Medicare records, it is a device capable of receiving and storing instructions. A computer used for receiving and storing data to be processed, transferring and editing data already stored,

making math computaions, making decisions of logic, and directing the action of the input and output units.

**central sterile supply**
See central supply.

**central supply**
The service or department of a hospital which washes, packages, and sterilizes materials, equipment, sheets, instruments, gowns, bandages and dressings for use in the operating rooms or parts of the hospital where sterile materials are required. Central supply may also distribute intravenous solutions.

**central tendency**
1. Average; middle. 2. Leaning to or tending to fall in the center, middle, or average part or area.

**C.E.O.**
Chief Executive Officer. A name that is synonymous with administrator or president of a health care facility, hospital, clinic or company.

**cephalo-**
Prefix meaning head.

**cerebral vascular accident (stroke)**
When the blood vessels serving the brain (usually the cerebrum) are blocked off causing the blood supply to not reach the tissue thus causing the tissue to die off. The part of the body controlled by the part of the brain affect is also affected.

**cerebro-**
Prefix meaning brain.

**certifiable**
Something that can be certified.

**certificate**
A printed or written statement; assurance or testimony that a formal requirement has been completed; promise kept or qualification met. To attest to or to verify.

**certificate of insurance**
A document delivered to the insured which summarizes the benefits and principle provisions of the group plan affecting the insured. In group insurance, a statement issued to a member of a group certifying that an insurance contract covering the member has been written and containing a summary of the terms applicable to that member.

**certificate-of-need**
A certificate issued by a governmental body to an individual or organization proposing to construct or modify a health facility, or offer a new or different health service, which recognizes that such facility or service when available will be needed by those for whom it is intended. Where a certificate is required (for instance for all proposals which will involve more than a minimum capital investment, change bed capacity, or

rate increase) it is a condition of licensure of the facility or service, and is intended to control expansion of facilities and services in the public interest by preventing excessive or duplicative development of facilities and services. The health systems agencies (local planning bodies under P.L. 93-641) are required to make recommendations to the State agencies regarding proposed new institutional health services within their areas.

**certificate-of-need controls**
Regulations intended to contain rising medical care costs.

**certification**
1. A mechanism by which a nongovernment agency or association (usually a professional association) grants recognition to an individual who has met certain predetermined qualifications specified by that agency. Such qualifications may include: 1) graduation from an accredited or approved educational program, 2) acceptable performance on an examination, and/or 3) completion of a given amount of work experience. 2. The process by which a governmental or nongovernmental agency or association evaluates and recognizes an individual, institution or educational program as meeting predetermined standards. One so recognized is said to be certified. Essentially synonymous with accreditation, except that certification is usually applied to individuals and accreditation to institutions. Certification programs are generally nongovernmental and do not exclude the uncertified from practice as do licensure programs. The process by which a nongovernmental agency or association grants recognition to an individual or organization who has met certain predetermined qualifications or requirements specified by that agency or association.

**certified**
Possessing a certificate; meeting the requirement of certification; officially passed, approved or vouched for.

**certified nurse-midwife (CNM)**
An individual educated in the two disciplines of nursing and midwifery, who possesses evidence of certification according to the requirements of the American College of Nurse-Midwives. See nurse-midwife.

**Certified Registered Nurse Anesthetist (CRNA)**
A graduate of an approved school of nursing who has met state requirements and earned current registration by state licensing authorities as a Registered Nurse. The person then must graduate from an approved school of nurse anesthesia accredited by the Council on Accreditation of Educational Programs of Nurse Anesthesia, the nationally recognized accrediting body for schools of nurse anesthesia, or its predecessor. While in this program the student receives education including in-depth studies of anatomy, physiology, biochemistry, pharmacology, and physics, and their relationship to anesthesia. The graduate must then evidence individual competency by passing a rigid qualifying examination which makes the person eligible for certification by the Council on Certification of Nurse Anesthetists, the nationally recognized certifying body for nurse anesthetists, or its predecessor. In order to ensure the high quality nursing and anesthesia care provided by a CRNA, he/she must be

recertified every two years by the Council on Recertification of Nurse Anesthetists, the nationally recognized recertifying body. This recertification is based on the fulfillment of continuing education requirements and other criteria. Due to his/her advanced education in the areas of respiratory and cardiopulmonary function, a CRNA often assists in the management and resuscitation of critical patients in intensive care, coronary care, and emergency room situations as well. The CRNA is responsible and accountable for the quality of services he/she provides to the public.

**Certified Respiratory Therapy Technician**
As used in JCAH accreditation, this is an individual who has been certified by the National Board for Respiratory Therapy, Inc., after successfully completing all education, experience, and examination requirements.

**certify**
To attest to or to verify.

**certiorari (Lat.)**
To make sure. A process that is similar to an appeal, wherein an appellate court; especially the United States Supreme Court, has the discretion to review a lower court's decision, but is not required to do so.

**cervico-**
Prefix meaning neck.

**cession**
1. To give something up. 2. To yield to force. 3. A voluntary giving up of a person's property to a court or to creditors in order to avoid legal consequences. 4. Abandonment.

**C.F.&I. or C.I.F.**
The price includes cost, freight and insurance paid by seller.

**C.F.R.**
Code of Federal Regulations; the publication containing federal administrative rules.

**chairside**
The dental equivalent of bedside.

**challenge for cause**
A challenge of a prospective juror, on the grounds of bias.

**chamberlain**
An officer who is a treasurer.

**champerty**
1. An illegal agreement to accept a lawsuit of another person by buying or sharing the winnings of the suit. 2. Joint power or authority.

**CHAMPUS**

Civilian Health and Medical Program of the Uniformed Services. See these words.

**CHAMPVA**

Civilian Health and Medical Program of the Veteran's Administration. See these words.

**chancre**

A lesion (sore) that occurs at the point of entry of an infection in some diseases; primarily a sore of the disease of syphilis.

**channels of infection**

The means through which infection enters the body and then causes the body to become infected by any of the disease-producing agents. The usual channels are the respiratory tract, the digestive tract, or breaks in the exterior surfaces of the body, with the mouth being the main portal of entry for the majority of infections.

**chaplain**

A clergyman, minister or layperson appointed to perform religious functions in a public institution such as a hospital, nursing home; also used in the armed forces to perform religious functions.

**chaplaincy service**

A service provided by some Health Care facilities in the form of spiritual support, pastoral care and religious counseling for patients.

**character**

The sum of personality traits and modes of responses of an individual.

**charge**

1. To blame or accuse; to place liability on; to burden. 2. An injunction; an order. 3. A claim or obligation. 4. The judge's instructions to a jury. 5. A formal accusation of a crime. 6. To take responsibility for.

**charge nurse (JCAH)**

According to JCAH accreditation of long term care facilities, this is a registered or licensed practical (vocational) nurse assigned to be in charge of a nursing unit.

**charge nurse (Medicare)**

A person who is: (1) licensed by the State in which practicing as a registered nurse or a practical (vocational) nurse who either is a graduate of a State-approved school of practical (vocational) nursing or has two years of appropriate experience following licensure by waiver as a practical (vocational) nurse, and has achieved a satisfactory grade on a proficiency examination approved by the Secretary, or on a State licensure examination which the Secretary finds at least equivalent to the proficiency examination, except that such determinations of proficiency shall not apply with respect to persons initially licensed by a State or seeking initial qualifications as a practical (vocational) nurse after December 31, 1977; (2) experienced in nursing service administration and supervision and, in areas such as rehabilitative or geriatric nursing, or acquires such preparation through formal staff development programs.

**charge-off**

1. Writing off of an item or money due to loss or depreciation. 2. Writing off the value of something in a health facility's records as a loss. When a debt becomes too difficult to collect, or becomes a bad debt, it may be written off or charged off. See bad debt.

**charges**

Prices assigned to units of medical service, such as a visit to a physician or a day in a hospital. Charges for services may not be related to the actual costs of providing the services. Further, the methods by which charges are related to costs vary substantially from service to service and institution to institution. Different third party payers may require use of different methods of determining either charges or costs. Charges for one service provided by an institution are often used to subsidize the costs of other services. Charges to one type or group of patients may also be used to subsidize the costs of providing services to other groups. See also actual, allowable, charges customary, charges prevailing, reasonable, and usual charge.

**charges, customary**

Generally, the amount which a physician normally or usually charges the majority of his patients. Under Medicare, it is the median charge used by a particular physician for a specified type of service during the calendar year preceding the fiscal year in which a claim is processed.

**charges, prevailing**

A charge which falls within the range of charges most frequently used in a locality for a particular medical service or procedure. The top of this charge establishes an overall limitation on the charges which a carrier . . .will accept as reasonable for a given service . . .Current Medicare rules state that the limit of an area's prevailing charge is to be the 75th percentile of the customary charges for a given service by the physicians in a given area.

**charitable immunity**

In malpractice, a doctrine in use in a decreasing number of States that nonprofit, or charitable, hospitals and other health facilities are not subject to suit for malpractice. The doctrine of charitable immunity relies on and involves: waiver of the patient's right to sue for negligence by accepting the charity; the basic unfairness, either assumed or stated, of applying a doctrine such as respondeat superior, which applies to commercial pursuits, to a nonprofit enterprise; and the increased financial demands upon the assets of the charity which might result from adverse judgments. There are exceptions to the rule of charitable immunity: a charity may be held liable for the negligence of an agent of the institution; a charity may be held liable to a stranger, i.e., one who is not a beneficiary; and, sometimes, a charity may be held liable only to the extent of its nontrust assets. The trend today is toward abolition of charitable immunity. This is based on the contention that there were illogical and conflicting bases upon which the doctrine was founded, the alleged unfairness of forcing the injured party to contribute indirectly to the charity by refusing him the opportunity to recover, and the availability of liability insurance. See also governmental immunity.

**charitable institution**
A nonprofit institution maintained by charity or by public funds, usually for the benefit of a specific class of persons or specific reason.

**charitable trust**
Property, money or real estate held by one party for the benefit of a hospital, school, nursing home, church, or charity.

**chart**
See medical record.

**charter**
1. Permission to start an organization; the document creating an organization. 2. Articles of incorporation and proper laws that give the right to incorporate that are written into a legal instrument. 3. A franchise. 4. To hire or lease a vehicle. 5. The contract used to create a lease.

**chattel**
Personal property other than land.

**chattel mortgage**
A mortgage on personal money, items, or property.

**chattel paper**
A legal document showing a debt secured by collateral.

**chattel, personal**
Any tangible personal article or personal property.

**check-off**
A method through which union dues are directly collected from worker's pay check.

**chemical equivalents**
Drug products from different sources which contain essentially identical amounts of the identical active ingredients in identical dosage forms, meet existing physiochemical standards in official compendia, and are therefore chemically indistinguishable. See also bioequivalence.

**chemical name**
The exact description of the chemical structure of a drug, based on the rules of chemical nomenclature. While long and cumbersome, this name is precise, serving as a complete identification of the compound to any trained chemist. It is related to the chemical formula of the particular drug.

**chemistry technologist**
Medical technologist, working under the supervision of a pathologist, physician, or qualified scientist, in performing qualitative and quantitative analyses of body fluids and exudates, utilizing quantitative equipment and

a wide range of laboratory instruments, to provide information for diagnosing and treating disease.

**chemo-**
Prefix meaning drug or chemical.

**chemoreceptor**
A specialized receptor which is sensitive to chemical agent.

**chemotherapy**
The therapeutic treatment of diseases or conditions through the use of chemical substances; sometimes used to identify treatment of infectious diseases or cancer with antimetabolites.

**chief executive officer**
The title of the individual appointed by the governing body of a health care facility to act in its behalf in the overall administration. Synonymous job titles may include administrator, president, superintendent, director, executive director, and executive vice-president.

**child abuse**
See battered child.

**child care worker**
Child care workers implement training programs and activities that provide therapeutic and preventive services for mentally ill and emotionally disturbed children. Specifically, they train children in self-help skills through intensive group sessions involving structured daily activities and reinforcement of other therapeutic experiences. They also record, evaluate, and report the progress of patients.

**Child Health Act**
A public law that amends the federal Social Security Act by authorizing funds for maternal and infant care and care for preschool and school age children. Items covered include dental care, crippled children's services, family planning services, and money for training and research.

**child psychiatrist, qualified**
According to JCAH for psychiatric, alcoholism and drug abuse facilities accreditation purposes, this is a doctor of medicine who specializes in the assessment and treatment of children and/or adolescents having psychiatric disorders and who is fully licensed to practice medicine in the state in which he or she practices. The individual shall have successfully completed training in a child psychiatry fellowship program approved by the Liaison Committee on Graduate Medical Education of the American Medical Association or have been certified in child psychiatry by the American Board of Psychiatry and Neurology, or have documented equivalent education, training, and/or experience.

**chimera**
1. A Greek mythical fire-breathing monster with a lion's head, a goat's body, and a dragon's tail. 2. Fanciful fantasy; imagination. 3. Impossible fantasy, absurdity.

**chimerical**
1. Fantastic; conceived fantasy. 2. Imaginary; unreal; impossible. 3. Participating or indulging in unrealistic visions.

**chiro-**
Prefix meaning hand.

**chiromancy**
Attempting to foretell future events through reading hands; fortune-telling by studying the palm of the hand; palmistry.

**chiropodist**
See podiatrist.

**chiropractor**
A practitioner of chiropractic, a system of mechanical therapeutics based on the principles that the nervous system largely determines the state of health, and that disease results from abnormal nerve function and conformity. Treatment consists primarily of the adjustment or manipulation of parts of the body, especially the spinal column. Some chiropractors also use physiotherapy, nutritional supplementation and other therapeutic modalities; radiography is used for diagnosis only. Operations, drugs and immunizations are usually rejected as violations of the human body. Chiropractic was founded in 1895 by D.D. Palmer and had grown by 1971 to 19,151 practitioners with 36 active chiropractic colleges (requiring four years of post high school education). Chiropractors are licensed by all States. Their services are covered in 27 State Medicaid programs. Manual manipulation of the spine is demonstrated on X-ray.

**chloral hydrate**
Knockout drops.

**choate**
Complete.

**choate lien**
A complete lien. A solid and legal lien; an enforceable lien in which both the lienor and the property under lien are definite and established.

**choice-of-law**
A situation or a case where a court must choose between a conflict of local laws and the laws of another jurisdiction.

**cholangiogram**
X-ray of the biliary tract involving the injection of a dye into this tract.

**cholecystogram**
An x-ray of the gall bladder.

**chose (French)**
Thing, article, personal property.

**chose in action**
An article, debt, damages, money or property wrongfully held by another party that is legally recoverable by a legal action such as a lawsuit.

**CHP (CHP a, CHP b)**
Comprehensive health planning agencies which were the predecessors to the present system of health planning in the nation which includes Health Systems Agencies. The "a" and "b" referred to state and local area groups respectively.

**Christian Science**
A religion, and system of healing through prayer and control of mind over matter. The services of Christian Science are covered under some health insurance programs including Medicare and, in some States, Medicaid, often with an exemption from standards applied by such programs to traditional medical providers.

**chronic brain syndrome**
See organic brain syndrome.

**chronic disease**
Diseases which have one or more of the following characteristics: are permanent, leave residual disability, are caused by nonreversible pathological alteration, require special training of the patient for rehabilitation, or may be expected to require a long period of supervision, observation or care. See also acute disease.

**chrono-**
Prefix meaning time.

**chronophobia**
Fear of time; often referred to as prison neurosis and is characterized by panic, anxiety, and claustrophobia.

**circadian rhythm**
Repetition of certain rhythmic phenomena every 24 hours.

**CircOlectric bed and Foster frame**
A bed-type device used to periodically change a patient from the prone to supine position or supine to prone with little or no effort on the part of the patient.

**circumstantial evidence**
Indirect proof of certain happenings or occurrences used to infer a fact. Possession of stolen drugs is circumstantial proof of the person being the thief.

**cite**
1. To summon. 2. To refer to. 3. To give legal notice. 4. To enjoin. 5. To name. 6. To prove through referring to a law.

**city/county hospital**
See hospital, city/county, city.

**civil action**
1. Any legal action between two or more individuals or parties. 2. Any legal action that is not a criminal action.

**Civilian Health and Medical Program of the Uniformed Services (CHAMPUS)**
1. A program, administered by the Department of Defense, without premium but with cost-sharing provisions, which pays for care delivered by civilian health providers to retired members, and dependents of active and retired members, of the seven uniformed services of the United States (Army, Navy, Air Force, Marine Corps, Commissioned Corps of the Public Health Service, Coast Guard, and the National Oceanic and Atmospheric Administration). 2. A government-sponsored program which provides hospital and medical services for dependents of active military service personnel, retired military service personnel and their dependents, and dependents of deceased members of the military who died on active duty.

**Civilian Health and Medical Program of the Veterans Administration (CHAMPVA)**
A program, administered by the Department of Defense for the Veterans Administration, without premium but with cost-sharing provisions to dependents of totally disabled veterans who are eligible for retirement pay from a uniformed service.

**civil law**
1. Law that was developed under the Roman Empire and survived in the European countries except Great Britain. Civil law is based on codes and statutes and is distinguished from the common law. 2. This also is used to refer to any legal proceedings that are not based on criminal law, statutes, codes or regulations, nor military law as in a civil lawsuit which is based on case law, tort law, etc. 3. Rules that regulate or control relationships between private parties rather than between private parties and governments. Also referred to as private law.

**civil malpractice**
Professional misconduct involving a criminal act. See malpractice.

**civil rights**
All rights of U.S. citizens guaranteed by the U.S. and State Constitutions.

**civil service**
All government employees except elected officials and judges who are selected by a controlled standardized method. Persons in military service are not considered civil service employees.

**C.J.**
Chief judge, chief justice.

**claim**
1. A statement or assertion of fact. 2. One's right to; entitled to. 3. To demand; to call for; to assert; urge; to insist. 4. One side of a case. 5. To seek to gain rights or fairness through the legal system, one must file a claim. 6. In insurance it is a demand for payment under an insurance

policy, contract or bond. 7. A request to an insurer by an insured person (or, on his behalf, by the provider of a service or good) for payment of benefits under an insurance policy.

**claimant**

A person who files a claim, asserts a right or applies for justice.

**claim for relief**

1. The first pleading in a complaint or lawsuit. 2. A summary statement that indicates that facts can be proven and the plaintiff should have the court's support in the claim against the defendant.

**claim review**

A review process conducted by a panel of physicians and administrators employed by the insurance carrier wherein the appropriateness of medical services provided are determined, which usually include cost and necessity of the services as stipulated by the health insurance program.

**claims incurred policy**

The conventional form of malpractice insurance, under which the insured is covered for any claims arising from an incident which occurred or is alleged to have occurred during the policy period, regardless of when the claim is made. The only limiting factors are the statutes of limitations, which vary from State to State. An alternative type of policy is the claims made policy.

**claims made policy**

A form of malpractice insurance gaining increasing popularity among insurers because it increases the accuracy of rate-making. In this type of policy the insured is covered for any claim made, rather than any injury occurring, while the policy is in force. Claims made after the insurance lapses are not covered as they are by a claims incurred policy. This type of policy was initially resisted by providers because of the nature of medical malpractice claims, which may arise several years after an injury occurs (see discovery rule). A retired physician, for example, could be sued and not covered, unless special provisions are made to continue his coverage beyond his years of practice. There are also retrospective problems for providers who switch from a conventional policy to a claims made policy, since the latter policy would not cover claims arising from events occurring during the years when the conventional policy was in effect. Insurers marketing such policies are now offering providers the opportunity to purchase insurance for both contingencies.

**claims review**

A review of claims by governments, medical foundations, PSROs, insurers or others responsible for payment to determine liability and amount of payment. This review may include determination of the eligibility of the claimant or beneficiary; of the eligibility of the provider of the benefit; that the benefit for which payment is claimed is covered; that the benefit is not payable under another policy (see coordination of benefits); and that the benefit was necessary and of reasonable cost and quality.

**claims status report**
A statement to the enrolled member which explains action taken on each claim.

**class action suit**
A lawsuit filed in the name of all persons having a common concern or in similar circumstances caused by a defendant's action.

**classifying**
The process of coding similar types of data, such as in medical record information.

**claustrophobia**
Fear of closed places.

**Clayton Act**
A Federal law, passed in 1914. This law extended the Sherman Act, which prohibits monopolies and price control and fixing.

**clean**
1. Free of disease-producing microorganisms. 2. No longer using drugs. 3. No longer breaking the law.

**clean hands**
1. Being fair and honest in all dealings and matters. 2. Being honest in a request for equitable relief.

**clean technique**
A technique that maintains a disease-free situation.

**clear and convincing proof**
Strong evidence, but not as strong as beyond a reasonable doubt.

**clear and present danger**
A legal test used to decide whether what has been said is protected by the First Amendment. A statement may be punishable by law if it could lead to violence or if it weakens national safety and security.

**clear title**
1. A title that has no liens or any other legal claims against it. 2. A document stating legal ownership that is free from all restrictions and debts.

**clemency**
A merciful act; giving leniency and forbearance. Showing mercy, giving lenient treatment or reducing the punishment for a criminal.

**clergy**
A person ordained to a position in a church that gives that person authority to conduct religious services. See chaplain.

**client**
1. A person engaged in a relationship to have someone act in another's behalf. 2. A person who employs a professional for service.

**climacteric**
Menopause. Sometimes used as a reference to the age period for men that women experience menopause.

**clinic**
Any facility used for diagnosis and treatment of outpatients. Clinic is irregularly defined, sometimes either including or excluding physicians offices, sometimes being limited to facilities which serve poor or public patients, and sometimes being limited to facilities in which graduate or undergraduate medical education is done.

**clinical dietitian, R.D. (Registered Dietitian)**
The clinical dietitian, R.D. is the member of the health care team that affects the nutritional care of individuals and groups for health maintenance. The clinical dietitian assesses nutritional needs, develops and implements nutritional care plans, and evaluates and reports these results appropriately. When functioning in an organization that provides food service, the clinical dietitian cooperates and coordinates activities with those of the department's management team.

**clinical equivalents**
See therapeutic equivalents and bioequivalence.

**clinical laboratory services**
The testing of specimens from the human body to aid in the diagnosis and treatment of physical diseases and other ill-health conditions.

**clinical pastoral counselor**
These health-oriented clergy work in health care settings with temporarily or permanently confined patients and their families. They provide individual and group counseling to assist patients in coping with temporary, chronic, and terminal illness.

**clinical privileges**
1. When permission is given by a health care facility to render medical care in the granting institution. What privileges allowed are within well-defined limits, based upon the physician or other health care provider's professional license and experience, skill, competence, ability, and judgment. 2. According to JCAH, for accrediting purposes, this is permission to render medical care in the granting institution within well-defined limits, based upon the individual's professional license and his experience, competence, ability, and judgment.

**clinical psychologist**
A health professional specializing in the evaluation and treatment of mental and behavioral disorders. A clinical psychologist generally has a doctoral degree in psychology, plus clinical training. Clinical psychologists are licensed by most States for independent professional practice and their services are reimbursed by many health insurance programs. They are not allowed to treat mental illness with drugs.

**clinic manager**
See administrator, clinic, chief executive officer.

**Clinico-Pathological Conference (CPC)**
The presentation and discussion of the physical examination and diagnostic test results to the medical staff; then a specialist or an expert analyzes the findings and provides his or her diagnosis. The pathologist then reports the diagnosis, based on tissue examination and opinion of the expert to proper authorities.

**close corporation**
A corporation in which the stock is held by a limited number of persons and not offered for public sale. Often refers to a corporation owned and operated primarily by a single family.

**closed panel group practice**
A dental care plan. The beneficiaries are allowed to go only to dentists who have agreed to work under and provide dental care under a prepayment plan.

**closed shop**
A union concept. A company or health care institution where only members of a particular union may work in or do certain jobs; where a worker must be a union member as a condition of employment; illegal under the National Labor Relations Act.

**closed shop contract**
A labor-management promissory agreement stipulating that only members of a certain union may be hired.

**closed staff**
Those physicians that have been approved by a hospital's governing board to practice medicine in their hospital and that may admit and care for patients. This is now the usual arrangement found in hospitals.

**closely held**
A company, hospital, or other health care facility or service that is owned by a family or by another company. See close corporation.

**cloture**
1. A formal closure. 2. The act of closing off a discussion or debate in a hearing. 3. A parliamentary procedure.

**CNS**
Central nervous system.

**cobol (Common business oriented language)**
A specific language by which business data processing procedures can be precisely described in a standard form. The language is intended not only as a means of directly presenting any business program to any suitable computer for which a compiler exists, but also as a means of communicating such procedures among individuals. This system is often utilized in health care enterprises business offices.

**code**
1. A complete body or set of laws of a nation, state, city, county, etc. 2. A set of rules and regulations pertaining to a specific area or subject. 3. The compilation and the arranging of laws in a systematic way. 4. The

arranging and organization of statutes, regulations and rules into books of law; as in the criminal code.

**Code of Judicial Conduct**
Rules of conduct created mostly for judges adopted by the American Bar Association and adhered to in many states.

**Code of Professional Responsibility**
The specific rules and regulations that govern the legal profession. Developed by the American Bar Association, it contains ethical guidelines and rules.

**codification**
1. To make into code. 2. The collecting and organizing of laws of a certain subject into a complete set of law. 3. To arrange laws by subject or area.

**codify**
To arrange laws by areas, subjects or topics.

**coercion**
1. Restraint by legal authority. 2. Force; making a person act against his free will. 3. Force by a government.

**coffin**
A thick-walled lead container used to transport radioactive materials.

**cognition**
1. The mental process of understanding, knowing and being aware. 2. The process of being aware or of knowing; mental awareness rather than emotional awareness.

**cognitive**
The process or mental state of comprehension, judgment, memory and reasoning, as contrasted with the affective or emotional domain.

**cognizable**
1. Within the jurisdiction of the court or other tribunal. 2. Capable of being understood, known, or recognized.

**cognizance**
1. The hearing of a case in a court; authority to hear a case or deal with a matter legally. 2. Judicial power to decide a matter; judicial decision; right to deal with a judicial matter.

**cognovit**
1. A written acknowledgement of one's liability especially made by a defendant in a civil suit in order to avoid the expense of going to trial. 2. A written statement of a debt. 3. A defendant's written acknowledgement of guilt.

**cohabitation**
Living together as man and wife, whether married or not.

**cohort**
Those who share a common characteristic. In demographics, all those persons born during a specified period.

**cohort study**
An inquiry in which a group (the cohort) is chosen for the presence of a specific characteristic at or during a specified time and followed over time for the appearance of particular related characteristics.

**coida de la mollera (Spanish)**
Fallen fontanel. A disorder occurring in the Mexican-American culture.

**coinsurance**
1. A cost-sharing requirement under a health insurance policy which provides that the insured will assume a portion or percentage of the costs of covered services. The health insurance policy provides that the insurer will reimburse a specified percentage (usually 80 percent) of all, or certain specified covered medical expenses in excess of any deductible amounts payable by the insured. The insured is then liable for the remaining percentage of the costs, until the maximum amount payable under the insurance policy, if any, is reached. 2. Insurance where the insured and the insurer carry the risk jointly. 3. Dividing the risk on all losses between an insurance company and its customers. 4. A plan under which the insured and the insurer share hospital and medical expenses resulting from illness or injury. Sometimes seen in major medical insurance. See cost sharing.

**coitus interruptus**
Sexual intercourse that is interrupted before the male ejaculates. Used as a form of birth control by withdrawal of the penis to prevent pregnancy. It is not a very effective form of birth control.

**cold turkey**
1. A common term for withdrawal from a drug. The immediate stopping or inability to get more of a substance that a person is addicted to. 2. Abrupt stoppage of drugs or smoking as a method to cease their use. Sometimes this results as the person is not able to get the drug. The term is based on drug addict's description of the chills and consequent gooseflesh experienced from going through withdrawal.

**collateral**
1. Additional; supplementary; complementary. 2. Property subject to a security interest. 3. Money or property put into security as a pledge to keep an obligation, as when taking out a loan.

**collateral assurance**
Assurance on a deal made beyond a regular deed.

**collateral attack**
Any effort to avoid a court's decision by requesting your case to be heard in a different court or different direction or through different channels.

**collateral estoppel**
An equitable doctrine which prevents a court from hearing a lawsuit involving issues which have already been determined in a prior and different proceeding.

**collection agency**
A business or service established for the main purpose of collecting overdue accounts receivable and bad debts. The services of a collection agency are usually utilized when all other internal means of collection have failed and after a specific amount of time has passed, as set by facility policy. A collection agency should not be used unless it is licensed, bonded, and can furnish references from other facilities or businesses.

**collection cycle (period)**
The amount of time from when a service is performed, the patient is billed, to when the cash is received for the service.

**collective bargaining**
The principle that allows or requires employers to bargain with official union representatives about wages, hours and other employment conditions. The process of negotiating employment benefits.

**collective bargaining agreement**
The contract and promise made between a union and its employer as a result of employment negotiations.

**collegial**
Equal power, responsibility and authority among peers or professionals.

**collegiate school of nursing**
A department, division, or other administrative unit in a college or university which provides primarily or exclusively a program of education in professional nursing and allied subjects leading to the degree of bachelor of arts, bachelor of science, bachelor of nursing, or to an equivalent degree, or to a graduate degree in nursing, and including advanced training related to such program of education provided by such school, but only if such program, or such unit, college or university is accredited.

**collusion**
1. Conspiracy; a secret agreement, or promise between two parties involving fraud against a third party. 2. Undisclosed agreements or acts by two or more parties taken to cheat or commit fraud against another; an agreement between two parties to act to the detriment of a third party.

**colonoscope**
A lighted optical type instrument used to visually examine the interior of the colon.

**colonoscopy**
The act of visually examining the interior of the colon with a lighted instrument.

**color**
1. A deceptive appearance that, while appearing to be one thing, represents another. Acting under color of law is an act that appears on the surface to be official but is not. 2. A sufficient warrant to cause action.

**colorable**
1. To cover or conceal; deceptive; false; counterfeit. 2. That which appears to be valid, but is not.

**colostomy**
A surgical opening where the colon has been opened to the body surface.

**colostomy care**
The specialized care of a colostomy, which is the diversion through surgery of the waste products of the body through an artificial opening on the abdomen. The care of the opening of the colon through the abdominal wall.

**coma**
1. An extensive degree of unconsciousness with little or no detectable mental or physical responsiveness. 2. A deep sleep, lack of observable motion, or unconsciousness due to surgery or injury or illness. See consciousness.

**co-maker**
A second or third party who signs a negotiable instrument, and is equally liable to the payment of the instrument.

**combat fatigue**
Physical and mental reaction to the stresses of combat or extreme military duty.

**comity**
Politeness; civility; courtesy and respect.

**command automatism**
A condition where a patient is open to the power of suggestion and follows it automatically.

**Commerce**
1. The exchange of goods and products. 2. To deal in trade. 3. To carry on the trafficking of goods. 4. To have social intercourse.

**commerce clause**
A clause in Article 1 of the United States Constitution that states the "commerce shall have the power . . . . to regulate commerce with foreign nations, and among the several states . . . ." (Article 1, Section 8, Clause 3, U.S. Constitution.)

**Commerce power**
See Commerce clause.

**commercial disability insurance**
See disability insurance.

**commercial health/medical insurance**
See major medical insurance.

**commercial term life insurance**
See life insurance.

**commercial whole life insurance**
See life insurance.

**commingle**
To mingle; mix together.

**Commission**
1. Authority to perform certain tasks or exercise certain powers. 2. A written grant of authority which allows particular powers to be given by the government, to one of its branches, or to an individual or organization. 3. Committing a crime. 4. Authority to act for another person.

**Commissioner**
1. One who has the authority to perform certain duties or acts. 2. The head of many public service boards or agencies. 3. The officer or chief in charge of agencies or branches of government.

**Commission on Heart Disease, Cancer and Stroke**
A special committee of people chosen to recommend public health service guidelines at the federal level for dealing with and eliminating or reducing the incidence of heart disease, cancer, stroke and other chronic diseases. The recommendations of this commission influence legislation and grant authorizations for types of research needed at universities and medical schools related to any aspect of these disorders.

**Commission on Professional and Hospital Activities (CPHA)**
A nonprofit, nongovernmental organization in Ann Arbor, Michigan established in 1955, for the purpose of collecting, processing and distributing information and data on hospital use for management, evaluation and research purposes. Two main programs of CPHA are the Professional Study (PAS) and the Medical Audit Program (MAP); a continuing study of hospital practice. The system abstracts and classifies information from medical records in a standard way. A computer-accessible data library at CPHA is available and is sponsored by the American College of Physicians, American College of Surgeons, American Hospital Association and Southwestern Michigan Hospital Council. See also discharge abstract.

**Commit**
1. Lawful authority to send a person to prison, a mental institution, reformatory or an asylum. 2. To do an act or crime. 3. To entrust; put into custody. 4. To offer or pledge services or obligations. 5. To consign a person to a mental hospital or psychiatric care facility.

**commitable**
Making a person legally capable of being committed.

**Commitment**
1. The formal legal process of putting a person into the official care of another person or placing one into a mental hospital or psychiatric hospital. 2. A court order, ordering a person to a mental hospital or prison.

**committal**
The act of committing as in committing a person to a psychiatric hospital.

**committee**
A group of people under one person's direction who are brought together for a special purpose which could include tasks such as: decision making, consideration of matters, the taking action or making reports on matters assigned to the group.

**Committee on Allied Health Education and Accreditation (CAHEA)**
A non-governmental agency that accredits educational programs which prepare individuals for entry into one of 26 allied health professions or occupations. CAHEA encompasses a broad range of review and evaluation activities of educational programs in allied health on behalf of the American Medical Association and 46 collaborating organizations composed of allied health professional organizations, medical specialty societies and other interest groups. As the final deliberative body for the assessment of compliance with established minimum acceptable standards for education in the allied health professions, CAHEA formulates its accreditation decisions on the basis of recommendations received from the 21 review committees that are sponsored by the collaborating organizations. Accrediting educational programs for the allied health professions began in 1933 through a cooperative agreement between the American Occupational Therapy Association and CAHEA's predecessor in accreditation, the Council on Medical Education of the American Medical Association. The growth in collaborative sponsorship for accreditation of allied health programs was moderate until the mid-1960's, when it accelerated to a rapid and sustained increase throughout the 1970's.

**committee report**
In congress, a formal report by a Congressional committee to the House of Representatives, Senate or both, concerning a proposed law or other matter. The report is a part of the legislative history and includes a summary of the proposed law, recommendations as to its passage and amendments and other relevant background information.

**commode**
1. A toilet. 2. A chair-like device that has a hole in the seat and is used as a portable toilet.

**commodity**
Articles or goods produced, bought or sold.

**commodum ex iniuria sua nemo habere debet (Lat.)**
No person should derive benefit from his own wrong.

**common**
Usual; ordinary; regular; applying to many persons or things.

**common law**
1. Law by judicial opinion or judge's decisions; judge-made law. 2. Law that originated from English law. 3. Case law which is different from statutory law enacted by legislatures and is a general body of principles derived from usage, custom, and from court decisions relating to governmental duties and security of individuals and their property. 4. Unwritten laws that are legally binding and are upheld by landmark or precedent cases rather than statutes or regulations. Derived from court decisions.

**common law action**
A civil lawsuit; a suit that is between private individuals and/or organizations.

**common law crime**
A crime that could be punished under common law, as distinguished from crimes punishable under statutes.

**common law marriage**
A couple living together as if married and holding themselves out publicly as if married and for a time period considered by law to be sufficient enough to create a legal marriage.

**common plan**
See common scheme.

**common pleas**
1. Civil lawsuits between two private parties. 2. The different types of civil trial courts.

**common scheme**
The planning or committing of two or more different crimes together.

**common stock**
Regular capital stock of a company or shares in a corporation that lack a definite dividend rate and are not preferred stock. The shareholders usually have voting rights at shareholder's meetings, depending on the amount of stock held.

**communicable disease**
A sickness or disease which can be transmitted by any means from person to person or from animal to man.

**community**
1. An entity for which both the nature and scope of a public health problem, as well as the capacity to respond to the problem, can be defined. Depending on the problem area and response capacity, the definition of community may vary. In most instances, the community can be defined as a geopolitical unit, geographical region, or a town, city or county. In certain areas, such as in a large metropolitan region, it may be necessary to evaluate major "communities" in the area for variations in the incidence of each public health problem, so that populations in

greatest need of services can be specified and scarce resources targeted effectively. 2. Also refers to a group of people or professions or situations that have many commonalities such as the medical community or the university community. 3. According to JCAH, for accrediting purposes it is the people, groups, agencies, or other facilities within the locality served by the long term care facility.

**Community Action Programs (CAP)**
An agency created in 1964 by the Economic Opportunity Act to provide federal monies to establish social service and health programs for special and needy populations. Programs created out of the CAP fund include, drug rehabilitation, elderly social service programs, neighborhood health centers and family planning services. Health related programs were supervised by the U.S. Public Health Services.

**community-at-large**
Includes all health care providers, services and programs and consumers, in a geographical, regional, rural, or metropolitan area. The systems or services provided in these areas, or the persons involved in the system or services.

**Community Development Program**
An Indian Health Service program which emphasizes the methods as well as the goals of Community Health Representative activity. The representative in this type of program strives toward the development of community organizations capable of identifying and solving health problems. The aim of programs emphasizing the Community Development approach is to bring about a greater degree of self-determination by the community and a greater role by the entire community in the decisions made by outside agencies that affect the community.

**community dietitian, R.D.**
The community dietitian, R.D., with specialized community dietetic preparation, functions as a member of the community health team in assessing nutritional needs of individuals and groups. The community dietitian plans, organizes, coordinates, and evaluates the nutritional component of health care services for an organization.

**community health care**
Activities and programs intended to improve the healthfulness of, and general health status in, a specified community. The term is widely used with many different definitions. It is variously defined, as above, in a manner similar to public health, synonymously with environmental health, as all health services of any kind available to a given community, or even synonymously with a community's ambulatory care.

**community health center**
An ambulatory health care program usually serving a catchment area with scarce or non-existent health services or a population with special health needs. Often known as neighborhood health centers. Grant support for such centers was originally provided on a research and demonstration basis from the Community Action Program of the Office of Economic Opportunity. Subsequently, the funding authority for these projects shifted

to section 314(e) of the Public Health Service Act. Community health centers attempt to coordinate Federal, State, and local resources in a single organization capable of delivering both health care and related social services to a defined population. Other ambulatory centers providing health services in areas of medical underservice and supported with 314(e) funds include family health centers and community health networks. P.L. 94-63, the Health Revenue Sharing and Health Services Act of 1975, incorporated neighborhood health centers, family health centers and community health networks under the single term, "community health centers," defined in section 330 of the PHS Act. While such centers may not directly provide all types of health care, they arrange for all medical services needed by their patients.

**community health education**
A process that bridges the gap between health information and health practices. Health education motivates one to utilize health information and to keep oneself healthier by avoiding actions that are harmful and by activating habits and behaviors that are beneficial. Community health education includes a set of activities which include: 1) Inform people about health, illness disability, and ways in which they can improve and protect their own health—including more efficient use of the health delivery system. 2) Motivate people to want to activate more healthful practices. 3) Help people to learn the necessary skills to adopt and maintain healthful behaviors and lifestyles. 4) Foster teaching and communication skills in all those engaged in educating consumers about health. 5) Advocate changes in the environment that facilitate healthful conditions and healthful behavior. 6) Advocate social and political changes that facilitate healthful conditions and behavior. 7) Add to knowledge through research and evaluation concerning the most effective ways of achieving the previous objectives. See community/public health educator, health education, community health promotion and protection.

**community health network (CHN)**
A community (State, county or city) health system for delivering medical care to the poor. Started by OEO in the early 1970's, the program was transferred to the Department of Health and Human Services and has now become part of the community health center program. A CHN usually consisted of several, centrally managed community or neighborhood health centers with necessary back-up hospital care.

**community health promotion and protection**
A major subsystem of the overall health system which includes those services delivered to the community as a whole in order to improve or maintain their health status. Major service categories within Community Health Promotion and Protection include: Health Education, Environmental Quality Management, Food Protection, Occupational Health and Safety, Radiation Safety, and Biomedical and Consumer Product Safety.

**community health promotion and protection services**
Services directed at the community level toward improving the personal health behavior of community residents and improving the quality of factors in the environment which affect their health.

**Community Health Representative**
A paraprofessional health worker employed by Indian tribal governments to function as a liaison between the community and health resources. These health workers work closely with physicians, public health nurses, sanitarians, medical social workers and other health team members to help improve the health conditions and health status of his or her tribe.

**Community Health Representative Program**
A program of the Indian Health Service conducted on Indian reservations and in Alaska that emphasizes Indian and Alaskan natives' involvement in community health. A product of the U.S. Public Health Services, it was developed in response to an emphasis upon Indians making decisions about themselves and their communities with two needs addressed: 1) greater involvement of native Americans in their own health programs and identification and solving of these problems; 2) greater understanding between native Americans and the Indian Health Service staff.

**community health worker**
These individuals work in the community in cooperation with medical personnel and social workers helping the client and the health community locate and utilize available sources of assistance.

**Community Liaison Program**
An Indian Health Service program which focuses upon the liaison role of the community health representative, but unlike the Health Liaison Program, emphasizes the representative as a link between the community and all outside resources, whether health related or not. The representative in this type of program works with reservation, city, and county agencies providing services in housing, education, employment assistance and general welfare assistance, as well as direct health care.

**community medicine**
The branch of medicine that concerns itself with community health care delivery, public health, preventive medicine or primary care to special populations. It also deals with assessing and evaluating needs and trends in disease, and health care delivery of groups or community populations. See preventive medicine.

**community mental health center (CMHC)**
An entity which provides comprehensive, ambulatory, mental health services, to individuals residing or employed in a defined catchment area. The term is defined in the Community Mental Health Centers Act (section 201) which specifies the services to be provided and requirements for the governance, organization and operation of the centers. The CMHC Act provides for Federal financial assistance for the construction, development and initial operation of CMHCs, and, on an ongoing basis, for the costs of their consultation and education services.

**community property**

All common or shared property acquired during the course of a marriage irregardless of who purchased it or whose name it is in.

**community psychiatry**

See community psychology.

**community psychology or community psychiatry**

That branch of psychiatry or psychology concerned with the delivery of mental health care to a specified population, usually residents of a designated geographical area. The purpose of community psychiatry or psychology is the acceptance of continuing responsibility for all mental health needs of a community, such as diagnosis, treatment, rehabilitation (often called tertiary prevention), and aftercare. Also included are early case-finding or secondary prevention and the promotion and mental health education and prevention of psychosocial disorders, which is primary prevention. The organization or facility for such services is typically the community mental health center. See community mental health center.

**community/public health educator**

Influences public attitudes toward achieving and maintaining high standards of health through teaching, community liaison and consultation, and dissemination of information. Alerts community groups and individuals to changing patterns of health care, to health hazards, and to activities which will promote community health safety. See Health Educator.

**community rating**

A method of establishing premiums for health insurance in which the premium is based on the average cost of actual or anticipated health care used by all subscribers in a specific geographic area or industry and does not vary for different groups or subgroups of subscribers or with such variables as the groups or subgroups of subscribers or with such variables as the group's claims experience, age, sex, or health status. The HMO Act (section 1302(8) of the PHS Act) defines community rating as a system of fixing rates of payments for health services which may be determined on a per person or per family basis "and may vary with the number of persons in a family, but must be equivalent for all individuals and for all families with similar composition." The intent of community rating is to spread the cost of illness evenly over all subscribers (the whole community) rather than charging the sick more than the healthy for health insurance. Community rating is the exceptional means of establishing health insurance premiums in the United States today. The Federal Employee's Health Benefits Program for example is experience rated, not community rated.

**community setting**

Settings in which community health promotion and health system enabling services, rather than personal health care services or patient-related support services, are provided. Voluntary or public agencies or schools for health professions/occupations typically provide services in community settings.

**commutation**

1. An alteration; a change. 2. In criminal law, it is the reduction in sentence; changing a criminal's punishment to one less severe.

**commute**

1. To stand in the place of another. 2. To reduce the sentence of one convicted of a crime. 3. Payment in kind or by compulsory duty.

**compact**

An agreement or contract between two parties, usually between governments or nations.

**company**

1. To be a companion to or to accompany. 2. An organization established to do business. 3. A number of persons united for the same cause, purpose or concern as a business; the members of a firm.

**comparability provision**

A provision in Medicare specifying that the reasonable charge for a service may not be higher than charges payable for comparable services insured under comparable circumstances by a carrier for its non-Medicare beneficiaries (see section 1842(b)(3)(B) of the Social Security Act.)

**comparative negligence**

A legal principle by which "fault" on each side of an accident is measured and the side with less fault is given money damages. In cases where the negligent acts of the plaintiff and the defendant are compared, damages are based on the degree of negligence of the defendant over and above that of the plaintiff. The degrees usually are "slight," "ordinary," or "gross." If negligence is concurrent and contributes to harm or injury, recovery is possible, but the plaintiff's damages are diminished proportionately as long as the plaintiff's fault is less than the defendant's, and if ordinary care was given, the injury could not have been avoided once it became apparent. (Rogers v. McKinley, 48 Ga. App. 262, 172 S.E. 663, 664) This rule does not exist in some states.

**comparative statements**

Different financial statements that provide information on the same organization or institution for different times (usually for two successive years).

**compelling state interest**

1. A concern that is serious or strong enough to enact a law at the state level which justifies the limiting of a person's constitutional rights.

**compendium**

A collection of information about drugs. Under the Federal Food, Drug, and Cosmetic Act, standards for strength, quality, and purity of drugs are those which are set forth in one of the three official compendia: the United States Pharmacopeia, the Homeopathic Pharmacopeia of the United States, the National Formulary, or any supplement to any of them. Since the Mid-1960's, publication by the FDA of a compendium has been proposed which would compile the labeling of all marketed drugs, to improve the amount and quality of information on drugs that is available to physicians or pharmacists as an aid in prescribing or dispensing. The compendium would consist of one or more volumes and would probably resemble an expanded version of the popular PHYSICIAN'S DESK REFERENCE, a private compendium in which drug manufacturers must purchase space and which does not provide information on all drugs. See also formulary.

**compensation**
1. The settlement of a debt. 2. A recovery payment for harm, damages, or loss. 3. In psychology, disguising an undesirable trait by exaggerating a positive, acceptable one. A mental mechanism in which a person substitutes a behavior for another which is less acceptable, and which the person believes will help him or her to cope better in life.

**compensatory damages**
Money or other means of remuneration given to a plaintiff to overcome damage, loss, or suffering.

**competency**
An acceptable level of skill proficiency required to carry out an activity.

**competent**
1. One qualified or suitably capable; one who is legally authorized and properly qualified; one possessing the right or legal qualifications meeting all requirements. 2. Of sufficient mental capacity as required by law. 3. One who is mentally able to control his or her life, to take care of his or her financial obligations, practice socially accepted behavior and whose judgment and behavior are reliable and controllable as to not be a danger to themselves or others.

**competent court**
A court having lawful jurisdiction.

**competent evidence**
1. Sound and solid facts and proof. 2. Evidence that is both relevant and proper. 3. Proof of a fact or point; evidence that is not excluded by any exclusionary rule.

**competent mind**
See compos mentis, competent.

**complainant**
1. One who makes an official complaint or files a complaint in court. 2. A lawsuit seeking legal remedy in the courts. 3. A plaintiff in a lawsuit.

**complaint**
1. The initial document filed in a civil lawsuit. 2. A formal charge or accusation which includes a statement of the harm done to the plaintiff by the defendant and a request for remedial actions from the court.

**complementary benefits (Medicare)**
A non-group agreement under which the insurance intermediary like Blue Cross, pays deductible and co-insurance for Medicare beneficiaries for hospital care.

**complex**

A psychiatric term for a group of associated ideas that have a common emotional relation. These are reviewed by some psychological theorists as unconscious and are believed to influence attitudes and associations.

**complex treatment**

Used in health insurance to refer to radiation therapy and oncology treatment of malignant disease requiring complex field localization or use of beam shaping devices (e.g., treatment of eyelid; mantle fields in Hodgkin's disease, etc.) or two or more fields per region or two or more regions per day, massive single dose treatment, intracavitary therapy applied with general anesthesia.

**compliance**

1. Yielding to a request; complying with wishes or demands. 2. Acting in a way that does not violate instructions; adhering to a prescribed treatment plan or drugs. Patient compliance is when the patient follows the doctor's orders or instructions. 3. To adhere to or fall within the scope of laws and regulations; to perform or act in a manner that does not violate rules, laws, regulations, or legal principles. See patient compliance.

**composition**

1. A formal agreement where a creditor will accept as full payment less than the total amount owed. 2. A bankruptcy agreement where the person in debt agrees to pay the creditors part of the money he owes.
compos mentis
Of sound mind; having use and control of all of one's mental facilities. See competent.

**compounding a felony**

Committing a crime in conjunction with another crime, such as accepting money or things of value in exchange for not prosecuting a crime which is also a felony.

**compound interest**

Interest paid on the principal or the main debt, and on the unpaid interest.

**comprehensive**

1. Comprehensive means broader coverage on diseases or accidents and higher indemnity payments in comparison with a limited clause; the insuring clause of contracts can be either comprehensive or limited. All inclusive, such as comprehensive health care, means that all medical and health care services are available.

**comprehensive care**

Total complete care and services provided beyond those offered by usual health insurance plans. Comprehensive care usually includes: dental care, eye care, mental health services, etc. This term is associated with prepaid group health plans, HMOs, Indian Health Services, military health services, etc.

**Comprehensive Health Insurance Plan (CHIP)**
National health insurance proposals.

**comprehensive major medical insurance**
A policy designed to give the protection offered by both a basic and a major medical health insurance policy.

**comprehensive service**
See services, also levels of service.

**compress**
A sterile pad or cloth that is applied to a wound or open sore; sometimes it is medicated.

**comptroller**
1. A top financial officer. 2. An employee in charge of fiscal affairs.

**compulsion**
An uncontrollable impulse to do certain acts or behaviors repetitively. See also obsession.

**compulsive personality**
A personality type characterized by overconscientiousness, controlling inhibition, inability to relax, rigidity.

**compulsory**
Used in connection with coverage under proposed national health insurance or other health insurance plans which require coverage to be offered or taken. A plan may be compulsory only for an employer (coverage must be offered to employees and a specified portion of the premium paid, if they opt to take it) or for individuals as well. Any universal public plan is necessarily compulsory in that the payment of taxes to support the plan is not optional with the individual.

**compulsory process**
To force a person to appear in court by an official action.

**computer**
An electronic machine that processes, analyzes and stores large amounts of data. This machine can perform preprogrammed computations and data analysis at high speeds, as well as produce reports and retrieve information quickly, effectively, accurately and economically.

**Computer Assisted Pathology Encoding and Reporting System**
See CAPER, MUMPS.

**computerized axial tomography (CAT)**
The first specialized radiological diagnostic technique in which a series of x-rays is taken from several points around a single plane or level of the body. From these x-rays a single, composite picture (scan) is developed by a computer. The scan represents a horizontal cross-section of the various tissues present at that level of the body. The machine used for this procedure is called an ACTA scanner. Another similar type instrument for reconstructing cross-sectional planes of the body is an

EMI scanner. "Axial"was dropped from the title and now it is referred to as a CT scan. See CT.

**con-**

**con**
Prefix meaning with; together.
against.

**concealment**
Hiding or withholding of information or evidence.

**C.O.N. -Certificate of Need**
See these words.

**conciliation**
1. To win over and bring together. 2. To soothe two sides of an argument and bring them together to a compromise.

**conclusion of fact**
A conclusion drawn or inference made from facts and evidence.

**conclusion of law**
The application of facts to particular principles of law to reach a final decision.

**conclusive**
1. Finishing a matter; completing an inquiry; finishing a debate. 2. Not allowing further evidence. 3. Plain; visible; obvious; clear. 4. Ended; final; decisive; no longer refutable.

**concur**
To unite in opinion; to agree. A concurring opinion is one in which two judges agree, but by using different reasoning.

**concurrent**
Having equal authority or jurisdiction.

**concurrent disinfection**
A protective measure taken to contain and control the spread of an infectious disease by or through a patient who is infectious.

**concurrently**
At the same time; to run together; concurrent sentences are prison terms that run at the same time.

**concurrent resolution on the budget**
In the Federal budget, a resolution passed by both Houses of Congress, but requiring the signature of the President, setting forth, reaffirming, or revising the Congressional budget for the United States government for a fiscal year. There are two such resolutions that must be completed each year: the first concurrent resolution by May 15, and the second concurrent resolution by September 15.

**concurrent review**

Review of the medical necessity of hospital or other health facility admissions upon or within a short period following an admission and the periodic review of services provided during the course of treatment. The intitial review usually assigns an appropriate length of stay to the admission (using diagnosis specific criteria) which may also be reassessed periodically. Where concurrent review is required, payment for unneeded hospitalizations or services is usually denied. The old HEW issued utilization review rules which would have required concurrent review (defined as review within one working day of admission) of all Medicare and Medicaid cases after July 1, 1975. Admissions which were found unnecessary would not have been reimbursed under either Medicare or Medicaid beyond three days after this finding. As a result of suit by the AMA against implementation of certain portions of these regulations, particularly the concurrent review requirement, implementation of the requirements was enjoined by temporary injunction. The old HEW rewrote the regulations. Under the enjoined regulations, review was to be conducted by a physician member or by a qualified nonphysician member of the committee or group assigned the utilization review responsibility in each hospital. Such individual was to be appropriately trained and qualified to perform the assigned review functions, and the review was to use criteria selected or developed by the hospital utilization review committee or group. Concurrent review should be contrasted with a retrospective medical audit which is done for quality purposes and does not relate to payment, and claims review, which occurs after the hospitalization is over.

**condemn**

1. To give a negative or adverse decision. 2. To blame; to sentence. 3. Found guilty of a criminal charge. 4. Official ruling that declares something unfit for use. This process is called condemnation. 5. To present a person as bad. 6. To convict.

**condition**

1. An uncertain future restriction or event that could create or destroy rights or obligations. A contract can have a condition written into it. 2. Anything required before performance or completion can be done; anything that could restrict or modify an occurrence; stipulations that may change or nullify a contract. 3. Any illness, injury, disorder, disease or congenital malformation.

**conditionally renewable**

A medical or health insurance contract which allows the insured person to renew the contract to a predetermined and stated date or advanced age. The insurer has the option of declining renewal only under conditions specifically set forth in the insurance contract.

**conditioning therapy**

See behavior therapy.

**conditions of enrollment**

In health insurance, those rules which determine eligibility for enrollment.

**conditions of participation**
The various conditions which a provider (e.g. hospital, skilled nursing facility) or supplier of services desiring to participate in the Medicare program is required to meet before participation is permitted. These conditions are specified in the statute and regulations and include compliance with title VI of the Civil Rights Act, signing an agreement to participate acceptable to the Secretary of HHS, meeting the definition of the particular institution or facility contained in the law (e.g., in order to participate as a hospital an institution must be a hospital within the meaning of section 1861 (e) of the Social Security Act and must further meet standards for health and safety specified in regulations), conformity with State and local laws, having an acceptable utilization review plan, and meeting appropriate PSRO requirements. Investigations to determine whether or not health care facilities meet or continue to meet conditions of participation are made by the appropriate State health agency, which is responsible for certifying that the conditions have been met and that the provider or supplier is eligible to participate.

**conference**
In Congress, a formal meeting of representatives of the House and Senate at which the differences between House and Senate versions of a single piece of legislation or policy are resolved. The members of the House and Senate chosen to conduct the conference are called managers and together form the conference committee. They jointly recommend a compromise version of the legislation, the text of which is the conference report. With the report comes an explanation of how the differences were resolved (the equivalent of a committee report, called the joint statement of managers) which becomes part of the legislative history. Since the compromise version is different from those originally passed, the conference report must be enacted by both the House and Senate before being sent for Presidential signature.

**confession**
1. Acknowledgement of guilt; disclosing of fault or committing a crime.
2. A statement by a person that he or she is guilty of a crime; admission of wrongdoing.

**confession and avoidance**
In common law, a form of pleading where a party confesses the allegation made is true and then presents new material that renders the charges legally void.

**confession of judgement**
1. When borrowing money, the borrower, if signing a statement or agreement in advance, can allow a lawyer for the lender to get 2. written promise by a debtor that upon default allows judgement to be entered against him. 3. A confession of judgement might be included as a clause in a contract.

**confidential**
Private or secret information, practices, or procedures. Confidentiality, as of a medical record, refers to the degree and circumstances in which information in such a record is private or secret. Information which is

held confidential may include medical, financial or other information about patients obtained in the course of medical practice, and information about the cost, quality and nature of the practice of individual and institutional providers obtained through payment and regulation programs. Confidentiality in practice is very hard to protect and various detailed efforts to do so in the health field have already been written into law. See Section 333 of the Comprehensive Alcohol Abuse and Alcoholism Prevention, Treatment and Rehabilitation Act. The circumstances under which information should be confidential are often controversial since confidentiality may well keep secret inappropriate acts by patients or providers, but its absence may well limit the freedom and confidence with which medicine is practiced or expose providers and patients to unnecessary embarrassement. See also Hippocrates of Cos.

**confidential communication**

Any communication that is conducted or passes between persons of a fiduciary relationship who have a duty not to reveal the contents of the information.

**confidentiality**

1. The requirement that a professional not disclose information received from a client or patient. This is also called privileged communication. 2. Medical ethics by which a health care provider is bound; a duty and expectation to keep secret all information provided to him by the patient. Some states do not legally recognize confidentiality and can require the health care professional to divulge any information needed in a legal proceeding. See fiduciary relationship.

**confidential relationship**

1. A relationship where a client or patient has a right to receive a high level of trust from a physician, psychologist, counselor, lawyer or other professional. 2. A relation in law that is created to prevent undue advantage due to unlimited confidential information being available to certain people, thus a duty is created which requires an ultimate degree of good faith between the parties in all interactions and transactions. 3. Any legal relationship that is recognized and definite, requiring trust and confidence, where a fiduciary relationship legally exists. See fiduciary relationship.

**confinement**

Any illness, disability, or injury that confines the insured person indoors (at home or hospital). Many policies specify that coverage is provided only if the insured is medically confined, as determined by the health care provider.

**confiscate**

1. To seize by proper authority; to appropriate. 2. The taking of private property without payment.

**conflict of interest**

1. When a government worker is in a position to sway business transactions for his own gain. 2. When one's own needs could violate a duty owed to those persons who have a right to depend on this duty.

**conflict of laws**
1. Contradiction and inconsistency in laws. 2. When a judge is forced to make a choice between laws of more than one state or country that may apply them to a case in order to make a decision.

**confrontation**
The right of a defendant (usually a criminal) through his lawyer to see and cross-examine all witnesses to be used against him.

**confused**
When a person appears bewildered; he or she may make inappropriate statements and give strange or incorrect answers to questions.

**confusion**
1. Failing to be able to distinguish between two or more items or facts. 2. A merger or blending together. 3. To confound facts; intermingling.

**confute**
To disprove or to prove a person or a statement to be wrong, false, or invalid.

**congenital**
Any condition, disorder, defect or occurrence that presents itself and exists from the time of birth; existing at or before birth.

**Congressional budget**
The Federal budget, as set forth by Congress in a concurrent resolution on the budget. These resolutions shall include: the appropriate level of total budget outlays and of total new budget authority, an estimate of budget outlays and new budget authority for each major functional category, for contingencies, and for undistributed intra-governmental transactions (based on allocations of the appropriate level of total budget outlays and of total new budget authority); the amount, if any, of the surplus or deficit in the budget; the recommended level of Federal revenues; and the appropriate level of the public debt.

**Congressional Record**
The record and account of the day-by-day proceedings of Congress. It is published daily.

**conjugal**
Having to do with marriage; belonging to or a part of the husband-wife relationship; arising from the husband-wife relationship.

**conjugal rights**
The rights of spouses to love, have companionship and sexuality.

**conjugal room**
A room set aside in an institution such as a hospital, nursing home or prison where a person may exercise his or her conjugal rights. See conjugal rights.

**connecting up**
To be put into evidence, information or facts have to "connect up" with other evidence or be relevant.

**consanguinity**
The degree of blood relationship or connection a person has with a common ancestor; blood relationship; kinship; a close relationship.

**consciousness**
A person's normal state of awareness.

**consciousness, levels of**
*Alert*: Awake and oriented to time, place, people, weather, environment, and surroundings. *Confused*: Awake but disoriented as to time, place, people, and surroundings. *Somnolent*: Drowsy or sleeps when alone; the patient may be confused when awake. *Stuporous*: Difficult to arouse; may be combative, aggressive, hostile at times. *Semicomatose*: Very little spontaneous movement or motion unless strong attempts to arouse the patient are made. *Comatose*: The patient may be or may not be responsive to painful stimuli; no spontaneous movements observable.

**consent**
1. Permission given; approval; voluntary and active agreement; voluntary compliance or acceptance of something done or proposed. 2. Purposeful agreement in the terms of a contract in a manner that the agreement is binding. 3. To give a health care provider through a written agreement, permission to do a certain procedure, treatment, or act. 4. Voluntary agreement by a person mentally capable of making an intelligent choice to do something proposed by another, such as a physician. Consent is implied in every agreement. Any act that is not distorted by fraud, duress or even a mistake. Submission does not necessarily suggest consent was given, as consent must be an active acquiescence or concurrence. See express consent, informed consent and implied consent.

**consent judgement**
An agreement by the parties to an action, entered into with the approval of the court.

**consequential damages**
Losses or injuries that are indirect or do not show up until later that are a result of a wrongful act.

**consideration**
The material aspects or ramifications of a contract. The price, motivation or reason to make a contract; something of value to convince a person to make a deal. Without "consideration" a contract is not valid; the motive for inducement of a contract. Also see valuable consideration.

**consign**
1. To give, send or deliver; to entrust things over for transportation or sale, while retaining ownership. 2. To leave in the custody of a third person. 3. To agree or consent to; to sign over to or to put in charge of.

**consignment**
1. To consign. 2. To have an item shipped or delivered. 3. Turned over to or entrusted to another person. The document by which an item is consigned.

**consolidation**

1. Treating separate lawsuits on the same subject and between the same persons as only one lawsuit. Uniting separate things into one. 2. To make solid. 3. To form into a firm; combining two benefices into one.

**consortium**

1. A partnership. 2. A joint effort of hospitals, health care or social organizations, institutions, associations, or societies to organize together in a common effort. 3. An organized partnership used to meet similar or common goals, when a single organization lacks its own base or ability to be successful on its own. 4. The right a spouse has to receive the other's love and services. 5. Joining together.

**conspiracy**

1. Persons joining together to do an unlawful act; sometimes, the planning itself is unlawful, even if the act is not. 2. An unlawful agreement between two or more parties.

**constitution**

A document which provides guidelines for and limitations to what a governing body, government, or organization can or cannot do.

**constitutional**

Consistent with the state or federal Constitution and is not in conflict with the basic constitution and laws of the state or a nation.

**constitutional law**

1. The law that determines the organization, structure, functions, principles and limitations of governments. 2. Laws created by federal, state, and/or provincial constitutions.

**constitutional right**

A right guaranteed by the Constitution.

**construct**

A mental process or a way an individual develops beliefs and values; how he interprets, construes, or determines the meaning of life. It is used to determine what and how thoughts and behaviors are perceived, remembered, learned or done. If a person has developed the construct that spiders are bad, he or she will avoid spiders. Constructs screen one's differentiation of beliefs and elements in life. They help determine good, bad, likes, dislikes, successes and failure and how to act because of these the next time they occur.

**construction**

A judge deciding the meaning of ambiguous words by looking at the surrounding circumstances and relevant laws.

**construction (cost of)**

This includes (a) the construction of new buildings, the expansion of existing buildings, and the acquisition, remodeling, replacement, renovation, major repair (to the extent permitted by regulations), or alteration of existing buildings, including architects' fees, but not including the cost of acquisition of land or offsite improvements, and (b) initial equipment of new buildings and of the expanded, remodeled, repaired, renovated, or altered part of existing buildings; but such term shall not include the construction or cost of construction of so much of any facility as is used or is to be used for sectarian instruction or as a place for religious worship.

**constructive**
1. Some factor or incident that is true legally; to establish by legal interpretation. 2. Inferred; implied.

**construe**
To arrive at a meaning of a statute, contract, or statement, by inference.

**consul**
One appointed by the government to reside in a foreign country to take charge of the person's country's needs, affairs and interests.

**consultant**
1. Any professional who provides expert or technical advice or services as requested. 2. According to JCAH, this is one who provides professional advice or services on request.

**consultation**
1. In medical or dental practice, the act of requesting advice from another provider, usually a specialist, regarding the diagnosis and/or treatment of a patient. The consultant usually reviews the history, examines the patient, and then provides his written or oral opinion to the requesting practitioner. Referral for consultation should be distinguished from referral for services, because responsibility for patient care is not usually delegated to the consultant. This definition distinguishes a consultation between providers from an encounter or visit between a provider and consumer. 2. In health insurance, a consultation is considered to include those services rendered by a physician whose opinion or advice is requested by another physician or agency in the evaluation and/or treatment of a patient's illness or problem. Consultations may be given in home, office, hospital, extended care facility, etc. There can be frequent occasions when the consultant may subsequently: 1) assume management in full or in part, or 2) need to see the patient on a repetitive basis for the purpose of further evaluation and/or treatment in a continuing consultative capacity. For insurance claims, this can only be determined in the individual case in question. In health insurance, there is no follow-up time assumed to be inherent in the rendering of a consultation. A referral may ensue after completion of a consultation, but such an event does not preclude the fact that the initial evaluation was a consultation. See referral.

**consultation and education services**
Services required of each community mental health center (CMHC) by section 201 of the CMHC Act which consist of consultation with, and education for, the staffs of programs and institutions in the CMHC's community which are likely to be responsible for or come in contact with people with mental illness (such as schools, prisons, bars and courts). Such services are specially subsidized by section 204 of the

CMHC Act because they are high priority preventive care, not usually reimbursed by the recipient institutions, and not covered under health insurance (which rarely covers services not directly delivered to insured individuals).

**consumer**

1. One who may receive or is receiving health services. While all people at times consume health services, a consumer as the term is used in health legislation and programs is usually someone who is never a provider, i.e., is not associated in any direct or indirect way with the provision of health services. The distinction has become important in programs where a consumer majority on the governing body is required, as is the case with community health centers and health systems agencies assisted under the PHS Act. 2. One who uses goods or services for his own use or needs rather than to use them for resale or make other products to sell. 3. A person who consumes something.

**consumer awareness**

Being aware of defective or unsafe products or misleading information related to the consumption or use of products.

**Consumer Credit**

The trade association created for the Insurers of Credit Insurance in the life, health/medical insurance areas.

**consumerism**

The consumer being aware of rights and expectations in his or her process of consuming.

**Consumer Price Index (CPI)**

An economic index prepared by the Bureau of Labor Statistics of the U.S. Department of Labor. It measures the change in average prices of the goods and services purchased by urban wage earners and clerical workers and their families. It is widely used as an indicator of changes in the cost of living, as a measure of inflation (and deflation, if any) in the economy, and as a means for studying trends in prices of various goods and services. The CPI is made up of several components which measure prices in different sectors of the economy. One of these, the medical care component, gives trends in medical care charges based on specific indicators of hospital, medical, dental and drug prices. The medical care component of the CPI characteristically rises faster than the CPI itself as do some other service components of the index. However, since the CPI measures charges, which are not always related to costs, the CPI may fail to accurately reflect changes in medical care costs.

**consummate**

1. To finish; a completion; carrying out an agreement; fulfill. 2. Finishing to the utmost degree what was intended; carrying out that which has merely begun.

**contaminate**

To make unsanitary, unclean or unsterile; to soil; to pollute.

**contamination**
Any unsanitary condition that results from contact with any object that has any pathogenic organisms on it.

**contemn**
1. To scorn, slight, or despise. 2. To treat as despicable. 3. To reject or scorn with disdain.

**contemner**
1. One who despises or scorns: a person who contemns. 2. The person committing contempt of court; one guilty of contempt.

**contempt**
Willful disregard for authority, whether judicial or legislative.

**contest**
To argue against or to oppose as in opposing a lawsuit.

**contingency fees**
Fees based or conditioned on future occurrences or conclusions, or on the results of services to be performed. Contingency fees are used by lawyers representing patients as plaintiffs in malpractice cases and are usually a set fraction (commonly a third) of any settlement awarded the patient. If no settlement is awarded, the lawyer is not paid. Such fees are said to give the lawyer incentives to try the case with full vigor, choose only cases which are likely to succeed, choose only cases which will have large settlements, and increase the amount of settlements sought. See also New Jersey rule.

**contingency reserves**
Reserves set aside by an insurance company for unforeseen or unplannable circumstances and expenses other than the normal losses incurred by the risks insured.

**continued stay review**
Review during a patient's hospitalization to determine the medical necessity, and appropriateness of continuation of the patient's stay at a hospital level of care. It may also include assessment of the quality of care being provided. Occasionally used for similar review of patients in other health facilities, see medical review. Used in the PSRO and Medicare programs where it is sometimes called extended duration review. See also concurrent review.

**continuing education**
Formal education obtained by a health professional after completing his degree and post-graduate training. Such education is usually intended to improve or maintain the professionl's competence. For physicians, some, but not all, States require a specified number of hours of recognized continuing education per year as a condition of continued licensure. The AMA conducts a voluntary program of recognition for physicians completing required amounts of recognized continuing education.

**continuing resolution**
In the Federal budget, legislation enacted by the Congress to provide budget authority for specific ongoing activities in a fiscal year in cases where the regular appropriation for such activities has not been enacted by the beginning of the fiscal year. The continuing resolution usually specifies a maximum rate at which the agency may obligate funds, based on the rate of the prior year, the President's budget request, or an appropriation bill previously passed by either House of the Congress.

**continuity**
1. Continuity refers to the degree of coordination present in the delivery of health care services to each consumer. Continuity is a measure of the extent to which the health system interrelates and integrates the various services delivered to a consumer over time and in various settings. 2. Continued, complete, total care from one health care practitioner or setting to another.

**contra (Lat.)**
Against; opposite.

**contraband**
Imported, exported, or goods held in violation of law; prohibited goods.

**contraception**
The prevention of fertilization of the ovum by the sperm by any means or method that is effective.

**contract**
1. A binding promissory agreement between two or more competent parties, upon sufficient consideration, that creates, modifies, or destroys a legal agreement to do or not do some act. See unilateral contract, bilateral contract, quasi contract. 2. In psychology, counseling, or psychiatry, a commitment by the patient or client to a specific course of action or change of behavior. In group or individual psychotherapy, the therapist-patient contract is created to attain the treatment goal or certain behavior change. 3. According to JCAH for psychiatric, alcoholism and drug abuse facilities accreditation purposes, this is a formal agreement with any organization, agency, or individual, approved by the governing body, that specifies the services, personnel, and/or space to be provided to, or on behalf of, the facility and the monies to be expended in exchange.

**contract clause**
Article 1, Section 10, Clause 1, U.S. Constitution: "No State shall...pass any...law impairing the obligation of contracts..."

**contract count**
Number of subscribers (excluding dependents) enrolled in a prepaid group health plan.

**contracted services**
Those services brought in from outside of the facility or institution and which are rendered by personnel who are not on the organization's

regular payroll. Money involved includes all related expense covered by the contract.

**contract law**
That area of law which deals with promissory agreements between two or more parties, thus creating a legal relationship between the parties.

**contribution margin (marginal income)**
Revenue less variable costs. The contribution margin may be expressed on a per-unit basis, as a total, or as a ratio.

**contributory insurance**
Group insurance in which all or part of the premium is paid by the employee, the remainder, if any, being paid by the employer or union. In this context, noncontributory insurance is insurance in which the employer pays all the premium. So called because the risk, or employee, contributes to the cost of the insurance as well as the insured. See also enrollment period.

**contributory negligence**
1. Conduct by an injured person that is below that of the standard expected of him or her for his or her own protection and for the protection of the rights and protection from harm of self or others. 2. Negligence on the part of the plaintiff, adding to or compounding the plaintiff's injury. The negligence of the plaintiff, if established, will eliminate the liability of the defendant.

**contributory program**
A method of payment for group coverage in which part of the premium is paid by the employee and part is paid by his or her employer or union.

**control group**
In research, it is part of an experimental design; the group in which an intervention treatment or factor being tested is deliberately omitted or not given.

**controllability**
In the Federal budget, the ability of the Congress or the President under existing law to control outlays during a given fiscal year. Uncontrollable and relatively uncontrollable describe outlays, and the programs (such as Medicare) in which they occur, that cannot be increased or decreased without changes in existing substantive law. Such spending is usually the result of open-ended programs and fixed costs, like social security and veterans benefits, and payments due under obligation incurred or commitments made during prior years.

**Controlled Substances Act (1970)**
Passed to establish a system of control over drugs of abuse and narcotics. A classification of abused substances was developed and restriction on their use was established. This law provided funds to develop programs related to drug addiction, treatment, rehabilitation and public health education related to drugs and their effects on the individual and society.

**controller**
Any institution's chief accounting officer who is responsible for planning and controlling the financial matters of the organization. Also called a comptroller.

**controversy**
A dispute between interests of adverse parties.

**controvert**
To dispute; contest; deny.

**convalescent centers**
Facilities utilized to care for convalescing patients on a short-term or intermediate length of stay or long-term care and are generally licensed as either skilled or intermediate care facilities. The basic services include medical supervision, rehabilitative programs, special diets and specialized medical services. Since patients are recovering, the center may help patients through rehabilitative services to regain health by providing a comprehensive care program. Some centers may discharge patients once a certain level of health and rehabilitation is achieved.

**conventional**
1. Arising from or created by an agreement between persons, not by a legal arrangement. 2. The common or usual way of doing things; ordinary; acceptable.

**conversion**
1. An illegal act that deprives a person of using his own property, for example, withholding a patient's personal belongings. 2. Unlawful seizing or appropriation and use of another's property.

**conversion privilege**
1. In insurance, this is the right of an individual covered by a group medical or dental insurance policy to continue his coverage on an individual basis (paying the full premium) when he terminates association with the insured group. In group health insurance, the right given the insured to change his group insurance to some form of individual insurance, without medical examination, upon termination of his group insurance (usually upon termination of employment or other source of membership in the group). Group insurance does not always offer a conversion privilege and, when it does, the available individual insurance is generally not of comparable scope of benefits or cost (usually being more expensive).

**conviction**
1. Having a firm belief. 2. To find a person guilty of a crime.

**Cooperative Health Statistics System (CHSS).**
A program of the National Center for Health Statistics in which Federal, State, ad local governments cooperate in collecting health statistics, so that any particular item of data is collected by that level which is best equipped to collect and distribute it to all levels. When in full operation, CHSS will collect data in the following seven subject areas: health manpower (inventories and surveys), health facilities (inventories and

surveys), hospital care, household interviews, ambulatory care, long-term care, and vital statistics. Legislative authority for the CHSS is found in section 306(e) of the PHS Act.

**cooperative hospitals**
Health care facilities controlled by the users of the health care services. These hospitals usually provide comprehensive care, have a prepayment system and utilize group practice. These prepaid comprehensive care programs are often referred to as HMOs (Health Maintenance Organizations).

**coordinated**
When used under Medicare and in conjunction with the phrase "home health services," means the integration of the multidisciplinary services provided by patient care team members directed toward meeting the home health needs of the patient.

**Coordinated Transfer Application System (COTRANS)**
A system begun in 1970 by the American Association of Medical Colleges in which the AAMC evaluates U.S. citizens receiving undergraduate medical education outside the United States and sponsors those it deems qualified for part one of the national board examinations. Students who take and pass the boards with this sponsorship may then apply to a U.S. medical school for completion of their training with advanced standing. Some students obtain sponsorship for the boards from an individual school without using COTRANS.

**Coordinating Council on Medical Education (CCME)**
A supervisory body established in 1972 to coordinate policy matters and accreditation at all levels of medical education. Among its organizational members are the AMA, the American Board of Medical Specialties, the AAMC, the AHA, and the Council of Medical Specialty Societies. It also has public and Federal members. See also Liaison Committees on Medical Education and Graduate Medical Education.

**coordination**
The process of assembling and synchronizing differentiated activities so that health care personnel can function effectively in the attainment of the health care organization's objectives and goals.

**Coordination Of Benefits (COB)**
1. Provisions and procedures used by insurers to avoid duplicate payment for losses insured under more than one insurance policy. For example, some people have a duplication of benefits, for their medical costs arising from an automobile accident, in their automobile and health insurance policies. A coordination of benefits or antiduplication clause in one or the other policy will prevent double payment for the expenses by making one of the insurers the primary payer, and assuring that no more than 100 percent of the costs are covered. There are standard rules for determining which of two or more plans, each having COB provisions, pays its benefits in full and which pays a sufficiently reduced benefit to prevent the claimant from making a profit.2.A clause written into some health insurance policies which means that if the member has other group

hospital, medical, or dental coverage with another company, the first company will take into account benefits that are payable by the other carrier in determining its own liability.

**coordination, types of**

In health care administration, there are four types of coordination approaches that have been identified. They are: *corrective coordination* — those coordinative activities which rectify an error or correct a dysfunction in an organization system after it has occurred; *preventive coordination* —those activities which are aimed at preventing the occurrence of anticipated problems of coordination or, at least, minimizing the impact of anticipated problems; *regulatory coordination* — those activities which are aimed at the maintenance of existing health care organizations structural and functional arrangements; *promotive coordination* — those activities which attempt to improve the articulation of the various parts of a health care organization.

**co-payer**

See co-payment, cost sharing, co-insurance, member co-payment.

**copayment**

1. A contract under which the insured party must pay a portion toward the amount of the professional services rendered. 2. A type of cost sharing whereby insured or covered persons pay a specified flat amount per unit of service or unit of time (e.g., $2 per visit, $10 per inpatient hospital day), their insurer paying the rest of the cost. The copayment is incurred at the time the service is used. The amount paid does not vary with the cost of the service (unlike coinsurance, which is payment of some percentage of the cost).

**coping**

1. Any rational, conscious, subconscious, intrapsychic, mental, emotional or social adjustment effort. Confronting, adjusting to, adapting to any conflict, change, stress, frustration or anxiety experienced in the process of carrying out one's daily activities. 2. Using defense or mental mechanisms to deal with or adapt to life and its constant state of change in a mentally healthy way.

**coping mechanisms**

See mental mechanisms.

**coprolalia**

The use of vulgar, obscene, or dirty words. It is characteristic in some cases of schizophrenia.

**coprophagia**

Eating filth or feces.

**coprophilia**

Excessive interest in filth or feces.

**copulation**

Sexual intercourse; a Latin derivative meaning "coupling or joining."

**copyright**
1. An author's exclusive right over the publication, copying and distribution of written or creative material such as trademarks, books, articles, etc. protected by law. 2. In written material, the copyright covers only the arrangement of words, but not the facts, experiences, thoughts or general ideas, provided they are not substantially copied in concrete form in which the circumstances and ideas have been developed, arranged and put into shape. (133F. 2d 889, 891). Right of first publication under common law copyright is that a copyright exists before a work is published and protects against unauthorized use. (39 N.E. 2d 249). © is the symbol for copyright.

**coram (Lat.)**
Before; in the presence of.

**coram nobis (Lat.)**
1. In our presence. 2. Calling the court's attention to errors of fact that would constitute a valid defense, and were not brought out in a previous trial where a conviction resulted. These facts presumable could have prevented the negative conviction.

**coram non judice (Lat.)**
In a court of incompetent jurisdiction.

**coronary care unit**
A special care unit in a hospital providing intensive care for patients with coronary disease. See special care unit.

**coroner**
1. A public official who holds inquests in regards to violent, sudden or unexplained deaths. 2. A public officer whose duty is to investigate any death which there is no reason to believe is not due to natural causes. 3. A county official whose duty it is to inquire into the manner and cause of deaths in cases where there is suspicion of foul play or violence.

**coroner's jury**
A jury that is involved in investigating a death that is not due to natural causes.

**corp**
Abbreviation of corporation.

**corporal punishment**
Physical punishment inflicted upon one's body, such as a beating or whipping. Used to distinguish types of punishment; physical from non-physical. Non-physical punishment would be something like a fine.

**corporate**
United or combined into a legal organization; unified with or belonging to a corporation.

**corporate bond**
A bond, payable by a corporation on a specified sum borrowed from bondholders.The bonds are payable on a fixed date and interest is payable at a fixed rate.

**corporate negligence doctrine**
The health care facility as an entity in case of a tort or lawsuit, would be held liable rather than its separate employees for the negligent act. It is the lack or failure of those entrusted with the task of carrying out the purpose of the corporation and the failure to follow, in a given situation, the established standards of conduct to which the corporation should conform.

**corporate responsibility**
A common, joint or unified responsibility commonly shared by those of a group or organization.

**corporate veil**
An assumption in law that the actions taken by a corporation are not a single action of one of its owners, thus single entities cannot be held responsible for those acts or things that occur in corporation.

**corporation**
1. An organization formed for legal purposes which is recognized by the law as an entity separate and distinct from its shareholders or promoters. 2. A group which obtains a charter granting it certain legal authorities, privileges, rights and liabilities. 3. A public or private organization set up to carry on a business or to perform business functions.

**corporeal**
1. Having objective physical substance or material existence. 2. Bodily; affecting a body. 3. Able to visibly see or be perceived by sight.

**corpus (Lat.)**
Body, a main body.

**corpus delicti (Lat.)**
1. The body of the crime. 2. The motive or reason for which a crime has been committed; proof that a crime has been committed.

**corpus juris (Lat.)**
Body of law; collection of laws. An encyclopedia of law, abbreviated as CJ or CJS (Corpus Juris Secundum).

**corrective therapist**
Provides medically prescribed programs of therapeutic exercise to physically and mentally ill patients to prevent muscular deconditioning resulting from inactivity and to attain resocialization and specific psychiatric objectives. See recreational therapy, physical therapy, and occupational therapy.

**corroborate**
To strengthen, confirm or add weight. In law this is done by confirming additional facts or evidence. To support credibility; to confirm or reinforce.

**co-signer**
A person who signs a document in conjunction with another person.

**cosmetic surgery**
Any operation directed at improving appearance, except when required for the prompt repair of accidental injury or for the improvement of the functioning of a malformed body member. The term would not apply to surgery in connection with treatment of severe burns or repair of the face following a serious automobile accident, or to surgery for therapeutic purposes which coincidentally serves some cosmetic purpose, but would include reshaping an ugly nose. Most health insurance plans and programs do not cover cosmetic surgery.

**cost**
1. The total level of economic investment required for the provision of health services. This level of investments includes all financial expenditures for capital and operating requirements. 2. Under Medicare, any reasonable costs of any services are determined in accordance with Medicare regulations establishing the method or methods to be used, and the times to be included.

**cost accounting**
One method of accounting. The accounting information is assembled and recorded for all the costs incurred to carry on an activity or operation, or to complete a unit of work or a specific job.

**cost-based reimbursement**
See cost-related.

**cost-base reimbursement**
One method of payment to a health care provider. It is mostly used by government health agencies and third-party payors, to pay for services rendered to patients. The amount of payment is based on the cost as defined by the third party for delivering the service.

**cost-benefit analysis**
A method of comparing the cost of a program with its expected benefits expressed in dollars. For example, the cost of establishing an immunization service compared with the total cost of medical care and lost productivity which will be eliminated as a result of more persons being immunized. Although there are exceptions, cost-benefit analysis generally excludes consideration of factors that cannot be ultimately measured in economic terms.

**cost center**
Accounting device whereby all related costs attributable to some "center" within an institution, such as an activity, department, or program (e.g., X-ray, a hospital burn center), are segregated for accounting or reimbursement purposes. Contrasts with segregating costs of different types, such as nursing, drugs or laundry, regardless of which "center" incurred them.

**cost containment**
The control of the overall cost of health care services within the health care delivery system. Costs are contained when the value of the resources committed to an activity are not considered to be excessive. For this

reason, the determination of cost containment is frequently subjective and dependent upon the specific geographic area of the activity.

**cost-effectiveness analysis**

A method of comparing alternative ways (e.g., alternative combinations of actions) for achieving a specific set of results. Alternatives are compared on the basis of the ratio of the cost of each alternative to its estimated future effects on objectives. Benefits and constraints are usually not expressed in dollars in a cost-effectiveness analysis.

**cost of capital**

The cost of money, including interest on debts and the cost of maintaining adequate owners' equity.

**cost of care**

1. The economic cost (includes out of pocket and insurance coverage) of the health service being provided to the individual. 2. The total capital outlay for a unit of service.

**cost of construction**

See construction.

**cost of insurance**

The amount which a policyholder pays to the insurer minus what he gets back from it. This should be distinguished from the rate for a given unit of insurance ($10 for a $1000 life insurance policy). Such costs, which may be difficult to obtain and are rarely compared, are roughly approximated by the loading or the ratio of amounts paid in benefits to income produced from premiums. See also expenses.

**cost or market, whichever is lower**

A method used in determining the cost and control and supplies for the financial statement. The inventory is set at the acquisition cost or current replacement cost, or market value, whichever is lowest.

**cost per patient day**

The cost of running a heath care facility divided by the number of inpatient days in a set time period. Various adjustments or corrections in the cost figures are made in order to compare cost per patient day between or among health care facilities.

**cost plus contract**

A contract that establishes the amount to be paid to a contractor plus a specified percentage of that price above cost of services provided.

**cost, reasonable**

1. Generally, the amount which a third party using cost-related reimbursement will actually reimburse. Under Medicare reasonable costs are costs actually incurred in delivering health services excluding any part of such incurred costs found to be unnecessary for the efficient delivery of needed health services (see Section 1861 of the Social Security Act). 2. For any specific service covered under Medicare, the lower of the customary charge by a particular physician for that service and the prevailing charge by physicians in the geographic area for that service.

Reimbursement is based on the lower of the reasonable and actual charges...Generally, the term is used for any charge payable by an insurance program which is determined in a similar, but not necessarily identical fashion.

**cost-related or cost-based reimbursement**
One method of payment of medical care programs by third parties, typically Blue Cross plans or government agencies, for services delivered to patients. In cost-related systems, the amount of the payment is based on the costs to the provider of delivering the service. The actual payment may be based on any one of several different formulae, such as full cost, full cost plus an additional percentage, allowable costs, or a fraction of costs. Other reimbursement schemes are based on the charges for the services delivered, or on budgeted or anticipated costs for a future time period (prospective reimbursement). Medicare, Medicaid, and some Blue Cross plans reimburse hospitals on the basis of costs; most private insurance plans pay charges.

**costs**
1. Expenses incurred in a lawsuit that the court can order the opposing side to pay. 2. Expenses incurred in the provision of services or goods. Many different kinds of costs are defined and used (see actual, allowable, direct, indirect, life, marginal and opportunity costs). Charges, the price of a service or amount billed an individual or third party, may or may not be the same as, or based on, costs. Hospitals often charge more for a given service than it actually costs in order to recoup losses from providing other services where costs exceed feasible charges. Despite the terminology, cost control programs are often directed to controlling increases in charges rather than in real costs.

**cost sharing**
Provisions of a health insurance policy which require the insured or otherwise covered individual to pay some portion of his covered medical expenses. Several forms of cost-sharing are employed, particularly deductibles, coinsurance and copayments. A deductible is a set amount which a person must pay before any payment of benefits occurs. A copayment is usually a fixed amount to be paid with each service. Coinsurance is payment of a set portion of the cost of each service. Cost-sharing does not refer to or include the amounts paid in premiums for the coverage. The amount of the premium is directly related to the benefits provided and hence reflects the amount of cost-sharing required. For a given set of benefits, premiums increase as cost-sharing requirements decrease. In addition to being used to reduce premiums, cost sharing is used to control utilization of covered services, for example, by requiring a large copayment for a service which is likely to be overused.

**co-surgeons**
In health insurance, under certain circumstances, two surgeons (usually with similar skills) may function simultaneously as primary surgeons performing distinct parts of a total surgical service (e.g., two surgeons

simultaneously applying skin grafts to different parts of the body or two surgeons repairing different fractures in the same patient.)

**cotenancy**
See cotenant.

**cotenant**
1. Two or more people sharing the same room or apartment. 2. One holding property by joint ownership.

**counsel**
1. A lawyer. 2. Professional advice. "Of counsel" can mean a lawyer assisting on a case.

**counsellor**
A lawyer; One who provides counsel or advise.

**count**
Each part of a criminal indictment or civil complaint. A count is a separate charge.

**counter**
To act in opposition to.

**counterclaim.**
An opposing claim used to offset an original complaint. In a civil lawsuit, a defendant presents a claim against the plaintiff. A counterclaim is usually related to the case at hand but is based on different charges than the plaintiff's original complaint.

**counterfeit**
1. Made without authority or right; forged copying or imitating without authority. 2. Passing off a false copy as an original.

**counteroffer**
A new offer made back, or an offer made to offset an original offer that was not adequate or satisfactory.

**counterphobia**
To prefer the very situation a person fears.

**countersign**
A second original signature used to approve or validate a document; a signature that is added to a document so to confirm or authenticate it.

**countertransference**
The therapist's conscious or unconscious emotional reaction to his client. See also transference.

**county hospital**
See hospital, city/county.

**course of employment**
Directly related to one's employment; during work hours.

**court**
1. The hall or chamber where law is practiced and justice is administered. 2. The assembling of persons and judges for hearing and trying cases. 3. Holding a judicial assembly.

**court day**
The day court is held.

**court of appeals**
The court that hears and decides appeals from a trial court. A middle level court. In some states, it is the highest court.

**court of claims**
A Federal court that hears complaints against the U.S. Government.

**court of common pleas**
A court of original and general jurisdiction over civil suits between private parties; in some states it is called the Superior Court or District Court.

**court of error**
A specialized court that has jurisdiction over cases that are alleged to have error.

**court of last resort**
A court from which there is no more appeal to a higher court.

**court of probate**
A court that is limited to the hearing of specialized problems such as wills and estates, problems of minors or concerns of legally incompetent persons.

**coutume (French)**
1. Custom. 2. A close equivalent for English "common law."

**covenant**
An agreement written into a deed or other document, promising performance or nonperformance of certain acts, or fixing certain uses or nonuses for property.

**covenantee**
One to whom a covenant is made.

**covenantor**
One making a covenant.

**cover**
1. In insurance, to shelter, shield, or defend from harm or injury. 2. To protect, as in insurance "coverage." 3. To include or compensate for, as in the travel expenses covered meals only.

**coverage**

**coverage**
The guarantee against specific losses provided under the terms

See benefit. of an insurance policy. Frequently used interchangeably with benefits or protection. The extent of the insurance afforded by a policy. Often used to mean insurance or an insurance contract. The specific types and amount of insurance. The extent of insurance benefits. Risks protected by insurance.

**coverture**
The rights, conditions, legal limitations or state of a married woman. The legal status or liability of a woman while married.

**C.P.A.**
Certified Public Accountant.

**creaming**
See skimming.

**credentialing**
The recognition of professional or technical competence. The credentialing process may include registration, certification, licensure, professional association membership, or the award of a degree in the field. Certification and licensure effect the supply of health manpower by controlling entrance into practice, and influence the stability of the labor force by affecting geographic distribution, mobility, and retention of workers. Credentialing also determines the quality of personnel by providing standards for evaluating competence, and defining the scope of functions and how personnel may be used.

**credentialism**
1. The requiring of a person or person to have a certain education, degree, certification of license to practice a profession. 2. Requiring a certain degree to be obtained prior to being allowed to take an exam for licensing. 3. Unnecessary requiring of a college degree to practice a profession. Credentialism has been successfully challenged in the courts, as skills and abilities have been found more important than a degree or license.

**credentials committee**
This body of physicians and administrative personnel reviews applications for staff membership with most efforts directed toward physician/medical staff selection.

**credibility**
1. To bring recognition or honor to someone. 2. The trust confidence and reputation has. 3. The truthfulness of a witness. 4. Ethical status of a professional.

**credible**
1. Believable. 2. Practicing a profession ethically. 3. Reliable; reputable; trustworthy.

**credit**
Confidence and trust in one's ability and integrity to pay one's debts.

**creditor**
The one to whom a debt or money is owed. The person with a legal right to collect a sum of money from another due to a financial or business transaction.

**credits**
In accounting, it is the records of money owed or money paid out. The opposite of debits.

**crime**
Criminal wrongdoings that have a negative effect on an individual or society. An act that is in violation of a government's penal laws. An offense or wrongdoing; an illegal act.

**crimen falsie (Lat.)**
Falsehood and fraud used to interfere with the administration of justice. Such offenses include deceit, forgery, fraudulent alteration of a document, or perjury.

**criminal**
1. An act that violates law, morality or a society's well-being; having to do with illegal or unlawful conduct. 2. One who has committed a crime; a person legally convicted of committing a crime.

**criminal action**
The process of litigation through which a person charged with a criminal offense is brought to trial to be tried and judged.

**criminal forfeiture**
Property seized by a government law enforcing agency because it was involved in a crime. A purse can be seized because it was used to smuggle drugs out of a health care facility. An airplane could be seized because it was illegally used to fly narcotics across the border into the United States.

**criminal law**
Those statutes, laws and regulations that deal with conduct offensive to society as a whole, or the state.

**criminal malpractice**
Professional misconduct involving a criminal act, or the breaking of criminal law.

**crippled child**
A female or male under the age of 21 who has an organic disorder, disease, condition or defect that hinders the normal growth and development of that person.

**crippled children's services**
Services provided by the Child Health Act were established when monies were authorized for identification, diagnosis and treatment of any child who is crippled or afflicted with a crippling condition. Title V of the Social Security Act comprises both the Maternal and Child Health and Crippled Children's Services Programs. The purpose of the Crippled Children's Services Program is to improve services for identifying children

who are crippled or who are suffering from conditions leading to crippling; and for delivering medical, surgical, corrective, and other services and care to these children; and for facilities for diagnosis, hospitalization, and aftercare.

**crisis of a fever**
The sudden reduction or passing of a fever.

**criteria**
1. Measures used to assess the performance characteristics of proposed or existing health system services. Criteria may include the measures used as health system indicators as well as additional measures related to the performance of specific services across all providers, or the performance of specific services offered by a particular provider. 2. Pre-determined elements of health care against which the necessity, appropriateness or quality of health services may be compared. For example, criteria for appropriate diagnosis of a urinary tract infection may be performance of a urine culture and urinalysis. Often used synonymously with guidelines. 3. For PSRO programs purposes, it is predetermined elements of health care, developed by health professionals relying on professional expertise, prior experience, and the professional literature, with which aspects of the quality, medical necessity, and appropriateness of health care services may be compared.

**criterion-referenced**
A clear description of a set of skills determined to be essential to performance of a role which can be used in a test situation to determine an individual's status with respect to those skills.

**critical care services**
Critical care includes the care of critically ill patients in a variety of medical emergencies that requires the constant attention of the physician at the bedside (cardiac arrest, shock, bleeding, respiratory failure, post-operative complications, critically ill neonate). Critical care is usually, but not always, given in a critical care area, such as the coronary care unit, intensive care unit, respiratory care unit, or the emergency care facility.

**CRNA**
Certified Registered Nurse Anesthetist. See these words.

**crock**
Deprecating housestaff term for a patient whose illness the housestaff (but not the patient) feels is unreal, nonphysical or insignificant. Use of the term should be discouraged since it often blinds the user to real patient needs, whether or not correctly perceived by the patient.

**cross-claim**
Similar to a counterclaim, wherein one defendant makes a complaint against another defendant in the same lawsuit, usually seeking indemnification for any damages owed to the plaintiff.

**cross-examination**
1. The process of questioning a witness. 2. The process of cross-examining, or being cross-examined. The close questioning of a witness called by the opposing party in a trial.

**cross-examine**
To question a witness already questioned by the other party during a trial or hearing. The questioning of a witness by a party other than the one who called the witness to the stand.

**cross-infection**
The contracting of a second communicable disease while already in the hospital for another primary condition or disease.

**cross tolerance**
When a person addicted to a drug can put off withdrawal by taking another, similar drug from the same drug group, i.e., one narcotic (heroin) can cause the same or similar effects of another narcotic (morphine).

**crude birth rate**
The number of live births in a specific period of time, usually a calendar year, per 1,000, 10,000, or 100,000 population.

**cryo-**
Prefix meaning cold.

**C.S.C.**
Civil Service Commission; regulates Federal employment.

**CT scanner**
"CT" stands for computed tomography, an x-ray technique which allows doctors to study cross-sectional views of the head and body through the use of an x-ray scanning device linked to a computer. This machine, called the CT scanner, makes it possible to directly visualize body tissue for the first time.

**cui bono**
For whose best interest, for whose good; for what good, for what useful purpose or benefit.

**culpable**
1. Deserving blame. 2. One who is guilty. 3. One who is at fault; one who has done a wrongful act.

**cultural shock**
The upset or disbelief which can occur when an individual moves from one social setting or culture to another.

**culture**
1. The cultivation of microorganisms, cells or tissues in a special growth medium. 2. The belief and value system of a group or of a society; acquired and transmitted standards in regard to judgments, rituals, and conduct.

**cum (Lat.)**
With.

**cum onere (Lat.)**
Taken on with burdens. With burden.

**cum testamento annexo (Lat.)**
With the will attached. A court appointed administrator who supervises the property of a person who died without having appointed someone to legally take care of his or her property.

**cumulative evidence**
Evidence that is used to prove what has already been proven.

**cunnilingus**
The oral stimulation of the female genitals by a partner.

**curador (Spanish)**
Healer, physician, curer, surgeon. See curandero.

**curandero (m.), curandera (f.) (Spanish)**
1. Curer. 2. Quack. 3. Medical charlatan. 4. A folk healer of the Mexican-American culture viewed as a lay healer practicing by virtue of a gift from God. A person awarded such a gift is given the title "Don." Such a divine gift is received through revelations and repeated dreams in which a personage who is known to have the power to intercede with the supernatural appears. Not all persons are allowed or honored with this calling. Dreams are necessary but are not sufficient criteria for divine election to the title or position of the curer. Curanderos have varied backgrounds, ranging from illiterate persons to physician's sons. Don Pedrite de Amarillo is the most famous and respected of all curanderos and is viewed as a saint by some. See bruja, curado.

**cure**
1. When a seller delivers goods, or products the buyer believes are unfit so he rejects them and the seller then delivers the proper goods in an acceptable form or state. 2. To heal through a system of medical treatment.

**curet**
A spoon-shaped medical instrument used for removing tissue or material from a body cavity.

**curettage**
Using a curet to remove tissue or material from the wall of a cavity such as the uterus.

**current assets**
The actual cash and assets that can be easily converted to cash in the normal course of the operations or within one year.

**current liabilities**
The debts and costs that will come due and require payment from current assets within the coming year.

**Current Procedural Terminology (CPT)**
A system of terminology and coding developed by the American Medical Association that is used for describing, coding and reporting medical services and procedures.

**current ratio**
The current assets divided by current liabilities. This is used to measure the current liquidity of a business, organization or facility.

**current services budget**
In the Federal budget a budget that projects estimated budget authority and outlays for the upcoming fiscal year on the continuance of existing programs without policy changes at the same levels of service as the fiscal year in progress. The Congressional Budget and Impoundment Control Act of 1974 requires that the President submit a current services budget to the Congress by November 10 of each year. To the extent mandated by existing law, estimates take into account anticipated changes in economic conditions (such as unemployment or inflation), different caseloads, pay increases, and benefit changes.

**custodial care**
Board, room, and other personal assistance services generally provided on a long-term basis, which do not include a medical component. Such services are generally not paid for under private or public health insurance or medical care programs, except as incidental to medical care which a hospital or nursing home inpatient receives. See also boarding homes.

**custodia legis (Lat.)**
1. In the custody of the law. 2. Property taken by legal process.

**custody**
1. Safekeeping, protection. 2. Care and keeping; parents have legal *custody* of their children. 3. To take into confinement and restraint as a suspect is taken into custody.

**custom**
1. Well established longterm practices. 2. Usual behavior and traditions of persons in an area, or in a particular business that take on legal meaning so that they influence a court's decision. 3. Related to common law or unwritten law used as it is a long established standard practice whereas common consent is backed by the force of the law.

**customary charges**
See charges, customary.

**CVP**
Central venous pressure.

**cyanosis**
A bluish color in the skin and mucous membranes due to lack of oxygen in the blood.

**cyclothymic personality**
A personality disorder characterized by regularly alternating periods of elation and depression, often not related to any experience or external circumstances.

**cystoscope**
A lighted optical instrument used to visually examine the interior of the urinary bladder.

**cystoscopy**
The act of examining the urinay bladder with a lighted optical instrument.

**cyto-**
Prefix meaning cell.

**cytotechnologist**
The primary responsibility of the cytotechnologist is to detect the presence of cellular disease through microscopic examination of cell samples. Upon examination of cell specimens, these professionals screen the nature and extent of disease (usually malignancies) and resultant cellular damage. To confirm their findings, they incorporate a variety of laboratory procedures including special staining techniques, enzymatic techniques, and electron microscopy. They must also familiarize themselves with physiological conditions in order to detect abnormal hormonal conditions. Cytotechnologists may also be involved in the supervision, administration, and teaching of other laboratory personnel in a cytology laboratory or department. They work closely with and report information to a pathologist. Most cytotechnologists work in hospitals or private laboratories. Some, however, may teach and/or conduct research in large medical centers.

# D

**damage, faisant**
Doing damage.

**damages**
1. Monetary awards granted by a court or hearing to a party or a person who has suffered harm, injury or loss. 2. A plaintiff's legal claim for money; recompense for a legal wrongdoing; monetary compensation or remuneration provided through the courts to a person sustaining harm, injury or loss through the unlawful or negligent acts of others. See recovery.

**damages, actual**
1. Any harm, loss or injury that can quickly and easily be shown to have occurred or been sustained for which the party or person who was injured can recover damages or be compensated as a matter of equity or rightness. 2. Compensation amounting to the actual loss, harm or damage sustained, incurred or suffered. Also called compensatory damages. See these words.

**damages, exemplary**
Punitive damages; damages paid to the plaintiff in excess of actual losses in a tort action to serve as punishment.

**damages, liquidated**
An established amount to be paid by the parties in a contract in the event of a default or breach by either side.

**damages, special**
Damages arising from actual out-of-pocket expenses paid by a plaintiff in a personal injury action.

**damnatus (Lat.)**
Prohibited by law.

**damnum (Lat.)**
Damage (singular).

**damnum absque injuria (Lat.)**
Damage or loss for which there is no legal remedy, thus, it cannot give rise to a civil action.

**dance therapist**
This therapist applies the principles and techniques of dance to the rehabilitation of mentally ill, mentally retarded, or physically disabled patients.

**D and C**
Dilation and curettage; surgically scraping the inside of the uterus after a miscarriage.

**dan et retiens nihil dat (Lat.)**
He who gives and retains; one who gives nothing.

**dangerous drugs**
See Harrison antinarcotic act.

**dangerous instrumentality**
Tools, devices, instruments, items or objects that are harmful in and of themselves, or can be harmful by nature of the design, such as surgical instruments, knives, guns, etc.

**dangerous per se**
An item dangerous in itself, which may cause harm without human cause, such as gasoline, bottled oxygen, or drugs.

**dangerous to life or health**
Any condition that poses an immediate threat to life or health, such as severe exposure to contaminants such as radioactive materials which have an adverse delayed effect on one's health.

**D.A.P.**
Draw-a-person. A psychological test using projective techniques.

**Darling case**
A landmark case—Darling v. Charleston Community Hospital (211 N.E. 2nd 53, Ill., 1965), a case where a trial court first allowed the Illinois Department of Public Health rules and regulations, the Charleston Community Hospital's bylaws, rules and regulations, and the Joint Commission on Accreditation's Standards for Hospital Accreditation to be admitted as documentary evidence in a court of law. This allowed the jury to utilize and review these documents as evidence in determining the standard of care the hospital and staff were to meet in caring for patients. The court decision found that the hospital failed to have an adequate number of professional nurses who were trained in recognizing the symptom of a progressive gangrenous condition of a patient's fractured leg in a cast. It was further found that the physician in charge failed to get an orthopedic consultation which was required by the medical staff bylaws.

**data bank**
A collection of data which is organized for rapid search and retrieval by computer.

**data base**
All basic information and known facts concerning a patient.

**data phone**
In computers, a system which transmits computer language over telephone circuits. The transmitting end receives data from punched cards, punched tape or magnetic tape, then converts these data into a transmission tone. The receiving end converts the tone into electrical

pulses that enter a computer or into a variety of other research, record, or business machines.

**data processing**
The recording, classifying, summarizing, computing, transmitting, and storing of information. Any hand or machine operation or combination of operations on data.

**data set**
A set of standardized and uniformly defined and classified statistics that describe an element, episode or aspect of health care, e.g., a hospital admission (see discharge abstract), ambulatory encounter, or a physician or hospital. Such data sets are used for evaluation, research and similar purposes.

**day care**
1. Care or treatment given in a health care facility, usually for surgical procedures done in the day and the patient leaving and returning home in the same day; synonymous with ambulatory surgery. 2. Adult day care is when an elderly person who spends nights and weekends with family or guardians is placed in a center for care during the work hours of the family. 3. Care and babysitting services for working parents.

**day care center/day health services**
Special services and treatment which address the health care needs of people in an ambulatory way rather than becoming a resident in a health care facility. See home health care.

**day certain**
A specific date or specified time in the near future.

**day hospital**
A situation where a hospital creates a setup whereby a patient spends the daytime in the hospital and returns home at night.

**day in court**
The right to be heard in court; the day your case comes up in court.

**de (Lat.)**
Of, by, concerning, from. The first word often used in old English statutes or writs.

**D.E.A.**
Drug Enforcement Administration.

**death**
1. Permanent cessation of all vital functions; the end of life (often called mortality). A simple concept whose actual occurrence medicine has made very difficult to define and measure. A consensus appears to be forming that death occurs when all measurable or identifiable brain functioning (electrical or any other kind) is absent for over 24 hours. 2. *Civil* death causes the loss of civil rights in some states; when a person is sentenced to life in prison. 3. *Presumptive* death or legal death results when an unexplained absence of life occurs for a length of time set by state law. See also hospice and euthanasia.

**death instinct**
See aggressive drive.

**death rate index**
To derive the adjusted death rate index, the following data are required:
O = occupancy rate for the hospital
O = mean occupancy rate for all hospitals in the sample
ALOS = average length of stay for the hospital
DR = death rate in the hospital
The death rate figure is determined as follows:

$$DR = \frac{\text{number of deaths excluding newborn deaths}}{\text{number of admissions excluding maternity admissions}}$$

**death rates**
Crude death rates are the number of deaths reported in a period of time, usually a year per 1,000, 10,000 or 100,000, population.

**debase**
To lower one's character, rank, or estimation.

**de bene esse (Lat.)**
Conditionally. Referring to the appearance of a witness; the presentation of evidence. Depositions or evidence may be accepted de bene esse.

**debenture**
A certificate acknowledging a debt. An unsecured bond; a corporate bond that contains a promise to pay its debt to the bondholder, although it is not supported by security.

**debit**
1. A sum of money owed and due; an amount owed as a debt. 2. Opposite of credits. 3. A bookkeeping term referring to the left page of a ledger.

**de bonis non (Lat.)**
Of the goods not taken care of. When an administrator has been selected to handle the property of a dead person whose executor is no longer available or has died.

**debt**
Goods, money or services owed by one person to another.

**debtee**
One to whom a debt is owed; a creditor.

**debtor**
One owing a debt; the party who owes money or goods to another.

**debt ratio**
The ratio of comparing long-term debts to a capital structure or comparing total debt to total assets. The debt ratio shows relative risk.

**debt service**

**debt service**
The payment of matured interest on and principal of debts;
The cost of ending uncollectable, old debts, including principal the amount needed, supplied, or accrued for meeting such payments and interest on such debt. The cost of ending a debt. during any given accounting period; a budget or operating statement heading for such items.

**decapitation**
The head being cut off; beheading.

**decedent**
1. A deceased person; one who has recently died. 2. One whose family or kin has died.

**deceit**
Any untrue, deceiving or false statement purposely made with the intention of fooling or misleading another party or person, which then causes harm.

**decision**
The formal results of the deciding of the dispute. A judge's resolution to a lawsuit.

**decisional law**
Those laws determined by courts; decisions which rule from case results rather than from statutes. See case law, common law.

**decision on the merits**
A decision reached and fully decided on an issue of a case so that no new or different lawsuits may be filed on the same issue by the same plaintiff.

**decision symbol**
In computerized business or medical records it is a symbol denoting the need for verifying the existence or non-existence of conditions or future actions.

**declaration**
1. An unsworn statement. 2. A formal statement. 3. A public proclamation.

**declaratory judgment**
A court decision outlining the rights and duties of parties in a dispute, but without coercing any performance or payment of damages.

**decree**
A judgment or order issued by a court or judge.

**decree nisi**
A provisional decree set by the court which can become final at a specified later time unless it is shown why it should not become final.

**decubitus ulcer**

A bedsore; a pressure sore produced by prolonged pressure or lying in one position. A serious problem for bedridden long-term care patients.

**deductible**

1. That which may be eliminated or subtracted, such as subtracting items from income for tax purposes. 2. In health insurance, it is the percentage of the total amount the insured person must pay as part of the care or before policy benefits begin. 3. Amount of loss or expense that must be incurred by an insured or otherwise covered individual before an insurer will assume any liability for all or part of the remaining cost of covered services. Deductibles may be either fixed dollar amounts or the value of specified services (such as two days of hospital care or one physician visit). Deductibles are usually tied to some reference period over which they must be incurred, e.g. $100 per calendar year, benefit period, or spell of illness. Deductibles in existing policies are generally of two types: (1) static deductibles which are fixed dollar amounts and (2) dynamic deductibles which are adjusted from time to time to reflect increasing medical prices. A third type of deductible is proposed in some national health insurance plans: a sliding scale deductible, in which the deductible is related to income and increases as income increases.

**deductible amount (Medicare)**

That amount of health care charges for which the Medicare recipient is responsible. For hospital charges, an amount roughly equal to the cost of the first day's care. For physician or other Part B charges, an amount set annually by the government.

**deductible liability insurance**

Coverage under which the insured agrees to pay up to a specified sum per claim toward the amount payable to the physician.

**deduction**

1. Reasoning from a known fact to an unknown; from general to specific. 2. Deducting; subtraction, such as items subtracted from income tax. 3. An abatement, as an amount deducted from a bill or charge.

**deed**

A written paper defining an interest in real estate and/or its transfer to another party. 1

**de facto (Lat.)**

Actual, in fact. A situation that actually or factually exists, whether or not it is within the scope of law.

**defalcation**

Defaulting. A failure to account for funds; not necessarily due to fraud or dishonesty, however, a suspicion usually exists that the money was wrongfully used.

**defamation**

1. The speaking of slanderous words. 2. The writing of degrading, harmful or slanderous statements; malicious false statements made against another. 3. Injuring a person's character; injury to one's reputation by

false and malicious utterances. This includes both libel and slander. See libel, slander.

**default**
1. An omission or a failure to perform a duty that one is legally bound to perform. 2. Failure to take the required steps or follow the correct procedures in a court action. 3. Failure to perform or take care of a legal obligation; failure to follow court processes in a lawsuit.

**default judgment**
1. A decision handed down from a judge or court against either party of a legal action for failure to follow due process, failure to answer claims, present a defense or appear in court. A judgment against the defendant due to his or her failure to appear in court, reply to legal documents or answer a plaintiff's complaint.

**defeasible**
That which can be divested or revoked if some contingency occurs; being defeated, ended, or undone by future action.

**defeasible fee**
A fee that may be no longer required due to the happening of some contingency. Defeated if certain conditions are not met.

**defeat**
To prevent, terminate or undo.

**defect**
1. An imperfection; a flaw. 2. The lack of something required by law. 3. Less than adequate or acceptable. 4. Lacking the legal principles which then makes an action insufficient, inadequate and not binding.

**defendant**
In a court action, the person defending; the one against whom an action is brought in a civil or criminal case; the person against whom recovery in damages is sought; the person being sued.

**defendant in error**
The party who won a judgment so that the losing party seeks to have it reversed in an appellate court by a writ of error. See appellee.

**defense**
The facts, laws and arguments presented by the defendant or the party against whom legal action is being heard.

**defense mechanisms**
Learned behaviors, attitudes or beliefs that are used by an individual to adjust to the environment, stress or challenging situations. Unconscious or conscious processes used to cope with or provide relief from emotional conflict and anxiety. Some common defense mechanisms are compensation, conversion, denial, displacement, dissociation, idealization, identification, incorporation, introjection, projection, rationalization, reaction formation, regression, sublimation, substitution, symbolization. See mental mechanisms.

**defensive medicine**
Using all tests and methods of diagnosis in medical practice, to reduce the threat of liability, for the principal purpose of deterring the possibility of malpractice suits by patients and providing a good legal defense in the event of such lawsuits.

**deference**
As used in assertiveness training, this is acting in a subservient way as though you are less important than others who are older, powerful, more experienced or knowledgeable.

**deferral of budget authority**
In the federal budget, any action or inaction of the executive branch, including the establishment of reserves under the Antideficiency Act, which temporarily withholds, delays, or effectively precludes the obligation or expenditure of budget authority. Under section 1013 of the Congressional Budget and Impoundment Control Act of 1974, the President is required to report each proposed deferral to the Congress in a special message. Deferrals may not extend beyond the end of a fiscal year and may be overturned by the passage of an impoundment resolution by either House of Congress. See also rescission.

**deferred payments**
Installment payments.

**deficiency disease**
Any specific disease or pathological state, with characteristic clinical signs, that is due to an insufficient intake of energy or essential nutrients; it is usually of dietary origin and can often be prevented or cured by bringing the intake up to an adequate level or otherwise changing the diet.

**deficiency judgment**
1. An action of foreclosure on a debt. 2. A decision by a court to cause a person to pay the difference between the amount gained by the judgment creditor by selling property and the amount of the judgment.

**deficit**
1. A shortage. 2. When a sum of money is not as much as expected or anticipated. 3. Something missing, due or lacking, something being less than it should be.

**definitive**
1. A final, conclusive and complete settlement of a legal question. 2. Absolute; complete; final.

**definitive care**
1. Medical or dental care provided by a physician or a dentist, generally in a medical or dental environment. 2. Diagnosis and treatment.

**deforce**
To wrongfully withhold property from the rightful possessor.

**defraud**
To cheat; deceive; deprive by deception.

**degree**
1. The seriousness of an act or crime. 2. A step, level or division. 3. A rank or diploma of recognition for educational attainment.

**dehors (French)**
1. Irrelevant to; foreign to; beyond; outside of. 2. Not contained within the record.

**Dei gratia (Lat.)**
By the grace of God.

**de jure (Lat.)**
1. Rightful; legitimate; lawful; by law. 2. Often contrasted with *de facto.* 3. Whether or not true in actual fact. An administrator may be the *de jure* head of a hospital even if the governing board takes actual power.

**del credere (Italian)**
One who works as an agent and who sells goods for another with the buyer paying for the goods.

**delectus personae (Lat.)**
The choice a person has; the legal right given to an original partner of a company, business, etc. to approve or disapprove or otherwise select other partners.

**delegate**
1. One who is authorized to act for another; a person chosen to represent another person or a group. 2. To select a person to represent you or to give responsibility to. 3. To entrust authority or responsibility to another to act as one's agent.

**delegated hospital**
For PSRO programs purposes, a hospital to which a PSRO has assigned the review functions of concurrent review and medical care evaluation studies. The PSRO monitors the hospital review committee to assure compliance with program requirements. Also known as a fully delegated hospital. See undelegated hospital.

**delegation**
1. The act of giving authority to another person. An administrator delegates responsibility to employees. 2. To commission authority, power and responsibility to another. 3. A group of delegates. 4. In the PSRO program, the formal process by which a PSRO, based upon an assessment of the willingness and capability of a hospital or other health program to effectively perform PSRO review functions, assigns the performance of some (partial delegation) or all (full delegation) PSRO review functions to the program. Delegation must be agreed upon in a written memorandum of understanding signed by both the PSRO and the program. The PSRO monitors the program's performance of the delegated functions without itself conducting them, and retains responsibility for the effectiveness of the review.

**delegatory law**
A law that states that physician extenders, such as physician assistants, are allowed to practice whatever procedure, therapy, or treatment that the supervising physician may see fit to delegate to the physician extender.

**deleterious**
Harmful; injurious.

**deliberate**
1. To carefully discuss and work through; to consider and discuss; carefully considered, planned and thought out. 2. Premeditated; intentional; an act done on purpose.

**delictum (Lat.)**
A wrongful or criminal act; a crime, tort, or wrongdoing. (singular)

**delinquency**
1. Failure; neglect; act of omission. 2. A violation of one's duty; misconduct. 3. Overdue monetary debts. 4. Failure in doing what the law dictates.

**delinquent**
1. Overdue; unpaid. 2. Neglecting to do what the law or duty requires. A juvenile delinquent is a minor who has broken the law or who has been seriously involved in illegal acts.

**delirious**
Mental confusion; restlessness; incoherence.

**delirium**
A mental disturbance characterized by restlessness, confusion, disorientation, bewilderment, agitation, and affective lability. It is associated with fear, hallucinations, and illusions.

**delirium tremens**
An acute psychotic mental state as a reaction to withdrawal from alcohol after a prolonged and severe period of drinking.

**delivery**
1. To hand over. 2. To legally transfer property or goods; transferring an item from one person to another.

**Delta Dental Plan**
An organizational name used to identify the first multistate dental service program coordinated by the National Association of Dental Service plans for the Northwest International Association of Machinists' Benefit Trust of Seattle; a professionally sponsored dental prepayment program.

**delusion**
An idea which has an irrational explanation, which is maintained by a person despite logical argument and objective reasoning and contradictory evidence or facts; clinging to an idea or belief that is not real.

**demand**
1. To seek what is due or claimed. 2. A valid claim that assumes that there is no doubt as to whom the claim belongs. 3. The claiming of a legal right as determined by the courts.

**demand for care**
The amount of health care service sought or needed by consumers in response to their perceived need for that service.

**demand note**
A note expressly stating that something is payable on demand.

**demand schedule**
In health economics, the varying amount of goods or services sought at varying prices, given constant income and other factors. Demand must be distinguished from utilization (the amount of services actually used), and need (for various reasons services are often sought which either the consumer or provider feels are unneeded). It is not always translated into use, particularly when queues develop. See also supply and elasticity of demand.

**demeanor**
Outward appearance and behavior; one's manner, conduct or air. It is not what a witness utters, but how he utters it; one's nonverbal actions and communication.

**demencia (Spanish)**
The loss of one's mind; insanity; dementia.

**dementia**
Organic loss of mental functioning.

**dementia praecox**
An old term used to describe what is now known as schizophrenia.

**de minimus (Lat.)**
Small, unimportant.

**de minimus non curat lex (Lat.)**
The law does not concern itself with trivial matters.

**de minis (Lat.)**
A writ of threats; where a person was threatened with bodily harm or destruction of property; to compel the offender to desist.

**demise**
1. Death. 2. Any lease. 3. A transfer or conveyance of property.

**demographic characteristics**
A concise narrative and description of the characteristics of the total population of a state, region, county, city etc.

**demography**
A sociological statistical analysis and study of a region, population or group.

**demonstrative evidence**
Evidence other than testimony; evidence physically shown or presented in court.

**demur**
1. To make a demurrer. 2. To object formally to a pleading. 3. To enter a demurrer. 4. To delay or postpone.

**demurrant**
One who demurs.

**demurrer**
1. A pleading for the dismissal of a lawsuit; a motion to dismiss a complaint due to failure to state a claim. 2. A legal pleading; the facts presented by one side of a case are not enough for a legal argument to stand up in court, thus it should be dismissed.

**denial**
1. A contradiction of statements made by the opposing party. 2. A plea against the facts claimed by the other side of a suit. 3. Refusal; rejection. 4. Deprivation or withholding. 5. In psychology or psychiatry, it is a conscious or unconscious defense or mental mechanism in which an aspect of external reality is rejected or when experiences, behaviors or actions are denied.

**de novo (Lat.)**
Once again. A writ *venire de novo* serves to summon a jury for a second trial on a case set up for a new trial. New from the start; for example, a *trial de novo* is a new trial ordered by a judge or by a court.

**dentacare**
A dental plan for groups under which a fixed monthly payment is made to a group of dentists who guarantee care for enrolled subscribers. Only offered as alternative to fee-for-service plan.

**dental appliance**
Any variety of devices or structures used to move irregularly placed teeth into proper position; orthodontic devices.

**dental assistant**
An individual who assists a dentist at the chairside in a dental operatory, performs reception and clerical functions, and carries out dental radiography and selected dental laboratory work. The actual number of active dental assistants is not known since most dentists train and employ dental assistants who are neither certified nor registered as members of an official organization. Dental assistants who have completed accredited educational programs are eligible for national certification examinations conducted by the Certifying Board of the American Dental Assistants Association. An accredited dental assistant program is usually conducted in a community college or vocational-technical school and must provide at least one year of academic training.

**dental auxiliary**
Any of a number of assistants to a dental surgeon.

**dental chart**
A diagram-type chart of the teeth on which clinical findings and results of examinations are recorded. See medical record.

**dental engine**
The motor and associated equipment such as continuous-cord belts over pulleys activated by a hand or foot switch that controls the drill.

**dental extender**
A dental hygienist or dental assistant who performs "expanded functions."

**dental geriatrics**
The branch of dentistry that treats dental related disorders and diseases peculiar to advanced age or the aged.

**dental health**
A state of complete normality and functional efficiency of the teeth and supporting structures, the surrounding parts of the oral cavity, and the various structures related to mastication and the maxillo-facial complex.

**dental health services**
All services designed or intended to promote, maintain or restore dental health including educational, preventive, and therapeutic services.

**dental hygienists**
Dental hygienists are oral health clinicians and educators who perform preventive and therapeutic services under the supervision of a dentist. Specific responsibilities vary, depending on state laws, but may include removing deposits and stains from patients' teeth, providing instructions for patient self-care, dietetic counseling, and applying decay preventing fluoride treatments. Hygienists take medical and dental histories, expose and process dental radiographs, make impressions of teeth for study casts, and prepare other diagnostic aids for use by the dentist. In some states, they are permitted to administer local infiltration anesthesia; place and remove dams, matrices, and sutures; and place, carve, and polish restorations in teeth after the dentist prepares the cavity. These latter functions, along with a limited number of others, are called expanded functions and require extended nontraditional training of the hygienist. Dental hygienists are licensed in all states. In addition, a few states have credentialing requirements for those dental hygienists who perform expanded functions. Graduation from an accredited program (except in Alabama) and licensing are required. The Commission on Accreditation for Dental and Dental Auxiliary Educational Programs established basic curriculum requirements and guidelines and accredits all approved dental hygiene programs. Individual states set requirements for licensing, but in all states these requirements include passing a written and clinical examination.

**dental insurance**
A form of insurance that provides protection against the costs of diagnostic and preventive dental care as well as oral surgery, restorative procedures, and therapeutic care.

**dental jurisprudence**
Also referred to as forensic dentistry. The area of law that encompasses dental knowledge and practice into applicable or related aspects of law. Statutes and codes that control and limit the professional practice of dentistry.

**dental laboratory technician**
See dental technician.

**dental laboratory technologist/technician**
Prepared to construct complete and partial dentures, make orthodontic appliances, fix bridgework, crowns, and other dental restorations and appliances, as authorized by dentists.

**dental service**
This is not a common hospital department, but is common to group health plans. Dental care is provided for ambulatory patients and sometimes for inpatients. The dental staff is organized as part of the hospital's medical staff.

**dental services (oral hygiene)**
According to JCAH long term care accreditation, services provided by a dentist. These services include, but are not necessarily limited to, annual oral examinations, routine and emergency dental care, and instruction to nursing personnel in routine oral hygiene.

**dental technician**
An individual who makes complete and partial dentures, orthodontic appliances, bridgework, crowns, and other dental restorations and appliances, as prescribed by dentists. Most dental technicians work in commercial dental laboratories. However, increasing numbers are employed by private dental practitioners and by federal, state and private institutions. Traditionally, dental technicians have been trained on the job, but the predominant method of training now is through formal programs offered by two-year post-secondary educational institutions. Upon completion of an aggregate of five years in dental technology training and experience, technicians are eligible to apply for examination and certification by the National Board for Certification in Dental Laboratory Technology. See also denturist.

**dental unit**
Equipment utilized in providing dental care, such as a dental engine, operatory light, worktable, water, compressed air, cuspidor, drills, etc.

**Denti-Cal**
A dental health plan in California sponsored by both the federal and state governments for people who are eligible for public assistance and low-income people.

**dentist**
1. A professional person qualified by education and authorized by law (usually by having obtained a license) to practice dentistry; the promotion, maintenance and restoration of individual dental health, and treatment of diseases of the teeth and oral cavity. 2. According to

JCAH, an individual who has received a Doctor of Dental Surgery or Doctor of Dental Medicine degree and is currently fully licensed to practice dentistry.

**denturist**
A dental technician who provides dentures for patients without benefit of a dentist's professional services. Denturists are rarely found in the United States and their practice is illegal in many states. They are increasingly common in Canada, particularly in Ontario where the provincial government has proposed legalizing their practice. See dental technician.

**deontology**
The study of acceptable behavior, duty and ethics, i.e. patient and doctor relations, disclosure to patients, etc.

**department**
A functional or administrative division of a hospital, health program or government agency. Sometimes also known as a program, division or service. A department within a hospital or medical school is typically headed by a responsible individual, either a chairman or director, has its own budget and admits its own patients, but is not a separate legal entity. They are frequently organized by medical specialty, i.e., a pediatric, radiology, or surgery department. There is no standard departmental organization for health programs. For JCAH accreditation purposes, this is an organizational unit of the hospital or the medical staff; a staff entity organized on administraive, functional or disciplinary lines.

**departmentation**
The structural framework of an organization, as compared to delegation, which is the assignment of authority. Four types of departmentation have been identified by management theorists: 1) functional departmentation—the grouping of activities according to a hospital's major tasks, i.e., nursing, pharmacy, central supply, etc. 2) departmentation according to process is the grouping of activities around equipment and machinery, such as radiology. 3) territorial departmentation is the grouping of activities on the basis of geography. 4) Product departmentation is the grouping of activities on the basis of output. It has the advantage of improved coordination. Organizational responsibility for end results can be readily identified and assigned. Its major disadvantage is the possible loss of central control.

**Department of Health and Human Services (HHS)**
The new name for the old Department of Health, Education and Welfare. In the federal government, this is a cabinet level department that is responsible for all national level concerns related to personal and community health, including but not limited to services, research, program development, regulations, etc. related to the nation's health and services to all the people of the United States and its territories.

**depecage (French)**
In conflict of laws, when a case presents more than one issue, laws of different jurisdictions are used to determine the dispute or conflicts.

**dependence**
See drug dependence.

**dependency**
The excessive reliance on another for psychological support. It reflects an unhealthy need for security, love, protection and mothering.

**dependency needs**
Vital needs of love, affection, belonging, shelter, protection, security, food and warmth. May be a manifestation of a form of regression when these needs appear openly in adults.

**dependent**
An individual who relies upon another individual for a significant portion of his support. In addition to the requirement for financial support there is often a requirement for a blood relationship. The Internal Revenue Code defines as dependents for the purposes of tax deductions any of the following over half of whose support for the calendar year was received from the taxpayer: children (biologic or adopted), grandchildren, etc.; stepchildren; brothers and sisters; stepbrothers and stepsisters; half brothers and half sisters; parents, grandparents, greatgrandparents, etc.; stepparents; nephews and nieces; uncles and aunts; inlaws (father, mother, son, daughter, brother or sister); nonrelatives living as members of the taxpayer's household; and a descendant of a brother or sister of the father or mother of the taxpayer who is receiving institutional care and who, before receiving such care, was a member of the taxpayer's household. The IRS Code provides that if the support of a dependent was furnished by several persons, one may claim the dependency deduction, if the others agree. In insurance and other programs the specific definition is quite variable, often being limited to the individual's spouse and children. Other dependents of the kinds recognized by the IRS are sometimes known as sponsored dependents.

**dependent child**
In health insurance, a natural or adopted child of the subscriber under 23 years of age, unmarried, and for whom the subscriber is allowed a tax exemption. This includes a physically handicapped or a mentally retarded child regardless of age provided the handicap existed before age 23, subject to verification.

**dependent contract**
A conditional contract where one party does not have to perform on the contract until the other party does something that it is required to do in regards to the contract.

**dependent nursing functions**
Activities carried out by a nurse as a result of following a physician's order.

**dependents**
Generally the spouse and children of an individual. Under some circumstances, parents or other members of the family may also be

dependents, such as an elderly person may depend on his or her family for finances, food, housing, clothing and medical care.

**deplete**
To reduce; lessen; exhaust; use up.

**deponent**
1. One who testifies under oath; one who deposes. 2. One who gives sworn testimony out of court as in a deposition.

**depose**
1. To testify under oath. 2. To unseat a person from public office. 3. To give sworn testimony out of court as in a deposition.

**deposition**
1. Written sworn testimony, made before a public officer for a court action, often it is answers to questions posed by a lawyer. Depositions are used for the discovery of information or evidence for a trial. 2. The process of taking sworn testimony out of court.

**depreciation**
The allocation of capital costs to the period in which the resources purchased for those capital costs will be used. Although depreciation can be computed using many approaches, the most common approach is straight line depreciation, or the even distribution of capital costs throughout the life of the asset. See capital depreciation.

**depression**
In psychiatry, a mentally unhealthy state characterized by sadness and loneliness; by low self-esteem associated with self-condemnation, by psychomotor retardation, occasional agitation; by withdrawal from interpersonal relations and occasional desires to die. Insomnia and anorexia are also often noted.

**derivative**
From another; owing its existence to something previous; being derived from. Originating from another or common source.

**derivative action**
A suit brought by a shareholder or stockholder on behalf of a corporation against a third party.

**derivative evidence**
Evidence, based on or derived from evidence that is illegally gathered, thus is not allowed in a trial.

**dermatology technician**
The dermatology technician prepares and administers materials which have been prescribed by a physician, usually a dermatologist, to cure or alleviate symptoms of skin problems.

**derogate**
To impair; to partially repeal; to reduce.

**derogation**
The lessening or weakening of an old law by a new law, thus limiting the effectiveness of the old law.

**desertion**
1. Abandoning with no intention of either returning or of reassuming one's responsibility. 2. The act of leaving or running away from.

**de son tort (Lat.)**
Of his own wrong. To take on a responsibility one has no right to assume, in which harm is done as a result of those actions.

**destroy**
The ending of contracts, or other legal commitments or documents, but it does not always mean actual destruction; to render a document's legal effect useless. The destruction of the legal effectiveness of a document by obliterating it or by cancelling it by tearing it up (valid only with wills) or by writing over it; i.e. writing "void" on it.

**desuetude**
Disuse. Laws fallen into disuse; to cease use.

**detail person**
A sales representative of a pharmaceutical manufacturer who promotes prescription drugs for use by physicians, dentists, and pharmacists. Such detailing includes personal presentations, advertising and provision of drug samples and educational materials prepared by the manufacturers to professionals in their offices. Many detail persons are now pharmacists.

**detainer**
1. Unlawful holding or keeping of another's possessions even if it was originally lawful, i.e., withholding a patient's diamond ring to insure that he or she pays a bill. 2. Detaining a person against his will. 3. A legal document issued by the court to continue to hold a person who is already being held.

**detection services**
Routine evaluation and screening of individuals without recognized symptoms for the purpose of identifying the individuals at risk who have certain diseases or conditions.

**detention**
Detaining or confining a person against his will.

**detention for questioning**
Holding a person in custody by the police for questioning without making a formal charge or arrest.

**deter**
To discourage; to stop. To discourage a person from doing something.

**determinable**
1. Liable to terminate if a predictable happening occurs. 2. To probably terminate; the potential to be ended. 3. Subject to being ended if a specific action occurs.

**determination**
The making of a final judgment or decision. This is usually done by a judge or other person designated as a decision maker, such as an arbiter.

**detinue**
1. Possessions or property unlawfully held by another person. 2. To sue for damages for the wrongful holding or detention of personal property. 3. A court ordered writ to get property back.

**detoxification**
1. To withdraw and remove the toxic effects of alcohol or a drug. Also known as detoxication. 2. According to JCAH for psychiatric, alcoholism and drug abuse facilities accreditation purposes, this is the systematic reduction of the amount of a toxic agent in the body or the elimination of a toxic agent from the body. See also cold turkey, methadone.

**detriment**
1. To cause injury, loss or harm. 2. Giving up a right, the result of which causes harm or damage.

**development**
A person's capacity and skill in functioning, related to size, age or growth.

**developmental disability (DD)**
A disability which originates before age 18, can be expected to continue indefinitely, constitutes a substantial handicap to the disabled's ability to function normally in society, and is attributable to mental retardation, cerebral palsy, epilepsy, autism, any other condition closely related to mental retardation because it results in similar impairment of general intellectual functioning or adaptive behavior or requires similar treatment and services, or dyslexia resulting from one of the conditions just listed.

**developmental tasks**
Skills and behavior patterns learned during development which a person should be able to do by certain age levels.

**development and review of patient care policies (Medicare)**
The facility should have policies which are developed with the advice of (and with provision for review of such policies from time to time, but at least annually, by) a group of professional personnel including one or more physicians and one or more registered nurses, to govern the skilled nursing care and related medical or other services it provides. See utilization review.

**devest**
To be lost or taken away. See divest.

**deviant**
1. Differing from what is considered normal or average. 2. Unusual or abnormal behavior; to do behaviors or acts that society disapproves of.

**deviation, statistical**
See average deviation, standard deviation.

**device**

An item or piece of equipment used in the healing arts that is not a drug. Device is defined in the Federal Food, Drug, and Cosmetic Act as including instruments, apparatus and contrivances, including their components, parts and accessories, intended for use in the diagnosis, cure, mitigation, treatment or prevention of disease in man or other animals; or to affect the structure or any function of the body of man or other animals. Among the products that are regulated as devices are crutches, bandages, wheelchairs, artificial heart valves, cardiac pacemakers, intrauterine devices, eye glasses, hearing aids and prostheses. The regulation of the marketing of devices is to assure that devices are safe and effective when properly used. See also pre-market approval.

**devise**

That which can be given by a will; to transfer property by will.

**devolution**

The transfer of a right or property by legal processes from one person to another.

**devolve**

1. To roll or fall upon. 2. To pass from one person to another.

**D.H.E.W.**

Department of Health, Education and Welfare, the old name of the Department of Health and Human Services. Education has been made a separate department. See Department of Health and Human Services.

**D.H.H.S.**

Department of Health and Human Services. The federal cabinet level department concerned with all aspects of health, health care and related activities as well as human services such as aging programs, welfare programs, etc.

**dia-**

Prefix meaning complete; through.

**diabetes**

A metabolic disorder characterized by excessive thirst and production of large volumes of urine. Often used to refer to diabetes mellitus.

**diabetes insipidus**

A metabolic disorder characterized by producing large amounts of dilute urine and a constant thirst due to a deficiency of vasopressin, a pituitary hormone, which regulates the levels of water allowed to remain in the blood or be passed off as urine.

**diabetes mellitus**

A metabolic disorder in which carbohydrates and sugars are not oxidized by the body to produce energy due to a deficiency of the hormone insulin.

**diagnosis**

The art and science of determining the nature and cause of a disease, and of differentiating among diseases.

**diagnosis and treatment services**
Services for evaluating the health status of individuals and identifying and alleviating disease and ill health or the symptoms thereof.

**diagnosis, behavioral health**
Determining a health "problem", health status and gathering information needed for program planning and evaluation or a prognosis. A health problem can be a symptom, an abnormal finding, or a threat to one's overall well-being or health status.

**diagnosis code**
The numerical classification of diseases, conditions, and injuries. The most common code used is the international classification of diseases adapted for use in the U.S. (ICD-9-CM) as compiled by the Commission on Professional Hospital Activities (CPHA). Adoption of the ICD-9-CM provides a uniform system of recording statistical data covering health services.

**diagnostic admission**
Admission to a hospital primarily for the performance of various lab and x-ray studies to establish a diagnosis.

**Diagnostic and Statistical Manual of Mental Disorders (DSM)**
A standardized handbook for the classification of mental illnesses. Formulated by the American Psychiatric Association, it was first issued in 1952 (DSM-I). The second edition (DSM-II), issued in 1968, correlates closely with the World Health Organization's *International Classification of Diseases.* It is now in its 3rd edition (DSM-III).

**diagnostic medical sonographer**
Uses acoustic energy for diagnosis, research, and therapy, operates ultrasound equipment to obtain diagnostic results, evaluates results for quality of technique, and in emergency situations, makes interim reports to medical staff.

**diagnostic radiology services**
The detection of physical diseases and other ill health conditions through the use of radiant energy.

**diagnostic related groups (DRGs)**
A diagnostic classification procedure developed by Yale University using 383 Major Diagnostic Categories (MDC), based on the ICD-8 code, which classifies patients into case types. The original purpose in the design was to improve the utilization review process. This classification procedure is now used in analyzing patient case mix, hospital reimbursement mechanisms, etc.

**diagnostic services**
According to JCAH long term care accreditation, any service (e.g., laboratory or radiological) designed to assist the practitioner in establishing a diagnosis.

**diagnostic studies**

Any test, x-ray, C.T. scan, visual exam, or procedure that is ordered by the physician to assist him or her in determining the seriousness, nature, and extent of a patient's pathological condition. Several types of tests are commonly conducted. Laboratory tests: a) Bromosulphalein test (BSP) (which is the injection of dye, intravenously, in order to study liver function); b) culture: (The growth of microorganisms under lab conditions on media using sputum, urine, wound drainage, etc.); c) Urine tests. Other diagnostic procedures include: abdominal paracentesis, angiogram, bone marrow biopsy, barium enema, bronchoscopy, cholecystogram, colonoscopy, cystoscopy, electrocardiogram (ECG), electroencephalogram, (EEG), electromyogram, gallbladder series (G.B.), gastric analysis, gastroscopy, intravenous pyelogram (IVP), laryngoscopy, myelogram, opaque cystogram, pericardial aspiration, pneumoencephalogram, proctoscopic examination, sigmoidoscopy, spinal tap or lumbar puncture, thoracentesis, upper gastrointestinal series (UGI). For definitions of these terms see a medical dictionary.

**dialysis technician**

Dialysis technicians operate and maintain renal dialysis equipment used in the treatment of patients with short- or long-term renal disorders and failures. The equipment removes toxic waste material from the blood that ordinarily would be removed by the patient's kidney. These individuals work under the direction of a physician, frequently an internal medicine specialist with a subspecialty in nephrology. They also schedule appointments for outpatient visits and maintain patient records or files.

**diastolic blood pressure**

The pressure of blood produced within the blood vessels when the ventricles of the heart relax.

**Diastolic pressure**

The lowest amount of pressure exerted by the blood being forced against the arterial wall during relaxation of ventricles of the heart.

**Dick-Read**

Based on theory of childbirth that fear is the main agent that produces pain. Women in labor have pain which increases fear which in turn increases tension. The increased tension causes more pain. The breaking of this self-destructive cycle includes slow abdominal breathing techniques and focusing on feelings and signals from your own body during labor.

**dicta (Lat.)**

Something a judge says that is not necessarily vital to the case; something said in passing. 2. Words in a written opinion not necessarily a part of the decision, but a general comment. The plural of dictum.

**dictionary**

A malevolent literary device for cramping the growth of language. (From *The Devil's Dictionary.*)

**dictum (Lat.)**

Singular of dicta. *Obiter dictum*, by the way.

**dietetic and nutritional services**
Translate nutritional needs into the selection, purchasing, preparation, and service of appropriate foods, along with maintenance of equipment, sanitation and cost control. They provide nutritional education to individuals and groups, and serve as nutritional consultants to health facilities and communities.

**dietetic assistant**
Writes food menus following dietetic specifications, coordinates food service to patients, orders supplies, maintains sanitation, and oversees the work of food service employees in health care facilities.

**dietetic educator R.D.**
Responsible for planning the curriculum of the dietetic practitioner and has responsibility for the nutrition education of medical, nursing, dental, and allied health personnel. The dietetic educator may be employed in medical centers, universities, or colleges.

**dietetics**
A profession concerned with the science and art of human nutritional care, an essential component of health science. It includes the extending and imparting of knowledge concerning foods which will provide nutrients sufficient to health and during disease throughout the life cycle and the management of group feeding.

**dietetic services**
According to JCAH for psychiatric, alcoholism and drug abuse facilities accreditation purposes, this is the provision of services to meet the nutritional needs of patients, with specific emphasis on patients who have special dietary needs, for example, patients who are allergic to certain foods or who cannot accept a regular diet.

**dietetic service supervisor (Medicare)**
1. A qualified dietitian. 2. A graduate of a dietetic technician or dietetic assistant training program, corresponding or classroom, approved by the American Dietetic Association. 3. A graduate of a State-approved course that provided 90 or more hours of classroom instruction in food service supervision and has experience as a supervisor in a health care institution with consultation from a dietitian. 4. Has training and experience in food service supervision and management in the military service. See qualified dietetic service supervisor.

**dietetic technician**
Dietetic technicians function as middle management and service personnel in health care facilities. Working with and under the direction of food service supervisors/dietetic assistants and dietitians, they assist with the planning, implementation, and evaluation of food programs, teach principles of nutrition, and provide dietary counseling. Their typical duties may include taking diet histories, calculating routine modified diets, teaching proper nutritional habits, and evaluating food programs for patients. They may counsel individuals and families in food selection, preparation, and menu planning as these relate to specific nutritional

deficiencies or needs. Where institutional policies permit, they may also train and supervise dietary aides.

**dietitian, (A.D.A.), R.D.**
A specialist educated for a profession responsible for the nutritional care of individuals and groups. This care includes the application of the science and art of human nutrition in helping people select and obtain food for the primary purpose of nourishing their bodies in health or disease throughout the life cycle. This participation may be in single or combined functions; in foodservice systems management; in extending knowledge of food and nutrition principles; in teaching these principles for application according to particular situations; or in dietary counseling. Being specially trained in applied nutrition and management of individuals in institutional and community settings, dietitians can be separated into five levels, administrative, clinical, community, research, or educators. See administrative dietitian, clinical dietitian, community dietitian, research dietitian. See qualified dietitian.

**dietitian (Medicare)**
A person who: 1) is eligible for registration by the American Dietetic Association under its requirements in effect on the publication of this provision; 2) has a baccalaureate degree with major studies in food and nutrition, dietetics, or food service management, has 1 year of supervisory experience in the dietetic service of a health care institution, and participates annually in continuing dietetic education. See qualified dietitian.

**dietitian, administraive, R.D.**
The administrative dietitian, R.D., is a member of the management team and affects the nutritional care of groups through the management of foodservice systems that provide optimal nutrition and quality food.

**dietitian, clinical, R.D.**
Applies the science and art of human nutrition to helping individuals and groups attain adequate nutrition. Diet prescription, food selection, and education and counseling of clients are the essential aspects of their service in hospitals, clinics, agencies, and community health programs.

**dietitian, community, R.D.**
Functions as a member of community health teams and plans, organizes, coordinates, and evaluates the nutritional component of health care services for a health agency or organization.

**dietitian, consultant, R.D.**
The consultant dietitian, R.D., with experience in administrative or clinical dietetic practice, affects the management of human effort and facilitating resources by advice or services in nutritional care.

**dietitian, qualified**
According to JCAH for psychiatric, alcoholism and drug abuse facilities accreditation purposes, this is an individual who is registered by the Commission on Dietetic Registration of the American Dietetic Association

or who has the documented equivalent in education, training, and/or experience, with evidence of relevant continuing education.

**dietitian, research, R.D.**
Evaluates and expands knowledge in nutrition, nutrition education, food management, food service, and the design of food equipment. The research dietitian is usually employed in a hospital or educational institution, or may be involved in research in community health programs.

**diet manual**
According to JCAH for psychiatric, alcoholism and drug abuse facilities accreditation purposes, this is an up-to-date, organized system for standardizing the ordering of diets.

**difficult feats**
Activities in school programs that by nature are dangerous, i.e., shop classes, athletics. Adequate instruction and warning should be directed to the student prior to performance.

**digital computer**
A special computer utilizing discrete data and logic processes on these data. This type of computer is contrasted with an analog computer. A computer using a number recording system, it works in units that can be counted and is the computer most often used by hospital or health care facility business offices for data processing.

**dilatory**
1. Intending to delay. 2. Delay used to gain time.

**dilatory defense**
An approach used by the defense that avoids the merits of the case, but instead attempts to delay the progress of the trial.

**diligence**
Care; carefulness; caution; prudence.

**dimunition**
1. Where an error has occurred or a fact omitted from the record but is certified in a writ of error. 2. Decrease; a reduction.

**diploma school**
A program which educates registered nurses or allied health professionals in a hospital, the diploma being given upon completion of the program. Classroom and laboratory teaching may be given under an arrangement with a college, but are the responsibility of the hospital and no college level degree is given. See associate degree and baccalaureate programs.

**diploma school of nursing**
A school affiliated with a hospital or university, or an independent school, which provides primary or exclusively a program of education in professional nursing and allied subjects leading to a diploma or to equivalent indicia that such program has been satisfactorily completed, but only if such program, or such affiliated school or such hospital or university or such independent school is accredited.

**diplomate**
Somebody who has a diploma; sometimes used to describe a board certified physician, because a diploma is given with certification.

**dipsomania**
An abnormal craving for alcohol; an uncontrollable impulse to become intoxicated.

**direct cost**
1. The costs of resources that are solely devoted to the operation of a specific activity. These costs do not include the distribution of costs to a cost center which are not specifically attributable to that cost center. 2. A cost which is identifiable directly with a particular activity, service or product of the program experiencing the cost. See also indirect cost.

**directed verdict**
The judge takes the judgment responsibility away from the jury by telling them what decision they must reach. A verdict rendered by the court, where the evidence is overwhelming for one party.

**direct evidence**
Facts showing proof or establishing factual material about an issue without the needing of other facts.

**direct examination**
The opportunity to do the first examination or questioning of a witness in a trial. Courtroom procedure allows the side which called that witness to do the first questioning.

**direction**
For JCAH accreditation purposes, this is authoritative policy or procedural guidance for the accomplishment of a function or activity.

**direct method**
Recording research, business, medical records or pharmacy input data on cards or tape by punching holes directly into the cards or tape by means of a card-punch or tape-punching machine.

**direct nursing activities**
Any treatment or care activities that a nurse provides in the presence of, or for a patient.

**director of nursing**
According to JCAH long term care accreditation, a registered professional nurse who is responsible for the full-time direct supervision of the nursing services and who is currently licensed by the state in which practicing. This person should have training and/or experience in rehabilitative, psychiatric, and/or gerontological nursing and one year or more of additional education and/or experience in nursing service administration. He or she shall attend continuing education programs at least annually.

**director of nursing services (Medicare)**
A registered nurse who is licensed by the state in which practicing, and has 1 year of additional education or experience in nursing service

administration, as well as additional education or experience in such areas as rehabilitative or geriatric nursing, and participates annually in continuing nursing education.

**direct patient care support services**
Those services which lend assistance to the prevention, diagnosis and treatment of disease or other ill health conditions, and to the restoration or habilitation of the ill or disabled.

**direct tax**
A tax that is directly paid to the government. Income tax is direct tax.

**disability**
1. Any limitation of physical, mental, or social activity of an individual as compared with other individuals of similar age, sex, and occupation. Frequently refers to limitation of the usual or major activities, most commonly vocational. There are varying types (functional, vocational, learning), degrees (partial, total), and durations (temporary, permanent) of disability. Benefits for disability are often only available for specific disabilities, such as total and permanent (the requirement for Social Security and Medicare). 2. The absence of adequate or competent physical or mental functioning, having a negative or diminishing effect on one's earning ability. 3. The lack of legal capability to do an act. 4. A condition that renders an insured person incapable of performing one or more of the duties required by his or her regular occupation. See also rehabilitation.

**disability days**
The number of productive days which are lost by a member of the work force due to accident or illness.

**disability income insurance**
A form of health insurance that provides periodic payments to replace the usual income while a person is unable to work as a result of illness, injury, or disease.

**disability insurance**
Compensation is paid to the employee for lost income and medical expenses due to limitation of usual or major activities resulting from injury or illness. The different payment approaches are: A) Commercial group disability: coverage for a group of persons, such as that provided by an employer. B) Commercial individual disability: coverage for a single person usually purchased by, or for that person. C) Workmen's compensation: compensation for lost income and medical expenses resulting from diseases or injuries experienced through employment. D) Social Security benefits: compensation for lost income for persons who have paid into Social Security for physical or mental disability following at least 12 months of disability.

**disaffirm**
1. To refuse to adhere to. 2. To set aside; repudiate; take back consent; refusing to abide by a former agreement.

**disallow**

1. To deny or refuse; to deny or reject a request; to refuse to allow. 2. The difference between what the physician currently charges and what Medicare or its intermediary allows to be paid (which often lags behind actual costs).

**discharge**

1. Release; dismiss; for example, to discharge a patient is to release him or her. To discharge a court order is to cancel or revoke it. 2. Do or perform a duty. 3. To end a contractual obligation. 4. To perform an act. 5. According to JCAH for psychiatric, alcoholism and drug abuse facilities accreditation purposes, this is the point at which the patient's active involvement with a facility is terminated and the facility no longer maintains active responsibility for the patient.

**discharge abstract**

A summary description of an admission prepared upon a patient's discharge from a hospital or other health facility. The abstract records selected data about the patient's stay in the hospital including diagnoses, services received, length of stay, source of payment and demographic information. The information is usually obtained from the patient's medical record and abstracted in standard, coded form. See also Uniform Hospital Discharge Data Set.

**discharge planning**

1. Planning that begins when a patient is admitted for treatment and is aimed at providing the patient the proper segments of the health care continuum. 2. The process of preparing a patient for another level of care and arranging the patient's release from the current health care setting.

**discharges and deaths**

The actual number of inpatients leaving a health care facility in a certain period of time. This usually does not include newborns.

**disciplinary rules**

1. Acts or performances a lawyer is not allowed to do. 2. A part of the Code of Professional Responsibility.

**disclaimer**

1. A denial of facts in question. 2. Rejection; repudiation of right, interest, or responsibility. 3. Renunciation of a claim, promise or responsibility.

**disclose**

To reveal; to tell all facts about a situation; to reveal the truth. See disclosure.

**disclosure**

1. Revelation. 2. That which is disclosed, told or revealed. 3. The impartation of information that is secret. See disclose.

**disclosure of ownership (Medicare)**
The facility supplies full and complete information to the survey agency as to the identity (1) of each person who has any direct or indirect ownership interest of 10% or more in such skilled nursing facility or who is the owner (in whole or in part) of any mortgage, deed of trust, note, or other obligation secured (in whole or in part) by such skilled nursing facility or any of the property or assets of such skilled nursing facility, (2) in case a skilled nursing facility is organized as a corporation, of each officer and director of the corporation, and (3) in case a skilled nursing facility is organized as a partnership, of each partner; and promptly reports any changes which would affect the current accuracy of the information so required to be supplied.

**discontinuance**
Dismissal; non suit.

**discount**
1. Reducing the amount of money; to lower the price. 2. To prove untrue.

**discount rate**
Interest rate used to discount future cash flows to their present value.

**discovery**
The formal inspection, reviewing, discussion and exchange of facts, evidence and information between the various parties to a legal action or a lawsuit. The process by which opposing parties obtain information from one another through adverse examination, interrogatories, depositions and inspection of pertinent documents.

**discovery rule**
In malpractice, a rule in use in some jurisdictions under which the statute of limitations does not commence to run until the wrongful act is discovered, or, with reasonable diligence, should have been discovered. The statute of limitations is the period of time, ordinarily beginning with the wrongful act, during which an injured party may sue for recovery of damages arising from the act. In some jurisdictions application of the discovery rule is limited to cases involving a foreign object left in the body of a patient. Some states have adopted statutory rules in malpractice cases which impose double time limits within which an action for malpractice may be brought. Typically these statutes provide that the action must be brought within a limited time after its discovery as well as within a limited time from the date the negligent act occurred.

**discrete**
Separate; individual; not part of a corpus.

**discrimination**
1. To make or observe a difference. 2. Failure to treat all people equally; illegally and unfairly treating people differently based on race, religion, sex, or age.

**disease**

An abnormal state in which the body is not capable of responsing or carrying on its required functions. Diseases have variations in seriousness, effect and extent. Diseases are also classified into 3 levels; 1) acute—relatively severe and of short duration, 2) chronic—less severe but of long and continuous duration and 3) subacute—intermediate in severity and duration; falls between acute and chronic. The cause of disease can be from disease-producing organisms, nutritional deficiencies, physical agents (i.e. heat, cold, blows by heavy objects), chemicals, birth defects, degeneration and neoplasms. Disease can be communicable (easily spread from one person to another, i.e. measles), or noncommunicable (occurs but is not easily spread from one person to another, i.e. cancer). 2. "Without ease." 3. A failure of the adaptive mechanisms of an organism to counteract adequately, normally or appropriately the stimuli and stresses to which it is subject, resulting in a disturbance in the function or structure of some part of the organism. This definition emphasizes that disease is multi-factorial and may be prevented or treated by changing any of the factors. Disease is a very elusive and difficult concept to define, being largely socially defined. Thus, criminality and drug dependence presently tend to be seen as diseases, when they were previously considered to be moral or legal problems. See also health, injury, acute, chronic and illness.

**disease code manual**

A listing of diseases by code based on Hospital Adaptation of International Classification of Diseases. See these words.

**disfranchise**

To take away one's rights, particularly one's right to vote.

**dishonor**

1. To refuse to accept. 2. To fail to respect a legal obligation.

**disinfectant**

Any substance, method or agent used to kill disease-producing microorganisms existing outside the body. Several approaches to killing diseases are used, such as heat for sterilization and incineration. Sunlight, chemical substances and agents are the most commonly used and they are also the most practical. The chemical agents phenol and carbolic acid are the standards by which new agents are measured for effectiveness.

**disinfection**

To render pathogens harmless through use of heat, antiseptics, antibacterial agents, etc.

**disinhibition**

Withdrawal of or lack of inhibition. Some drugs and alcohol can remove inhibitions. In psychiatry, disinhibition leads to the freedom to act on one's own needs, rather than to submit to the demands of others or adhere to the expectations of law or society.

**disinter**

To exhume; to take out of the grave.

**disinterested**
1. Having no personal interest or opportunity for personal gain; indifferent. 2. Impartial; a nonbiased opinion; One having no vested interests.

**disjunctive allegation**
Two mutually exclusive yet alternative charges connected with the conjunction "or."

**disk-set storage**
A storage device used in computerized medical records or insurance forms which permits the use of interchangeable disk sets or packs.

**dismemberment**
The loss of a limb or of one's sight.

**dismissal**
A court order that removes a suit from litigation.

**dismissal without prejudice**
Dismissal of an action while not barring subsequent action on the same concern.

**dismissal with prejudice**
A final decision on an action, that bars the right to bring any other action on the same cause.

**disorderly conduct**
Actions that disturb the peace or public morality and well being.

**disorientation**
To lose one's orientation and sense of direction. Inability to judge time, space, and personal relations. This can occur in most acute and chronic brain disorders.

**disparagement**
1. Anything that degrades, disgraces or detracts. 2. Discrediting or belittling something or someone.

**dispensary**
1. A place where medicines are dispensed. 2. A treatment facility similar to an outpatient clinic where free primary care is delivered and medications are provided to patients. 3. An outpatient treatment facility used for sick call in the military.

**dispensing fee**
A fee charged by a pharmacist for filling a prescription. One of two ways that pharmacists charge for the service of filling a prescription, the other being a standard percentage markup on the acquisition cost of the drug involved. A dispensing fee is the same for all prescriptions, thus representing a larger markup on the cost of an inexpensive drug or a small prescription than on an expensive drug or large prescription. However, it reflects the fact that a pharmacist's service is the same whatever the cost of the drug. Some pharmacists combine the two approaches, using a percentage markup with a minimum fee.

**dispensing optician**
A technologist who makes and fits glasses or lenses prescribed by opthalmologists or optometrists. Opticians measure facial contours and assist in frame and lens selection. Optical laboratory technicians grind lenses according to prescription. Some opticians grind lenses and adjust and fit the frame to the customer. There are 2 year associate degrees in opthalmic dispensing. Three to four years of on-the-job training in an apprenticeship program can also qualify individuals for this field. Additional training is necessary to fit contact lenses.

**displacement**
A defense or mental mechanism, in which an emotion or experience is transferred from its original object to another object; an emotional reaction that is transferred from one object to another.

**disposable earnings**
One's total pay less deductions.

**disposition**
1. A final settlement decision, resulting from a court's judgment. 2. In psychiatry, a person's inclinations as determined by his mood.

**dispositive facts**
Facts that clarify and settle a legal issue.

**dispossession**
1. Ousting wrongfully; removing a person from his or her property by force, deception or illicit use of the law. 2. To dispose.

**dispute**
1. To debate or argue; a disagreement between two parties. 2. To doubt; to question the truth of a matter.

**disqualify**
1. To make ineligible. 2. To make disabled or unfit. 3. To declare unqualified.

**disseisin**
1. The dispossession. 2. The wrongful putting out of the rightful owner. 3. A deprivation of possession.

**dissemble**
1. To conceal. 2. To disguise the appearance of.

**dissentiente (Lat.)**
Dissenting.

**dissenting opinion**
A judge's formal disagreement with the majority decision of a lawsuit. If it is recorded, it is a *dissenting opinion.*

**dissociation**
A defense or mental mechanism, through which one's emotions are separated and detached from an idea, situation, or object. Dissociation may defer an emotional experience.

**dissociative neurosis**
A breakdown in mental functioning, possibly a defensive response to psychological stressors which may be too overwhelming to cope with. Perceived loss of identity is one possible symptom.

**dissolute**
Lewd; profligate; wanton.

**dissolution**
To dissolve or terminate; to end. The dissolution of a contract is when there is mutual agreement to end it.

**dissolution of marriage**
The end or legal termination of a marriage, except for annulments. See divorce.

**dissolve**
Terminate; end; cancel or do away with.

**distinguish**
1. To show differences. 2. To distinguish a case is to prove the issue at hand as applicable or why it is not essential or applicable.

**disto-**
Prefix meaning far.

**distortion**
False presentation of reality.

**distrain**
To unlawfully or legally seize another person's personal property; to seize goods or property.

**distress**
1. In law it means to take property or goods, without legal process, away from a wrongdoer in order to procure payment. The seizing of personal property in order to force the payment of taxes. 2. In psychology, when referring to stress, it is a troubled or suffering of the or mind; worry; anguish.

**distributive law**
Deals with the distribution of funds and services by government agencies or bodies, such as health agencies.

**district**
A sub-division of different geographical areas, created for judicial, political or administrative purposes. See hospital district.

**district attorney (D.A.)**
The head criminal prosecuting lawyer of a Federal or state district. County or city attorneys are also equivalent to a district attorney.

**district court**
Trial courts of the U.S., or low-level state courts.

**diuretic**
Any drug that promotes excretion of urine.

**divers**
Many or several. Different.

**diversion**
1. To turn aside. 2. Placing criminals or juvenile delinquents into special rehabilitation programs, rather than jail. 3. To divert; to refocus attention.

**diversity of citizenship**
A constitutional doctrine requiring the parties on opposite sides in a lawsuit to reside in different states as a prerequisite to the federal courts taking jurisdiction.

**divest**
To strip or dispossess; to take away; to deprive someone of authority, property, a right, or title. Also called devest.

**dividend**
1. A policyholder's share in the divisible surplus funds of an insurance company apportioned for distribution, which may take the form of a refund of part of the premium on the insured's policy. 2. A share of profits or property of a corporation which is distributed to its stockholders.

**Division of Emergency Medical Services.**
A subagency of the U.S. Health Service Administration that administers programs at state and local levels which are supported by federal grants to develop local emergency medical care programs.

**Division of Manpower Analysis**
Now called the Division of Health Professions Analysis.

**Division of Manpower Training Support**
Now called the Division of Health Professions Training Support.

**divorce**
Legally ending a marriage by a court order, also called dissolution of marriage. See these words.

**dizziness**
Vertigo; the sensation that one is whirling around; loss of equilibrium.

**DNA**
Deoxyribonucleic acid. The genetic matter contained in most living organisms and which is responsible for the control of heredity.

**docket**
A calendar or agenda of scheduled court proceedings, usually prepared by a clerk of the court. The schedule of cases for trial in court.

**doctor**
Usually used synonymously with physician, but actually means any person with a doctoral degree.

**doctor-patient relationship**
The confidential and personal interaction that exists between one who is ill and one who is selected to heal or cure a disease or disorder.

**doctrine**
A common law principle or policy followed by the judiciary.

**document**
A written legal paper or record; a printed record or recorded record that serves as proof. For example, a contract, medical records, an x-ray. A public document is a written paper that is open for public inspection.

**documentary evidence**
Written evidence; important written information that could be used to prove certain facts or have important legal meaning.

**document of title**
1. A written record used in business as proof of a right to possess goods. 2. A bill of lading; a receipt.

**doing business**
1. The management of business within a jurisdiction, as a continuous effort, so as to render the business subject to the jurisdiction of the local courts. 2. Carrying on business for profit within a state so that another person could sue if need be. 3. It also means that the state can tax the company and hold it legally responsible for its business transactions.

**domain**
Ownership or control; ultimate ownership.

**domestic**
1. Belonging or relating to home, state, or country. 2. Pertaining to one's place of residence.

**domestic corporation**
Created in one's own nation, state or area. A corporation created and incorporated under the laws of that state, as opposed to a foreign corporation.

**domicile**
1. A person's permanent official and legal residence, home or main residence. 2. Residing within a jurisdiction with no present intention to live elsewhere.

**domiciliary**
Relating to one's domicile, or permanent home.

**dominant**
Having rights, responsibility or control over another.

**dominant cause**
See proximate cause.

**dominion**
Control, domination, ownership or power over others, positions, property or land.

**domitae naturae (Lat.)**
Domestic animals. Animals that are generally tame and occasionally wander at large. Opposite of ferae naturae.

**donatio causa mortis**
See causa mortis.

**donatio inter vivos (Lat.)**
A gift between living persons.

**donative**
Related to old canon law. A donation or benefit given; a gift. A donative trust is a gift given to another person.

**donee**
1. One to whom a gift or grant is made or power given. 2. One who receives the gift of an organ to be transplanted; the one in which a donated organ or other body part is transplanted.

**donor**
1. A person giving a grant or gift to another or granting another power to do something. 2. Giving of an organ or body part, for use by another person. 3. One who donates or bestows a donation.

**dormant**
Sleeping, latent, inactive, silent or concealed.

**dormant partner**
Silent partner.

**dosage**
The control of the number, amount, size and frequency of a dose. See dose.

**dose**
The quantity, amount or portion of a substance, drug or agent to be given in one administration.

**dose, booster**
A quantity of a vaccine given to a person at a predetermined time interval once a primary dose has been given. The second or third dose is the booster dose. It is usually in smaller amounts and is to work to continue the immune response of the primary dose.

**dose, fatal**
A quantity or amount of a substance that can cause death.

**dose, lethal**
The amount of a drug, substance or agent that is a large enough quantity to cause death.

**dose rate**
The dose delivered or administered in a specific period of time or frequency.

**dose, skin**
The amount or quantity of radiation at the skin level, including primary and back scatter radiation.

**dose, tolerance**
The greatest amount of a drug, substance or agent that is safely administered to a patient without any risk of harm.

**double blind technique**
A method used in research to study a drug, or other medical procedure in which both subjects and investigators are kept unaware of (blind to) who is actually getting which specific treatment. The method is one of the few ways of eliminating bias, conscious or unconscious, in both subjects and investigators. Classically, in drug studies the method involves the use of a look-alike placebo. In "triple blind" studies the people analyzing the data are also unaware of the treatment used.

**double entry**

**double entry**
A bookkeeping method where every transaction made is recorded.
One system of accounting which requires that for every entry Entries are made as a debit and a credit, so it is easy to check made on the debit side of an account, an entry must be made for by using both rows and columns of numbers, with one balancing the the corresponding amount on the credit side of another account other. or accounts.

**double indemnity**
Insurance that pays off double the amount if something happens in a certain way. A policy provision usually associated with death, which doubles the payments of certain benefits when certain kinds of accidents occur.

**double insurance**
A person holding life or health/medical insurance from two or more companies that covers the same risk. It may be illegal or against the insurance contracts to collect from more than one company the total amounts, as you can be paid for an injury or death only once, or be paid more than each policy states that the risk was worth.

**double jeopardy**
Being prosecuted twice for the same crime. This is protected against by the U.S. Constitution.

**doubt**
To have strong disbelief, mistrust or uncertainty about the proof of facts; to fluctuate or appear uncertain about the truth or the facts.

**down payment**
A large sum of money paid at the time that something is purchased on time (in installment payments).

**D.P.**
Doctorate of Podiatry.

**D.Phar**
Doctorate of Pharmacy.

**DPH or Dr. P.H.**
Doctorate of Public Health.

**DPT**
A vaccine containing diphtheria, pertussis and tetanus; a triple-antigen immunization.

**Draconian law**
Related to the Athenian law-giver Draco. Related to or in reference to a code of laws that is especially cruel, harsh, severe and rigorous, based on Draco of 7th century B.C. (Greece).

**draft**
1. The first writing; a sketch. 2. A bill of exchange, a check. A written negotiable instrument from one party to another which is used for the payment of money; the drawing of money.

**draw**
1. To write a check; to prepare a written demand for payment of a sum of money; take money out of the bank or out of an account. 2. To create a legal document. 3. To take out of one's body, as to draw blood.

**drawee**
One on whom a bill of exchange, an order or draft is drawn, and who is expected to pay the bill for the amount presented.

**drawer**
The one drawing or preparing a bill of exchange, draft or order, or one who signs a draft or order.

**drawing tests**
Any psychological projective test in which the subject is asked to draw objects and such things as people, trees, and houses, which are used to assess their attitudes, feelings and perceptions.

**draw sheet**
A bed sheet that is purposely shortened. It is placed over the bottom sheet and covers the area between the chest and the knees of the patient. The draw sheet protects the mattress and lower sheet while helping to keep the patient dry and comfortable.

**drayman**
One who transports goods.

**dread**
Anxiety related to or created by fear of a specific danger, as opposed to anxiety, which is usually regarded as objectless.

**dread disease insurance**
See specific disease insurance.

**dread disease rider**
A clause added onto a health insurance policy which provides supplemental benefits for certain conditions, diseases or disorders.

**dressing**
The sterile, clean bandaging material used to directly cover and protect a wound while aiding in the control of bleeding.

**Drinker respirator**
A special type device that allows controlled automatic breathing in a patient who suffers paralysis of the muscles which control breathing.

**drip**
The continuous slow drop by drop administration of a liquid into a patient via an IV.

**drip, Murphy**
The slow continuous drop by drop administration of saline solution into the rectum.

**droit (French)**
Right, justice, or law.

**drug**
Any substance intended for use in the diagnosis, cure, mitigation, treatment or prevention of disease, or intended to affect the structure of function of the body (not including food), or components of these substances. Substances recognized in the official U.S. Pharmacopeia, the official Homeopathic Pharmacopeia of the U.S., or the official National Formulary are drugs. See also device and biologic, safe and effective, compendium and formulary, new and not new (and "me too"), over-the-counter and prescription, labeling and package insert, established and brand, NDA and MAC, DESI and IND, and drug monograph and drug dependence.

**drug abuse**
Persistent or sporadic drug use inconsistent with or unrelated to acceptable medical or cultural practice. The definition of drug abuse is highly variable, sometimes also requiring excessive use of a drug, unnecessary use (thus incorporating recreational use), drug dependence, or that the use be illegal. See also alcoholism.

**drug addiction**
Generally used synonymously with drug dependence, often wrongly assumed to be synonymous with drug abuse, and very irregular in meaning.

**drug administration (Medicare)**
1. An act in which a single dose of a prescribed drug or biological is given to a patient by an authorized person in accordance with all laws and regulations governing such acts. The complete act of administration entails removing an individual dose from a previously dispensed, properly labeled container (including a unit dose container), verifying it with the physician's orders, giving the individual dose to the proper patient, and

promptly recording the time and dose given. 2. For JCAH accreditation purposes, this is the act in which a single dose of an identified drug is given to a patient.

**drug compendium**
See compendium.

**drug dependence**
A state, psychic and sometimes also physical, resulting from the interaction between a person and a drug, characterized by behavioral and other responses that always include a compulsion to take the drug on a continuous or periodic basis in order to experience its psychic effects, and sometimes to avoid the discomfort and other physical effects of its withdrawal or absence. Tolerance for the drug may or may not be present. A person may be dependent on more than one drug. Its characteristics will vary with the agent involved, and this must be made clear by designating the particular type of drug dependence in each specific case—for example, drug dependence of narcotic type, of cannabis type, of barbiturate type, of amphetamine type, etc. As defined here, drug dependence may or may not be dangerous to the dependent individual or the public, severe, or illegal.

**drug dispensing**
1. According to JCAH accreditation, this is the issuance of one or more doses of a prescribed medication in containers that are correctly labeled to indicate the name of the patient, the contents of the container, and all other vital information needed to facilitate correct patient usage and drug administration. 2. Under Medicare, an act entailing the interpretation of an order for a drug or biological and, pursuant to that order, the proper selection, measuring, labeling, packaging, and issuance of the drug or biological for a patient or for a service unit of the facility.

**Drug Efficacy Study Implementation (DESI)**
The plan of the Food and Drug Administration for implementing the evaluations and recommendations of the Drug Efficacy Study Group of the National Academy of Science-National Research Council respecting the effectiveness of drugs marketed prior to 1962 under approved new drug applications. The Drug Efficacy Study was undertaken in 1966 to evaluate all of the drugs the FDA had approved as safe prior to 1962, when Congress first required that drugs also be proved effective before marketing. The Drug Efficacy Study Group evaluated nearly 4,000 individual drug products, finding many of them ineffective or of only possible or probable effectiveness. The FDA is still in the process of implementing those judgments by removing some of the drugs from the market.

**druggist**
Sombody who operates a drug store. Sometimes considered synonymous with pharmacist, but is not always limited to people with a pharmacy degree (or even to operators of drug stores in which prescription drugs are dispensed) and is usually applied only to pharmacists who operate, or at least work in, drug stores,

**drug habituation**

Generally used synonymously with drug dependence, sometimes used to mean psychic drug dependence, often wrongly assumed to be synonymous with drug abuse, and very irregular in meaning.

**drug history**

According to JCAH for psychiatric, alcoholism and drug abuse facilities accreditation purposes, this is a delineation of the drugs used by a patient, including prescribed and unprescribed drugs and alcohol. A drug history includes, but is not necessarily limited to, the following: drugs used in the past; drugs used recently, especially within the preceding 48 hours; drugs of preference; frequency with which each drug is used; route of administration of each drug; drugs used in combination; dosages used; year of first use of each drug; previous occurrences of overdose, withdrawal, or adverse drug reactions; and history of previous treatment received for alcohol or drug abuse.

**drug holiday**

Discontinuing the administration of a drug to patients or residents in long-term care for a limited period of time in order to evaluate and determine baseline behavior, behavior effects of drugs and to determine the correct dosage of psychoactive drugs and their side effects.

**drug interaction**

The effects or reaction of two or more drugs taken simultaneously. Often they produce a different effect than if either drug was taken alone. The interaction of two drugs may have a potentiating and/or additive effect with possible serious side effects resulting. An example of drug interaction is alcohol and sedative drugs taken together and causing additive central nervous system depression. See synergistic effect.

**drug monograph**

A rule which prescribes, for a drug or class of related drugs, the kinds and amounts of ingredients which it may contain, the conditions for which it may be offered, and directions for use, warnings and other information which its labeling must bear. Drug monographs established by FDA state conditions under which drugs may be marketed as safe and effective and not adulterated or misbranded, and thus without an approved new drug application.

**drug therapy**

The use of drugs to treat physical and mental illness. Also known as chemotherapy. See also maintenance drug therapy.

**DSM-I**

Abbreviation for the first edition of the American Psychiatric Association's *Diagnostic and Statistical Manual of Mental Disorders* published in 1952. See these words.

**DSM-II**

Abbreviation for *Diagnostic and Statistical Manual of Mental Disorders,* second edition (1968). See these words.

**DSM-III**
Abbreviation for *Diagnostic and Statistical Manual of Mental Disorders,* third edition (1980). See these words.

**dual choice (dual option)**
Refers to federal legislation that requires employers to give their employees the option to enroll in a local health maintenance organization or in the conventional employer-sponsored health insurance program. The practice of giving people a choice of more than one health insurance or health program to pay for or provide their health services. Usually done by employers who offer employees more than one group health insurance program, or a health insurance program and a prepaid group practice to choose from as a benefit of their employment. Characteristic of the Federal Employees Health Benefits Program. Required by the HMO Act, PL 93-222, of employers with respect to qualified HMOs (section 1310 of the PHS Act).

**dual coverage**
A plan under which the insured has insurance coverage by more than one carrier.

**dubitante (Lat.)**
Doubting. This term is fixed to a judge's name in court reports, showing that he doubts the correctness of the decision.

**duces tecum (Lat.)**
Bring with you. A subpoena requiring a person summoned to court to bring certain documents or evidence to court. A physician may be required to bring medical records or x-rays to court to be used as evidence.

**due**
Suitable; proper; owed; usual; regular; sufficient or reasonable. "Due care" is ordinary or expected care that is at the level sufficient for the situation. Payable, owed and already matured, as a note is due. See due care.

**due care**
That amount or degree of care that would be exercised by an ordinary person in the same situation. See reasonable man, ordinary person, negligence. See due.

**due date**
Day a debt must be paid. The date that something is due or is to arrive.

**due notice**
Reasonable or sufficient notice.

**due process**
The right to proper litigation procedures in the event a legal action should occur, such as a right to a hearing or a fair trial. The Due Process Clause of the Constitution of the United States provides that no person shall be deprived of life, liberty, or property without due process of law. A person should have enough advance notice and a chance to

present his side of a legal complaint. No law or any governmental legal process should be arbitrary, biased, rushed or unfair.

**dum fervet opus (Lat.)**
In the heat of the action.

**dummy**
Fake, a sham; set up as real. A front.

**dummy corporation**
A corporation that meets legal requirements but is really acting as a tool of or is secretely controlled by another.

**dun**
1. To urge or demand payment. 2. To loudly, persistently and insistently demand payment of a debt. Literally means "with a loud noise."

**duo-**
Prefix meaning two.

**duplication of benefits**
Occurs when a person covered under more than one health or accident insurance policy collects, or may collect, payments for the same hospital or medical expenses from more than one insurer. Individual health insurance policies, under state laws, sometimes include antiduplication clauses against overinsurance due to two similar policies issued by the same insurer; loss-of-time coverage in excess of the insured's monthly earnings; and duplicate coverage with other insurers, if the insurer has not been given written notice of such duplicate coverage prior to the date of loss. Because of this notice limitation, many individual insurance policies do not include antiduplication clauses. Since the limitation does not apply to group insurance, it usually does contain such clauses, especially in major medical policies. However, most states will not allow group policies to apply such clauses to individual insurance. Where duplication exists with a group antiduplication clause, the group insurer responsible for paying its benefits first is the primary payer. See also coordination of benefits.

**duration of visit**
As used in health services research, this usually is the time the physician spent in face-to-face contact with the patient, not including time the patient spent waiting to see the physician, time the patient spent receiving care from someone other than the physician without the presence of the physician, or time the physician spent reviewing records, test results, etc. In cases where the patient received care from a member of the physician's staff, but did not see the physician during the visit, the duration of visit is recorded as zero minutes.

**duress**
Coercion; threats; pressure or force put on a person to do what he or she would not otherwise do, such as commit a misdemeanor.

**Durham Rule**
A test for criminal responsibility, based on concept of irresistible impulse. If it is shown that a defendant was diseased and had a defective mental state when he committed a crime, and that the crime was due to the mental state, the Durham Rule maintains that he cannot be held criminally responsible.

**duty**
1. Any moral or legal obligation to another person. 2. Conduct owed to a person or a patient, especially if he has a right to expect something from another person, therefore, it is insured that the expectation is carried out in a competent manner. 3. Any obligation, moral or ethical, to perform or follow a specific order of conduct.

**D.V.M.**
Doctor of Veterinary Medicine.

**DWI**
1. Driving While Intoxicated. 2. Also, died without issue; childless.

**Dyer Act**
A federal law making it an offense to take a stolen motor vehicle across a state line. (Passed in 1919)

**dying declaration**
Words of a dying person about a crime. Under usual conditions, such testimony is not considered good evidence, but words of a dying person are usually allowed or believed.

**dys-**
Prefix, meaning bad, malicious, hard, painful, difficult.

**dyslexia**
Reading disability in which one is unable to comprehend or understand the written word. It is not related to one's intelligence level.

**dyspareunia**
Physical pain in sexual intercourse experienced by women; usually accompanied by emotional concerns with sexual intercourse.

**dysphagia**
Difficulty in, or inability to swallow.

**dyssocial behavior**
Also known as sociopathic behavior; that is, behaviors that are marginally criminal, such as sadists, racketeers, prostitutes, and illegal gamblers. See antisocial personality.

**dystressor**
Any occurrence, event, experience, life change, loss, difficulty, pain, that causes mental or emotional upset, physiological changes, wear and tear on the body or any deviation from positive conditions that causes stress and to which a person cannot easily adapt, cope or adjust.

**dysuria**
Difficulty urinating, or pain upon urination.

# E

**Early and Periodic Screening Diagnosis and Treatment Program (EPSDT)**
A program mandated by law as part of the Medicaid program. The law (section 1905(a) (4) (B) of the Social Security Act) requires that by July 1, 1969, all states have in effect a program for eligible children under age 21 to ascertain their physical or mental defects, and such health care, treatment, and other measures to correct or ameliorate defects and chronic conditions discovered thereby, as may be provided in regulations of the Secretary. The state programs are not just to pay for services but also to have an active outreach component to inform eligible persons of the benefits available to them, actively to bring them into care so that they can be screened, and, if necessary, to assist them in obtaining appropriate treatment. EPSDT should properly refer only to programs which have all of these elements.

**earned income**
Personal money gain derived from personal work or services rendered as distinguished from other kinds of income, such as income for the facility or business.

**earnest money**
An amount paid by a buyer in order to hold or to bind a seller to a deal or to the terms of an agreement; a deposit to show a buyer's good faith.

**earnings test**
A formula used to determine and assess retirement benefits in which payments are reduced according to one's current earnings as determined by a preestablished schedule.

**easement**
1. A right, privilege or convenience which an owner of land has over the adjacent parcel by prescription, grant or necessary implication and without profit, such as a roadway, gate, waterway, etc. 2. A privilege or right an owner of a parcel of land has to use the land of another for a special reason as long as it is not inconsistent with the owner's general use.

**E.B.T.**
Examination before trial. A part of the discovery process. See deposition.

**ECG**
Electrocardiogram. See these words.

**echo-**
Prefix meaning sound.

**echocardiography**
An ultrasound diagnostic method using echo or a sound reflecting technique used to determine the presence or absence of fluid in the sac surrounding the heart, or the position and motion of the heart walls.

**echoencephalography**
An ultrasound or ultrasonic diagnostic method in which sound waves are beamed through the head and echoes are recorded graphically to determine any change in brain structure.

**echogram**
The record made by the echoes of echography.

**echography**
The use of ultrasound or ultrasonic sound waves as a diagnostic method. Ultrasonic waves are beamed at the tissue to be diagnosed and the echoes are recorded on a graph, or an oscilloscope, which helps determine density, structure, etc. See ultrasonography.

**ecological fallacy**
The common erroneous assumption that because two things are associated one must be caused by the other. See also Hawthorne and Halo effects.

**ecology**
The study of man's relationship with the environment.

**economic characteristics**
The economic condition of the state and its residents.

**economic issues/constraints**
Those economic aspects that might hinder the implementation of the Health Systems Plan.

**Economic Opportunity Act of 1969**
See Community Action Program.

**economic order quantity**
In materials management considering time and cost, it is the best mix of cost and amount of inventory or supplies to be ordered when the inventory is reduced to a level where it is wise to replenish the supply.

**Economic Stabilization Program (ESP)**
A federal program established to control wages and prices. On August 15, 1971, all wages and prices were frozen for a period of ninety days. During that period a system of wage and price controls administered through a Cost of Living Council was implemented. Controls continued, with periodic changes in the flexibility and the intensity with which they were enforced until their legislative authority ultimately expired in April 1974. Wages and prices in the health care industry were controlled through a specialized series of regulations. The 32½ months the controls were in effect is the only period in which medical care price increases have slowed markedly since the enactment of Medicare and Medicaid; during that period increases in medical care prices were limited to 4.3 percent.

**economies of scale**
Cost savings resulting from aggregation of resources and/or mass production. In particular, it refers to decreases in average cost when all factors of production are expanded proportionately. For example, hospital costs for a unit of service are generally less in 300 than 30 bed hospitals. (There is some evidence that they may be greater in 1,000 bed than 300 bed hospitals, a diseconomy of scale.) Frequently used, less accurately, to refer to savings achieved when underused resources are used more efficiently. For example when many individuals use the same product, or when health care facilities share in the costs and use of expensive equipment (e.g. automated laboratory equipment) or otherwise underused and highly trained personnel (e.g., open-heart surgery teams).

**E.C.T.**
Electroconvulsive therapy. See electroconvulsive therapy, shock treatment.

**edentulous**
Without teeth.

**edict**
An official public order announced or proclaimed by a public official or a head of state.

**Educational Commission for Foreign Medical Graduates (ECFMG)**
An organization sponsored by the AMA, AHA, AAMC, Association for Hospital Medical Education, and Federation of State Medical Boards of the U.S. which operates a program of educating, testing and evaluating foreign medical graduates who seek internships and residencies in the U.S. The ECFMG was formed in 1974 by merger of the Educational Council for Foreign Medical Graduates, incorporated in 1956, and the Commission for Foreign Medical Graduates. Certification of FMGs is granted by the ECFMG after receiving documentation of their education, and passage of an examination of their medical competence and comprehension of spoken English. Such certification is necessary for full licensure of FMGs in 47 states and territories. See also federation licensing examination.

**educational diagnosis**
As used in health education, it is the determining of factors that predispose, enable, and reinforce certain health behaviors.

**educational therapist**
A person who works with mentally ill, mentally retarded, or disabled patients. He/she instructs patients in academic subjects to further medical/mental recovery and prevent mental deterioration.

**educational tool (aid)**
Any material, method, approach or activity (such as a bulletin board, leaflet, or videotape, etc.) that aids in learning and teaching.

**E.E.G.**
Electroencephalogram. A recording device used for recording electrical impulses of the brain.

**E.E.O.**
Equal Employment Opportunity.

**E.E.O.C.**
Equal Employment Opportunities Commission

**effect**
1. The power to produce results. 2. To be operative or in force. 3. To produce. 4. A result; to begin or to show results.

**effective date**
In health insurance, the date on which a membership goes into effect, making benefits available.

**effectiveness**
The degree to which diagnostic, preventive, therapeutic or other action or actions achieves the intended result. Effectiveness requires a consideration of outcomes to measure. It does not require consideration of the cost of the action, although one way of comparing the effectiveness of actions with the same or similar intended results is to compare the ratios of their effectiveness to their costs. The Federal Food, Drug, and Cosmetic Act requires prior demonstration of effectiveness for most drugs marketed for human use. No similar requirement exists for most other medical action paid for or regulated under federal or state law. Usually synonymous with efficacy in common use. See also safety, quality, efficiency and DESI.

**effects**
Personal property or one's personal belongings.

**efferent**
Moving away from the center.

**efficacy**
Commonly used synonymously with effectiveness, but may usefully be distinguished from it by using efficacy for the results of actions undertaken under ideal circumstances and effectiveness for their results under usual or normal circumstances. Actions can thus be efficacious and effective, or efficacious and ineffective, but not the reverse.

**efficiency**
The relationship between the quantity of inputs or resources used in the production of medical services and the quantity of outputs produced. Efficiency has three components: input productivity (technical efficiency), input mix (economic efficiency), and the scale of operation. Efficiency is usually measured by indicators such as output per man hour or cost per unit of output. However, such indicators fail to account for the numerous relevant dimensions (such as quality) of both inputs and outputs and are, therefore, only partial measures. Colloquially, efficiency measures the "bang for the buck" but, as the above suggests, it is a difficult concept to define and quantify. Ultimately, efficiency should probably be measured in terms of the costs of achieving various health outcomes; defining it in terms of productivity assumes that what is produced is efficacious and used in an effective manner.

**effluent**
Flowing out of or flows forth, like sewage out of a pipe, an outflow of a sewer, storage tank, pipe, canal or channel, which causes pollution.

**e.g. (Lat. abbrev.)**
Exempli gratia. Used in writing to mean "for example."

**ego (Lat.)**
Self. In psychoanalytic theory, ego is one of the three major divisions of the psychic apparatus, the others being the id and superego. The ego represents certain mental mechanisms and serves to mediate between the demands of primitive instinctual drives (the id), of internalized parental and social prohibitions (the superego), and reality.

**egocentric**
One who is self-centered, preoccupied with his or her own needs, lacking in concern or interest for others, and very selfish.

**egomania**
Serious or pathological self-centeredness or preoccupation with one's self.

**egregious**
Negatively exceptional; known for negative qualities; infamous.

**ejectment**
An old legal action to regain possession of premises; to win damages for unlawful retention. Now generally provided by forcible entry and detainer statutes.

**ejusdem generis (Lat.)**
Of the same kind of class or type.

**elasticity of demand**
In health economics, a measure of the sensitivity of demand for a product or service to changes in its price (price elasticity) or the income of the people demanding the product or service (income elasticity). Price elasticity is the ratio of the resulting percentage change in demand to a given percentage change in price. Price elasticity of demand for health services allows one to predict the effect on demand of different cost sharing provisions in proposed NHI programs and thus aids in predicting the differing stress their enactment would place on the health system.

**elation**
Emotion characterized by enjoyment, confidence, and euphoria; an emotional high.

**el doctor (Spanish)**
Physician. Also referred to as medico.

**elective**
When applied to health care service, service that can be delayed without substantial risk to the patient and is not necessary immediately, to prevent imminent death or serious impairment of the health of the individual.

**elective benefit**

An insurance benefit payable in lieu of another. For example, a lump sum benefit may be allowed for specified injuries in lieu of weekly or monthly indemnity.

**elective surgery**

Surgery which need not be performed on an emergency basis, because reasonable delays will not affect the outcome or surgery unfavorably. It should be understood that such surgery is usually necessary and may be major.

**Electra complex**

The female child's attraction to her father; as compared with the Oedipus complex.

**electro-**

Prefix meaning electricity.

**electroanesthesia**

Anesthesia caused by use of electric current passed through tissue either on a local or general basis.

**electrocardiograph**

An electronic device which measures and records the heart's impulses on a graph which is called an electrocardiogram (ECG, EKG).

**electrocardiographic effect**

Changes shown in the electrical activity of the heart, usually caused by the patient taking drugs.

**electrocardiographic technician**

Generally, these individuals maintain and operate electrocardiographic machines, both in clinical settings and in private offices. The data are used by the physician, frequently an internist or cardiologist, to diagnose, treat, and monitor the change in a patient's heart over time. Electrocardiographic (EKG) technicians also may conduct other tests, such as vectorcardiograms and phonocardiograms. They may schedule appointments and maintain EKG files, depending on the health care setting. This is the largest occupational category in the group.

**electrocardiography services**

Most major health care facilities offer this service. The EKG or ECG technician assists in recording the electrical impulses produced by the heart muscles. The graph recordings are reviewed and interpreted by a physician cardiologist to assess heart conditions.

**electrocautery**

The destruction of tissue for medical reasons through the use of a needle or snare that is made hot electrically and is inserted into warts, polyps, or other tumorous growths to burn them off.

**electroconvulsive therapy**

1. A psychiatric treatment procedure used to treat depression when other methods have failed. It involves the use of electric current directed to the brain to induce unconsciousness or convulsive seizures which may reduce

or eliminate depression. 2. According to JCAH for psychiatric, alcoholism and drug abuse facilities accreditation purposes, this is a form of somatic treatment in which electrical current is applied to the brain producing uncoordinated muscle contraction in a convulsive manner.

**electroencephalograph (EEG)**
An electrical instrument that records the electrical activity of the brain on a graph which is called an electroencephalogram.

**electroencephalographic technician/technologist**
Electroencephalography (EEG) is the scientific field devoted to recording and studying the electrical activity of the brain. The EEG technician or technologist operates and helps maintain encephalographs, which record tracings of the brain's electrical activity. Tracings obtained from the electroencephalograph are used to help physicians, usually neurologists, diagnose and monitor the progress of such disorders an epilepsy, tumors, cerebral vascular strokes, and head injuries. The use of EEGs in determining cessation of brain function also has made these functions important in vital organ (heart, kidney, liver) transplant operations. Depending upon the health care setting, the EEG technician/technologist may schedule appointments and maintain EEG patient files.

**electroencephalography (EEG)**
A therapeutic service provided in many health care facilities. An EEG technician uses an electroencephalograph to record a patient's brain waves. Electrodes are attached to the patient's head and then recordings are made and interpreted by a physician.

**electromyograph (EMG)**
An electrical instrument that records the electrical activity of the muscles.

**electromyographic technician**
These individuals assist physicians in recording and analyzing bioelectric potentials originating in muscle tissue. This information is used to diagnose and monitor various disease processes. The electromyographic technician operates and helps maintain the various electronic equipment used to gather this information and assists in patient care and record keeping.

**electronic-computer system.**

**electronic data processing (EDP)**
Accumulation, analysis, processing of data through electronic computers.

**eleemosynary**
Charitable.

**element**
The first and most fundamental principal or part; a basic part.

**elephant policy**
See trolley car policy.

**elevator**

A device used to raise a broken bone of the skull or cheek. A plier/lever like device used to lift a tooth up and out of its socket during extraction.

**eligibility**

To be eligible for benefits under Medicaid, the individual has to meet the minimum guidelines which are established by each state as directed by federal guidelines. The four categories include: A.B.—Aid to the Blind, A.P.T.D.—Aid to the Permanently and Totally Disabled, O.A.A.—Old Age Assistance, A.F.D.C.—Aid to Families with Dependent Children. Medically needy recipients includes people in these categories whose incomes are enough to not meet public assistance eligibility, but it is still not sufficient to pay the medical bills. Medically needy also includes any person 21-64 years old who has a similar financial situation as provided in the previous sentence. What is covered by Medicaid is usually determined on a state by state basis and thus varies. The coverage, benefits and those needing assistance have changed to allow more health care to be provided to those in need medically. But the goals of a uniform program and to have the barriers of access to primary health care removed have not been totally met. However, a set of minimum benefits are available to those in need and access to health care has been increased.

**eligibility, Home Health Care (Medicare)**

In establishing Medicare eligibility for home health coverage, two major criteria must be substantiated: 1. The patient must be homebound; 2. The patient must be homebound because of medical necessity. Both criteria must be met in order to meet Medicare requirements. See homebound.

**eligibility period**

1. In insurance, this is the time allotted during which potential members may enroll in group life or health insurance programs without providing evidence of insurability. 2. The time period under a major medical policy during which reimbursable expenses can be accrued.

**eligible**

Legally qualified; eligibility for Medicare or Medicaid benefits means meeting all the legal requirements. Worthy of receiving. See eligibility.

**elimination period**

In insurance, the period of time after the beginning of a disability for which no indemnities are payable.

**elixir**

A liquid preparation usually containing alcohol, glycerin or syrup, which is used as a medium or vehicle to carry medicine or drugs.

**emancipated**

No longer under the control of another.

**emancipation**
1. Removal of control or influence. 2. Setting free; a child is emancipated when he is old enough so that the parents have no further control over or parental duties to him or her.

**embalming**
The process of preserving a dead body through the use of chemical compounds in order to delay putrefaction.

**embezzlement**
The fraudulent appropriation of money or goods entrusted to one's care by another.

**embolism**
The obstruction of a blood vessel; e.g., a blood clot, an air bubble.

**embracery**
Attempted corruption of a juror; jury fixing.

**emergency**
Any threat to life or health that is sudden and immediate.

**emergency admission**
Any emergency or surgery that needs to be cared for or treated immediately, as compared to elective admission or elective surgery which can be delayed without harm to the patient's health.

**emergency care**
Care for patients with severe, life-threatening, or potentially disabling conditions that require intervention within minutes or hours. Most hospitals and programs providing emergency care are also asked to provide care for many conditions which providers would not consider as emergencies, suggesting that consumers define the term more nearly synonymously with primary care and use such programs as screening clinics. See also emergency medical service system; care; emergency.

**emergency hospital services**
Also commonly referred to as emergency room (ER), emergency department, casualty ward, emergency ward (EW). This service or department provides immediate emergency care on a 24-hour basis for acutely ill or injured patients. Many patients using this service may not be acutely ill. Nurses, clerks, aides, technicians and other personnel also work in the emergency room. Some hospitals may have their own ambulance service to augment their emergency services. Emergency medicine is now a new medical specialty. Some hospitals contract emergency services out to a group of emergency physicians.

**emergency kit**
According to JCAH for psychiatric, alcoholism and drug abuse facilities accreditation purposes, this is a kit designed to provide the medical supplies and pharmaceutical agents required during an emergency. In compiling emergency kits, staff should consider the patients' needs for psychotropic, anticholinergic, and adrenalin agents.

**Emergency Medical Services System Act of 1973 (PL 93-154)**

Through PL 93-154, Congress mandated that emergency medical care must utilize a systems approach to providing emergency medical care. Fifteen elements of an emergency medical system were provided in this law, which include: 1) enough manpower to provide 24-hour care, 2) adequate training programs for all levels of EMS care on a regional level, 3) an emergency medical communication system, 4) transportation capabilities be made available on a regional level, 5) develop specialized emergency facilities, 6) critical care units be advanced, 7) integrate EMS with public safety agencies, 8) consumer participation, 9) insure availability and accessibility of care, 10) continuity in transfer of patients, 11) standardization of medical records, 12) consumer education be advanced, 13) review and evaluation be ongoing, 14) linkage to disaster programs, 15) regional and inter-regional mutual aid agreements be created.

**emergency medical service system (EMSS)**

An integrated system of appropriate health manpower, facilities and equipment which provides all necessary emergency care in a defined geographic area. The development of such systems is federally assisted under the Emergency Medical Services Systems Act of 1973, PL 93-154, in which the term is defined and the necessary components of the system listed (sections 1201 and 1206 of the PHS Act). One characteristic of such a system is a central communications facility using the universal emergency telephone number, 911, and having direct communications with all parts of the system with planned dispatching of cases to properly categorized facilities.

**emergency medical technician (EMT)**

Working as a member of an emergency medical team, the emergency medical technician (EMT) responds to and provides immediate care to the critically ill or injured and transports them to medical facilities. The EMT determines the nature and extent of illness or injury and establishes either first-aid procedures to be followed or need for additional assistance. EMTs administer prescribed first-aid treatment at the site of the emergency or in specially equipped vehicles. They communicate with professional medical personnel at emergency treatment facilities to obtain instructions regarding further treatment and to arrange for reception of victims at the treatment facility. EMTs have been classified into several levels: the EMT-A, EMT-1, or EMT-1A who provide basic life support outside of the hospital. EMT-Z is a rural paramedic who is qualified to provide advanced, as well as basic life support. EMT-T or EMT-3 is qualified to provide advanced cardiac and trauma life support under medical supervision. EMT-3 is also used synonymously with paramedic. Due to the confusion of trying to establish levels of EMTs, some states simply have EMTs, intermediate EMTs and paramedics, all based on levels of training.

**emergency services**

The rendering or administering of temporary medical help by responding to, evaluating, and assisting in emergency situations.

**emesis**
Vomiting.

**emetic**
Any substance that causes vomiting.

**eminent domain**
Right of the government to take private property for public use upon payment of compensation for it.

**emission standards**
The maximum amount of a pollutant allowed to be discharged from a single source.

**emolument**
Profits from employment or serving in an office, in the form of a salary, advantages, fees, or other gain.

**emotional deprivation**
Lack of sufficient and appropriate interpersonal relations and love, especially in the early developmental years. Separation from one's mother or poor mothering can contribute to this.

**emotional support**
Encouragement, hope and inspiration given to a person.

**empacho**
A Spanish term for a disease that occurs mostly in children. Characterized by a swollen abdomen as a result of intestinal blockage; surfeit, indigestion.

**empanel**
To have citizens serve as members of a jury. See impanel.

**empathy**
Ability to emotionally place oneself in another person's place, his frame of reference, and understand his feelings.

**empirical**
Based on or relying upon observation, experiment or research.

**emplead**
To accuse; to bring a charge.

**employee**
One who works for another in return for pay.

**employee benefit program**
Any or all work benefits not included in the employee's gross salary, provided by the employer. Medical/health insurance, disability income, retirement, and life insurance which is paid for all or in part by the employer.

**employee benefits**
The extra cost-related factors that offset employee salaries, including the amounts paid by the employer on behalf of the employees that are not

included in the gross salary. Such payments are usually considered overhead payments and are fringe benefits. While not paid directly to employees, they are a part of the cost of salaries and benefits; such as: group health or life insurance, contributions to employee retirement, professional fees, educational benefits, etc.

**Employee Health Insurance Plan (EHIP)**
One of the three parts of a national health insurance proposal.

**Employee Retirement Income Security Act (ERISA)**
An Act affecting the financial position of employees covered by a retirement plan. The act prescribes federal standards for funding, participation, vesting, termination, disclosure responsibility of fiduciary and tax treatment of private retirement plans. See Pension Reform Act of 1974.

**employer**
A person or organization that selects employees, pays their salaries, retains the power over dismissal and directs the employees' conduct during working hours.

**emptor (Lat.)**
A buyer; a purchaser.

**EMSS Act of 1973**
Emergency Medical Services System Act of 1973.

**E.M.T.**
Emergency medical technician. See these words.

**en (French)**
In.

**enable**
To give authority or power or opportunity to act.

**enabling clause**
The portion of a law that provides officials with power to put a statute into effect and to enforce it.

**enabling factor**
In health education planning, it is any environmental factor, skill or resource required to attain the desired health behavior.

**enabling statute**
A law that provides power to a public official or public office.

**enact**
1. To make into. 2. To put a law into effect; a bill passed by a legislature. 3. To establish a law; to decree.

**en banc (Lat.)**
On the bench. With all judges sitting in the court. See in banco.

**enceinte (French)**
Pregnant.

**encoding**
The use of specific signs and symbols to communicate a message.

**encopresis**
Involuntary passage of feces, usually during sleep.

**encounter**
A contact between a patient and health professional in which care is given. Some definitions exclude either telephone contacts or home visits. An encounter form records selected demographic diagnostic and related information describing an encounter.

**encounter group**
A sensitivity group conducted on the emotional insight level rather than on intellectual insight. It is often oriented to the here and now, with emphasis on developing awareness and improving coping behavior.

**encroach**
1. To gradually intrude; to advance beyond acceptable or prescribed limits. 2. The extending of one's rights over another person's rights. 3. To go beyond customary limits; inroads beyond proper or original limits.

**encumber**
1. To hold back an action. 2. To burden and load down with claims or debts. Making property subject to a charge. See also incumber.

**encumbrance**
To put a claim or lien on an estate; a claim or lien against property. Also see incumbrance.

**endemic**
A disease or disorder that is native to, limited to or restricted to a particular area.

**endogenous**
1. Coming from within. 2. Derived from within the body.

**endorse**
The writing of a name on a document. Also see indorse.

**endorsement**
1. Recognition by a state of a license given by another state, when the qualifications and standards required by the original licensing state are equivalent to or higher than those of the endorsing state. The licensee is relieved by endorsement of the full burden of obtaining a license in the endorsing state. There is not necessarily any reciprocity between the two states. 2. In health insurance this is a provision added to a subscriber contract whereby the scope of coverage is enlarged or modified; a rider.

**endoscope**
An instrument used to visually examine the interior of the rectum and sigmoid colon.

**endowment**
A fund, usually consisting of donations, set up for a public institution such as a hospital.

**enema**
The introduction of a solution into the rectum and sigmoid colon.

**enfranchise**
To make free; to naturalize; to allow political privileges.

**engage**
1. To promise or pledge. 2. Take part in or to do; to be involved in; to encounter.

**engagement**
A contract or an obligation; a promise; an agreement.

**en gros (Lat.)**
1. In gross. 2. Wholesale. 3. To buy in bulk or by the gross.

**engross**
Make a final or official copy of a document.

**enhancement**
To augment; to make higher; increasing or making larger; to make greater or better.

**enjoin**
1. To forbid; to prohibit; to stop by injunction; to command or require. 2. A court order to stop a person from doing something. 3. Directing a person or persons to refrain from doing certain acts or to begin doing some acts.

**enroll**
To agree to participate in a contract for benefits from an insurance company or health maintenance organization. A person who enrolls is an enrollee or subscriber. The number of people (and their dependents) enrolled with an insurance company or HMO is its enrollment. See also open enrollment.

**enrolled bill**
A bill that is in the process of becoming a law by passing it through the proper legislative process.

**enrolled member**
In health insurance, a subscriber, spouse or dependent child who has been enrolled in a program by completing the proper application and for whom payment has been received.

**enrollee**
1. One who is enrolled. 2. One who is entitled to receive a specific set of services from a group health plan or from insurance with prepayment usually a part of the plan accompanying enrollment.

**enrollment period**
Period during which individuals may enroll for insurance or health maintenance organization benefits. There are two kinds of enrollment periods, for example, for supplementary medical insurance of Medicare: the initial enrollment period (the seven months beginning three months before and ending three months after the month a person first becomes eligible, usually by turning 65); and the general enrollment period (the first three months of each year). Most contributory group insurance has an annual enrollment period when members of the group may elect to begin contributing and become covered. See also open enrollment.

**enter**
1. To introduce; to admit. 2. To put in writing. 3. To file. 4. To go into; to become a part of; to formally write in the court record.

**enteric-coated**
In drugs, a special coating used on tablets and capsules which delays release of the drug until it is in the intestines.

**entering judgment**
The formal recording of a court's final decision in the court's permanent records.

**entirety**
All; completely; a whole.

**entitle**
1. To give a title to; to be honored by a title. 2. To give claim to. 3. Right to something once you meet the legal requirements to get it.

**entitled**
One who has established eligibility. Any elderly person, 65 years or over, must apply, and establish with the Social Security Agency, before he or she is entitled to benefits before any benefits are payable. In cases where the person failed to establish eligibility by age 65, benefits may be made retroactive, but not to exceed one year. Protection begins at age 65, but has been interpreted to begin on the first calendar day of the month in which one becomes 65. Dependents may quality for benefits as well as the survivors of the deceased. Even aliens who have met certain resident requirements may qualify. See eligibility, medical eligibility.

**entitlement authority**
In the federal budget, legislation that requires the payment of benefits or entitlements to any person or government meeting the requirements established by such law. Mandatory entitlements include social security benefits and veterans' pensions. Section 401 of the Congressional Budget and Impoundment Control Act of 1974 placed restrictions on the enactment of new entitlement authority.

**entity**
An existence. A real item.

**entrapment**
An act by a law enforcement officer to induce a person to commit a crime that the person would not have done otherwise.

**entrust**
To deliver something to another with a mutual understanding as to its use, with the belief that the understanding will be honored. Also see intrust.

**entry-level health educator**
The point at which an individual is capable of performing the specifications of the role identified. Skills and knowledge necessary to perform the role can be obtained through successful completion of a bachelor's degree program at an accredited university or college with a major emphasis in health education. See health educator.

**entry, writ of**
A writ to recover real property wrongfully withheld.

**enure**
1. To take effect. 2. To a person's advantage. Also see inure.

**enuresis**
Bed wetting.

**envidia (Spanish)**
1. Envy; a grudge; emulation. 2. An emotional disorder existing among the Mexican-American culture, caused by envy, fear and anger, based on natural, emotional and supernatural forces.

**environment**
Any or all aspects, conditions and elements that make up an organism's surroundings and influence its growth, development, survival and behavior.

**environmental factors affecting the health of the residents**
A description of the environment in which the individual operates and how it affects his health.

**environmental health**
The field of environmental health is the process of health hazard identification, detection, management, and control. As this field has expanded over the past 20 years, so have the breadth and depth of knowledge required and the degree of responsibility conferred upon environmental health practitioners. These practitioners are known by the title sanitarians or environmentalists. Environmental personnel are involved in inspections and regulatory activities, overseeing interpretation and enforcement of laws related to health and safety of the public.

**environmental health engineer**
Applies engineering principles to the control, elimination and prevention of environmental hazards such as air pollution, water pollution, solids pollution and noise pollution. (sanitary engineer)

**environmental health technician**
Having completed training at the associate degree level, the technician assists in the survey of environmental hazards and performs technical duties under professional supervision in many areas of environmental health such as pollution control, radiation protection, and sanitation protection. (sanitary technician)

**environmentalist**
Minimum education at the baccalaureate level is required. Plans, develops, and implements standards and systems to improve the quality of air, water, food, shelter, and other environmental factors, manages comprehensive environmental health programs, and promotes public awareness of the need to prevent and eliminate environmental health hazards. (sanitarian)

**environmental quality management**
Those measures taken to protect the community from environmental hazards causing or contributing to disease, illness, injury or death. Environmental hazards include air, water, and noise pollution, as well as hazards related specifically to unsafe residential and community environs.

**environmental services**
Inspect, evaluate, and gather data for their use in the design, operation, and control of systems for prevention and elimination of environmental hazards.

**E.O.**
Executive order.

**eo nomine (Lat.)**
Under that name.

**E.P.A.**
Environmental Protection Agency.

**epidemic**
The outbreak of a disease or disorder that affects significant numbers of persons in a specific population at any time. High occurrence of a disease in many people for a given disease at a specific time or in rapid succession in an area.

**epidemiological diagnosis**
The process of determining the extent, distribution and causes of disease or health concerns in a specified population.

**epidemiology**
The study of the nature, cause, control and determinants of the frequency and distribution of diseases and disability in human populations. This involves characterizing the distribution of health status, diseases or other health problems in terms of age, sex, race, geography, etc.; explaining the distribution of a disease or health problem in terms of its causal factors; and assessing and explaining the impact of control measures, clinical intervention and health services on diseases and other problems. The epidemiology of a disease is the description of its presence in a

population and the factors controlling its presence or absence. See also incidence, prevalence, morbidity and mortality.

**epistaxis**
Nosebleed.

**E.P.S.D.T.**
Early and Periodic Screening Diagnosis and Treatment Program.

**Equal Employment Opportunity Act (EEO)**
See Equal Employment Opportunity Commission.

**Equal Employment Opportunity Commission**
United States agency created in 1964 to end discrimination based on race, color, religion, sex or national origin in employment and to promote programs to make equal employment opportunity a reality. The Commission reviews charges of discrimination and investigates accordingly. If there is a basis for the charge, the Commission will attempt to remedy the situation through conciliation, conference, persuasion, and, if necessary, through appropriate legal action.

**equal protection of laws**
A constitutional requirement. The government shall treat all people equally. It is restricted from setting up illegal categories to justify treating a person unfairly, based on race, religion, age or origin.

**equitable**
Just, reasonable, fair, honest, right; having equity.

**equity**
1. Fair treatment. 2. When the law is lacking, or does not cover an issue, then fairness is used to make the judgment; a court's power to use fairness where specific laws do not cover the situation. 3. Fairness; moral justness; fairness in a particular situation. 4. The owner's net value in property.

**equity court**
A special court which administers justice according to a sense of fairness.

**equivalency testing**
Testing intended to equate an individual's knowledge, experience and skill, however acquired, with the knowledge, experience and skill acquired by formal education or training. Successful completion of equivalency tests may be used to obtain course credits toward an academic degree without taking the courses, or a license which requires academic training without having the training. See also proficiency testing.

**E.R.**

**-er**
Emergency room. See emergency hospital services.
Suffix meaning one who.

**eremophobia**
Fear of being by oneself.

**ergo (Lat.)**
Therefore.

**erogenous**
Sexually sensitive to touch.

**erogenous zone**
Any sensitive, sensuous area of the body—principally the genitals, anus, and mouth—capable of being stimulated sexually.

**eros**
1. The god of love. 2. Referring to love, sexuality or sex drive.

**erotic stimuli**
Any stimuli or sensations that cause sexual excitement or arousal.

**erotomania**
Unhealthy preoccupation with sexual activities or fantasies.

**erratum (Lat.)**
Mistake. (singular) (errata, plural).

**error**
A serious enough mistake to entitle the losing party to have the case reviewed by an appellate court. A mistake made by a judge in the litigation process either in fact or in law. A mistake in judgment. An opinion that is or was wrong.

**error, law of**
See law of error.

**error, writ of**
See writ of error.

**erytophobia**
Fear of blushing.

**escalator clause**
A contract clause that allows rent or prices to be raised with rises in costs, expenses, inflation, or shortages.

**escheat**
The taking over of property by the state because of abandonment or lack of ownership.

**Escobedo Rule**
Escobedo v. Illinois, 378, U.S. 478 (1964). The case which gave rise to the ruling that a suspect must be warned of his right to remain silent and his right to an attorney.

**escrow**
To trust a document or money to a third party, to be delivered to the benefited party upon satisfaction of certain specified conditions or agreements.

**espanto**
A Spanish term for a disorder in which the individual is frightened as he or she claims to have seen supernatural spirits or events.

**esq.**
Esquire, a title given to lawyers.

**establish**
1. To appoint. 2. To demonstrate or prove; to prove a point. 3. Set up or create; to create a precedent.

**established name**
Name given to a drug or pharmaceutical product by the United States Adopted Names Council (USAN). This name is usually shorter and simpler than the chemical name, and is the one most commonly used in the scientific literature. It is the name by which most physicians and pharmacists learn about a particular drug product in their professional training. An example would be penicillin, a well-known antibiotic. Also known as the generic name or official name. An established name for drugs is required by section 502(e) of the Federal Food, Drug, and Cosmetic Act.

**established patient**
One known to the physician and/or whose records are normally available.

**Establishment Clause**
The First Amendment of the Constitution guarantees that "Congress shall make no law respecting an establishment of religion . . ."

**estate**
The extent, degree, nature or quality of interest in ownership of land.

**estate by the entireties**
A joint-tenancy between husband and wife with right of survivorship.

**estate for years**
An estate that terminates after a specified period of time or years; a leasehold.

**estate in severalty**
An estate held by a single person, with no one else holding an interest.

**estop**
To bar, preclude, or prevent.

**estoppel**
1. A bar. 2. A statement or admission that prevents the person making it from producing evidence to the contrary.

**estoppel by judgment**
Being barred from raising an issue against a person in court because a judge had already decided the issue.

**estoppel certificate**
A written statement by a mortgage company on the amount due on a particular date on a mortgage.

**estro-**
Prefix meaning female.

**ethical drug**
A drug which is advertised only to physicians and other prescribing health professionals. Drug manufacturers which make only or primarily such drugs are referred to as the ethical drug industry. Synonymous with prescription drug.

**ethical malpractice**
Any professional misconduct or negligence that is considered improper or immoral by a profession as a whole. See malpractice.

**ethics**
A system of morals, expectation and behaviors for all professionals, especially health care providers. Professional standards of conduct.

**ethnic**
Relating to cultures or races or to groups of people with similar traits and customs that are unique, yet common to the culture.

**ethnoscience**
Systematic approach to the study of the customs of a designated race or group in order to obtain accurate data regarding behavior, beliefs, perceptions, values and interpretations of life.

**etio-**
Prefix meaning cause.

**etiology**
The study of the causes of disease. The science of causes or origins; the study of beginnings or causes. See cause.

**et non (Lat.)**
And not. A phrase used in pleading, introducing negative arguments.

**et ux (Lat.)**
Et uxor. And wife.

**et vir (Lat.)**
And husband.

**euphoria**
An exaggerated feeling of well-being that is inappropriate for the actual experience at hand. It is often associated with opiate, amphetamine, and alcohol abuse.

**eustress**
Positive stressful events; euphoria. See benestressor.

**euthanasia**
1. Painlessly putting a person who suffers from a painful and incurable disease to death. 2. The act or practice of killing individuals (active) or allowing them to die without giving all possible treatment for their disease (passive), because they are hopelessly sick or injured, for reasons of mercy. See also hospice and death.

**evaluation**
The process of determining the degree to which an objective has been completed or met. It usually includes a review of the objectives, establishing the criteria used to measure degree of success; contrasting an object of interest with a standard or known expectancy.

**evasion**
1. Artful avoidance; to avoid a duty or a question by cleverness or deceit. 2. The act of not facing up to something or of avoiding it.

**eviction**
A landlord, hospital, nursing home, or other institution removing a tenant from the property either by taking direct action using force if needed or by going to court to get an order for removal.

**evidence**
1. Information, facts, observation, objects, recollections, papers, medical records, x-rays or other documents, records or forms presented at a trial or hearing. 2. Any facts, information or testimony that might be used in a trial to prove the alleged claims.

**evidence law**
The rules and principles controlling the testimony or documents that can be admitted or accepted as proof in a trial.

**evidence of insurability**
Any statement or proof of a person's physical condition or occupation affecting his acceptability for insurance.

**evidentiary fact**
A fact that is learned from evidence.

**ex-**
Prefix meaning out.

**ex (Lat.)**
A prefix, meaning: forth, out of, away from, no longer, from, thoroughly, because of, by, with, it appears as if.

**ex aequitate (Lat.)**
From or in equity.

**examination**
To examine, the act of searching or inquiring for facts or truth; questioning a witness in court.

**examine**
To inspect, scrutinize, investigate, and question.

**examiner**
Physician appointed by the Medical Director of a life or health insurer to examine applicants prior to purchasing a policy.

**except**
To eliminate or omit from consideration; to make an exception of; to take exception to, to exclude; to not include; to object to.

**exceptant**
One taking an exception during a proceeding.

**excepted period**
Time after the beginning date of a policy during which sickness benefits will not be payable. Also known as "waiting period."

**exception**
A formal disagreement with a judge's ruling. A statement that the lawyer does not agree with the judge's decision, and will save the objections until later.

**excise tax**
A single-stage commodity tax (i.e. a tax levied on a commodity only once as it passes through the production process to the final consumer). An excise tax is narrowly based; enabling legislation specifies precisely which products are taxed, as well as the tax rate. Sales taxes are more broadly based; their tax base comprises many commodities and legislation designates those commodities not subject to tax. Excise taxes are commonly assessed on automobiles, cigarettes, liquor or gasoline. They are sometimes levied in hopes of discouraging the use of the product taxed. Revenues from such taxes may also be set aside from general revenues and used for some purpose related to the taxed product. For example, an excise tax on cigarettes might discourage smoking by raising its cost and revenues from it might be used to fund cancer screening programs.

**exclusionary clause**
A part of a contract that restricts the legal remedies for one side if the contract is broken.

**exclusionary rule**
A rule to keep relevant but illegally obtained evidence out of a trial. The exclusionary rule often means that illegal evidence may not be used in a trial.

**exclusions**
1. Specific hazards, perils or conditions listed in an insurance or medical care coverage policy for which the policy will not provide benefit payments. Common exclusions may include preexisting conditions, such as heart disease, diabetes, hypertension or a pregnancy which began before the policy was in effect. Because of such exclusions, persons who have a serious condition or disease are often unable to secure insurance coverage, either for the particular disease or in general. Sometimes excluded conditions are excluded only for a defined period after coverage begins, such as nine months for pregnancy or one year for all exclusions. Exclusions are often permanent in individual health insurance, temporary (e.g., one year) for small groups in group insurance, and uncommon for large groups capable of absorbing the extra risk involved. 2. Specified illnesses, injuries, or conditions listed in an insurance policy for which the insurance company will not pay. Other common exclusions are self-inflicted injuries, combat injuries, plastic surgery for cosmetic reasons, and on-the-job injuries covered by Worker's Compensation.

**exclusions and limitations**
In health insurance, services, supplies, benefits or conditions that are excluded from or limited in an agreement.

**exclusive**
1. Limited; sole: one only. 2. Excluding or shutting out others; keeping out all but what was called for or specified.

**exclusive jurisdiction**
A jurisdiction in one court to the exclusion of all other courts.

**ex colore officii (Lat.)**
By color of office. An erroneous assumption of a right to perform an act by authority of one's office, status or position.

**ex contractu (Lat.)**
From a contract. One of the two sources of obligations and causes of action, the other is ex delicto—see this word.

**excreta**
Feces; urine; waste products eliminated by the body.

**exculpate**
1. To clear from a charge; to prove guiltless; to provide an excuse or justification.

**exculpation**
1. The act of exculpating. 2. The removal of a burden or duty.

**exculpatory**
1. To exculpate. 2. Excusing blame or actions; diminishing or extinguishing guilt or blame.

**exculpatory clause**
A provision in or stipulation in a document by which one party is relieved of responsibility or has the burden removed for things that go wrong or for losses incurred.

**excuse**
1. An explanation of justification for an act. 2. A plea offered in defense of one's unintentional act or conduct. 3. A false or pretended reason for one's acts.

**excuser**
One who pardons or excuses.

**ex delicto (Lat.)**
From a tort. One of the two sources of obligations and causes of action, the other is ex contractu (q.v.)—see these words.

**execute**
1. To fulfill; to put into effect; to complete; make valid. 2. To carry out; to perform all necessary formalities. 3. To make valid by signing and delivering a document.

**execution**
1. Making a document valid. 2. Carrying out or completing; carrying into effect. An official carrying out of a court order; effective action and completion. A writ of the court, allowing authority to place a decision into effect. 3. Putting someone to death.

**execution sale**
A sale made under proper court authority following a levy on property of a debtor.

**executive**
1. The branch of government empowered to carry out and administer the laws. 2. The administrative branch. 3. A high official in a branch of the higher levels of government, a hospital, company, or other organization.

**executive committee**
This is made up of the chiefs of departments and service, elected members of the staff, and other administrative officers, and is the major decision-making body for the medical staff.

**executive order**
1. A law or policy ordered by the chief officer of an organization. 2. A law set forth by the president or a governor that need not be passed by the legislature.

**executive session**
A meeting which is closed to the general public, being open only to the committee members, their staff and others specifically invited. Sometimes used synonymously with mark-up, especially in the House of Representatives where mark-ups are now rarely held in private.

**executor, executrix**
One with proper authority; one who is designated to administer and settle an estate.

**executory**
That which has yet to be performed; still to be carried out; incomplete.

**exemplary damages**
See damages, exemplary or punitive damages.

**exemplification**
An official transcript of a public document used as evidence.

**exempli gratia (Lat.)**
For the sake of example; for example. Abbreviated e.g. and used in writing.

**exemption**
Freedom from service, burden or tax.

**exercise physiologist**
Works with clinicians in hospitals with rehabilitation programs to provide exercise stress testing and cardiovascular rehabilitation for patients.

**ex gratia (Lat.)**
By grace; gratuitous.

**exhibit**
1. Any object or document offered to a court as evidence. 2. To administer a drug or other treatment as a cure or remedy.

**exhibitionism**
A form of sexual deviation characterized by a compulsive need to expose one's genitals.

**exhume**
1. To disinter; dig out of the ground or unbury. 2. To disclose or reveal.

**exigency**
A situation requiring immediate aid or attention.

**ex necessitate (Lat.)**
By necessity.

**ex officio**
1. By the power of office. 2. According to JCAH, it is position by virtue of, or because of, an office, with no reference to specific voting power. When a person is an ex officio member of a board or committee, he or she is allowed to attend and listen to all proceedings but has no say, input or vote.

**exoneration**
1. To unburden; to relieve or take away a charge or obligation. 2. Clearing a crime, a harm done, or wrongdoing.

**exorcism**
A spiritual practice where demons which are supposed to have entered a person's mind or body are removed.

**expanded functions**
Dental care clinical procedures formerly done solely by dentists that dental hygienists are now allowed to do depending on state laws. It varies from state to state according to individual state laws covering the practices of dental hygienists, such as delivery of local anesthesia, root planing, curretage, packing of amalgams, etc.

**expanded functions training program**
An educational program which has as its objective the education of individuals who will, upon completion of their studies in the program, be qualified to assist in the provision of dental care under the supervision of a dentist.

**ex parte (Lat.)**
With only one side present; partly; on behalf.

**expatriation**
Voluntarily giving up one's country to become a citizen of another.

**expectancy**
1. Something hoped for. 2. An interest in property which is vested, but possession is deferred until a future time.

**expectant right**
A right contingent on a set of circumstances that can occur in the future.

**expected date of confinement (EDC)**
Expected date of the birth of a baby.

**expected morbidity**
Expected incidence of sickness or injury within a given group during a given period of time as shown on a morbidity table.

**expected mortality**
Expected incidence of death within a given group during a given time period as shown in a mortality table.

**expedite**
To facilitate; to hasten.

**expediter**
One who expedites.

**expense**
1. Money laid out or expended; money paid out for needed goods or services. 2. Any great or undue cost or drain on the finances of a person or organization. 3. In insurance, the cost to the insurer of conducting its business other than paying losses, including acquisition and administrative costs. Expenses are included in the loading.

**experience rating**
A method of establishing premiums for health insurance in which the premium is based on the average cost of actual or anticipated health care used by various groups and subgroups of subscribers and thus varies with the health experience of groups and subgroups or with such variables as age, sex, or health status. It is the most common method of establishing premiums for health insurance in private programs. See also community rating.

**experimental group**
In research using an experimental design, the group to which the treatment under study is administered. See also control group.

**Experimental Health Service Delivery System (EHSDS)**
This was a system developed under a program supported by the Health Services and Mental Health Administration under general health services research authorities to develop, test and evaluate the organization and operation of coordinated, community-wide health service management systems (EHSDS) in various kinds and sizes of communities. EHSDS sought to improve access to services, moderate their costs and improve their quality.

**Experimental Medical Care Review Organization (EMCRO)**
An organization assisted by a program initiated in 1970 by the National Center for Health Services Research and Development (now the NCHSR). The program, a forerunner of the PSRO program, was set up to help medical societies in creating formal organizations and procedures for reviewing the quality and use of medical care in hospitals, nursing homes, and offices throughout a defined community. The use of explicit criteria and standard definitions were required of all EMCROs but the particular approach to organizing the review was determined by the individual organization. Ten such organizations were initially supported. The program was phased out after enactment of the PSRO program.

**expert witness**
A special person or professional possessing particular knowledge, expertise or experience who is called in to testify at a trial, presenting facts, specialized information and drawing professional conclusions based on facts concerning a case, or circumstances related to a case.

**expire**
1. A term somewhat inappropriately used by the health care community meaning "died" or "death" as in "the patient expired at 10:15 p.m.;" to conclude; to come to an end. 2. To close or conclude something that is renewable such as driver's license. 3. To give off; breathe out.

**explanation of benefits**
In insurance, it is a recap sheet that accompanies a Medicare or Medi-Cal check, showing breakdown and explanation of payment on a claim.

**explosive personality**
A personality disorder in which the person shows extreme anger and hostility.

**expository statute**
A law that explains the meaning of a previously enacted law.

**ex post facto (Lat.)**
After the fact.

**express**
1. Clear, direct or actual. 2. Unambiguous; definite; stated explicitly.

**express assumpsit**
An undertaking to perform some act, manifested in unmistakable terms.

**express consent**
Consent that is given directly either orally or in writing. Express consent is positive, honest, direct and unequivocal; no inference or implication to supply its meaning. (Pacific Nat. Agricultural Credit Corp. v. Hagerman, 40 N.M. 116, p. 2d 667, 670).

**expressio unius est exclusio alterius (Lat.)**
The expression of one thing rules out the other. A rule used for interpreting documents.

**express trust**
A trust created by express intent and terms of the settlor, as opposed to an implied trust.

**expropriation**
The taking of private property for public use.

**expunge**
To strike out; the blotting out of. Refers to police records when an inference might be drawn. To wipe it off the books.

**ex relatione (Lat.)**
Upon relation, when a case is titled "State ex rel. Doe v. Roe" it means that the state is bringing a lawsuit for Doe against Roe.

**ex tempore (Lat.)**
Without preparation.

**extended benefits**
Insurance coverage supplemental to either a basic hospital plan or a basic hospital-surgical-medical plan. Sometimes diagnostic x-ray and laboratory (DXL) examinations are covered on an outpatient basis.

**extended care**
Care provided in a nursing or convalescent home as opposed to care provided in a residence or hospital.

**extended care benefits (Medicare)**
Benefits in a skilled nursing facility that is approved by Medicare.

**extended care facility (ECF)**
1. A medical facility used for treatment of a patient after he or she is discharged from a hospital and still needs further specialized and continued care. 2. Previously used in Medicare to mean a skilled nursing facility which qualified for participation in Medicare. In 1972, the law was amended to use the more generic term skilled nursing facility for both Medicare and Medicaid. Medicare coverage is limited to 100 days of post hospital extended care services during any spell of illness; thus Medicare coverage in a skilled nursing facility is limited in duration, must follow a hospital stay, and must be for services related to the cause of the hospital stay. These conditions do not apply to skilled nursing facility benefits under Medicaid. Thus, the continued use of the term "extended care facility benefits" is a kind of shorthand to refer to the benefit limitations on skilled nursing facility care under Medicare.

**extended care services**
As used in Medicare, services in a skilled nursing facility provided for a limited duration (up to 100 days during a spell of illness) after a hospital stay, and for the same condition as the hospital stay was for. As defined under Medicare, the following items and services furnished to an inpatient of a skilled nursing facility are included: nursing care provided or supervised by a registered professional nurse; bed and board associated with the nursing care; physical, occupational, or speech therapy furnished by the skilled nursing facility or by others under arrangements with the

facility; medical social services; such drugs, biologicals, supplies, appliances and equipment as are ordinarily used in care and treatment in the skilled nursing facility; medical services provided by an intern or resident of a hospital with which the facility has a transfer agreement; and other services as are necessary to the health of the patients.

**extended coverage**
Provision in certain health policies, usually group policies, that allows the insured to receive certain benefits for specified losses sustained after termination of coverage; for example, maternity expense benefits incurred for a pregnancy in progress at the time of the insured's termination.

**extended duration review**
See continued stay review.

**extended family**
Includes the central or nuclear family plus other relatives such as uncles, aunts, grandparents, cousins, etc.

**extended service**
See service, also levels of service.

**extension**
1. An agreed-upon postponement of a planned legal proceeding. 2. A lengthening of time; allowing more time to pay a bill, pay off a loan, meet a contract, etc.

**extenuate**
To reduce; to mitigate; to diminish; to underrate or lessen.

**extenuating circumstances**
1. Circumstances that tend to diminish the severity of a crime and its punishment. 2. Facts that make a crime less awful or bad. It may not lessen the crime, but it does tend to lower the punishment.

**extern**
According to JCAH, this is a student in a recognized medical school who is employed by a hospital to perform specific supervised duties, with the approval of the dean of his school; or a student in a recognized dental school who is employed by a hospital with an organized dental service to perform specific supervised duties, with the approval of the dean of his school.

**external disaster**
According to JCAH for psychiatry, alcoholism and drug abuse facilities accreditation purposes, this is a catastrophe that occurs outside the facility and for which the facility, based on its size, staff, and resources, must be prepared to serve the community.

**externality**
In health economics, something that results from an encounter between a consumer and provider, which confers benefits or imposes costs on others, and is not considered in making the transaction (its value, the external cost, not being reflected in any charge for the transaction). Pollution is the classic example. In health, an externality of immunizations is the

protection that they give the unimmunized, since that protection is not considered when an individual immunization is obtained or priced.

**external reporting**
The reporting of financial activities to stockholders and the public.

**externship**
An educational training experience that occurs outside or external from the mother educational institution, such as a radiologic technologist student going into a hospital to gain practical experience taking x-rays and doing related work. This is similar to an internship. See internship.

**extinguishment**
1. To put an end to; to nullify. 2. The ending or stopping of a right, authority or power. 3. To wipe out or end, such as ending a contract or a vested interest.

**extort**
1. Misuse of authority to obtain something. The getting of something illegally. 2. To compel; coerce; for example, to force a confession by depriving a person of food. To get something by illegal threats of harm.

**extortion**
The illegal forceful taking of money by threats, force, or misuse of public office; blackmail or the selling of protection.

**extra cash policy**
An insurance policy which pays cash benefits to hospitalized individuals in fixed amounts unrelated to the individual's medical expenses or income. Such policies are usually sold to individuals separately from whatever other health insurance they have, and typically have high loadings.

**extradition**
A state turning over a person to another state when the second state requires the person for a criminal charge and trial.

**extrajudicial**
Unconnected with the business of the court or the litigation system.

**extrajudicial confession**
A confession made out of court. Whether or not it was made to an official of the court, it is still a confession.

**extra judicum (Lat.)**
Out of court; beyond jurisdiction.

**extraordinary remedy**
Actions a court will take if necessary. These can include habeas corpus and mandamus.

**extremis (Lat.)**
Last illness.

**extrinsic evidence**

Facts drawn from things outside a contract or document in question; evidence not found within a document, contract or agreement.

**eyewitness**

1. One who saw an illegal act occur; someone with first hand knowledge of an act. 2. Someone who can testify as to what he saw, heard or witnessed.

# F

**face of instrument**
The factual information of a document as expressed by the language used in the document, without any modification, interpretation or explanation or extrinsic facts added.

**face value**
1. The actual and obvious amount of value an instrument, item, goods or note has, as determined by the language used in the note itself. 2. The amount written on a financial document.

**facilities**
Buildings, including physical plant, equipment, and supplies, used in providing health services. They are one major type of health resource and include hospitals, nursing homes, and ambulatory care centers. Usually it does not include the offices of individual practitioners. According to JCAH accreditation, facilities are building(s), equipment, and supplies necessary for implementation of services by personnel. See health facilities.

**facility**
According to JCAH for psychiatric, alcoholism and drug abuse facilities accreditation purposes, this is an organization that provides psychiatric, substance abuse, and/or mental health services to patients.

**facsimile**
An exact copy.

**fact**
1. An act or an actual event or occurrence that took place; an actual happening. 2. Something that exists and is real; not what should be, but what is or has been; that which has taken place. 3. A physical object or appearance as it actually was at the time of the incident.

**facta sunt potentiora verbis (Lat.)**
Deeds are stronger than words.

**factor**
A broker; a commercial agent or servant utilized to sell goods entrusted to him by a principal or master. One who is provided with goods or items of value for the express purpose of marketing and selling them, thus receiving a commission for his business activities.

**factoring**
The practice of one individual or organization selling its accounts receivable (unpaid bills) to a second at a discount. The latter organization, called the 'factor,' usually but not always, assumes full risk of loss if the accounts prove uncollectible. In health services delivery, the

expression generally refers to a hospital's or physician's sale of unpaid bills to a collection agent. Factoring has sometimes been used in Medicaid because of the delays that hospitals and physicians experience collecting from the state Medicaid agency. In these cases, the improved cash flow is worth the discount in the amount received by the provider. Because factoring is subject to fraud and abuse, Congress has sought to prohibit some of its uses.

**fact situation**
A summary of the facts of a case or dispute without any legal conclusions drawn or interpretations or comments made.

**factum (Lat.)**
Act; fact; a central fact or an act, as distinguished from a legal concern which a question focuses on or can change a question.

**Fahrenheit (F)**
The temperature scale in most common usage in which the freezing point of water is 32° and the boiling point of water is 212°.

**failure**
1. Inadequate performance; abandonment or defeat. 2. Lack or deficiency. 3. An unsuccessful attempt or neglect of duty.

**failure of consideration**
1. Consideration once contemplated and paid for, loses or diminishes in value or is not completed. 2. A want for or lack of consideration; a contractual obligation unperformed. 3. Consideration that was once good which has become worthless or no longer exists, either all or in part.

**failure of evidence**
Failure to offer proof or to establish all the evidence related to an issue.

**failure of good behavior**
Reason for removal of a civil service employee, for doing behavior that is against recognized standards of conduct, morality and propriety.

**failure of issue**
How a will or deed is viewed in the event the person making it has no surviving children or never had any children.

**failure to cooperate**
Any intentional, material or fraudulent changes or variations of statements as given before or at a trial.

**failure to look**
Failing to see an object, item or event that was obvious, clear and within the range or normal vision of any ordinary person.

**failure to perform**
When reciprocal promises have been made and a person has not fulfilled the promise, it is viewed as a refusal to perform unless it is based on a previous set condition or circumstance.

**fainting**
A temporary loss of consciousness as a result of a diminished supply of blood to the brain; syncope.

**fair and impartial trial**
The safeguarding of and respect for an accused person's rights, with opportunity for a trial and the rights guaranteed by the Constitution.

**fair and reasonable compensation**
Paying full compensation.

**fair comment**
Under libel law and the First Amendment, the right to comment upon the conduct of public figures or officials without being held liable for defamation of character, slander or libel, as long as the statements made by the writer are done with an honest belief that they are true, even though they may contain comments not completely true.

**fair damages**
Recovery that is more than nominal damages so as to compensate for injury suffered.

**fair hearing**
1. Administrative agencies use this word to describe the trial-like decision-making process hearings which they use when a party appeals an administrative policy or decision. The hearing does not have to use full trial rules or procedures, but is supposed to be fair because authority is fairly exercised and accepted procedures and rules are used. 2. Under Medicare, it is an opportunity to be heard, as in judicial proceedings, upon request from a Medicare beneficiary when a request for Part B payment is denied or not acted upon within a reasonable length of time, provided the amount in controversy is over $100. The hearing is conducted by an impartial party and the decision of the hearing officer is final.

**fair knowledge and skill**
Health care providers are expected to have a reasonable level of knowledge or degree of skill.

**fair persuasion**
Argument, debate, exhortation and convincing conversation addressed to a patient without threat of physical harm, financial loss or persistent molestation, harassment or misrepresentation.

**fair use**
The limited use of something copyrighted without infringing on the copyright or committing plagiarism, usually the material is used in education or teaching and not used for moneymaking purposes.

**faith**
Confidence, trust, belief, unquestioning belief, reliable trust; good faith is showing honesty and sincerity.

**faith cure**
A religious or folk belief approach to healing or curing an illness. Curing through prayer and confidence and the laying-on-of-hands.

**faith healer**
A person or member of a religious group who assists in the curing of disease through faith and/or the laying on of hands. Also referred to as a faith curer.

**false**
Untrue; fake; unreal; phony; wrong.

**false arrest**
1. The unlawful restraint or deprivation of one's liberty; a tort. 2. Arrest without authority, authorization or a real reason.

**false imprisonment**
1. To hold a person against his will. 2. Unlawfully detaining, or constraining a person. 3. Arrest without authority, or justification. 4. To restrain or put restraints on a patient against his or her will.

**false negative**
A person wrongly diagnosed as not having a disease or condition which in fact he does have. See also false positive.

**false positive**
A person wrongly diagnosed as having a disease or condition when in fact he does not. When doing a medical screening or other diagnostic procedure it is important to know both how many false positives and false negatives the procedure gives in normal use. See also sensitivity and specificity.

**false pretense**
Deceit; a lie used to cheat a person out of his money, property or an item of value.

**falsus in uno (Lat.)**
In one false part. If a jury believes that one part of what a witness says is deliberately false, it may disregard all of the testimony or regard all previous statements as false.

**family**
1. A collective body of people living in one household related by blood, marriage or other legal arrangement. 2. A group of persons living together as a single unit. 3. Parents and their children. 4. Being related by blood or marriage. 5. For U.S. census purposes, a group of two or more persons related by blood, marriage, or adoption who are living together in the same household. 6. Group insurance and some national health insurance proposals offer coverage for eligible individuals and their families. In this context family usually refers to an individual and his dependents, which, since dependents do not necessarily have to be related to or living with the individual, is quite a different definition. The specific or detailed meaning is quite variable.

**family car doctrine**
The parent or legal guardian who owns a car will be liable for damage done by a family member driving the car.

**family expense policy**
A policy which insures both the policyholder and his immediate dependents.

**family ganging**
The practice of requiring or encouraging a patient to return for care to a health program with his whole family, even if the rest of the family does not need care, so that the program can charge the patient's third-party for care given to each member of the family. The practice and term originated and is most common in Medicaid Mills, which frequently have the mother of a sick child bring in all her other children for care whether or not they need it.

**family member**
In health insurance, spouse or any eligible children of the subscriber or the spouse who have been enrolled by the subscriber.

**family physician**
A physician who assumes continuing responsibility for supervising the health and coordinating the care of all family members regardless of age. Often in the past viewed as low-level generalists, however such physicians are now highly trained specialists whose work demands specific skills. These skills include functioning as medical managers, advocates, educators and counselors for their patients. See also personal physician, primary care, and general practitioner.

**family planning**
The use of a range of methods of fertility regulation to help individuals or couples to avoid unwanted births; bring about wanted births; produce a change in the number of children born; regulate the intervals between pregnancies; and control the time at which births occur in relation to the age of parents. It may include an array of activities ranging from birth planning, the use of contraception and the management of infertility to sex education, marital counseling and even genetic counseling. Family planning has succeeded the older term, birth control, which is now felt to be too negative and restrictive in meaning. Birth control can be separately defined as the prevention of pregnancy by contraception, abortion, sterilization or abstinence from coitus.

**fantasy**
1. An imagined mental picture or daydream. 2. An unrealistic belief or imagined occurrence that a person may actually think is real.

**farmer's lung**
A lung disorder caused by occupational exposure to fungal spores that grow in hay stored prior to proper drying. An acute form is reversible, but the chronic form can cause irreversible breathlessness. Prevention and avoidance is the best medical advice.

**fas (Lat.)**
Right; justice.

**fast**
1. To abstain from food for a long period of time. Secure or held firmly.

**fastigium**
The highest point of a disease or fever.

**fatal**
1. Causing death; capable of causing death. 2. An end. 3. A serious mistake in a legal procedure that could unfairly hurt the party who complains about it. 4. An error in the legal process which could cause a new trial or a default to occur.

**fatality ratio**
See case fatality ratio.

**fault**
1. To fail. 2. To be incorrect or wrong. 3. Guilty of an improper act, mistake or error; negligence; lack of care; failure to perform duty. 4. A defect or imperfection. 5. A wrongful act, omission or breach of duty. 6. Want of care. 7. Determining or fixing blame; to blame. See negligence.

**favorable selection**
See skimming.

**F.D.A.**
Food and Drug Administration. The branch of the U.S. Department of Health and Human Services regulating the safety of food, drugs, cosmetics, etc. See Food and Drug Administration.

**fear**
Unpleasurable or painful feelings with accompanying psycho-physiological response to a real or perceived threat or danger. See also anxiety.

**feasance**
To carry an obligation, duty or condition into effect. To perform an obligation.

**fecal impaction**
A mass of hardened, mostly dry feces packed into the folds of the rectum.

**feces**
The body waste discharged by the large intestine. The solid waste material that is eliminated and passed out through the anus. Also referred to as stool.

**federal**
1. Having to do with the major or central government. 2. Created and supported by a central authority in common affairs, such as the United States Federal Government.

**Federal Employees Health Benefits Program (FEHBP)**
The group health insurance program for Federal employees; the largest employer-sponsored contributory health insurance program in the world. It is voluntary for the employees; about 80% of those eligible being covered. At present it covers 8.8 million persons—2.8 million federal employees and annuitants and their 6 million dependents. It was established under the Federal Employees Health Benefits Act of 1959 (P.L. 86-382, codified in chapter 89, title V, U.S. Code), began operation in July, 1960, and is administered by the United States Civil Service Commission. Every employee may choose between two government-wide plans: a service benefit plan administered by Blue Cross and Blue Shield, and an indemnity benefit plan offered by the insurance industry through the Aetna Life Insurance Company. In addition to the two government-wide plans, there are fifteen employee organizations offering indemnity type plans to their members. An additional choice is available to employees residing in certain geographic areas where prepaid group practice plans are in operation.

**Federal Health Insurance Plan (FHIP)**
One of three health insurance proposals for national health insurance, also called the Comprehensive Health Insurance Plan.

**federalism**
Rules, constitutions or principles of a central controlling government.

**federalist**
One who works for or supports a central controlling government.

**Federal question**
A legal issue concerning the U.S. Constitution of any statute enacted by the U.S. Congress.

**federal questions**
Cases or disputes directly involving the U.S. Constitution or U.S. statutes.

**Federal Register**
1. A newsletter in which the rules and regulations of U.S. administrative agencies are published. Abbreviated "Fed. Reg." 2. An official, daily publication of the federal government providing a uniform system for making available to the public proposed and final rules, legal notices, and similar proclamations, orders and documents having general applicability and legal effect. The Register publishes material from all Federal agencies.

**federation**
A formal organization league or government united in a central power for a common goal or purpose.

**Federation Licensing Examination (FLEX)**
A standardized licensure test for physicians developed by the Federation of State Medical Boards of the U.S. for potential use on a nationwide basis. In fact, some 48 states now use the FLEX as their test for licensure, although they vary in the score required for licensure. The

FLEX exam is based on test materials developed by the National Board of Medical Examiners. See also national board examinations.

**feds**
Slang for any governmental agency and its employees.

**fee**
Payment requested for professional services. A monetary charge for services.

**feedback**
1. A positive or negative response to a system's output for the purpose of influencing a process. 2. In communication, it is the response.

**fee for service**
A method of charging patients for services or treatment whereby a physician or other practitioner bills for each patient encounter or treatment or service rendered. This is the usual method of billing by the majority of the country's physicians. Under a fee for service payment system, expenditures increase not only if the fees themselves increase, but also if more units of service are charged for, or more expensive services are substituted for less expensive ones. This system contrasts with salary, per capita or prepayment systems, where the payment is not changed with the number of services actually used or if none are used. While the fee-for-service system is now generally limited to physicians, dentists, podiatrists and optometrists, a number of other practitioners, such as physician assistants, have sought reimbursement on a fee for service basis. See also fee schedule, fractionation and capitation.

**fee schedule**
A listing of accepted charges or established allowances for specified medical or dental procedures. It usually represents either a physician's or third party's standard or maximum charges for the listed procedures. See also relative value scale.

**fee screen**
A term used by the Social Security Administration to describe the customary, prevailing, and reasonable charge amounts established for physician services by the carrier at the beginning of each fiscal year. It implies that charges (or fees) in excess of these computed rates are "screened out" thus providing payment to the physician by the carrier at a level lower than the actual charge. As a general term, fee screens is used synonymously with "prevailing charges" or "prevailings."

**fee simple absolute**
Real property wherein ownership is unconditional and without limitation.

**fee splitting**
An unethical practice referring to a physician, surgeon or consultant returning part of his fee to the referring physician for making the referral.

**fellatio**
Use of the mouth or tongue to externally stimulate the male genitalia.

**fellow**
The banding or associating together of persons with equal rank or position in a profession; a member of a professional or learned society or profession having the same standards and ideas, such as a Fellow in the American College of Hospital Administrators.

**fellow (mid or post residency)**
A graduate of a medical, osteopathic, or dental school who has had an advanced period of graduate training and is in a fellowship program in a subspecialty or in a clinical research program.

**fellow servant rule**
An employer is not responsible for injuries that one employee does to another if the employees were carefully chosen or if proper care was exercised to avoid the mishap.

**fellowship**
1. Being an associate; mutual association of professional persons on an equal basis who have the same occupations or interests. 2. A special endowment of money to provide support of a graduate student in a college or university; the rank of a fellow in a university.

**felon**
One who commits a felony or has been convicted of committing a felony.

**felonious**
1. Of the magnitude or extent to be felony. 2. With intent to commit a felony or major crime.

**felony**
A crime for which a person can be sent to a state prison. Usually based on the extent of seriousness of the crime, such as a specified dollar amount, which may vary in different states.

**felony murder**
A homicide committed while attempting a felony. A crime usually having a prison sentence of one year or more.

**felony-murder rule**
An accidental killing while committing a felony may make the accidental killing a murder.

**feme covert**
A married woman. Used to describe the legal disabilities of a married woman.

**feme sole**
A single woman, including those previously married.

**ferae naturae (Lat.)**
Wild animals. Animals that are naturally wild. The opposite of domitae naturae.

**fertility rate**

This rate is determined by comparing the fertility of different populations and standardized birth rates. These are often used to eliminate the effect on the birth rate of differences in structure of the population (most commonly the age and sex structure). A measure of the general fertility rate is computed by dividing total live births occurring in one calendar year by the mid-year population of women aged 15 to 44.

**fetal heart monitor**

A specialized electronic instrument with highly sensitive sensors that are attached to the outside of a mother's stomach in the last hours of labor. The sensors pick up the fetal heartbeat and this activity is recorded on a graph and/or is shown on an oscilloscope. From watching the readout on the graph or on the oscilloscope, ths physician can tell if the baby is going through the stress of labor in a normal way, or if the baby is in distress.

**fetishism**

Achieving sexual excitement from an inanimate object—such as a piece of underwear. An article of clothing that is a sex symbol. A deviant form of sexual behavior.

**fetus**

The unborn developing baby from the third month of pregnancy until birth.

**fever**

A rise in the body temperature above the normal temperature of 98.6°F or 37°C (oral temperature). Also referred to as pyrexia.

**ff. (abbrev.)**

Following (pages).

**fiat (Lat.)**

"Let it be done"; a command or order given through legal authority; an authorization or directive.

**F.I.C.A.**

Federal Insurance Contributions Act; the Social Security tax taken out of one's pay check or income.

**fiction, legal**

To use something that is false or non-existent as if it is true or real. Legal fictions are created and used to help do justice.

**fictitious**

Fake; false; not real; made up; imaginary; counterfeit; not genuine.

**fictive**

Fictitious.

**fidelity bond**

A guarantee of a person's honesty; indemnity against dishonesty and negligence.

**fides (Lat.)**
Faith, *bona fides* means good faith; *mala fides* means bad faith. See these terms.

**fiduciary**
Relating to or founded upon a trust or confidence. A fiduciary relationship exists where an individual or organization has an explicit or implicit obligation to act in behalf of another person's or organization's interests in matters which affect the other person or organization. A physician has such a relation with his patient and a hospital trustee with a hospital. Because a — relationship with a provider obligates one to act in the interests of the provider, people with such relationships are defined as providers by P.L. 93-641, rather than as consumers, for such purposes as determining whether a health systems agency governing board has a consumer majority. Any relationship based on trust and confidence. A relationship and commitment between two persons in which one person acts for another in a position of trust; these can include a physician and patient or psychotherapist and client; parent and child; minister and members of his church. See trust, trustee.

**fiduciary relationship**
See fiduciary.

**field experience**
An on-the-job educational and training experience in a health agency, institution or facility. Synonymous with internship and externship. See these words.

**FIFO**
"First in, first out," a method of calculating merchandise or inventory.

**Fifth pathway**
One of the several ways that an individual who obtains all or part of his undergraduate medical education abroad can enter graduate medical education in the United States. The fifth pathway provides a period of supervised clinical training to students who obtained their premedical education in the United States, received undergraduate medical education abroad, and pass a screening examination approved by the CCME. When these students successfully completed a year of clinical training sponsored by a U.S. medical school they then become eligible for an AMA approved internship or residency.

**filiation proceeding**
Same as a paternity suit. See these words.

**filibuster**
Stopping or slowing legislative action by the making of long speeches or the introduction of irrelevant information.

**film badge**
A piece of photographic film that is darkened by nuclear radiation. Radiation exposure can be checked by inspecting the film, which is worn like a badge by nuclear workers, radiologists and radiological technologists.

**final argument**
In a trial, when each side delivers their final statement to the jury, presenting how they perceive the facts and how they think law, fairness and justice applies to these facts.

**final decision**
1. The last decision of a court; the one upon which an appeal can be based. 2. The last decision of a court from which there are no more appeals.

**final disposition**
A final judgment before the court; a final decision establishing the rights and obligations of the parties involved in a dispute or action.

**financial feasibility**
The evaluation of a proposed health care service in terms of its ability to pay the costs of its operation. The analysis of the financial feasibility of an addition to the health care system is measured by matching the reasonable revenues to be received to the costs of the activity.

**finder's fee**
A fee paid to a person for finding business or referring business to another person.

**finding**
1. A determination of a question of fact. 2. A decision about evidence. 3. A conclusion of law.

**fire participation/wall**
For JCAH longterm accreditation, it is a wall or barrier constructed to resist the passage of both fire and smoke for a minimum of two hours under fire conditions. Such walls are required to separate patient/resident-occupied areas from other areas or to separate conforming and nonconforming structures.

**firm offer**
A written offer or agreement between a customer and a merchant that will be held open for a certain period of time. An offer in which terms of a deal give assurance that it will be held unrevokable for lack of consideration for a reasonable time.

**first aid**
The first and immediate emergency care and treatment given to a person who has been injured or is suddenly ill. It includes self-help and home emergency care. Emergency care is given until advanced and complete medical care is secured.

**first-dollar coverage**
Coverage under an insurance policy which begins with the first dollar of expense incurred by the insured for the covered benefits. Such coverage, therefore, has no deductibles although it may have copayments or coinsurance. See also last dollar coverage.

**first impression, case of**
A case presenting a question of law never previously considered for which no precedent has been set.

**first intention healing**
Primary or the first healing that occurs in an injury or wound when the tissues have been closed or pulled together.

**fiscal**
Pertaining to financial matters or budget periods. A fiscal year is a budget year. Related to the management of money. See fiscal year.

**fiscal agent**
1. An agent or insurance company that processes claims and issues payment for state or federal health insurance agencies or other insurance companies. 2. A contractor who is responsible for processing claims for health care services provided by health care practitioners and institutions to Title XVIII beneficiaries or Title XIX recipients. Title XVIII fiscal agents are known specifically as intermediaries and carriers.

**fiscal intermediary**
A contractor that processes and pays provider claims on behalf of a state Medicaid agency. Fiscal agents are rarely a risk, but rather serve as an administrative unit for the state, handling the payment of bills. Fiscal agents may be insurance companies, management firms, or other private contractors. Medicaid fiscal agents are sometimes also Medicare carriers or intermediaries. See intermediary

**fiscal management**
According to JCAH for psychiatric, alcoholism and drug abuse facilities accreditation purposes, These are procedures used to control a facility's overall financial and general operations. Such procedures may include cost accounting, program budgeting, materials purchasing and patient billing.

**fiscal resources**
The financial disbursements needed to accomplish the goals and objectives stated in the HSP.

**fiscal year**
Any twelve month period for which annual accounts are kept. Sometimes, but by no means necessarily, the same as a calendar year. The federal government's fiscal year was from July 1 to the following June 30 for years, but changed in 1976 to be from October 1 to the following September 30.

**fishing expedition**
1. Using the courts or questioning a witness to uncover information or facts that are suspected but have not been brought out or proven. Using a court to get information that is not actually a part of a lawsuit. 2. Irrelevant questioning of a witness. 3. A broad and probing use of the discovery process.

**fixed asset**
A physical and tangible item like a building, machine, vehicle etc. essential to the operation of a business, and to which a dollar value can be fixed.

**fixed charges**
Set fees; set costs or expenses. 2. Hospital operation costs that continue whether or not profits come in; such as rent.

**fixed costs**
Costs which are constantly incurred regardless of the volume of income or business and which do not vary with utilization rates; such as rent, leases, utilities. Also called constant costs.

**flagellantism**
Sexual arousal or gratification achieved from whipping or being whipped.

**flagrante delicto (Lat.)**
In the act of commiting a crime.

**flat maternity**
A single inclusive maternity benefit for all charges incurred as a result of pregnancy, childbirth, and complications arising therefrom. A limit (such as $1,000) may be applied per pregnancy or per year. See also switch and swap maternity.

**flatulence**
The presence of excessive gas in the intestines.

**flatus**
Gas or air in the stomach or intestines.

**flexible budgeting**
An accounting method that uses the concept of fixed and variable costs and is adjusted for actual level of operations.

**flexion**
Decreasing the angle of a joint in a limb; the act of bending.

**flight of ideas**
Rapid succession of thoughts without any logical association.

**flim-flam**
A trick or game aimed at deceit. Trickery.

**floating capital**
The capital at hand that is used to meet current or due expenses.

**flora; microflora.**
Microorganisms present in certain situations such as intestinal flora.

**flow chart**
1. A diagram used to show an organizational structure, a staffing procedure or steps in a process, method or system in planning, or a health care management procedure. 2. In computerized business or medical records, it is a diagram showing the sequence of data processing

operations. In data processing it is a graphic representation for the definition, analysis or solution of a problem in which symbols are used to represent data processing operations, data flow, and equipment.

**flow chart symbol**
A symbol used to represent operations, direction, data flow, or equipment in a problem. Used in flow charting and data processing.

**flow line**
Used in data processing and flow charting; a line representing a connecting path between symbols on a flow chart.

**fluorescein angiography**
A photographic technique formulated by Novotney and Alvis in 1961 that uses injection of an intravenous bolus of sodium fluorescein, then taking rapid sequential photographs of the vasculature of the retinal areas as the dye enters the vascular system.

**fluoridation**
The addition of controlled, small amounts of fluoride to public water supplies for the purpose of reducing the incidence of dental cavities in the public using the water.

**fluoroscopy**
Radiologic or diagnostic study using a fluorescent screen rather then x-ray film.

**flush**
Redness of the skin, usually of the face and neck.

**F.O.B.**
Free on board. (See these words) The price of merchandise including freight and transportation.

**focus**
1. The point of convergence of light rays or sound waves. 2. The principal site of an infection. 3. The main emphasis of treatment or therapy.

**fomite**
Any inanimate object which carries, spreads or harbors pathogens and is capable of transmitting a disease.

**fontanel, fontanelle.**
A baby's soft spot; one of the spaces in the skull of an infant, which has a membrane and skin covering.

**Food and Drug Administration (FDA)**
An agency of the Department of HHS with responsibility for protecting the public against poisoning, contamination or any other health hazards in foods, food substances, food additives. This agency also assumes the safety and effectiveness of drugs and drug substances. The FDA has six subagencies 1) Foods, 2) Drugs, 3) Biologics, 4) Radiological Health, 5) Medical and Diagnostic Products, 6) Veterinary Medicine. The National

Center for Toxicological Research is also a separate subagency of the FDA.

**food poisoning**
The eating or consuming of food products contaminated by microorganisms or toxins resulting from bacteria or insecticide residues. Most common bacterial food poisonings are salmonella, staphylococcus, clostridium welchii, and clostridium botulinum (botulism).

**food protection**
Those measures taken to assure wholesome and clean food free from unsafe bacteria and chemical contamination, natural or added deleterious substances, and decomposition during production, processing, packaging, distribution, storage, preparation and service; and to assure that marketed foods comply with established nutritional quality and packaging identification guidelines.

**foodservice systems management**
An array of components formed into a unified whole to perform a systematic, purposeful activity. When used in conjunction with foodservice, it would be the components that make up the production and service of food.

**footboard**
A board placed at the foot of a bed so a patient can brace his feet against it.

**forbearance**
1. A delay in enforcing rights. 2. Refraining from action on a case.

**force**
1. Co compel; a binding power. 2. Violence that is unlawful. 3. To strengthen power, authority or validity.

**forced sale**
A sale made to pay off a judgment ordered by the court, and done according to rules set by the court.

**force majeure (French)**
A major force; superior power or force; irresistible force.

**forcep**
A surgical instrument with two blades and handle used to handle sterile supplies or to compress or grasp tissues.

**foreclosure**
Forcing the payment of a debt through seizing and selling the property or security for the debt, usually related to a mortgage.

**foreign corporation**
Distinguished from a domestic corporation. An alien corporation is incorporated outside the United States, its territories or a state.

**foreign jurisdiction**
A jurisdiction other than the one in which the court sits.

**foreign medical graduate (FMG)**
A physician who graduated from a medical school outside of the United States and, usually, Canada. U.S. citizens who go to medical school outside this country are classified as foreign medical graduates (sometimes distinguished as USFMGs), just as are foreign-born persons who are not trained in a medical school in this country, although native Americans represent only a small portion of the group. The term is occasionally defined as, and nearly synonymous with, any graduate of a school not accredited by the LCME. See also COTRANS, ECFMG, fifth pathway, J visa, labor certification, schedule A, medical graduate, foreign.

**forensic**
Having to do with law. The legal aspects of a profession other than the legal profession, such as forensic psychiatry.

**forensic dentistry**
See dental jurisprudence

**forensic medicine**
Medical knowledge related to law and to the solving of legal issues in health care and medicine. Medical jurisprudence; health care law.

**forensic pathologist**
A medical doctor who specializes in the legal ramifications of an unnatural death. He is often a coroner or works with a coroner and investigates unnatural or suspicious deaths through autopsy, testing and other medical modalities.

**forensic psychiatry**
The branch of psychiatry that is concerned with legal aspects of mental illness and mental health care.

**foreplay**
Purposeful sexual contact or sensual petting that increases sexual arousal prior to intercourse; precoital stimulation.

**foreskin**
The loose skin covering the shaft of the penis; also referred to as prepuce.

**forfeit**
1. To lose or give up. 2. To lose a right due to some fault, crime, error, being negligent in a duty, or breach of contract.

**forgery**
1. Making a fake or fradulent document. 2. Intent to commit fraud by fabricating or altering something like a record or signature.

**formal party**
Involved in a lawsuit in name only; having no interest in a legal proceeding, but named in it.

**formication**
The sensation of ants running over the skin. It is commonly experienced in delirium tremens and cocainism.

**forms of action**

1. The special and technical way each different type of lawsuit formerly was filed. 2. Classes or types of private or common law related to personal actions.

**formula grant**

A grant of federal funds, usually to states but sometimes to other governmental units or private organizations, authorized by law for specified purposes in which the amount of the grant is based on a formula which divides the total funds available among the eligible recipients according to such factors as the number and average income of the population to be served.

**formulary**

1. A listing of drugs, usually by their generic names. A formulary is intended to include a sufficient range of medicines to enable physicians or dentists to prescribe medically appropriate treatment for all reasonably common illnesses. A hospital formulary normally lists all the drugs routinely stocked by the hospital pharmacy. Substitution of a chemically equivalent drug is filling a prescription by brand name for a drug in the formulary is often permitted. A formulary may also be used to list drugs for which a third party will or will not pay, or drugs which are considered appropriate for treating specified illnesses. 2. According to JCAH for psychiatric, alcoholism and drug abuse facilities accreditation purposes, this is a catalog of the pharmaceuticals approved for use in a facility. A formulary lists the names of the drugs and information regarding dosage, contraindications, and unit dispensing size. See compendium, National Formulary.

**fornication**

Sexual intercourse between unmarried persons which can be viewed as unlawful.

**for-profit hospital**

See hospital, proprietary.

**forseeability, doctrine of**

1. A person is responsible and liable to know about potential natural and proximate results of any act to another person to whom a duty is owed. 2. Ability to predict or see beforehand. 3. What a prudent, careful, ordinary and thoughtful person or professional under similar circumstances, with similar training and skills, would expect or predict to happen. 4. Alertness to possible future hazards that could exist in a certain behavior, event or act. See ordinary person, reasonable man.

**forswear**

1. To falsely swear to; similar to perjury. 2. To make an oath to or to swear to that which a person knows is untrue or false.

**forthwith**

Immediately or as soon as possible.

**Fortran (formula translation)**
In computers, any of several programming languages, closely resembling the language of mathematics.

**fortuitous**
By chance; an accidental occurrence.

**forum. (Lat.)**
A court; the court in which an action is heard.

**forum non conveniens (Lat.)**
Court of inconvenience. A court may refuse to hear a case if it is believed that by doing so it might cause an undue hardship to the defendant. Forum non conveniens assumes that there is a competent jurisdiction where the case may be heard.

**forward funding**

**foundation for medical care (FMC)**
When an agency or organization obligates or sets funds aside in the same year for anticipated needs in subsequent fiscal years. See advance appropriation.
An organization of physicians, sponsored by a state or local medical association, concerned with the development and delivery of medical services and the cost of health care. See medical foundation.

**four corners**
1. Refers to all information in a document but excludes all other related material not in the document. 2. In reference to the face of a written document. 3. The examination, writing and construction of the document as a whole. See face.

**Fowler's position**
A bed-sitting position where the head of the bed is raised and the knees elevated.

**fractionation**
The practice of charging separately for several services or components of a service which were previously subject to a single charge or not charged for at all. The usual effect is that the total charge is increased. The practice is most commonly seen as a response to limiting increases in the charge which is fractionated.

**fracture board**
A support board placed under the mattress of a bed to provide added support.

**franchise**
A special privilege granted by the government to operate a regulated monopoly by corporations to use trade names in marketing a product.

**franchise insurance**
A form of insurance in which individual policies are issued to the employees of a common employer or the members of an association

under an arrangement by which the employer or association agrees to collect the premiums and remit them to the insurer.

**frank**
Freely speaking or admitting; free.

**franking privilege**
Sending materials or mail through the U.S. mail service without paying postage.

**fraternal insurance**
A cooperative type of insurance provided by social organizations for their members.

**fraud**
1. Something done or said to deceive. 2. An act of deceit, deception or trickery. 3. Knowingly using a means to cheat someone. 4. Intentional misrepresentation by either providers or consumers to obtain services, obtain payment for services, or claim program eligibility. Fraud may include the receipt of services which are obtained through deliberate misrepresentation of need or eligibility; providing false information concerning costs or conditions to obtain reimbursement or certification, or claiming payment for services which were never delivered. Fraud is illegal and carries a penalty when proven. See also abuse.

**frauds, staute of**
Statutes patterned after an English law (statute) of 1677, which required certain instruments and sales of some goods, to be in writing to avoid fraud and perjury.

**fraudulent**
Cheating; deceitful; under false pretense.

**fraudulent concealment**
Hiding or suppressing a fact or circumstances which a party to a lawsuit is legally or morally bound to provide or disclose.

**fraudulent conveyance**
A transfer of property to someone else in order to cheat the person who has a right to it out of the property.

**F.R.C.P.**
Federal Rules of Civil Procedure.

**free clinics**
Neighborhood clinics or health programs which provide medical services in relatively informal settings and styles to, generally, students, transient youth, and minority groups. Care is given at no or nominal charge by predominantly volunteer staffs.

**freedom of speech**
A Constitutional right guaranteed by the First Amendment. Freedom to speak as long as it does not interfere with or infringe upon others' rights.

**free exercise clause**
The First Amendment of the U.S. Constitution guarantees that "Congress shall make no law . . . prohibiting the *free exercise* of religion, speech . . ."

**free floating anxiety**
Unfounded or unrealistic fear or worry that is not associated with any specific idea or attached to an object or event.

**free noncontractual patient**
A patient for whom a facility, physician or clinic agrees to provide facilities and services for which no bill is rendered.

**free on board**
Goods for shipment are to be loaded without expense or charge. Abbreviated F.O.B.

**free-standing support setting**
A location where health services are provided which support the delivery of personal health care services without providing direct patient care, and which is not a component of an organization which delivers personal health care services in another setting. Example: pharmacy.

**frequency distribution**
A table used in statistics which shows the number of observations in a group; for example, the numbers of persons with a specific disease in certain age groups.

**friction**
Rubbing; that force which opposes motion; when two objects are rubbed together.

**friendly suit**
A legal proceeding initiated by a friendly agreement; a lawsuit used to settle a point of law affecting opposing parties who are friendly.

**frigidity**
Coldness toward sexual activity; lack of sexual desire; inability to have an organism or sexual excitement. May affect either sex, but usually refers to the female.

**frivolous**
Having no legal value or meaning. Being of little legal worth.

**frolic**
An act by an employee or health care provider that has nothing to do with what he is employed to do.

**frotteur**
One who is sexually aroused by bumping into or rubbing against someone in a crowd; not necessarily associated with touching or contact of the genitals.

**fructus industriales (Lat.)**
Industrial fruits. Products of labor and industry; i.e. drugs produced by pharmaceutical manufacturers. Opposed to *fructus naturales,* the products of nature—minerals; fruit from trees.

**fructus naturales (Lat.)**
Natural fruits or products of nature, such as minerals or orchard fruit from trees. Opposed to *fructus industriales.*

**frustration**
In psychiatry, an emotional upset state caused by stopping a drive or by blocking an attempt to accomplish. This can lead to hostility.

**frustration of contract**
When the chance for completing an agreement has become impossible due to a change that is not the fault of the persons establishing the contract.

**F.Supp.**
Federal Supplement. See National Reporter System.

**F.T.C.**
Federal Trade Commission. The federal agency that enforces prohibitions against unfair competition and unfair or deceptive acts and trade practices.

**F.T.E.**
Full time equivalents. See staffing ratio, full time equivalent.

**fugitive from justice**
One who has committed a crime and flees to avoid prosecution.

**fugues**
A state where a person unconsciously wanders about, performing involuntary acts. Also see ambulatory automatism.

**full costs**
Total costs incurred to provide a service, accomplish an activity or complete a program.

**full disclosure**
In finances it is a procedure requiring that all significant information on a health care facility's financial positions and operations be presented in the financial statements.

**full faith and credit**
1. Each state must recognize and respect laws and cases from other states when appropriate. 2. A judgment rendered in a foreign jurisdiction has the same effect and obligation and force in other states as it has in the state where it was handed down. U.S. Constitution; Article IV, Section 1.

**full-time equivalent (FTE)**
The number of physicians or employees who work for or provided service to a hospital, facility, college, clinic, etc. during a specific period. One

person working full time for a full year equals one full time equivalent. One person working full time for a six month period equals .50 FTE, while one person working half time for one full year also equals .50 FTE.

**full-time staff**
Physicians and other health care professionals and support personnel who work full-time in the health care facility, paid by the hospital, facility, or medical school, and are distinguished from the visiting staff, who are physicians or allied health care providers who are in private practice earning their livelihood through charges to patients.

**fully delegated hospital**
See delegated hospital.

**function**
1. A collection of related activities that must be performed to fulfill an area of responsibility. 2. A specific or special duty or performance required of a professional in the course of his work. A normal or expected action.

**functional age**
A measure of one's age based on ability and performance capacities rather than chronological age.

**functional classification**
In the federal budget, a means of presenting budget authority, outlay, and tax expenditure data in terms of the principal purposes which federal programs are intended to serve. Each specific account is generally placed in the single function (e.g., national defense, health) that best represents its major purpose, regardless of the agency administering the program. The Congressional Budget and Impoundment Control Act of 1974 requires the Congress to estimate outlays, budget authority, and tax expenditures for each function. Functions are subdivided into narrower categories called subfunctions.

**functional illiterate**
One who is not able to read at the level needed to exist and function in a complex society.

**functional maintenance services.**
Equivalent to rehabilitation services. (JCAH)

**functional obsolescence**
A need to replace equipment of facilities because they have become inefficient due to new developments being discovered or invented since its original purchase or construction.

**fund**
1. Any sum of money kept available for use upon demand; a collection of money allocated for a specific use. 2. Having a store or stock of something.

**funded**

In insurance, having sufficient funds to meet future liabilities. Can also be used in speaking of trust funds for social insurance programs. Capital depreciation is said to be funded if the amounts included in an institution's reimbursements for capital depreciation are set aside in a fund used for capital purposes rather than being spent on current operating costs. Few third party payers which reimburse capital depreciation require that it be funded as a condition of reimbursing it.

**fund-raising**

Also called development or hospital development. It is a temporary or permanent department that solicits gifts, money and other donations for the hospital. Some hospitals have this position as a top administrative position while others put less status on it.

**fungible goods**

Goods that are to be uniform; one unit is equivalent to any other of the same product; e.g., a liter of plasma is interchangeable with another.

**futures**

1. Speculative transactions. 2. For delivery at a future time. 3. Related to contract law in that an agreement is made to buy or sell at a set price and by a certain date.

**F.Y.**

Fiscal year.

# G

**gainful**
Profit producing, advancing, productive, as in gainfully employed.

**gamophobia**
Fear of marriage.

**G.A.O.**
General Accounting Office. The office that assist the U.S. Congress in financial matters.

**gaol**
Jail.

**garisher**
One who garnishes or serves garnishment on another.

**garnishee**
One who holds money or property of a defendant and is ordered to hold it until a lawsuit is settled, or in order to pay to a judgment creditor.

**garnishment**
1. Legal summons to a person not involved in a legal proceedng to appear in a lawsuit. 2. A legal proceeding through which a person's wages are withheld and given to a person to whom a debt is owed. 3. A legal notice to hold and not dispose of a defendant's property until a lawsuit is settled.

**gastric**
Pertaining to the stomach.

**gastric decompression**
The aspiration or removal of gastric contents, fluids or gas using a syringe or suction machine.

**gastric gavage**
A method of artificial feeding using gastric intubation.

**gastric intubation.**
To insert a tube into the stomach for therapeutic or diagnostic purposes.

**gastric lavage.**
To administer and then siphon back a liquid or solution through a catheter that has been introduced into the stomach.

**gastroenteritis**
Inflammation of the stomach and the intestines.

**gastroscope**
A lighted endoscope used to visually examine the stomach.

**gastroscopy**
The examination of the stomach with an endoscope/gastroscope.

**gavage**
A method of feeding through a tube. Usually it refers to the artificial feedng through a tube inserted down into the stomach. This is not a common method of tube feeding and is used mostly on patients who are unwilling or unable to eat food in the normal manner.

**Geiger counter**
A gas-filled electrical instrument used to count the presence of atomic particles or rays.

**gender role**
All that a person says or does to indicate a person's role as a male or female. One's maleness or femaleness.

**gene**
The biologic unit that is the determiner of one's heredity located on a chromosome.

**general adaptation syndrome (GAS)**
The body's general response or coping to stressors.

**general denial**
Used in a pleading to deny every allegation set forth in a complaint.

**general execution**
A court order to seize personal property of a defendant to be used to pay off a judgment brought against the defendant. This is executed by an official of the court.

**general hospital**
See hospital, general.

**general issue**
An answer to a complaint. See general denial.

**general jurisdiction**
A court's ability to rule over any controversy that may be brought before a court within legal bounds of a person's rights or the court's responsibility, authorization or geographical boundaries.

**generally accepted accounting principles**
The prominent rules and procedures used in accepted accounting practice as set by the Accounting Principles Board and the Financial Accounting Standards Board to include both general guidelines and the detailed practices and procedures.

**generally recognized as effective (GRAE)**
One of the conditions which a drug must fulfill if it is not to be considered a new drug, and thus not subject to the pre-market approval requirements of the federal Food, Drug, and Cosmetic Act. To be

generally recognized as effective, the drug must be so considered by "experts qualified by scientific training and experience to evaluate the safety and effectiveness of drugs" and have been "used to a material extent or for a material time." FDA determines that a drug is GRAE, subject to judicial reversal if its determination is arbitrary or capricious. The Supreme Court has held that for a drug to be generally recognized as effective, its sponsor must supply the FDA with the same kind of evidence consisting of adequate and well-controlled investigations by qualified experts that the law requires in order to secure approval of a new drug application. See also generally recognized as safe.

**generally recognized as safe (GRAS)**
One of the conditions which a drug must fulfill if it is not to be considered as a new drug: or a food must fulfill if it is not to be considered as a food additive. A drug which is GRAS and GRAE need not go through the pre-market approval procedures prescribed in the federal Food, Drug, and Cosmetic Act for new drugs. General recognition of safety of a drug must be "among experts qualified by scientific training and experience to evaluate the safety and effectiveness of drugs", and to acquire general recognition of safety and effectiveness a drug must be "used to a material extent or for a material time."

**general medical services**
The diagnosis and treatment of non-emergent physical diseases and other ill-health conditions or their symptoms by techniques distinct from those used in obstetric, surgical, diagnostic and therapeutic radiology and clinical laboratory services.

**general paresis.**
Organic brain syndrome caused by a chronic syphilitic infection.

**general partner**
The member of a partnership who has the authority to bind the partnership, who shares in the profits, and who has unlimited liability for the losses. A partnership must have at least one general partner and may have more than one general partner as well as limited partners.

**general power of appointment.**
1. Authority by which a person in a position of authority or power appoints anyone he chooses. 2. The authority given by a testator to a third person to dispose of the testator's estate.

**general practitioner (GP)**
A practicing physician who does not specialize in any particular field of medicine (e.g. is not a specialist). A family physician has specialized in general practice and is subject to specialty board examination, in the care of families; a primary care physician may be a specialist in any of several specialties.

**general revenue.**
Government revenues raised without regard to the specific purpose for which they might be used. Federal general revenues come principally

from personal and corporate income taxes and some excise taxes. State general revenues come primarily from personal income and sales taxes.

**general verdict**
A verdict by a jury without elaboration on the specific facts of the case.

**generic equivalents**
Drug products with the same active chemical ingredients sold under the same generic name but often with different brand names. Generic equivalents are often assumed to be, but are not necessarily, therapeutic equivalents.

**generic name**
The established, official, or non-proprietary, name by which a drug is known as an isolated substance, irrespective of its manufacturer. Each drug is licensed under a generic name, and also may be given a brand name by its manufacturer. The generic name is assigned by the United States Adopted Names Council (USAN), a private group of representatives of the American Medical Association, American Pharmaceutical Association, United States Pharmacopeia and Food and Drug Administration, plus one public member. See also maximum allowable cost program and antisubstitution law.

**genetic assistant**
The genetics assistant works with the genetics counselor in providing services to patients. Specifically, he/she obtains complete genetic case histories from patients and families with inherited diseases or birth defects.

**genetic counseling**
The presentation of the scientific facts involved in inherited pathological conditions. Showing the prospective parents the likelihood of transmitting certain characteristics to any offspring. See genetic counselor.

**genetic counselor**
A person trained to offer coordinative and supportive care to the patient with potential or actual genetic disease, and to counsel patients concerning the origin, transmission, and development of hereditary characteristics that have a relationship to birth abnormalities. The genetic counselor obtains a complete genetic history from patients and families with inherited diseases or birth defects and counsels them about the probability of transmitting these characteristics to their offspring.

**genitalia.**
The reproductive organs of both sexes, usually the external parts.

**genocide**
The mass killing of human beings judged to be inferior, defective or handicapped.

**geographic characteristics**
As used in health planning, it is a description of the topography of the state and its relationship to health and health care.

**geriatric care worker**
An individual who works in skilled nursing facilities, especially those providing care to infirm, elderly patients. They administer to the various physical and social needs of the elderly patient in the institutional setting. They bring to the task an understanding of the problems of institutionalization, economic needs, and attitudes toward the elderly as these concepts relate to this specific population.

**geriatrics**
A specialty in medicine that deals with the aged and the problems of aging; the medical aspects or concerns of growing older or being old.

**germane**
Native to; related; appropriate; pertinent.

**germicide**
Any agent or substance that kills pathogenic microorganisms.

**gerodontics.**
The branch of dentistry that deals with diagnosis, treatment and research related to dental disorders and conditions peculiar to elderly persons. See dental geriatrics, gerontology.

**gerontocracy**
A political situation where the elderly citizens constitute the political ruling group by virtue of their age, wisdom, loyalty and dedication to the country.

**gerontology.**
The sociological, psychological, health and biological study of aging; social and health aspects of growing old.

**geropsychiatry**
A branch of psychiatry that deals with mental health problems of being old or growing old.

**gerrymandering**
1. The purposeful changing of political boundaries or districts to assure one political party continued majority control of a legislature. 2. In hospital administration, the dividing of responsibilities so as to take executive power and responsibility from the administrator. This is done by the governing board when it wishes to retain direct control as well as policy responsibility, either because they feel that they can run the hospital better than the administrator or because the administrator has been incompetent and ineffective. In the process of gerrymandering, usually the administrator's responsibilities are limited to the housekeeping and hotel functions only. A business manager may be appointed to be responsible for the financial aspects of the hospital, reporting directly to the treasurer of the governing board. These acts put hospital responsibilities on the governing board, thus its members effectively become not only the board but also the executives of the hospital. A large number of committees can be appointed to cover every hospital function, and tend to take over executive functions, thus bypassing the administrator.

**gestalt (German)**
A specific, existing, concrete, organized entity with definite shape or form. Whole, or wholeness.

**gestalten (German)**
Common and familiar objects as perceived in one's mind.

**gestalt psychology.**
A psychology that studies natural configurations and patterns due to direct experience instead of searching for mental elements and discounts the stimulus-response theories. It emphasizes perceptual wholes and that behavior takes place in an environment full of organized stresses and strains.

**Gestalt therapy**
A type of psychotherapy that emphasizes the treatment of the person as a whole—his physical, mental and emotional areas; his perceptual configuration, and his interrelationships with people and the environment.

**gift over**
A gift made from person A to person B for life and then it is given to person C—this constitutes a gift over.

**G.I.G.O.**
Garbage in-garbage out. An expression used by computer specialists referring to the fact that if incorrect data or information (garbage) is entered into a computer, then the results or answers will also be incorrect and useless (garbage).

**globus hystericus**
A hysterical response where a person feels as if he has a lump in his throat.

**gloss**
An annotation; an interpretation; an explanation. An explanation of a statement in a document that is usually on the same page.

**glossolalia**
Terminology or jargon that is not understandable.

**G.M.E.N.A.C.**
Graduate Medical Education National Advisory Committee.

**gnoso-**
Prefix meaning knowledge.

**G.N.P.**
Gross national product. One indicator of the health status of a country is how much of the gross national product the country spends on its health care. Even though no true correlation between high health status and the amount of money spent on health care exists, it is still one of the useful measures of health status.

**goal**

1. The highest attainable health status and the optimum health system performance technically achievable and consistent with community ideals. Goals are expressed with reference to a specified time period. 2. In health planning, a quantified statement of a desired future state or condition, such as an infant mortality of less than 20 per thousand live births, a physician to population ratio greater than four per thousand. Health planning formulates goals and seeks to achieve them. A goal differs from an objective by lacking a deadline, and usually by being long range (five to ten years) rather than sort (one to two years). 3. According to JCAH for psychiatric, alcoholism and drug abuse facilities accreditation purposes, this is an expected result or condition that takes time to achieve, that is specified in a statement of relatively broad scope, and that provides guidance in establishing intermediate objectives directed towards its attainment.

**goal level**

The quantitative level with respect to a particular indicator specified in a goal to express the desired level of a goal achievement.

**goal/need analysis.**

In health planning, as the second major phase of the Plan Development Process, goal/need analysis begins with a review of the health status and health system reference projection. Goal setting consists of defining the highest attainable levels of quality and excellence—with respect to health status and health system indicators—toward which the community may reasonably aspire. Because health status and health system goals are expressed quantitatively wherever possible—as desired indicator levels—it is possible to calculate the gap between projected indicator levels (from the reference projection) and the desired or goal level. THis gap represents either a health status improvement need or a health system need. Goal/need analysis ends with the establishment of objectives and priorities. It should be noted that health status and health system assessment, together with goal/need analysis—up to but not including the establishment of objectives and priorities—is sometimes referred to as need assessment.

**gonad**

An ovary or testicle.

**gonorrhea**

A sexually transmitted venereal disease caused by the Neisseria gonorrhoeae.

**good**

1. Valid. 2. Lawfully sufficient; collectible. 3. Legal.

**good cause**

With justification; to have a sufficient legal reason; not arbitrary.

**good consideration**

1. Natural duty. 2. Consideration of love and affection.

**good faith**
Honest; having standards of fair dealing.

**goods**
Personal belongings; personal property; merchandise, freight, wares.

**Good Samaritan act.**
A law that most states have to protect physicians, nurses and citizens when rendering first aid to a person in an emergency. See Good Samaritan statutes.

**Good Samaritan Doctrine**
When giving first aid care to an injured person in an emergency, a person may not be held liable for any harm caused to an injured person except as such harm may be the result of his negligence.

**Good Samaritan statutes.**
These laws create immunity from liability so health care providers, and in some states, lay persons, will be willing to render first aid in an emergency. These statutes protect those who render aid in an emergency situation from a civil redress suit and compensation to the injured. It provides limited protection even if harm results, as long as he acts as a reasonable and prudent person.

**good title**
A valid title, free from liens, charges, claims and encumbrances.

**gork**
Originally an acronym for "God only really knows," and then used by housestaff for patients whose problems were so mysterious as to defy diagnosis. It has now lost all connection with its original meaning and is used negatively to describe patients who are, and are likely to remain, comatose.

**gout**
A crippling physical disorder affecting one's joints, caused by excessive uric acid in the blood.

**governance**
The controlling or directing of an organization through a group of persons chosen to serve as a governing body.

**governing board (or body)**
A group of representative people who make important final decisions, direct, rule, manage and administer policy and rules over a company, or corporation, such as a hospital, nursing home or HMO. See board of directors

**governing body**
According to JCAH long term care accreditation, it is the individual, group, or governmental agency that has the ultimate responsibility and authority for the operation of the facility. See board of directors

**governing body and management (Medicare)**
A skilled nursing facility should have an effective governing body or designated persons so functioning, with full legal authority and responsibility for the operation of the facility. The governing body adopts and enforces rules and regulations relative to health care and safety of patients, to the protection of their personal and property rights, and to the general operation of the facility. The governing body develops a written institutional plan that reflects the operating budget and capital expenditures plan.

**governmental function**
Since health care involves public benefit, governmental health agencies duties imposed upon them as a corporate subdivision of the state.

**governmental immunity**
In malpractice, a doctrine providing that, despite the general proposition that a negligent act gives rise to tort liability for that act, the government, subject to certain qualifications, cannot be sued for the negligent acts of its officers, agents, or employees unless it consents to such a suit. This concept of governmental immunity had its origin in ancient common law doctrine and the principle has been firmly established that a state cannot be sued without its consent. However, the individual can still be held liable for his or her own acts. As with charitable immunity, the trend is towards an increasing willingness of the courts to impose liability as the states and the federal government enact statutes to waive their immunity in tort suits.

**government de factor**
The actual government in power.

**government de jure**
The rightful government.

**government instrumentality doctrine**
Any organization run by a branch of the government cannot be taxed.

**grace period**
A specified period after a premium payment is due, in which an insurance policyholder may make a payment. The period of time during which the protection of an insurance policy continues.

**graduated lease**
A special lease which calls for varying the rental charges, usually based on a periodic appraisal or the passage of time.

**graduate medical education.**
Medical education given after receipt of the M.D. or equivalent degree, including the education received as an intern, resident or fellow, and continuing education. This use contrasts with that in general education where graduate education refers to graduate school education leading to a masters, doctoral or equivalent degree (called undergraduate medical education in medicine). It is sometimes limited to education required for specialty board certification. Education at this level usually includes

supervised practice, research and even teaching, as well as didactic learning.

**graduate training program, bi-lateral**
Program conducted in a medical school department and a teaching hospital service (or the same clinical services in two hospitals where there is no medical school involvement).

**graduate training program, independent**
Operates with no relationship to a medical school for graduate training. The hospital administration and medical staff determine the number of house officers to be trained, select the candidates, and supervise the training programs.

**graduate training program, integrated**
Program stems from medical school academic department with department chairman playing an integral role in the determination of the number of house staff in the clinical services in two or more hospitals. Residents rotate from hospital to hospital. The hospital may pay the house officer salaries directly or they may pay the salary amounts into a central fund (usually administered by a medical school department of a nonprofit organization).

**-gram**
Suffix meaning record.

**grammatica falsa non vitiat chartam (Lat.)**
Bad or false grammar does not invalidate a need.

**grandfather clause**
1. Used in licensing and certification. This clause provides an exception to new laws and requirements for a person entering a field or profession that requires minimum education and standards for licensing. It is unrealistic to demand that a person already successfully working in a field should have to meet new requirements and qualifications. New criteria and requirements apply only to people newly applying for admission. 2. An exception to a new law or rule that allows those already practicing their profession to continue doing so, otherwise they would be stopped by the new legal restriction.

**grandfather provision**
A clause or provision of law that permits continued eligibility or coverage for individuals or organizations receiving program benefits under the law despite a change in the law which would otherwise make them ineligible; or in some other manner exempts a person, organization or thing from a change in law which would otherwise affect it. For example, the federal Food, Drug and Cosmetic Act exempts certain drugs from the Act's pre-market approval requirements on the basis of their longstanding use.

**grand jury**
A special jury put together to determine whether or not there is sufficient evidence to prove that a crime has been committed and to

justify bringing charges and a case to trial. A separate jury is called to try the case.

**grand larceny**
The theft of property that is valued at more than a specified dollar amount which constitutes a felony.

**grand mal**
The type of epilepsy in which the person has gross seizures accompanied by the loss of consciousness.

**grand rounds**
In a medical school or teaching hospital, the weekly review and discussion of a patient as the presentation of a case or educational material, in an auditorium, to all the medical staff of the hospital for the purpose of learning.

**grant**
1. To provide money for special purposes. 2. To give; convey; bestow or confer a gift. 3. A subsidy.

**grantee**
The person or organization to whom a grant is made.

**grantor**
The organization or person making a grant.

**-graph**
Suffix meaning instrument for recording.

**-graphy**
Suffix meaning process of recording.

**gratuitous**
Freely given without stipulation or consideration; voluntarily given or done without payment.

**gratuitous guest**
A person riding in a vehicle such as a bus or an ambulance without payment, but with permission and knowledge of the operator, i.e., a loved one accompanying an injured family member in the ambulance is not charged, but the injured person is.

**gratuitous licensee**
A visitor who is not a trespasser, i.e., visitors in a hospital. A non-business visitor.

**gratuitous transfer**
A free transfer made without payments, limitation or consideration.

**gravamen**
The foundation, basis, gist or parts of a complaint.

**grief**
Extreme sadness appropriate to an actual loss; emotional or mental suffering due to loss and bereavement.

**grievance procedure**
A special administrative procedure or policy establishing a proper or accepted way of dealing with employment problems or hearing complaints between employees and employers.

**gross**
1. Total amount. 2. Great. 3. A large amount together. 4. Flagrant or shameful. Extremely distasteful or ugly to look at.

**gross income**
All money and income; expenses and cost included in the total amount of income. See net income.

**gross lease**
Any lease which requires the lessor to pay all or most of the expenses of the leased property, which could include items such as taxes, insurance, maintenance, utilities, etc.

**gross negligence**
The performing of care or expected duty in a reckless manner, having no concern or regard for the consequences of the acts; willful and wanton disregard for rights or care of others. The want of level of care which a prudent person would take if personal health or property were the concern. Such negligence as is shown by a reckless disregard of another's life, limb, happiness or health, or ignoring the safety of persons involved who are exposed to dangerous circumstances. Indifference to one's legal duty so far as patients or clients would be affected in a serious manner; much more serious or higher in magnitude than simple inadvertence, but is not an intentional wrong. Gross negligence occurs when a person knows the results of his or her acts, but is wanton and indifferent to the results, but did not intentionally perform the acts to purposefully cause harm. However, the person may have had some intent.

**gross weight**
A total weight, including the weight of containers.

**ground rules**
In health insurance it is the basic and introductory material provided in the procedure coding manual to help with the filing of insurance claims by the health care provider. Ground rules in the procedure coding manual include: general information and instructions, special services and modifiers, as well as codes for services and procedures.

**grounds**
Basic facts; the foundation, or points of a case or dispute. The basic reason for a cause of action.

**group**
In group insurance, a body of subscribers eligible for group insurance by virtue of some common identifying attribute, such as common employment by an employer, or membership in a union, association or other organization. Groups considered for insurance are usually larger than nine persons.

**group agreement**
A method of providing coverage under one master plan for a number of individuals comprising a group by virtue of employment or other associations.

**group certificate**
A special document given to each member of a group health program to show benefits provided under the group plan's contract. It is issued to the employer or other insured person.

**group contract**
In insurance, it is a contract made with an employer that covers a group of persons.

**Group Health Association of America (GHAA)**
Founded in 1959. Its national headquarters are in Washington, D.C. and is to assist and represent health maintenance organizations. GHAA has relationships with HMO plan personnel and is familiar with management needs of HMOs.

**group health plans**
These health care services and facilities are comprehensive, prepaid HMO type health care services, providing health care to those members who have enrolled and prepay for use of the services. Many group health plans charge a small additional fee. Drugs and other health care items and services are usually provided at a reduced cost. See prepaid group practice plan. See health maintenance organization.

**group insurance**
Any insurance plan by which a number of employees of an employer (and their dependents) or members of a similar homogeneous group, are insured under a single policy, issued to their employer or the group with individual certificates of insurance given to each insured individual or family. Individual employees may be insured automatically by virtue of employment, only on meeting certain conditions (employment for over a month), or only when they elect to be insured (and usually to make a contribution to the cost of the insurance). Group health insurance is usually experience rated (except for small groups, all of which insured by an individual company in the same area are given the same rate by that company) and less expensive for the insured than comparable individual insurance (partly because an employed population is generally healthier than the general population, and partly because of lower administrative costs, especially in marketing and billing). Note that the policyholder or insured is the employer not the employees. See also contributory insurance.

**group legal services**
Legal aid given to members of an organization or employees of a company. It is prepaid on a group basis, similar to prepaid health insurance.

**group practice**

A formal association of three or more physicians or other health professionals providing services with income from medical practice pooled and redistributed to the members of the group according to some prearranged plan (often, but not necessarily, through partnership). Multi-specialty groups offer advantages to the patient by their ability to provide several kinds of services on an integrated basis. Groups vary a great deal in size, composition and financial arrangements. See also solo, private and prepaid group practice, Group Medical Management Association.

**group psychotherapy**

A type of psychiatric or psychological treatment that involves several patients participating together in therapy with one or two psychotherapists, who facilitate emotional and rational cognitive interactions in the members of the group in order to change maladaptive behavior of each member.

**growth**

1. A normal or natural increase in weight and height; a normal increase in physical size. 2. The multiplication and proliferation of cells.

**G.S.A.**

General Services Administration—manages the property of the United States Government.

**guarantee**

A promise that goods are of a certain high quality, will be fixed if broken, will last for a certain time period; can be a part of a contract to replace or fix certain items if they fail to function properly within a certain time period. Also correctly spelled guaranty.

**guaranteed continuable**

See guaranteed renewable.

**guaranteed renewable**

Contracts that an insured person has the right to continue in force due to paying the premiums, during which period the insurer has no right to make any unilateral changes in any provision of the contract. Premiums may not be changed for an individual but only for classes of insureds.

**guardian**

1. One who has the legal right and duty to take care of another person because he legally cannot take care of himself, i.e., a child, or in some cases, an elderly person. 2. For JCAH long term care accreditation, it is an individual who has legal authority to act on behalf of another individual. 3. According to JCAH for psychiatric, alcoholism and drug abuse facilities accreditation purposes, this is a parent, trustee, committee, conservator, or other person or agency empowered by law to act on behalf of, or have responsibility for, an applicant or patient.

**guardian at litem**

A lawyer, appointed by a court to handle the interests of another person, usually a minor or other person under legal disability, during the process of a lawsuit in which the person is involved.

**guest statute**
In some states, a person who rides as a guest in another person's car cannot sue the driver if there is an accident unless it involved more than ordinary negligence.

**guidelines**
General directions, criteria or policy. A standard, principle or instructions by which a judgment can be made, policy determined, an action taken or a grant application filled out.

**guilt**
1. The act of having done wrong. 2. Having done a wrong or a crime, usually with intent. 3. Shame; the painful, emotional feeling associated with the violation of one's value system or a transgression of moral-ethical beliefs. 4. In psychiatry, an emotional state filled with self-reproach and need for punishment. Guilt can provide normal psychological and social functions. Guilt with special intensity or the absence of guilt characterizes many mental disorders, such as depression and antisocial personality, respectively.

**guilty**
1. Deserving of blame. 2. One responsible for doing harm or committing a crime. 3. Proven to have committed a crime or a civil wrong; the opposite of being innocent.

**gyneco-**
Prefix meaning female.

**gynecology**
The branch of study and medicine which deals with the female reproductive tract and associated conditions and processes.

**gynephobia**
Fear of women.

**gynosperm**
Sperm bearing an x chromosome.

# H

**H.A. (Lat.)**
Hoc Anno. In this year.

**habeas corpus (Lat.)**
You have the body. A court order to secure the release of a person who is being held unlawfully. The principle implies neither guilt nor innocence, but speaks to the issue of due process for detaining a person.

**habilitability**
The legal principle that requires a rented place or residence or apartment to be fit to live in.

**habilitation**
See rehabilitation.

**habilitation and rehabilitation services**
Services to restore the ill and disabled individual to, or assist the developmentally disabled individual to achieve the fullest physical, mental, social, vocational and economic usefulness of which he is capable. See rehabilitation.

**habitual**
1. On a regular basis. 2. Something done so often it is by habit, not chance; occurring more than just occasionally; doing a behavior so frequently that it occurs by compulsion rather than by chance.

**habitual intemperance**
Drunkenness that is continual and interferes with family life or one's job. It can be grounds for divorce in many states. In some states, drug addiction falls under this rule.

**habituation**
See drug habituation, abuse and dependence.

**H.A.C.**
Health Advisory Council. A local advisory council to the Health Systems Agency. In some areas these are called Sub Area Advisory Councils (SAC).

**half-life**
A method used to classify the rate of decay of radioisotopes or chemicals according to the time it takes them to lose half their strength or intensity.

**halfway house**
A community based facility for patients with mental or emotional problems who no longer need the full facilities of a mental hospital but

are not yet ready to go out on their own. The term is also used to describe minimum security penal institutions.

**hallucination**
A false experience or an experience that exists only in one's mind. It can be brought on by emotional factors, or by drugs or alcohol. Common hallucinations involve sights, sounds and tastes, however a reaction by any of the senses is possible. See also auditory, gustatory, hypnagogic, hypnopompic, kinesthetic, lilliputian, tactile and visual hallucinations.

**hallucinogen**
Any drug which causes distortion of one's emotions, perceptions, sensations or fantasies.

**hallucinogenic drug**
See psychotomimetic drug.

**hallucinosis**
A state where a person experiences hallucinations while being fully conscious.

**halo effect**
The effect (usually beneficial) which the manner, attention and caring of a provider have on a patient during a medical encounter regardless of what medical procedures or services the encounter actually involves. See also Hawthorne effect and placebo.

**halt symbol**
A symbol that stops a computer when a job is completed.

**haphephobia**
Fear of being touched.

**haplology**
A disorder where a patient has rapid speech in which syllables are left out. Certain manias and schizophrenic conditions exhibit this symptom.

**harass**
To badger; to trouble or bother; to disturb persistently; to weary; to fatigue.

**harbor**
1. To feed and shelter; conceal, keep or detain a person for illegal purposes. 2. To hide something. 3. To keep a person from law enforcement officers.

**hard case or hardship case**
A case where fairness requires a loose interpretation of legal principles due to hardships experienced by the party of the case.

**hard money**
Money set aside to run a program, organization or institution that is from a firm, assured and ongoing source. Money that will flow regularly into an organization or a program on a continuous basis and that will

not end. Sources of hard money usually are state government, local government or private business. See soft money.

**hardware**

1. The equipment and materials making up a data processing system. 2. In media and telecommunications, it is the machinery and equipment such as projectors and videotape machines. Software is the items that are played or used on the hardware. See software.

**harm**

Any injury, wrong or damage done to either a person, to a person's rights, or to property that warrants legal consideration.

**harmless error**

1. An error of a lower court that has little effect on an appellant's basic rights or on the decision or the merits of the case. 2. An error that does not merit a review or reversal of a judgment.

**Harris flush**

Irrigation of the lower bowel to promote the expulsion of gas from the intestines. This is used with post-operative patients, whose intestinal tracts have not been functioning and need assistance in reestablishing normal peristaltic function.

**Harrison Antinarcotic Act**

A law established by the U.S. government to restrict the use and distribution of dangerous drugs. Drugs controlled by this law include opiates and their derivatives, such as morphine and heroin, plus many stimulants such as amphetamines and cocaine, and hallucinogens such as LSD and marijuana. This law also provides certain limitations and requirements for writing prescriptions for the drugs controlled by this act. See schedule of drugs

**Hawthorne effect**

The effect (often beneficial, almost always present) which an encounter with a provider, health program or other part of the health system has on a patient which is independent of the medical content of the encounter. The Hawthorne effect is similar to the placebo effect, but is not obtained intentionally and is the effect of the encounter with a provider or program on the patient rather than of what they do for him. The effect may be changed (intentionally or not) by changing the provider or program (for instance by painting a clinic or changing its appointments system). Since health services research usually changes the services being studied simply by being done or in unintentional ways, the resulting change in the Hawthorne effect may well confound the results of the research. The name comes from classic industrial management experiments at the Hawthorne plant of the Western Electric Company.

**hazard**

A situation or event which introduces, or increases the probability of, occurrence of a loss arising from a peril, or that increases the extent of a loss; such as slippery floors, unsanitary conditions, or congested traffic.

**hazardous area**

In JCAH longterm care facilities accreditation this is a room that contains combustible or flammable materials of such a nature as to increase the potential hazards of a fire. Hazardous areas include kitchens with commercial cooking ranges, maintenance and repair shops, handicraft and gift shops, and boiler rooms. They also include rooms used to store combustible supplies, flammable gases or liquids, or oxidizing agents in significant quantities.

**hazardous procedures**

According to JCAH for psychiatric, alcoholism and drug abuse facilities accreditation purposes, these are procedures that place the patient at physical or psychological risk or in pain.

**hazard surveillance program**

In JCAH longterm care facilities accreditation, this is a program involving routine periodic surveys by personnel or staff to identify unsafe conditions or practices occurring at the facility.

**H.B.**

House Bill. A bill introduced in the House of Representatives to become law.

**headnote**

An abstract of a case placed at the beginning of the case when it is finally published.

**head of family**

The person who financially and morally supports a family or group of related persons who live together. See family.

**health**

Defined by the World Health Organization as "a state of complete physical, mental, and social well-being and not merely the absence of disease or infirmity." Experts recognize, however, that health has many dimensions (anatomical/physiological, emotional, spiritual, social, and mental) and is often culturally defined. The relative importance of various disabilities will differ depending upon the cultural milieu and the role of the affected individual in that culture. Most attempts at measurement have taken a negative approach in that the degree of ill health has been assessed in terms of morbidity and mortality. In general, the detection of changes in health status is easier than the definition and measurement of the absolute level of health.

**health administration**

1. Health administration is a generic term covering the activities of a broad range of individuals: health planners and policy analysts in federal, state, regional, and local agencies; hospital and clinic administrators; and administrators of group practices, health maintenance organizations, or long-term care facilities, among others. Health administrators are involved in planning, coordinating, organizing, evaluating, and directing the resources and procedures necessary to provide health services. Administrators work in hospitals, rehabilitation centers, ambulatory health

care centers, group practice plans, health maintenance organizations, voluntary health agencies, state and local health departments, home health services, nursing homes, and health planning agencies. Health administrators are also employed by private health insurance firms and research agencies to design, implement, and evaluate health programs. Administrators may also teach or conduct research in educational programs which train health service administrators at both graduate and undergraduate levels. Some positions in government service utilize health administrators in areas such as health manpower, health statistics, health services research, health planning, program evaluation, and program planning. 2. Planning, organizing, directing, controlling, and coordinating the resources procedures by which needs and demands for health and medical care and a healthful environment are converted to specific services for individual clients, organizations and communities. (The Commission of Education for Health Administration)

**Health Aide Program**

Characterizes programs which emphasize the role of the representative as one of assistance to specific Indian Health Service personnel in both clinical and field health programs. Representatives in programs of this type work closely with physicians, public health nurses, sanitarians, medical social workers, and other health team members.

**Health and Human Services, Department of (HHS)**

The new title of the old Department of Health, Education and Welfare. A Federal level agency established for the furthering of the good health of American citizens and for providing essential human and health services. The major goal of HHS is to provide health related service to the U.S. public that protect and advance the quality of life for all Americans with special emphasis placed on those least able to help themselves such as poverty level or minority groups.

**Health and Human Services, Department of (HSS)**

The Federal government's cabinet level agency established for furthering of the good health of American citizens and for providing essential human services. The major purpose of HHS is to provide health related services that protect and advance the quality of life for all Americans with special emphasis placed on those least able to help themselves.

**health belief model**

1. A systematic method of reviewing one's beliefs, values and expectancies in regards to health status, health behaviors, health practice and utilization of the health care system. 2. A paradigm used to predict and explain health behavior based on value-expectancy theory.

**health card**

An identification card, similar to a credit card, proposed in several national health insurance bills, which would be issued to each covered individual or family unit. This card would be presented at the time services were rendered in lieu of any cash payment. The individual would subsequently receive a bill for any cost-sharing not covered under the insurance plan. Health cards would be used to simplify eligibility determination, billing and accounting, and the study of use of services.

The idea presents interesting confidentiality problems particularly under the Federal Credit Disclosure Act.

**health care administration**
See health administration.

**health care administrator**
See health services administrator.

**health care corporation (HCC)**
An organization proposed by the American Hospital Association in its NHI proposal which would assume overall management responsibility for providing all needed personal health services in a defined catchment area.

**health care system goals and objectives**
Describe the desired state of the health services which are provided for the people of a state to improve their health status.

**health care team**
A group of health care professionals who provide coordinated services to achieve optimal health care of the client. See health team.

**health continuum**
A continuum with a high health status on one end and extreme illness or death at the other.

**health education**
1. A process with intellectual, psychological, and social dimensions relating to activities which increase the abilities of people to make informed decisions affecting their personal, family, and community well-being. This process, based on scientific principles, facilitates learning and behavioral change in both health personnel and consumers, including children and youth. 2. In its orientation to the consumer, health education is comprised of activities which do the following: 1) Inform and educate people about health, illness, disability, and ways in which they can improve and protect their own health, including more efficient use of the delivery system. 2) Motivate people to want to change to more healthful practices. 3) Help them learn the necessary skills to adopt and maintain healthful practices and lifestyles. 4) Foster teaching and communications skills in all those engaged in teaching consumers about health. 5) Advocate changes in the environment that facilitate healthful conditions and healthful behavior. 6) Add to knowledge via research and evaluation concerning the most effective ways of achieving the above objectives. 3. The process of assisting individuals, acting separately and collectively, to make informed decisions about matters affecting individual, family and community health. Based upon scientific foundations, health education is a field of interest, a discipline and a profession.

**health education services**
Those services directed toward forming, educating and motivating the public to adopt personal life styles and nutritional practices which will promote optimal health, avoid health risks, and make appropriate use of health care services in the community.

**health education settings**
The variety of organizational entities in which health educators are found working.

**health educator**
An individual prepared to assist individuals, acting separately or collectively, to make informed decisions regarding matters affecting their personal health and that of others.
Role: Set of related responsibilities which depict the nature of the services health educators perform in society.
Role Delineation: The process of clarifying the role performed by health educators through specifying responsibilities and functions and identifying requisite skills and knowledge.
Role Specification: The identified responsibilities and functions of a professional role which must be carried out through application of identified skills and knowledge. See entry-level health educator.

**health facilities**
Collectively, all buildings and facilities used in the provision of health services. Usually limited to facilities which were built for the purpose of providing health care, such as hospitals and nursing homes, and, thus, does not include an office building which includes a physician's office. Health facilities, with health manpower are the principal health resources used in producing health services. See also beds, boarding homes, capital, capital depreciation, certificate-of-need, clinic, Hill-Burton, institutional health services, institutional licensure, JCAH, inpatient, length of stay, Life Safety Code, modernization, outpatient, per diem cost, proprietary hospital, and hospital.

**health hazard appraisal**
See health risk appraisal.

**health insurance**
1. All types of insurance reimbursing costs of hospital and medical care. In some cases, a person is reimbursed for lost income arising from illness or injury. Also known as medical insurance, accident and health insurance, disability income insurance. 2. Insurance against loss by disease or accidental bodily injury. Such insurance usually covers some of the medical costs of treating the disease or injury, may cover other losses (such as loss of present or future earnings) associated with them and may be either individual or group insurance.

**Health Insurance Benefits Advisory Council (HIBAC)**
An advisory council to the Department of Health and Human Services, whose primary role, pursuant to section 1867 of the Social Security Act and as detailed in its charter, is to provide advice and recommendations on matters of general policy in the administration of Medicare and Medicaid. This role was reaffirmed after Departmental review, and the Council was rechartered on December 13, 1974, to continue the provision of such advice to the Secretary for two additional years. The Council consists of nineteen non-governmental experts in health related fields who are selected by the Secretary and hold office for terms of four years. In recognition of the broad impact of Medicare and Medicaid on health care

delivery throughout the country, the management and staff support for the Council has been transferred to the Office of the Assistant Secretary for Health. Organizationally, this is to enable information on policy issues to be more directly channeled to the Council and provides the Assistant Secretary for health ready access to, and analysis of, HIBAC issues.

**health insurance claim number (HIC) (Medicare)**
An identification number assigned to Medicare beneficiary. It is a seven or nine digit number (which may be the Social Security Number) with either an alpha prefix or suffix. The number must appear on all documents related to a beneficiary.

**Health Insurance for the Aged and Disabled**
The social insurance program authorized by title XVIII of the Social Security Act and known as Medicare.

**health interview survey**
An information collecting system used by the U.S. Public Health Service for gathering data on health-related issues. On a periodic or special care basis, interviewers from the Public Health Service visit homes in the U.S. to interview residents about diseases, illness, abnormal conditions, disabilities and utilization of health services.

**Health Liaison Program**
Emphasizes the liaison role of the Community Health Representative (CHR) but views this role as a link primarily between the community and health resources such as the Indian Health Service, county medical agencies, medical welfare programs and local voluntary medical agencies. See Community Health Representative.

**health maintenance**
Preventive, diagnostic, curative, and restorative health services available to a client, group or community.

**health maintenance organization (HMO)**
1. A health care organization that provides a wide range of comprehensive health care services for a specified group at a fixed or prepaid periodic payments. 2. An entity with four essential attributes: 1) an organized system for providing health care in a geographic area, which entity accepts the responsibility to provide or otherwise assure the delivery of 2) an agreed upon set of basic and supplemental health maintenance and treatment services to 3) a voluntarily enrolled group of persons, and 4) for which services the HMO is reimbursed through a predetermined, fixed, periodic prepayment made by or on behalf of each person or family unit enrolled in the HMO without regard to the amounts of actual services provided. (From the report of the Committee on Interstate and Foreign Commerce on the HMO Act of 1973, P.L. 93-222, in which the term is legally defined, section 1301 of the PHS Act.) The HMO must employ or contract with health care providers who undertake a continuing responsibility to provide services to its enrollees. The prototype HMO is the Kaiser-Permanente system, a prepaid group practice located on the West Coast. However, medical foundations sponsored by groups of physicians are included under the definition.

HMOs are of public policy interest because the prototypes appear to have demonstrated the potential for providing high quality medical services for less money than the rest of the medical system. Specifically, rates of hospitalization and surgery are considerably less in HMOs than occurs in the system outside such prepaid groups, although some feel that earlier care, skimping or skimming may be better explanations. See also prepaid healthplans (PHPs), individual practice associations, qualified and group practice. See group health plan.

**health manpower**
Collectively, all men and women working in the provision of health services whether as individual practitioners or employees of health institutions and programs; whether or not professionally trained; and whether or not subject to public regulation. Facilities and manpower are the principal health resources used in producing health services. See also capitation, CCME, FMG, graduate and undergraduate medical education, professional, practice, credentialing, internship and residency, and proficiency and equivalency testing. See schedule A.

**health manpower education initiative award (HMEIA)**
A grant or contract under section 774 of the PHS Act (added by the Comprehensive Health Manpower Training Act of 1971, P.L. 92-157) which authorizes awards to health or educational entities for health manpower programs which will improve the distribution, supply, quality, utilization, and efficiency of health personnel and the health services delivery system. Support has been provided for the development of area health education centers (AHECs), the training of physician assistants, and the identification and encouragement of disadvantaged students with a potential for training in the health professions, among other activities.

**health manpower plan**
That plan which concerns itself with the health manpower needs of a state.

**health outcomes**
In health education planning, this refers to any change in health status in a group or population that results from health promotion or health care utilized as measured at one point in time; a cross-sectional epidemiological study of health concerns or health status. A measure of the results of health activation, health education and health promotion.

**health physicist**
Requires minimum education at the baccalaureate level. Directs research, training, and monitoring programs to protect hospital patients and laboratory personnel from radiation hazards, inspects and evaluates standards and decontamination procedures and develops new methods to safeguard man and the environment against unnecessary radiation exposure.

**health physics technician**
Required training is below the baccalaureate level. Monitors radiation levels, gives instruction in radiation safety, labels radioactive materials,

and assists the health physicist in conducting experimental studies in radiation.

**health planning**

1. A process which establishes desired future levels for health status and health system performance, designs and selects among alternative actions aimed at modifying the health system so future levels of health status and health system performance conform to desired levels, and suggests steps for implementation of the recommended actions. 2. Planning concerned with improving health, whether undertaken comprehensively for a whole community (see CHP) or for a particular situation, type of health service, or health program. Some definitions clearly include all activities undertaken for the purpose of improving health (such as education, traffic and environmental control and nutrition) within the scope of responsibility of the planning process; others are limited to including conventional health services and programs, public health, or personal health services. See also goals and objectives, state health planning and development agency, health systems agency, and policy, management and budget.

**health policies**

The definite course or method of action selected by the Health Systems Agency Governing Body to guide and determine present and future decisions affecting the health status of its areas.

**health practitioner**

Any person who provides a health care service.

**health professional**

See professional.

**health promotion**

Any combination of health education and related organizational, political and economic interventions designed to facilitate behavioral and environmental adaptations that will improve or protect health.

**health resources**

Resources (human, monetary or material) used in producing health care and services. They include money, health manpower, health facilities, equipment and supplies. Resources, available or used, can be measured and described for an area (see medically underserved and catchment area), population (see medically underserved population), or an individual program (an HMO) or service.

**health risk appraisal**

A newly developed preventive medicine tool which seeks to identify and reduce major risks to continued good health. A questionnaire is filled out and physical exam type tests such as blood tests are conducted. Some programs are computer assisted. The purpose of doing an appraisal is to determine one's health risks and to assist in changes and/or develop treatment programs. An appraisal provides answers to the following questions: 1) What are the major causes of death for people in my age, race, and sex grouping? 2) How do my risks of dying in the next ten years compare to average? 3) What can I do to reduce my risks?

**health service area**
A geographic area appropriate for the effective planning and development of health services. Section 1511 of the PHS Act requires that health service areas be delineated throughout the United States. The governors of the various states designate the areas using requirements specified in the law respecting geography, political boundaries, population, health resources and coordination with areas defined for other purposes. See also catchment area and locality.

**health service plans**
Those plans of state agencies that address the provision of health services to the residents of a state.

**health services administrator**
Health services administrators occupy middle and top-level management positions in a variety of settings: hospitals, public and private health agencies, social service agencies, and government health agencies. Minimum education at the baccalaureate level is required for job entry. Those who serve as administrators range from executives who have major responsibility in policy formation to managers who direct the internal operations of a health organization to staff specialists such as health planners, systems analysts, or fiscal experts. The functions of the positions are broadly based and include planning, organizing, staffing, budgeting, directing, and coordinating. See health administration.

**health services research**
Research concerned with the organization, financing, administration, effects, or other aspects of health services; rather than with human biology, and disease and its prevention, diagnosis and treatment. In a sense, health services research concerns itself with the form, and biomedical research with the content of medicine.

**health statistician**
Uses statistical theory, techniques, and methods to determine useful measurements or meaningful relationships of information relating to health or disease. Also referred to as a biostatistician.

**health status**
The state of health of a specified individual, group or population (such as a state, an HMO membership, or a work organization). It is as difficult to describe or measure as the health of an individual and may be measured with people's subjective assessment of their health, or with one or more indicators of mortality and morbidity in the population, such as longevity, maternal and infant mortality, and the incidence or prevalence of major diseases (communicable, coronary, malignant, nutritional, etc.). These are measures of disease status, but have to be used as proxies in the absence of measures of either objective or subjective health. Health status conceptually is the proper outcome measure for the effectiveness of the specific population's medical care system, although attempts to relate variations in health status and the effects of available medical care have

proved difficult and generally unsuccessful. It cannot be measured with measures of available health resources or services (such as physician to population ratios) which, in this context, would be process measures. See also vital statistics National Health Survey, health risk appraisal.

**health status and health system assessment**
That part of the plan development process involving the selection of health status and health system indicators, collection (or estimation) of past and current data for the selected indicators, and a reference projection of how those indicators will change over a five- to ten-year period if there are no changes in current plans or programs. Assessment is the first major phase of activities in plan development and ends just prior to the selection of goals.

**health status goals and objectives**
These statements specify in quantitative and qualitative terms, a desired achievement in the personal health of a population and the time frame for this achievement.

**health status indicator**
A quantitative measure used to reflect the health status of the community. Health status indicators may be general measures of quality of health such as indicators of longevity and functional ability, or measures of disease or disorder which comprise or account for dysfunction or mortality.

**health status of the residents**
A description of the wellness level the residents of a state are at a particular point in time. It should present the current health of the residents, the factors affecting their health, and the existing health delivery system.

**health status priorities**
The ranking of desired changes in the personal health of a population according to their amenability to intervention.

**health survey**
A program for studying a group or population, in order to assess its health status, the conditions influencing or influenced by its health, and the health services and medical care available to and used by it. See also National Health Survey.

**health system**
All the services, functions and resources in a geographic area whose primary purpose is to affect the state of health of the population. The health system may be considered to include three major subsystems: community health promotion and protection, personal health care, and health system enabling services.

**health system enabling services**
A major subsystem of the overall health system which includes those services provided by various governmental and nongovernmental agencies in order to insure the availability, accessibility and acceptability of quality health services in the most cost-effective manner possible. Major service

categories within health system enabling include: health planning, resources development, financing, regulation and research.

**health system indicator**
A measure to represent how well the health system is performing. Health system indicators usually measure broad, general characteristics of the health system such as the availability, accessibility, acceptability, quality, continuity and cost-effectiveness of health services.

**health system plan (HSP)**
A long range health plan prepared by a health systems agency for its health service area specifying the health goals considered appropriate by the agency for the area. The HSPs are to be prepared after consideration of national guidelines issued by the Department of Health and Human Services and study of the characteristics, resources and special needs of the health service area. Section 1513 of the PHS Act requires and specifies the nature of an HSP. See also annual implementation plan.

**health systems agency (HSA)**
A health planning and resources development agency designated under the terms of the National Health Planning and Resources Development Act of 1974, P.L. 93-641 requires the designation of an HSA in each of the health service areas in the United States. HSAs are to be non-profit private corporations, public regional planning bodies, or single units of local government, and are charged with performing the health planning and resources development functions listed in section 1513 of the PHS Act. The legal structure, size, composition and operation of HSAs are specified in section 1512 of the Act. HSA functions include preparation of a health system plan (HSP) and an annual implementation plan (AIP), the issuance of grants and contracts, the review and approval or disapproval of proposed uses of a wide range of federal funds in the agency's health service area, and review of proposed new and existing institutional health services and making of recommendations respecting them to state health planning and development agencies. HSAs replace areawide CHP agencies but with expanded duties and powers. See comprehensive health planning.

**Health Systems Agency activities**
Functions of the Health Systems Agency in the accomplishment of the goals and objectives stated in the HSP. See Health Systems Agency.

**health system services**
Related activities which utilize health resources whose primary purpose is to contribute to the improvement or protection of health status of the population or the environment affecting their health.

**health system settings**
Sites in which health resources are utilized in order to deliver health system services.

**Health Systems Plan facilities component**
That portion of the Health Systems Plan (HSP) of the Health Systems Agency that concerns itself with health care facilities. Refers to that segment of the HSP describing the existing health facilities in a state.

**health systems priorities**
The ranking of desired changes in a characteristic of the health delivery mechanism according to importance and amenability to intervention.

**health team**
A group of individuals with varying skills who provide health care services, whose cooperative efforts are designed to assist people with their health.

**hearing**
A court or trial-like proceeding that takes place in a legislative body or an administrative agency and held in a court-like manner.

**hearing examiner or hearing officer**
A judge-like official who directs hearings.

**hearsay**
Second-hand evidence; evidence or facts not from or based on personal knowledge of a witness, but based on information from other persons.

**hearsay evidence**
Statements used as evidence that are not from the personal knowledge of the witness.

**hearsay exception**
Certain evidence based on hearsay can be admitted in a trial if it falls under the special evidence rule that provides for an exception. Hearsay exceptions are based on the probability under the circumstances that the evidence is accurate.

**hearsay rule**
A rule of evidence law restricting the admission of evidence which is not the personal knowledge of a witness. Hearsay evidence is allowed but only under certain situations and governed by strict rules.

**heart attack**
See cardiac arrest, myocardial infarction.

**Heart-balm Act**
State laws eliminating or restricting civil lawsuits for breach of promise to marry.

**heat of passion**
1. A state of violent and uncontrollable anger that is provoked. 2. A state of mind that may reduce a homicide from murder to manslaughter.

**hebephrenia**
A type of schizophrenia, characterized by shallow, inappropriate emotions, with childish behavior and mannerisms that are unpredictable. Delusions may also be present.

**hedonism**
Seeking after pleasure and avoiding pain.

**heebie-jeebies**
An attack of nervousness.

**heed**
To regard with care; to give careful notice; to pay close attention to; to take special care or notice; to consider; to take notice.

**heedily**
Cautiously.

**heedless**
Inattentive; unmindful; careless.

**held**
Decided in court; a final decision of a court.

**hematocrit**
Determination of the amounts of plasma and corpuscles in the blood.

**hematology technologist**
Medical technologist, working in a hospital under supervision of a hematologist or laboratory director, in performing quantitative, qualitative and coagulation tests on cellular and plasma components of blood for use in the diagnosis and treatment of disease.

**hematoma**
Blood collecting in a tissue, organ, or body space due to a break in the wall of a blood vessel.

**hemiplegia**
Paralysis of one side of the body. This is usually the result of a cerebral vascular accident (stroke). Because some of the nerve cells of the brain have been damaged and cannot function, the part of the body controlled by the damaged tissue cannot function. There may be loss of sensation as well as a loss of motor ability. The amount of loss in either of these areas will vary with individual patients.

**hemoglobin**
The oxygen carrying pigment in red corpuscles. A compound made up of hematin and globin.

**hemorrhage**
Excessive bleeding; large amounts of blood escaping from the blood vessels.

**hemostat**
A surgical clamp used to stop the flow of blood from blood vessels. See Kelly forcep.

**henceforth**
From this time forward; now and in the future; from now on.

**herb**
A plant which is valued for its medicinal, drug, savory or aromatic qualities.

**herbalist**
A healer who uses herbs for treatment; an herb doctor; one who prescribes herbs to heal illnesses.

**hereafter**
In the future; in the time to come; following this.

**herein**
In this document.

**hereinabove**
Before this.

**hereinafter**
After this.

**hereto**
To this.

**heretofore**
Before, or in times past.

**herewith**
In this, or with this.

**hermaphrodite**
A person born with both female and male sexual organs, usually one sex dominates.

**hermeneutics**
The science or art of interpretation; the art of interpreting legal documents.

**heroin**
An addicting opiate drug. It is the drug most commonly used by narcotics addicts.

**hertz**
Frequencies as measured in cycles per second. 1 cps = 1 Hz.

**heterosexuality**
Sexual attraction to and contact with opposite-sex persons. The capacity for heterosexual arousal and attraction is probably innate and biologically programmed.

**H.E.W.**
The old Department of Health, Education and Welfare: one U.S. Cabinet department. Now called the Department of Health and Human Services.

**hex**
A jinx; a supernatural spell imposed through witchcraft.

**H.H.S.**
The Department of Health and Human Services, see these words.

**H-ICDA**
Hospital Adaptation of the "International Classification of Diseases". It is a numerical coding system used to identify diagnosis on admission and discharge. This international code was adapted for use by hospitals in the United States.

**hierarchy**
The ranking of persons or ideas by levels, usually with more personnel at the bottom and gradually getting fewer in numbers at the top levels. Most bureaucracies and health organizations are arranged this way.

**high crimes and misdemeanors**
The basis for impeachment as provided by the U.S. Constitution. The exact meaning of the phrase is not clear.

**high hazard area**
In JCAH longterm care facilities accreditation, this is a room in which combustible and flammable supplies are stored in such a manner as to increase the hazard potential. These areas include soiled linen and trash collection rooms and paint shops.

**high option**
In a Federal Employees Health Benefits Plan, and some other insurance policies, denotes one of two or more levels of insurance which may be chosen by the subscriber. Under such options the benefits covered are usually essentially the same except that the high option provides lower deductibles and other cost-sharing requirements and more generous time or quantity limits than the low option. The premium for the high option is higher than the low option to reflect the more generous coverage.

**Hill-Burton**
Legislation, and the programs operated under that legislation, for federal support of construction and modernization of hospitals and other health facilities, beginning with P.L. 79-725, the Hospital Survey and Construction Act of 1946. The original law, which has been amended frequently, provided for surveying state needs, developing plans for construction of hospitals and public health centers, and assisting in construction and equipping them. Until the late 1960s, most of the amendments expanded the program in dollar amounts and scope. More recently, the administration has attempted to terminate the program while the Congress has sought to restructure it toward support of outpatient facilities, facilities to serve areas deficient in health services, and training facilities for health and allied health professions. Under P.L. 93-641, the National Health Planning and Resources Development Act of 1974, the Hill-Burton program will be administered by the state health planning and development agency. The purpose of the existing Hill-Burton programs was modified by P.L. 93-641 to allow assistance in the form of grants, loans or loan guarantees for the following purposes only: modernization of health facilities; construction of outpatient health facilities; construction of inpatient facilities in areas which have

experienced recent rapid population growth; and conversion of existing medical facilities for the provision of new health services.

**Hippocratic Oath (late 5th century B.C.)**

I swear by Apollo the physician, by Aesculapius, Hygeia and Panacea, and I take to witness all the gods, and all the goddesses, to keep according to my ability and my judgment the following Oath:
To consider dear to me as my parents him who taught me this art; to live in common with him and if necessary to share my goods with him; to look upon his children as my own brothers, to teach them this art if they so desire without fee or written promise; to impart to my sons and the sons of the master who taught me and the disciples who have enrolled themselves and have agreed to the rules of the profession, but to these alone, the precepts and the instruction. I will prescribe regimen for the good of my patients according to my ability and my judgment and never do harm to anyone. To please no one will I prescribe a deadly drug, nor give advice which may cause his death. Nor will I give any woman a pessary to procure abortion. But I will preserve the purity of my life and my art. I will not cut for stone, even for patients in whom the disease is manifest; I will leave this operation to be performed by practitioners (specialists in this art). In every house where I come I will enter only for the good of my patients, keeping myself far from all intentional ill-doing and all seduction, and especially from the pleasures of love with women or with men, be they free or slaves. All that may come to my knowledge in the exercise of my profession or outside of my profession or in daily commerce with men, which ought not to be spread abroad, I will keep secret and will never reveal. If I keep this oath faithfully, may I enjoy life and practice my art, respected by all men and in all times; but if I swerve from it or violate it, may the reverse be my lot.

**Hippocratic theory of bodily humors**

Humors are blood, phlegm, black bile and yellow bile, which vary both in temperature and moistness. Health is a state of balance within the four humors, evidenced by a somewhat warm, wet body. Sickness is believed to be a result of humoral imbalance, which causes the body to become excessively dry, cold, hot, wet, or a combination of these. Herbs, food and medications are also classified as wet or dry, hot or cold. To restore balance to the body, a "cold" disease is treated by administering "hot" foods, herbs or medications. In folk medicine practice, the hot-cold (caliente-frio) application has been a somewhat useful system of diagnosis and treatment.

**hirsutism**

Abnormal hairiness, particularly in women.

**histogram**

A bar graph that is similar to a line graph except that it uses perpendicular rectangles to indicate levels or points.

**histologic technician**

Works under supervision of a pathologist or other qualified physician in sectioning, staining, and mounting human or animal tissues and fluid for microscopic study. Requires one year of training. Job skills are primarily technical; tissue evaluation and screening are not involved at this level.

**histo-technologist**
Conducts microscopic study of human and animal tissue for diagnostic, research, or teaching purposes. Serves in a supervisory capacity to the histologic technician. May perform preliminary tissue evaluation and screening prior to tissue examination by the pathologist. Requires a baccalaureate degree.

**hitherto**
Of the past; in the past.

**HMO**
Health Maintenance Organization. See these words.

**Hobson's choice**
1. Choosing between two or more objectionable or devastating choices. 2. Freedom to choose when no meaningful choice exists, such as an option between having a breast removed because of cancer or not having it removed and eventually dying of cancer.

**hoc (Lat.)**
This.

**hold**
1. To retain or detain. 2. To have in safe keeping. 3. To own something lawfully. 4. To decide; a final decision of a court. "The court holds that . . ." 5. To conduct or take place—to hold a hearing. 6. To bind by contract.

**holder**
1. One who holds. 2. A person with legal authority to detain or hold something. 3. One legally possessing a negotiable instrument. 4. The legal owner of an item.

**holder in due course**
Any person or holder who obtains a negotiable instrument in good faith and without knowledge or information that it is bad or overdue.

**hold harmless**
1. Promising to cover any claims that could arise against another party. 2. A provision of law that prevents a governmental entity, institution or other party from suffering additional expenses or loss of benefits as a result of a change in a statute or regulations. Without such a provision such an entity or institution would be responsible for expenses not previously anticipated due to an expanded caseload, more generous coverage provisions, or both. On the other hand, the use of hold harmless provisions often creates substantial confusion, heterogeneity and inequity in eligibility, coverage and responsibilities under a statute. 3. In insurance, a provision offering the insured protection in disputes between the insurer and the provider of a covered service.

**holding**
1. A court's ruling upon the admissibility of evidence or issues raised during a trial. 2. Ownership of stocks, or shares.

**holding company**
A company created to control or have a dominant interest in other companies through owning or controlling their stock or to create a tax shelter.

**hold over**
1. To keep possession after the period of agreement ends. 2. To stay in office after the term of office is up.

**holism**
A theory of healing or therapy that views the body as a whole and must be viewed as the sum of its parts; in health, the whole person—physical, social, mental, spiritual and emotional parts, must be treated as having equal importance. See wholistic.

**holistic**
A term derived from holism, which relates to organic or functional relationships between parts and wholes; whole entities making up reality and exist more than the mere sum of their parts. See wholistic.

**holograph**
A handwritten and signed legal document. A document written entirely in the hand of the person who executed it and signed it; usually a will.

**holographic will**
A handwritten will by the testator.

**homebound**
A vague term that is open to interpretation, but under Medicare and health insurance programs, when referring to home health care, it generally means there must be a normal inability to leave home, consequently requiring exceptional effort to do so. If the patient does in fact leave home, he could still be considered homebound if the absences are: infrequent, of short duration, for the purpose of receiving medical treatment, or for occasional supportive personal care (barber, beautician), and if the absences do not indicate that the patient has the capacity to obtain the health care provided outside rather than in the home.

**home care**
No skilled nursing service, but help with bathing, housekeeping, meal preparation, transportation, financial matters, etc. Not home health care.

**home care department/service/program**
According to JCAH for accreditation purposes, it is a formally structured organizational unit of the hospital that is designed to coordinate the effective provision of physician-directed nursing and other therapeutic health care services in the patient's residence, and that provides at least one therapeutic service directly.

**home health agency**

A non-profit organization which provides home health care. To be certified under Medicare an agency must provide skilled nursing services and at least one additional therapeutic service (physical, speech or occupational therapy, medical social services, or home health aide services) in the home. Services are provided as determined by and adapted to the health needs of individuals and families in all age groups, all diagnostic categories, and all economic situations. These services must be ordered by a licensed physician or one who is federally employed. Direct reassessments followed by renewal of orders is mandatory.

**home health aide**

A specially trained paraprofessional who helps public health nurses, home health nurses and other health care providers with bedside care of patients in the patient's own home.

**home health care**

An essential component of comprehensive health care, includes skilled and supportive services necessary to maintain a person in his place of residence. Services are planned and coordinated to promote, maintain, restore health or minimize the effects of illness or disability. Health services are rendered to an individual as needed in the home. Such services are provided to aged, disabled, sick or convalescent individuals who do not need institutional care. The services may be provided by a visiting nurse association (VNA), home health agency, hospital or other organized community group. They may be quite specialized or comprehensive (nursing services, speech, physical, occupational and rehabilitation therapy, homemaker services and social services). Under Medicare, such services must be provided by a home health agency. Under Medicaid, states may, but do not have to, restrict coverage of home health care to services provided by home health agencies.

**home health care eligibility**

See eligibility, home health care.

**home health services**

1. An array of services provided singly or in combination to individuals and families in their place of residence or in ambulatory care settings for the purpose of preventing disease; promoting, maintaining or restoring health; or minimizing the effects of illness, disability and the normal process of aging. 2. Services appropriate to the needs of the individual and his family are planned, coordinated and made available by an organized health agency—through the use of agency-employed staff, contractual arrangements or a combination of administrative patterns. Medical services are primarily provided by the individual's private or clinic physician, although in some instances, agencies will employ or contract for physician's services. 3. Those health services which can be safely and effectively rendered in the patient's home or place of residence on an intermittent basis. Home health services shall include skilled nursing services and at least one of the following services: physical, respiratory, occupational or speech therapy; medical social work, home health aide services. See home health care, Home Health Agency.

**homemaker aide**
These individuals work under the professional supervision of appropriate health professionals or social workers and assist elderly, ill, or disabled persons with meals, shopping, household chores, bathing, and other daily living needs, both physical and emotional.

**homemaker services**
Non-medical support services (e.g., food preparation, bathing) given a homebound individual who is unable to perform these tasks himself. Such services are not covered under the Medicare and Medicaid programs, or most other health insurance programs, but may be included in the social service programs developed by the states under title XX of the Social Security Act. Homemaker services are intended to preserve independent living and normal family life for the aged, disabled, sick or convalescent. See also alternatives to long term institutional care.

**homeo**
A prefix denoting like, similar.

**Homeopathic Pharmacopeia of the U.S.**
One of the three official compendia in the United States recognized in the federal Food, Drug, and Cosmetic Act.

**homeopathy**
A system of medicine expounded by Samuel Hahnemann based on the simile phenomenon (similia similibus curantur). Cure of disease was said to be effected by minute doses of drugs which produce the same signs and symptoms in a healthy person as are present in the disease for which they are administered. This was said to stimulate bodily defenses against the signs and symptoms. This system of medicine is no longer practiced in the United States. The Hahnemann Medical College now trains allopathic physicians. See also osteopathy, allopathy.

**homeostasis**
A balance. The maintaining of a constant balance in bodily process in order to continue optimal functioning.

**home plan**
A term used by both the Blue Cross Inter-Plan Band and reciprocity programs to identify the plan which provides coverage for a subscriber. See host plan.

**home rule**
Local government, self-governing.

**home setting**
A person's usual or temporary place of residence (except where such place of residence is the health care institution), with the result that the patient does not travel in order to receive services.

**homes for the aged**
Institutions from skilled nursing facilities to private homes offering custodial care. The most basic services a custodial care home usually provides are clean, well-maintained rooms; good meals; assistance in

personal care; some recreational programs; a courteous, concerned and pleasant staff; and a system for emergency treatment.

**hometown medical and dental care**
In the Veterans Administration health care program, outpatient medical or dental treatment paid for by the program and provided eligible veterans in their own communities by VA approved doctors or dentists of their own choice. Such treatment is furnished when the care cannot be given by VA clinic facilities, or when the health of the patient or distance to be traveled gives sufficient justification.

**home visit**
See housecall and visit, home health care, home health services.

**homicide**
The killing of another person; the killing of a human being; not always a crime.

**homosexuality**
Sexual attraction to or contact with the same-sex persons. There are two types of homosexuals: overt and latent. See also bisexuality, heterosexuality, inversion, lesbianism.

**homosexual panic**
Sudden and severe anxiety, precipitated by fear that one may be a homosexual or carry out homosexual impulses. See also homosexuality.

**Hon.**
Abbreviation for "honorable," a title used to address a judge.

**honesty**
Forthrightness of conduct and uprightness of character; truthfulness.

**honor**
1. To accept and pay when due. 2. To accept or pay a negotiable instrument; to honor a check. 3. Integrity, credibility, uprightness.

**horizontal exit**
In JCAH longterm care facilities accreditation, this is an exit that leads from one area of refuge from fire and smoke on a given floor of a building to another area of refuge on the same floor of the building or at the same level in an adjoining building. Both areas of refuge must be of sufficient size to accommodate the number of people expected to occupy both areas at any given time, and both areas must be separated by a fire partition extending from the top of the building to the floor that provides exit to the outside.

**hormone**
A chemical substance produced by various organs of the body that provides specific regulatory effects.

**hornbook**
A book on the basic principles of one subject of law. A basic book or primer on law.

**hospice**

A program which provides palliative and supportive care for terminally ill patients and their families, either directly or on a consulting basis with the patient's physician or another community agency such as a visiting nurse association. Originally a medieval name for a way station for crusaders where they could be replenished, refreshed and cared for; used here for an organized program of care for people going through life's last station. The whole family is considered the unit of care and care extends through the mourning process. Emphasis is placed on symptom control and preparation for and support before and after death. Hospices originated in England (where there are about 25) and are now appearing in the U.S.

**hospital**

1. An institution whose primary function is to provide inpatient services, diagnostic and therapeutic, for a variety of medical conditions, both surgical and nonsurgical. In addition, most hospitals provide outpatient services, particularly emergency care. Hospitals are classified by length of stay (short-term or long-term); as teaching or nonteaching; by major type of service (psychiatric, tuberculosis, general and other specialties, such as maternity, children's or ear, nose and throat); and by control (government, federal, state or local, for-profit (or proprietary), and non-profit). The hospital system is dominated by the short-term, general, non-profit community hospital, often called a voluntary hospital. 2. A facility with at least six beds that is licensed by the state as a hospital or that is operated as a hospital by a federal or state agency and is therefore not subject to state or local licensing laws.

**hospital, acute care**

1. A short stay hospital with an average length of stay of less than 30 days. 2. For PSRO programs purposes, a health care institution or distinct part of a health care institution providing health care services in the PSRO area, as defined in Section 1861(e)-(g) of the Act, except that the institution shall not be a Christian Science Sanatorium operated or listed and certified by the First Church of Christ Scientist, Boston, Massachusetts. For the purposes of gathering data about hospitals, the PSRO may use the following definition: a health care institution in which the average patient stay is less than 30 days. See hospital, acute care hospital.

**hospital-based physician**

A physician who spends the predominant part of his practice time within one or more hospitals instead of in an office setting, or providing services to one or more hospitals or their patients. Such physicians sometimes have a special financial arrangement with the hospital (salary or percentage of fees collected), and include directors of medical education, pathologists, anesthesiologists and radiologists, as well as physicians who staff emergency rooms and outpatient departments.

**hospital beds**

The average number of beds, cribs, and pediatric bassinets (excluding bassinets for newborn babies) that are regularly maintained and used for inpatients in a health care facility during a certain time period which is usually a period of one year; one basic measure of the size of a hospital.

**hospital benefits**
Benefits provided under an insurance policy for hospital charges incurred because of an illness or injury.

**hospital, city**
A hospital that is administered, financed and controlled by a municipal government and managed by an appointed board of consumers and citizens. These hospitals primarily serve the indigent but some provide care for both indigent and paying patients.

**hospital, city-county**
A hospital that is jointly financed and controlled by municipal and county governments, often for indigent patients. See hospital, county.

**hospital, community**
Independent, nonprofit hospital corporations governed by citizens interested in establishing and providing hospital care for their community. Community hospitals are nonprofit corporations which have an elected board of trustees or directors.

**hospital corner**
One method of securing the corner of sheets around a mattress so they do not come loose. Also called mitered corner.

**hospital, county**
A hospital under the administration of a county board of supervisors or a county commission. Large urban county hospitals provide care for the indigent and medically indigent. Smaller, rural hospitals provide care for both private patients and indigent patients.

**hospital district**
This is when several hospitals are organized on a regional basis similar to school districts. Hospital districts are governmental subdivisions established for the purpose of supporting and administering hospitals through the power of taxation of the population in the district. The hospitals are governed by a board of directors elected by the district residents. This makes the district independent of city, county, or state government. This is an uncommon form of health care organization except in a few states, e.g., Texas and California.

**hospital emergency department**
The facilities and services found in acute care hospitals which provide for the management of outpatients who come to the hospital for treatment of conditions considered by the patient or his representative to require immediate medical care in the hospital environment. The term is synonymous with emergency room, accident room, and casualty room.

**hospital expense insurance**
Health insurance protection against the costs of hospital care resulting from the illness or injury.

**hospital fatality ratio**
See case fatality ratio.

**hospital, general**
An establishment that provides—through an organized medical staff, permanent facilities that include inpatient beds, medical services, and continuous nursing services—diagnosis and treatment, both surgical and nonsurgical, for patients who have any of a variety of medical conditions. It has: an administrator to whom the governing authority delegates the full-time responsibility for the operation, patients admitted on the medical authority of the medical staff, a medical record maintained for each patient, pharmacy services maintained in or by the institution and supervised by a licensed pharmacist, diagnostic x-ray services, with facilities and staff, clinical laboratory services with facilities and staff, anatomical pathology services, operating room services with facilities and staff, and food served to patients to meet their nutritional requirements.

**Hospital Insurance Program (Part A, HI)**
The compulsory portion of Medicare which automatically enrolls all persons aged 65 and over, entitled to benefits under OASDHI or railroad retirement, persons under 65 who have been eligible for disability for over two years and insured workers (and their dependents) requiring renal dialysis or kidney transplantation. The program pays, after various cost-sharing requirements are met, for inpatient hospital care and care in skilled nursing facilities and home health agencies following a period of hospitalization. The program is financed from a separate trust fund funded with a contributory tax (payroll tax) levied on employers, employees and the self-employed. Under the program each hospital nominates an intermediary which reviews and pays claims from that hospital for the program.

**hospital insurance protection**
See Medicare benefits, hospital insurance program.

**Hospital International Classification of Diseases Adapted for use in the United States (H-ICDA)**
See International Classification of Diseases, adapted for use in the United States.

**hospital, investor-owned**
This is usually a chain of hospitals owned by a corporation. The corporation also provides management contracts to other hospitals. Some are not-for-profit corporations while others provide stock that is offered for public sale.

**hospital, long term**
Each state has one or more state hospitals providing institutional care of the mentally ill, blind, deaf, retarded and tuberculosis patients. These hospitals are administered by departments, boards, or administrative agencies of state governments, such as a department of health and welfare or health services. The state operates schools for the blind, deaf, and mentally retarded, and infirmaries or hospitals in or supportive of reform schools, detention centers and prisons.

**hospital-medical insurance**
Protection that provides benefits toward the cost of any or all health care services normally covered under various health insurance plans.

**hospital privileges**
See staff privileges.

**hospital, proprietary (for-profit)**
These types of hospitals can be owned by one individual owner or a group (of physicians) as a partnership or corporation. Usually these hospitals are used for the care of their own patients referred by physicians who are part owners or stockholders. Profits in this type of hospital are turned over to stockholders or the owners.

**hospital service charge**
The price per day for inpatient care, which usually includes food, nursing care, overhead, administration and any services used by most patients.

**hospital, short term**
Acute care general hospital. See hospital, general.

**hospital-sponsored ambulatory care department/service/program**
According to JCAH for accrediting purposes it is one or more organizational units, or components thereof, of the hospital, regardless of location, that are under the responsibility of the governing body and through which nonemergency health care services are provided to patients who do not remain in the hospital overnight. This shall not be construed to include individual diagnostic studies performed by the hospital as a service, or those services performed by practitioners in their offices through a written agreement. See ambulatory care, ambulatory setting.

**hospital, teaching**
See teaching hospital.

**host**
Any live organism that harbors another as a parasite or as an infectious agent.

**hostile witness**
One with an obvious prejudice and hostility towards the party who called him or her. See adverse witness.

**host plan**
A term used by the Blue Cross Inter-Plan Bank program to identify the plan in the area where services are provided to a subscriber who is a member of another Blue Cross plan.

**hot and cold applications**
Any hot or cold packs that are applied to an area of the patient's body to cause change in temperature for a therapeutic purpose.

**hot cargo clause**
Used in a contract between an employer and a union. It usually states that the employer will not allow anyone to handle materials

manufactured or to be transferred by a body with whom there is a labor dispute.

**hot line**
A crisis telephone service to provide assistance for people in distress or need of help (e.g., suicide prevention). It is staffed by trained lay people and professionals with professionals also used in an advisory or a back-up capacity. Most hot lines operate 24 hours a day, seven days a week. The number is widely publicized.

**housebreaking**
The breaking into and entering a building or house to commit a crime. It is called burglary if done after dark.

**housecall**
A visit by a physician or other provider to a patient's home. Now considered by some to be an obsolete practice of physicians.

**household**
A group of related people or family living together. See family.

**housekeeping**
The department that provides support services and is responsible for cleaning the hospital floors, walls, and does window-washing, trash disposal, etc.

**house officer**
A medical, osteopathic, or dental school graduate who is an intern, resident, or fellow in a program of clinical training, service, and research.

**housestaff**
1. Generally, the physician staff in training at a hospital, principally comprised of the hospital's interns, residents, and fellows. Members of the housestaff are called house officers. Occasionally also applies to physicians salaried by a hospital who are not receiving any graduate medical education. 2. According to JCAH for accrediting purposes, it is those individuals, licensed as appropriate, who are graduates of medical, dental, osteopathic, or podiatric schools; and who are appointed to a hospital professional graduate training program that is approved by a nationally recognized accrediting body approved by the Commissioner of Education; and who participates in patient care under the direction of licensed practitioners of the pertinent clinical disciplines who have clinical privileges in the hospital and are members of, or affiliated with, the medical staff.

**Hoyer lift**
A portable and movable lift that utilizes a sling to lift handicapped or aged persons into and out of bathtubs or whirlpools.

**H.R.**
House of Representatives.

**HSA**
Health Systems Agency. The statewide health planning agency established under P.L. 93-641. See Health System Agency.

**HSP (Health Systems Plan)**
The document developed by a Health Systems Agency that becomes part of the state health plan and is a detailed statement of goals, objectives, and recommendations for improving the health of the state's residents and increasing the accessibility, acceptability, continuity and quality of health services, while restraining costs.

**H.U.D.**
Department of Housing and Urban Development. The U.S. Cabinet department that coordinates federal housing and land use policy and funds housing construction through a variety of programs.

**humanism**
The interest a person has in or one's devotion to human welfare.

**humanistic**
Being sensitive to another's total needs. Being sensitive to a person's health, social, mental, emotional, spiritual, cultural and economic needs by treating them with fairness, kindness and understanding, with a view of the person being a good, capable and positive person.

**humanistic medicine**
Medical practice and culture which respects and incorporates the concepts that: the patient is more than his disease, the professional more than a scientifically trained mind using technical skills, both are whole human beings interacting in the healing effort; a person is more than his body, he is a unique, interdependent relationship of body, mind, emotions, culture and spirit; each person has the capacity to define and be increasingly responsible for himself, the professional seeks to assist the patient in taking and fulfilling his responsibility for himself; health and disease are not matters of the moment but have an intricate past, present and future; physical disease, pain, suffering, aging and even death can frequently be valuable, meaningful events in an individual's life and effective practice requires not just conventional skills but also effective development and use of human qualities such as intuition, inventiveness and empathy.

**humanistic psychology**
A recent development in the field of psychology, which is a combination of existential psychology and traditional psychology. Humanistic psychology believes man is basically good, is capable of healing himself, stresses the positive aspects of life and personal growth while maximizing one's abilities, self-worth, capacity for choice and one's responsibility for one's self in life.

**human services/mental health technologist**
Requires minimum education at the associate degree level. Employs skills as a generalist, based upon knowledge of human behavior and social and emotional problems in settings providing mental health and social rehabilitation services. Employs a holistic, non-custodial approach to the individual, treating the symptomatic and causative elements that affect the individual's ability to respond to his environment.

**human subject research**
According to JCAH for psychiatric, alcoholism and drug abuse facilities accreditation purposes, this is the use of patients receiving services in the systematic study, observation, or evaluation of factors related to the prevention, assessment, treatment, and understanding of an illness. This involves all behavioral and medical experimental research that involves human beings as experimental subjects.

**humidity**
The degree of moisture in the air.

**humiliation**
Sense of disgrace, guilt and shame often experienced by depressed persons.

**hunger**
The unpleasant physical feelings as a result of deprivation of something, such as food or drugs.

**hung jury**
When a jury is unable to reach a verdict or decision; no consensus can be reached among jurors.

**hygiene**
An antiquated term for the science of health and its preservation; refers more to personal health.

**hyper-**
Prefix meaning above; up.

**hyperactivity**
Increased muscular activity. A disturbance found in children that is manifested by constant restlessness and rapid movements.

**hyperalgesia**
Unusual sensitivity to pain.

**hyperalimentation**
The administration of nutrients intravenously.

**hyperbaric chamber**
A specialized treatment room designed to utilize compressed air. The compressed air is introduced into the sealed chamber to raise the atmospheric pressure several times above normal with the patient being given pure oxygen at the same time. The chamber is used by patients who need more oxygen than can be gotten under normal conditions.

**hyperkinesis**
See hyperactivity.

**hyperopia**
Farsightedness. Occurs when the focal plane is behind the retina and is therefore never reached. It may be caused by an abnormally biconvex lens or by an eyeball which is too short. The person with hyperopia has

difficulty seeing near objects unless he or she uses glasses with convex lenses.

**hyperorexia**
Extreme hunger. See also bulimia.

**hyperpragia**
Excessive thinking, self-talk and mental activity. It is often a part of the manic phase of manic-depressive illness.

**hypersensitivity**
An acute response by the body to a foreign substance, drug, food etc.

**hypersomnia**
Uncontrollable drowsiness or sleepiness.

**hypertension**
Persistently high arterial blood pressure; it may have no known cause or can be associated with other diseases; high blood pressure.

**hypertrophy**
An increase in the size of tissues or organs as a result of an increase in the size of the cells.

**hyperventilation**
Excessive breathing or overbreathing often associated with stress or anxiety. It is characterized by reduction of blood carbon dioxide, complaints of light-headedness, feeling faint, tingling of the extremities, palpitations, and respiratory distress.

**hypnosis**
Using techniques of suggestibility to alter the consciousness of another. The subject responds with a high degree of suggestibility, both mental and physical, during the trance-like state.

**hypnotic**
A drug used for the sole purpose of producing sleep.

**hypo-**
Prefix meaing below; under.

**hypoglycemia**
A low level of glucose in the blood.

**hypothermia**
A reduced body temperature sometimes induced as a therapeutic measure or caused by exposure to the cold, due to being inadequately dressed for cold weather.

**hypothesis**
A supposition used to explain phenomena; a theory, assumption or a calculated guess.

**hypothetical question**
Combining a group of facts in such a manner as to create a logical situation or question which has not been shown to actually be true.

Hypothetical questions are often asked of expert witnesses to elicit an opinion based upon facts that the expert does not personally know, but which the examining attorney hopes to prove.

**hypoventilation**
A reduced amount of air entering the lungs, usually caused by shallow respirations.

**hysterectomy**
The surgical removal of the uterus.

**hysterical neurosis**
A neurosis that is a response to emotional stress. It often involves a sudden loss of function. This neurosis may have one of two reactions: 1) the conversion type, in which the senses of the voluntary nervous system are involved, or 2) the dissociative type, in which the person's state of consciousness is affected.

# I

**iatro-**
Prefix meaing physician.

**iatrogenesis**
A secondary illness, injury, infection or disease produced inadvertently as a result of treatment for some other disorder or illness.

**iatrogenic**
Resulting from the activity of a physician. Originally applied to disorders induced in the patient by autosuggestion based on the physician's examination, manner or discussion (see halo effect). It is now applied to any condition in a patient occurring as a result of treatment by a physician or surgeon, such as a drug reaction.

**iatrogenic illness.**
Any illness or condition that was unintentional, precipitated, or secondarily induced by heath care examination.

**ibid (Lat.)**
From the same place, the same.

**I.C.D.A.**
The International Classification of Diseases, adapted for use in the United States (ICDA), is used mainly by governmental agencies and the World Health Organization. This reference book is classified either anatomically or by type of disease.

**I.C.T. (insulin coma therapy)**
One form of shock treatment therapy using large amounts of insulin, given to a depressed patient, usually a schizophrenic, to induce a therapeutic coma.

**I.C.U.**
Intensive care unit. See these words.

**id**
According to psychoanalytic theory, it is the unconscious part of the person that controls primitive desires and urges. It is ruled by pleasure.

**idealization**
A mental mechanism where self-confidence is carried to an unrealistic level; being blind to one's own faults, mistakes, shortcomings or to wrongly place another in a position of being perfect or overestimating them.

**ideational shield**
An intellectual and rational defense against anxiety that could be caused by being subjected to criticisms and rejection. Often a result of a fear of being rejected and feeling threatened if he criticizes another person, which he usually dislikes in himself. In both group and individual therapy, patients are allowed to lower this ideational shield.

**idee fixe**
A recurring idea that is associated with obsessional states.

**idem (Lat.)**
Exactly alike or the same.

**identifiable medical services**
In health insurance these services are provided prior to or during a surgical procedure or in the post-operative period (e.g., diabetic management, operative monitoring of cardiac or brain conditions, management of post-operative electrolyte imbalance, prolonged patient or family counseling, psychological support, etc.)

**identification**
A mental mechanism that is a form of hero worship; to feel, act and wish to be another person; identifying and having excessive admiration for someone you admire.

**identification number (I.D.#)**
A subscriber's six (6) or nine (9) digit Blue Cross number. Also called the agreement number.

**identification with the aggressor**
When a person creates, dwells on and incorpoates within himself the behaviors of a person who is a source of anger and frustration from the outside world.

**identity crisis**
A loss of the sense of oneself to accept the role expected of him by society; characterized by isolation, withdrawal, extremism, rebelliousness and negativism.

**idiopathic**
1. Without known cause. 2. Disease that originates in itself.

**idiosyncratic effect**
An unusual and unexpected effect from a medication where abnormal and unpredictable symptoms occur.

**idiot**
An obsolete term to distinguish the degree of mental retardation. See mental retardation.

**idiot-savant**
A retarded person able to perform mental feats unusual for his capability, such as solving complicated puzzles or calculations.

**i.e. (Lat.)**
Id est. That is.

**ignominy**
Dishonor; public disgrace.

**ignorantia legis non excusat (Lat.)**
Ignorance of the law is no excuse.

**illegal**
Against the law; contrary to the law; breaking a city, county or state's statutes.

**illegitimate**
1. No logical; an incorrect deduction. 2. Not having any legal authorization. 3. Bastard; a child born to parents who are not legally married. 4. Actions that are against the law; unlawful; contrary to law. 5. Actions not in keeping with accepted behavior or use.

**illicit**
Unauthorized, unlawful; against; prohibited, illegal; not allowed by law; improper acts, unauthorized conduct.

**illness**
Usually used synonymously with disease. Can be differentially defined by saying illness is present when an individual perceives himself as diseased and disease is present when identifiable by objective, external criteria.

**illuminism**
A hallucination in which the patient carries on conversations with imaginary supernatural creatures.

**illusion**
Any mental picture that is false; unreal perception and misinterpretation of an occurrence.

**illusory**
Deceptive; having false appearances.

**illusory promise**
An agreement that has the appearance of a promise or contract, but depends upon the intent of the promisor. Usually this is not a contract and is not legally binding.

**imbecile**
Obsolete term for a level or degree of mental retardation. See mental retardation.

**imitation**
The following, mimicking, or copying the behaviors and values of another person.

**immaterial**
Unnecessary; unimportant; trivial; irelevant; not of concern.

**immediate cause**
The final cause or end event that caused injury, harm or danger without any further related happenings. This is related to proximate cause. See proximate.

**immediate issue**
A child or children.

**imminent**
Impending, likely to occur without delay; about to happen, threatening to occur.

**immobility**
Restricted movement of a patient.

**immobilization**
1. The rendering of a limb, injured part of the body or the total body by applying a splint or cast or weights. 2. To strap down or secure a patient to a stretcher or ambulance bed for transportation to a hospital, nursing home or other health care facility. 3. To restrain or restrict or incapacitate a hostile or violent person through physical devices or drugs.

**immunity**
1. Freedom from obligation; exempt from duty. 2. Freedom from a duty required by law. 3. Freedom from prosecution on items you have given testimony about. 4. When governmental boards are exempt from performing duties that generally are required of other persons. 5. Resistance to or protection from a disease.

**immuno-**
Prefix meaning safe; protection.

**impaction**
A condition often found in some older long-term care patients of mostly dry, hardened and lodged feces. Also referred to as impacted stool.

**impair**
To diminish in acceptance or quality; to hinder; to lessen one's power; to make worse, lessen or otherwise limit.

**impanel**
The selecting and retaining of jurors for a trial. See empanel.

**impeach**
1. To remove a public official from office for misconduct. 2. To establish the untruthfulness of a witness.

**impeachment**
The removal of a public official from public office, such as a governor, judge, or president.

**impediment**
A disability to the making of a legal contract.

**impertinence**
1. Irrelevant. 2. Not pertinent to the trial or issue at hand. 3. Without relationship to the matter. 4. Proof or evidence presented that is not relevant to the issue.

**implead**
1. To bring a third party into a lawsuit. 2. To accuse. 3. To bring suit; to sue at law.

**implementation plan**
The process by which an agency promotes the accomplishment of the recommendations in its plan. Plan implementation utilizes a combination of methods including advocacy, financial and/or technical assistance to providers, and regulatory controls.

**implied**
1. Suggested, expected or understood but not actually expressed. 2. Known indirectly; assumed to be known. 3. Obvious due to the facts.

**implied consent**
Implied consent differs from expressed consent as it is not written or orally agreed upon but is derived by acts, signs, behaviors, facts, inaction or silence or any action to cause the other party to assume that consent has been given.

**implied contract**
A contract not created by an expressed or written agreement, but implied, as it may legally be deduced from assumptions, and circumstances of a transaction and/or the relationship of the parties.

**implied remedy**
A lawsuit brought to protect a Constitutional right. A right being violated shows that a remedy through a lawsuit is justified.

**implied trust**
1. A trust that is inferred from circumstances rather than expressed in writing. 2. A trust that is implied by law.

**implied warranty**
A legal inference of quality when something is sold by a merchant.

**imposed consent**
An involuntary submission to treatment as authorized by law. Some public health statutes allow the state to require that children be inoculated or immunized against specific diseases prior to being allowed to enter school. Adults may also be required to have certain vaccinations prior to embarking on foreign travel or returning to the United States.

**imposibilium nulla obligatio est (Lat.)**
There is no obligation to do the impossible.

**impossibility of contract completion**
See impossible.

**impossible**
1. Not capable of happening or being completed. 2. That which cannot be finished. 3. A contract is not binding and is an impossibility if it objectively cannot possibly be completed.

**imposts**
Taxes; usually duty on goods or import taxes. Any tax imposed by proper authority or power.

**impotence**
Inability to achieve an erection of the penis.

**impound**
1. To take into legal custory. 2. To legally seize, secure or take an item into custody until any legal disputes or questions about it are decided.

**impoundment**
In the federal budget, any executive branch action or inaction that precludes the obligation or expenditure of budget authority provided by the Congress. An impoundment resolution is a resolution of the House of Representatives or the Senate which expresses its disapproval of a proposed deferral of budget authority set forth in a special message ordinarily transmitted by the President. Passage of an impoundment resolution by either House of Congress has the effect of overturning the proposed deferral and requires that such budget authority be made available for obligation. See also rescission.

**impression, case of first**
A dispute involving a new question, never dealt with before by the courts, and lacking precedent.

**imprimatur (Lat.)**
Let it be printed.

**imprisonment**
1. Restraint of liberty or involuntary confinement. 2. To deprive a person of his liberty or freedom.

**improper venue**
1. A wrongly selected or incorrectly designated city, county or area to hear a case in court; has nothing to do with a court's jurisdiction, only the location of a court. 2. Not correct, fair, convenient or just to hold a trial in a territory, place, geographical area. See venue.

**improvident**
Lacking foresight.

**improvidently**
Diminishing the effectiveness of a court.

**impugn**
To refute; to show as untrue; to oppose to challenge.

**imputed**
1. To be accountable for. 2. If a person does not know a fact, he or she should have known it; to attribute to in a negative sense.

**imputed knowledge**
It is the person's duty to know certain available facts. Knowledge may be imputed to a person and he will be legally held accountable for it as if the facts are or were known.

**imputed negligence**
If a physician is negligent and an RN is responsible for carrying out the physicians's orders or his actions, the physician's negligence is *imputed,* carried over or attributed to the RN.

**imputed notice**
If a person is given notice of a court appearance or a fact or a lawsuit, and the physician is a nurse's agent, master, manager, then notice to the physician can be imputed as notice to the nurse.

**inadequate personality**
Emotional and physical instability where a person is unable to cope with the normal demands of life.

**inadmissible**
Facts or items that cannot be admitted into evidence in a trial.

**inadvertence**
1. Lack of attention. 2. Carelessness. 3. A mistake or oversight.

**inalienable**
Cannot be given away, taken away, bought, transferred or sold. Constitutional rights are inalienable rights that cannot be taken away.

**inappropriate affect**
1. When emotions and behavior are not congruent or are out of harmony with ideas and thought processes. 2. Having emotions not appropriate for the situation.

**in articulo mortis (Lat.)**
At the point of death.

**inattentive**
Lacking the ability to concentrate or focus one's thoughts upon a specific idea or object.

**in banco (Lat.)**
1. In bank. 2. On the bench. Court proceedings before all the judges of the court, as opposed to proceedings at *nisi prius,* which is with only a single judge and a jury.

**inc.**
Abbreviation for incorporated.

**in camera (Lat.)**
In chambers. 1. A hearing or court in session with spectators and reporters not allowed in the room. 2. In the judge's private office.

**incapacity**
The lack of the legal ability or power to do something. An injury serious enough to prevent working.

**incarceration**
1. Confinement. 2. Shut in. 3. Imprisonment.

**inception**
Beginning; commencement.

**incest**
Sexual intercourse between a closely related man and woman. Such activity or a marriage of such is against the law. 2. Sexual activity between close members of a family. Common patterns include are father-daughter, mother-son, and between children. Incest may also be done homosexually.

**inchoate**
1. Not completed; unfinished. 2. An incomplete or invalid document; a partial or part of a legal document, thus lacking completeness.

**incidence**
In epidemiology, the number of cases of disease, infection, or some other event having their onset during a prescribed period of time in relation to the unit of population in which they occur. It measures morbidity or other events as they happen over a period of time: the number of accidents occurring in a manufacturing plant during a year in relation to the number of employees in the plant; or the number of cases of mumps occurring in a school during a month in relation to the pupils enrolled in the school. Usually refers only to the number of new cases, particularly of chronic diseases. The incidence of common colds is high relative to their prevalence. In health economics, the distribution of a tax among groups, usually income groups, in the population. Nominal incidence is the distribution mandated by law, such as a specified division of a payroll tax between employers and employees. Ultimate incidence is the distribution after the income effects of the tax are allowed for. For example, most economists feel that the employer's share of a payroll tax is ultimately borne by the employees in lower wages or consumers in higher prices.

**incident**
According to JCAH for accrediting of long-term care facilities it is an action or occurrence of minor significance.

**incidental**
Occurring in connection with something else or depending upon something else more important.

**incident report**
1. According to JCAH for accrediting of long-term care facilities it is a written report by either a patient/resident or a staff member that documents any unusual problem, incident, or other situation for which the patient/resident or staff member wishes to have follow-up action taken by appropriate administrative or supervisory personnel. 2.

According to JCAH for psychiatric, alcoholism and drug abuse facilities accreditation purposes, this is documentation of events or actions that are likely to lead to adverse effects and/or that vary from established policies and procedures pertaining to patient care.

**incident to**
Belonging to, a part of; dependent upon some other thing.

**incised wound**
A cut that is smoothly and cleanly made, usually by a knife, metal edge, glass or other very sharp object.

**incision**
A surgical cut.

**incite**
Provoke; encourage; stir up. Cause, create or start something.

**incoherence**
Communication that is disconnected, illogical and incomprehensible.

**income**
The return, often measured in money, from one's business, labor, or capital invested. As one example of the complexity of defining income in operational terms the I.R.S. 1040 should be considered as a specific definition of income. Welfare programs attempt to distinguish earned income (wages or net earnings from employment) and unearned income (support or maintenance furnished in kind or cash; annuities pensions, retirements or disability benefits; prizes, gifts, and awards; proceeds from insurance policies, support and alimony payments; inheritances; and rents, dividends, interest and royalties). Note that fringe benefits of employment (such as the employer's contribution to the cost of health insurance) are often not considered as income for tax purposes thus enhancing their real value (and creating, for example, an indirect federal subsidy of group health insurance). See also resources.

**income approach**
An appraisal method used to determine the value of rental or lease property by using the estimated net income over the life of the equipment or property, discounted to determine its current value.

**income averaging**
Reducing taxes by showing that income in prior years was far lower than the present income and thus, pay taxes on the average income for previous years.

**income distribution plan**
A finance program which establishes how income will be paid to its recipients. Various factors of a distribution plan include: a) equal distribution, b) production incentive, c) seniority, d) administrative functions, e) developmental activities, f) outside income, g) length of service, and h) new members. Income distribution plans that include production incentives are more widely used.

**income statement**
A financial statement that evaluates operating performance by comparing financial gains with incurred costs over a given period of time.

**income tax**
Taxation on profits from business, work, or investments.

**in common**
1. Several people having one thing together. 2. More than one person sharing in an endeavor.

**incommunicado**
Cut off from communication, such as a prisoner who is kept from communicating with his attorney, family, friends, or others outside the jail or prison.

**incompatibility**
Incapable of legally existing together.

**incompetence**
A psychiatric legal term suggesting that perceptions and thought processes are not totally adequate to make sound judgments and may lead to abnormal behavior or harm to the person or others.

**incompetency**
1. Lack of a legal right to do something. 2. Lacking the mental ability to take charge of and manage one's own affairs. 3. Inability to perform and do something that is normally expected.

**incompetent**
One who is unfit to do a job because of morality, insanity, a mental deficiency or some other disabling reason. Not legally qualified. See incompetence.

**incompetent evidence**
Evidence that is lacking in facts and thus may not be admitted into a legal proceeding.

**inconsistent**
1. Lacking consistency and predictability. 2. Contradictory; if an event takes place one way and it does not occur the same way the next time. 3. Not dependable.

**incontinence**
The loss of control of either bowel or bladder or both. Some of the common causes of incontinence are spinal cord injury, disease, infection, loss of sphincter (muscle) power, loss of bladder tone, disorientation due to drugs, or lack of interest on the part of the patient or nurse in maintaining or establishing control.

**inconvenience**
1. Posing a minor hardship. 2. From a trivial to a serious injustice.

**incorporate**
To formally and legally create a corporation.

**incorporeal**
Legally meaning without body.

**incorporeal hereditament**
Something intangible capable of being inherited.

**increment**
1. A step by step gain or increase. 2. The process of adding to something. 3. A step upward.

**incriminate**
To expose facts or information about oneself or another so that it could lead to being charged with a crime.

**incriminatory**
Showing guilt.

**incubation**
Microorganisms under conditions favorable to their growth.

**incubation period**
The time it takes for growth of a pathogen between the time of entrance of the pathogen into a medium conducive to growth and the onset of the symptoms of the infection.

**incubus**
To take on something oppressive or burdensome.

**inculpatory**
To accuse. To establish or fix blame or guilt.

**incumbent**
One who presently occupies a public office.

**incumber**
See encumber, encumbrance.

**incur**
1. Acquire; get; to obtain or inherit something bad. You incur a liability when a court decides a judgment against you that forces you to pay money. 2. In insurance, to become liable for a loss, claim or expense. Cases or losses incurred are those occurring within a fixed period for which an insurance plan becomes liable whether or not reported, adjusted and paid.

**indecent**
Offensive to the morality of the public or society.

**indefeasible**
A right that cannot be revoked, or taken away; that which cannot be voided.

**indefinite term**
A jail or prison sentence given for an indefinite time period up to a certain maximum number of years.

**indemnified**
Made whole again; reimbursed.

**indemnify**
To compensate or reimburse a person who has suffered a loss or damages due to injury or harm done.

**indemnity**
1. An insurance contract to compensate a person for losses of a limited or particular type. 2. One party is compensated for loss by another party. 3. A benefit paid by an insurer for a loss insured under a policy.

**indemnity benefits**
Under health insurance policies, benefits in the form of cash payments rather than services. The indemnity insurance contract usually defines the maximum amounts which will be paid for the covered services. In most cases, after the provider of service has billed the patient in the usual way, the insured person submits to the insurance company proof that he has paid the bills and is then reimbursed by the company in the amount of the covered costs, making up the difference himself. In some instances, the provider of service may complete the necessary forms and submit them to the insurance company directly for reimbursement, billing the patient for costs which are not covered. Indemnity benefits are contrasted with service benefits.

**indenture**
A deed to which two or more persons are signatories and parties.

**independent contractor**
A separate contractor hired to do a particular piece of work using his own skills and by his own control.

**independent medical evaluation (medical review) (Medicare)**
The governing body of a nursing home or hospital adopts policies to ensure that the facility cooperates in an effective program which provides for a regular program of independent medical evaluation and audit of the patients in the facility to the extent required by the programs in which the facility participates including at least annually, medical evaluation of each patient's need for skilled nursing facility care.

**independent professional review (IPR)**
Another name for medical review required by Medicaid for inpatients in long-term care facilities.

**indeterminate**
An indefinite time period; with an exact time period not set.

**indexed**
Describes an amount which is regularly adjusted in proportion to changes in some index, e.g. social security payments are now indexed to (or adjusted to reflect changes in) the Consumer Price Index. Some proposed NHI plans index premiums, cost-sharing, catastrophic thresholds, income levels, or reimbursement rates to the CPI.

**indexing**

In financial matters it is a procedure for using a formula with a fixed payment or rate of return to compensate for the devaluation caused by inflation.

**Indian Health Service**

The Bureau in HHS which is responsible for delivering public health and medical services to Indians throughout the country. The federal government has variable but direct and permanent legal obligations to provide health services to most Indian peoples undertaken in treaties written with the Indian Nations in the last two centuries. The Indian Health Service is responsible for trying to fulfill these obligations within its very severe budgetary restrictions.

**indicator**

A quantitative measure chosen to reflect the health status of the population or to represent how well the health system is performing, and by which the level and change in community health and in health system performance are judged.

**indicia**

1. Signs; circumstances. 2. A fact that is probable, but not certain as shown by some indication or circumstance.

**indictment**

1. A legal formal accusation of crime made by a grand jury. 2. A written accusation from a grand jury.

**indigent**

A person of poverty status; a poor person. A person without property or money.

**indirect cost**

1. An assessment of cost as provided by office space, heat, lighting, office equipment, security, etc. 2. A cost which cannot be identified directly with a particular activity service or product of the program experiencing the cost. Indirect costs are usually apportioned among the program's services in proportion to each service's share of direct costs.

**indirect evidence**

Circumstantial evidence; or evidence from facts that are not obvious or easily observed.

**indispensable party**

A person, group of people or organization who have a vested interest in the outcome of a lawsuit, thus a final decision cannot be made unless they are formally included in the lawsuit.

**individual health insurance**

Health insurance covering an individual (and usually his dependents) rather than a group. Individual insurance usually offers indemnity benefits and has higher loadings than group insurance.

**individual health protection services**
Individual education, routine examination and use of drugs, substances or devices in order to render an individual protected against disease and promote his optimum health.

**individual insurance**
Insurance policies which provide protection to the policyholder and/or his family (as distinct from group insurance). Sometimes called personal insurance.

**individual practice**
See solo practice.

**individual practice association (IPA)**
A partnership, corporation, association, or other legal entity which has entered into an arrangement for provision of their services with persons who are licensed to practice medicine, osteopathy, dentistry, or with other health manpower (a majority of whom are licensed to practice medicine or osteopathy), which arrangement provides: that such persons provide their professional services in accordance with a compensation arrangement established by the entity; and to the extent feasible 1) that such persons use such additional professional personnel, allied health professions personnel, and other health personnel as are available and appropriate for the effective and efficient delivery of the services 2) for the sharing by such persons of medical and other records, equipment, and professional, technical and administrative staff, and 3) for the arrangement and encouragement of the continuing education of such persons in the field of clinical medicine and related areas. The term originated and is defined in the Health Maintenance Organization Act of 1973, P.L. 93-222, section 1302(5) of the PHS Act. IPAs are one source of professional services for HMOs and are modeled after medical foundations. See also individual practice plan.

**individual practice plan**
Usually synonymous with a medical foundation. Sometimes used to refer specifically to a health maintenance organization, which obtains its professional services from an individual practice association.

**Individual Responsibility Program (IRP)**
A private medical relationship entered into by a patient and physician. The doctor undertakes to provide the patient with the best medical services possible, and the patient assumes the responsibility of compensating the physician for his efforts.

**individual therapy**
A form of psychotherapy where a professional psychotherapist treats only one patient at a time. See also group psychotherapy, psychotherapy.

**indivisible**
That which cannot be divided; inseparable.

**indorse**

The signing of a name on the back of a document, such as a check, whereby the property or money of the name written is given to another. To sign a paper or document. See endorse.

**indorsement**

1. The actual process of signing a negotiable instrument or document. 2. To support, reinforce or back up a cause.

**indorso (Lat.)**

On the back.

**inducement**

1. Convincing another person to enter into a proposition or to get involved in a situation. 2. In the pleading stage, it is an explanatory introduction about the complaint allegations. 3. A motive or reason for something happening.

**industrial health services**

Health services provided by physicians, dentists, nurses, or other health personnel in an industrial setting for the appraisal, protection, and promotion of the health of employees while on the job. Occupational health services is now the preferred term.

**industrial hygiene**

1. A health profession, science and art devoted to the recognition, evaluation and control of environmental factors or stressors arising from the workplace, which may cause sickness, impair health and well-being or cause significant discomfort and inefficiency among workers or citizens of the community. 2. Control of environmental health hazards that arise out of employment. 3. An essential program in industrial health programs, and may be a function of a medical department or a separate parallel organization under environmental health, engineering, safety or research, and concerns itself with loss control and accident prevention as found in health care institutions.

**industrial hygienist**

Conducts programs in industry to measure and help control, eliminate and prevent occupational hazards and diseases.

**ineluctable**

Inevitable; not to be avoided.

**iner alios (Lat.)**

Among other persons.

**in esse (Lat.)**

In being; existing.

**in evidence**

1. Proof; facts or items that have been presented and accepted in a trial as evidence. 2. Facts or items that are already presented to the court as evidence; facts already proven.

**in extremis (Lat.)**
In the final illness before death. 2. At the very end. 3. About to die.

**infamy**
Loss of one's reputation due to conviction of a major crime.

**infant**
1. A person under the age of majority. 2. A very young child. 3. A minor.

**infant mortality**
The death (mortality) of live-born children who have not reached their first birthday, usually measured as a rate: number of infant deaths per 1,000 live births in a given area or program and time period. The infant mortality rate is one common measure of health status. Infant mortality varies among countries at least partly because the definition is somewhat variable. See also neonatal and perinatal mortality.

**infarct**
Death of heart muscle in a localized area usually caused by an obstructed artery in the heart.

**infection**
The invasion of an organism by pathogens and the reaction of the body to the harmful organisms.

**infection control committee**
The Joint Commission on Accreditation of Hospitals (JCAH) and the American Hospital Association in 1958, recommended the organizing of an infection control committee to be responsible for the investigation, control, and prevention of infections within each hospital. Guidelines for the infection control committee include: all hospitals and other health care facilities shall establish a committee on infection control, the committee shall meet regularly (monthly or bimonthly) and at special times as the need arises. (The committee should include the infection control coordinator, hospital administrative person, internal medicine, surgery, pathology and nursing service.) Small hospitals and nursing homes must develop some form of disease surveillance program and if it is not feasible for smaller institutions to employ a full-time infection control coordinator, they may meet the requirement in several ways. 1) Private qualified consultants in infection control practices. 2) Infection control coordinators of large health care facilities may serve as consultants. 3) Interhospital infection control committees.

**infectious agent**
Any microorganism that is capable of producing infectious disease through a host or an environmental condition that is favorable to the transmission of the pathogenic organism.

**infectious disease**
A disease which is caused by the invasion and multiplication of microorganisms in body tissues, especially that causing local cellular injury.

**in fee**
1. In fee simple. 2. An unqualified freehold estate. 3. Unconditional ownership.

**inference**
To show a fact or circumstance to probably be true through reasoning based on other proven facts or propositions.

**inferior court**
1. Any lower court. 2. A court with limited or special responsibilities and jurisdictions. 3. The relationship of a court within the hierarchy of a court system. 4. A court whose decisions could be reviewed by a higher court, such as a superior or supreme court.

**infestation**
The invasion of one's body by parasites, mites or ticks.

**infirm**
Ill; feeble; weak; suffering from a disease.

**infirmary**
A term more commonly used in the past for a health care facility, hospital or institution where sick or infirm patients are housed or treated.

**infirmity**
1. An ailment or disease of character substantial enough to cause an insurer to not issue a policy. 2. An unsound or unhealthy state of one's body; feebleness. 3. A defect or moral weakness.

**inflammation**
The reddening, heating, swelling and pain that comes to tissue when injured or infected.

**informa pauperis (Lat.)**
As a pauper. Allowing a person to have subpoenas issued and have a counsel provided without having to pay any legal fees, due to poverty.

**information**
1. A criminal accusation issued by a public officer with authority to do so. This differs from an indictment which is issued by a grand jury. 2. A sworn written acusation of a crime.

**information processing system**
In compuers it is the procedure of determining, classifying, assessing, sorting, recording, summarizing, communicating, and storing information.

**informed consent**
1. An agreement by a patient to allow some physical treatment procedure to take place, such as surgery, that is based on a full disclosure of facts to the patient so he or she can make the decision intelligently, to allow or not allow it to take place. The facts have to be understood and complete. 2. A doctrine which requires that no diagnosis, treatment or therapeutic procedure be performed on a patient without being informed in clear understandable terms, of risks, dangers, procedures and alternatives prior to giving consent. Unless a patient is given clear

understandable adequate information about tests, procedures, treatments, therapeutic interventions, drugs to be given and what will happen to his body in a language and a manner that he can clearly and competently understand, then informed consent has not been completed and it may not be valid. 3. Consent, preferably in writing, obtained from a patient to all on the doing of something to or on the patient utilizing specific medical, surgical or research procedures after the proposed procedure and risks involved have been fully explained in non-technical terms and understood. If the patient is a minor, or is incapable of understanding or communicating, such consent must be obtained from a close adult relative or legal guardian.

**in foro conscientiae (Lat.)**
In the forum of the conscience. From a moral point of view.

**infra-**
Prefix meaning below or inferior.

**infra (Lat.)**
Below; within; beneath or under.

**infraction**
1. Violation. 2. A violation of a minor law. 3. A breach or violation of duty or contract.

**infrared heat**
A radiant type of heat used to penetrate body tissues by using infrared rays, heat lamps and incandescent light bulbs for therapeutic reasons.

**infringement**
1. A violation of a right. 2. The illicit or unauthorized using, selling, manufacturing or distributing of something protected by law. 3. Encroachment.

**ingestion**
The taking in of food, water or medication.

**in gross**
See easement in gross.

**ingrossing**
Making a document in its final, official form by producing a perfect copy.

**in haec verba (Lat.)**
In these words. By these words.

**inhalation therapist**
A respiratory technologist trained in specialized therapies and treatments used to care for patients with respiratory problems.

**inhalation therapy services**
Most major health care facilities offer this service. The inhalation therapist administers oxygen and therapeutic gases and mists to patients under the direction of the physician. A separate department and facilities

for inhalation therapy are set aside and are separate from the operating room.

**inherent**
1. Built in, a part of the item itself. 2. Derived from and inseparable. An *inherent danger* is a built-in danger. See inherently dangerous.

**inherently dangerous**
An object that has in itself the potential for causing harm, injury or destruction against which precautions must be taken. See dangerous per se.

**inherent vice**
A basic defect.

**inhibition**
The abnormal suppression or depression of a normal function or behavior, such as sexual desire.

**in invitum (Lat.)**
1. Against the unwilling. 2. Initiating proceedings against an unwilling, non-consenting party.

**initiative**
1. A motivation, power or driving force from within. 2. The power of the people to enact laws by voting.

**injunction**
1. A court order prohibiting a person from performing some act, (a preventive injunction), or demand that he start to do some act (mandatory injunction). 2. An injunction may be preliminary or temporary until the charge can be fully heard in court or the dispute passes. 3. It can become permanent or final once the case has been decided.

**injunctive relief**
Redress for a wrong done by an injunction against the party causing the harm.

**injure**
1. To hurt or harm. 2. To violate the legal rights of another person.

**injurious falsehood**
A false or untrue statement that leads to intentional harm, even if it is not a defamation of character.

**injury**
1. Wrong, harm, or damage done to a person's rights, body, reputation or property. 2. Traumatic (in insurance) or iatrogenic (in malpractice) damage to the body, of external origin, unexpected and undesigned by the injured person.

**injury independent of all other means**
An injury resulting from an accident, provided that the accident was not caused by an illness.

**in-kind**

1. A term used in grants to identify a type of matching funds. In-kind usually refers to a dollar value given to office space, desks, office machines, vehicle, etc., to be used as matching funds to acquire a grant. 2. The same type of thing. 3. A closely similar, but not identical object. 4. In law, to restore or provide the protection of the law to a situation. In lieu of, instead of; to replace; in place of; in its stead.

**in litem (Lat.)**

For a lawsuit.

**in loco parentis (Lat.)**

In place of the parent. Acting as a parent as far as legal concerns, care, supervision and discipline of a child is concerned.

**in medias res (Lat.)**

1. In the middle of the thing. 2. To the heart of the matter, without introduction.

**innocent**

Not guilty. Not involved with or responsible for an act or harm done or a crime. Without knowledge of legal problems involved.

**inoperative**

1. Not presently in effect. 2. Not active or effective. A law no longer used or in effect is *inoperative.*

**inorganic**

Having no organic origin; used to describe acids or compounds that do not contain carbon.

**in paid**

1. In the country; meaning, not in a court or record. 2. An act done informally.

**in pais (French)**

Anything done on an informal basis and not with proper legal authority.

**in pari delicto (Lat.)**

In equal fault; equally to blame, having an equal portion of the fault.

**inpatient**

1. A person who is a bed patient in a hospital. 2. A patient who has been admitted at least overnight to a hospital or other health facility (which is therefore responsible for his room and board) for the purpose of receiving diagnostic, treatment or other health services. Inpatient care means the care given patients staying in a healthcare facility.

**inpatient programs**

According to JCAH for psychiatric, alcoholism and drug abuse facilities accreditation purposes, these are programs that provide services to persons who require an intensity of care that warrants 24-hour supervision in a hospital or other suitably equipped setting. Such programs are usually located in facilities classified as institutional occupancies in Chapter 10 of the 1973 edition of the Life Safety Code (NFPA 101).

**in perpetuo (Lat.)**
In perpetuity. Forever.

**in personam (Lat.)**
The bringing of a legal action or lawsuit to enforce rights against another person, but not against society as a whole.

**input**
The putting of data into a computer to be processed. The transferring of computer data from an external storage unit to an internal storage unit.

**input and output symbol**
A symbol used in computers to identify either input or output functions.

**input measure**
A measure of the quality of services based on the number, type and quality of resources used in the production of the services. Medical services are often evaluated by measuring the education and training level of the provider, the reputation and accreditation of the institution, the number of health personnel involved, or the number of dollars spent, as proxy measures for the quality of the service. Input measures are generally recognized as inferior to process and outcome measures because they are indirect measures of quality and do not consider the actual results, or outcomes, of services. They are often used nonetheless because people are accustomed to their use, and they are easily obtained. See also output measure.

**input media**
In computers it is the forms on which data is recorded which is to be processed.

**inquest**
An official inquiry. A coroner's hearing into the cause of a person's death especially when the death was due to violence or was suspicious.

**inquisitorial system**
The process by which a judge finds facts to represent the state's interest in a trial. It is the opposite of the adversary system used in the U.S. trial courts.

**in re (Lat.)**
Concerning; in the matter of. A title used in judicial proceedings in which there are no opponents, but an item of concern requiring a court's attention. Commonly used in appellate case titles, i.e., In re Polemis. (Polemis was the owner of a destroyed steamship in a landmark case on foreseeability).

**in rem (Lat.)**
Judgment. A judgment against the property within a court's jurisdiction. A judgment in rem can be enforced against any person controlling the object of the judgment.

**insane**
See insanity.

**insanity**
1. A legal, not a medical word referring to an individual who is incapable of managing or unable to control his life, take care of his finances, practice socially acceptable behavior, and unable to distinguish right from wrong. 2. A disorder of the mind, abnormal behavior. 3. Denoting certain kinds of mental illness or disturbance. 4. Legally incompetent. 5. The legal term for psychosis; where a person can be legally determined incompetent if that person's judgment and behaviors are so unreliable and uncontrollable as to cause that person to be a danger to himself or others. A person determined insane can be committed to a mental hospital or a psychiatric ward of a hospital for observation, therapy and other treatments. Insanity is not inherited and usually is temporary and is not feeblemindedness.

**insecurity**
Feelings of helplessness and inadequacy. Unable to comfortably face anxieties about one's place, future, goals and relationships.

**insecurity clause**
A clause in a contract purposefully included so that a creditor can cause a debt to come due if there is reason to believe that it is necessary.

**insight**
1. Become aware of and having an understanding of one's own emotions, psychological and maladaptive behavior. Two types of insight are possible: 1) intellectual insight—knowledge and awareness without any change of behavior; 2) emotional insight—knowledge and understanding of one's own feelings, values and behavior, providing positive changes in personality and behavior. 2. Self-understanding. 3. The extent one understands the mechanisms of his attitudes and behavior; acceptance by a patient that he or she is ill.

**in solido (Lat.)**
As a whole; for the whole. When two or more parties are in solido, each party is liable for the entire payment.

**insolvency**
The inability of a person to pay his debts as they become due. See insolvent.

**insolvent**
A person who cannot pay his debts, or whose assets are less than his liabilities.

**insomnia**
An inability to sleep, which can be caused by mental, emotional or physical problems.

**in specie (Lat.)**
1. In the same way. 2. A specific, similar or same act.

**inspection**
A part of discovery; the right to see, review, question and copy the opposing party's documents in order to view their information and case and to gather evidence.

**installment**
1. Any part of or partial payment of a debt on a regular basis. 2. To be placed into an office. 3. Parts appearing at intervals.

**instance**
1. A forceful request. 2. Any situation or occurrence. 3. To offer an example. Cause of instance is a cause that proceeds the request of a party. Court of first instance is the first court to hear a case.

**instant**
1. Present; soon to happen; current. 2. Without delay; urgent, immediate. 3. A split second or moment in time.

**instant case**
The present case at hand; the case being discussed.

**instigate**
1. To incite; to provoke into action. 2. To prompt or to urge on. 3. Push into action; abet. 3. To start.

**instinct**
A basic, inborn drive.

**institution**
1. A health care facility. 2. A public organization such as a hospital, nursing home, prison, college or church. 3. The starting of a process. 4. A basic system of laws. 5. The act of establishing new rules or laws.

**institutional health services**
Health services delivered on an inpatient basis in hospitals, nursing homes or other inpatient institutions and by health maintenance organizations; but may also refer to services delivered on an outpatient basis by departments or other organizational units of or sponsored by such institutions. The National Health Planning and Resources Development Act of 1974, P.L. 93-641 (section 1531(5) of the PHS Act) defines them as services and facilities subject under HHS ruls to section 1122 review, and requires that all institutional, but not non-institutional, health services be subject to certificate-of-need review and periodic review for appropriateness.

**institutional licensure**
A proposed licensure system (not presently in use in any state) under which medical care institutions would be generally licensed by the state and would then be free to hire and use personnel as each saw fit, whether or not they met usual, individual licensure requirements. Using this system, formal education would become only one of many criteria used in assigning employees to particular positions. Institutional licensure is a suggested remedy to the alleged rigidities of the individual personnel licensing and certification programs presently in use in the health field.

Other criteria could include job experience, and in-service training. Arguments in is favor are that it would allow increased job mobility within the health care field, and greater institutional efficiency. It would perhaps also foster teamwork, and require only one licensing body at the state level rather than the many health licensing agencies presently functioning in each state. Such a system would not end the need for separate licensure of independent practitioners assume that licensure can assure the quality of an institution's services deprives the patient of any assurance that the individual serving him has met individual licensure requirements, and indentured individuals providing care to the institutions through which they are licensed.

**institutional neurosis**

A form of psychological railroading, characterized by an erosion of individual personality traits, increased dependency, emotional distance and an increase in attentiveness to one's self. A result of institutionalization and a failure of the staff to treat the elderly or mentally ill with appropriate respect and in a humane manner.

**institutional planning (Medicare)**

A plan that provides for an annual operating budget which includes all anticipated income and expenses related to items which would, under generally accepted accounting principles, be considered income and expense items (except that nothing in this paragraph shall require that there be prepared, in connection with any budget, an item-by-item identification of the components of each type of anticipated expenditure or income). It also provides for a capital expenditures plan for at least a 3-year period (including the year to which the operating budget described in paragraph 1 of this section is applicable) which includes and identifies in detail the anticipated sources of financing for, and the objectives of each anticipated expenditure in excess of $100,000 related to the acquisition of land, the improvement of land, buildings, and equipment, and the replacement, modernization, and expansion of the buildings and equipment which would, under generally accepted accounting principles, be considered capital items. Review and updating is done at least annually, and is prepared, under the direction of the governing body of the institution, by a committee consisting of representatives of the governing body, the administrative staff, and the organized medical staff (if any) of the institution.

**instructions**

The rules and directions provided by a judge to a jury; a judge explaining procedure, rules, expectations as to how a jury should go about reviewing and deciding a case, including questions to be considered, issues to be decided, the laws, burden of proof and how they need to be considered in order to reach a final decision.

**instrument**

1. A legal written document or paper. 2. A questionnaire used in research; a form, questionnaire or information gathering tool.

**instrumentality**
The legal situaton created when a minor corporation is completely controlled by another major corporation.

**insufficiency**
In equity pleading, an answer that fails to reply to the allegations of a complaint.

**insulin coma therapy**
A form of psychiatric therapy in which insulin is administered to the patient to produce a coma. It is used in certain types of depression and schizophrenia in which other therapies have not been successful. This is not used much anymore. See electroshock therapy.

**insurable interest**
1. A financial interest in another person, organization, goods or items. 2. An insurance contract must include an interest or activity that is insurable. A person can suffer a financial loss if the object is lost as a person dies, thus this interest has to be insured.

**insurable risk**
A risk which has the following attributes: it is one of a large homogeneous group of similar risks; the loss produced by the risk is definable and quantifiable; the occurrence of loss in individual cases is accidental or fortuitous; the potential loss is large enough to cause hardship; the cost of insuring is economically feasible; the chance of loss is calculable; and it is sufficiently unlikely that loss will occur in many individual cases at the same time.

**insurance**
The contractual relationship which exists when one party, for a consideration, agrees to reimburse another for loss to a person or thing caused by designated contingencies. The first party is the insurer; the second, the insured; the contract, the insurance policy; the consideration, the premium; the person or thing, the risk; and the contingency, the hazard or peril. Generally, a formal social device for reducing the risk of losses for individuals by spreading the risk over groups. Insurance characteristically, but not necessarily, involves equitable contributions by the insured, pooling of risks, and the transfer of risks by contract. Insurance may be offered on either a profit or nonprofit basis, to groups or individuals. See also social insurance and prepayment.

**insurance clause**
The clause which indicates theparties to a health or other insurance contract, sets forth the type of losses, benefits or services covered, and defines the benefitr to be paid.

**insurance commissioner**
The state official charged with the enforcement of laws pertaining to insurance in the respective states. The commissioner's title, status in government and responsibilities differ somewhat from state to state but all states have an official having such responsibilities regardless of his title. Sometimes called superintendent or director.

**insurance company**
Any corporation primarily engaged in the business of furnishing insurance protection to the public.

**insurance pool**
An organization of insurers or reinsurers through which particular types of risk are shared or pooled. The risk of high loss by any particular insurance company is transferred to the group as a whole (the insurance pool) with premiums, losses, and expenses shared in agreed amounts. The advantage of a pool is that the size of expected losses can be predicted for the pool with much more certainty than for any individual party to it. Pooling arrangements are often used for catastrophic coverage or for certain high risk populations like the disabled. Pooling may also be done within a single company by pooling the risks insured under various different policies so that high losses incurred by one policy are shared with others. See also assigned risk.

**insured**
The individual or organization protected in case of loss under the terms of an insurance policy. The insured is not necessarily the one at risk, but the one who is protected from accident or sickness. In group insurance the employer is the insured, the employees are the risks.

**insurer**
1. The organization, agent or company that provides and writes insurance. 2. The party to an insurance policy who contracts to pay losses or render services.

**intake**
According to JCAH for psychiatric, alcoholism and drug abuse facilities accreditaton purposes, this is the administrative and assessment process for admission to a program.

**intangible**
Rights rather than physical properties; that which has no physical quality.

**intangibles**
Things that have no physical properties, such as rights, rather than objects; bank accounts, patents, copyrights, etc.

**integrated**
To complete. Combined together into one; made whole.

**integrated agreement**
An agreement made in a document as the final and complete explanation of the agreement. This written document is labeled the "integration."

**integrating services**
The coordination of services in a continuum in order to provide the maximum efficiency and utilization while minimizing duplication and cost.

**integration**
1. In contract law, a document that is accepted by both parties as final. 2. The process of making whole or complete. 3. Bring together. 4. The

balancing of ratios of races and to give all races equal treatment. See integrated.

**intelligence**
Capacity for understanding, recalling, mobilizing, being successful in school and integrating what one has learned and using it in new situations; ability of the mind, specifically the ability to make good and rational judgments plus its memory, imagination, reasoning, perception and ability to distinguish and recall.

**intemperance**
Want of moderation of self-control; excess.

**intensity of service**
The quantities of services provided to patients in a hospital or some other identifiable setting. Intensity can be expressed in terms of a weighted index of services provided, or in terms of a set of statistics indicating the average number of laboratory tests, surgical procedures, X-rays, etc., provided per patient or per patient day. Intensity is a function of the type of program and its case-mix.

**intensive care unit**
A special care unit in a hospital providing special equipment and specially trained personnel for the concentrated care of critically ill patients. See special care units.

**intensive care unit (ICU)**
A specialized nursing unit which concentrates in one area within a hospital, seriously ill patients needing constant nursing care and observation. Some intensive care units limit their services to certain types of patients such as coronary care, surgical intensive care, and newborn intensive care units. See also progressive patient care.

**intent**
1. To commit an act with a purpose or reason; to purposefully do an act or behavior. 2. The aim or purpose of using certain means to reach a particular goal.

**intention**
1. To do something with intent; the doing of an act on purpose. 2. That which is intended or planned.

**intentional tort**
When someone commits injury, harm or wrong on purpose and it is other than a crime. Whenever damage or harm is done to another person willfully, intentionally and without just cause or excuse, yet it is no explicitly covered by a law. Some intentional torts can be treated as a crime rather than a civil wrong.

**inter-**

**inter**
To bury; place in the earth.
Prefix meaning together; among; between.

**inter (Lat.)**
Among or between; *inter se* means among themselves.

**inter alia (Lat.)**
Among other things.

**interdiction**
Prohibition.

**interest**
1. A person's personal or financial involvement in an action. 2. Any right in property. 3. Extra money received for lending money. 4. Money paid for the use of money; another person's money. 5. The cost incurred for borrowing funds. These costs are only the value of funds received for loans given to the entity. They are expressed as a percentage of the total loan.

**interest charge**
An additional charge made on unpaid bills after a certain period of time. Some health facilities believe that charging finance charges provides additional revenue to the health facility and allows for the competition for the patient's dollar with other businesses. Many administrators of health facilities believe that finance charges are inappropriate in health care.

**interference**
When two different parties make a claim on what may be the same discovery, invention or production.

**interim**
1. In the middle or between. 2. A temporary, or intermediate period; meanwhile. 3. Intervening period.

**interim facilities**
Facilities designed to provide teaching space on a short-term (less than ten years) basis while facilities of a more permanent nature are being planned and constructed.

**interlineation**
Inserting written words between printed lines.

**interlocking directorates**
When a person serves as a director of two or more corporations.

**interlocutory**
1. Intermediate; provisional. 2. Discussion or dialogue going on while a lawsuit is in progress. 3. Presented or announced during the course of a lawsuit. 4. Not a final or definitive.

**intermediary**
A public or private agency or organization selected by providers of health care which enters into an agreement with the Secretary of HHS under the Hospital Insurance Program (Part A) of Medicare, to pay claims and perform other functions for the Secretary with respect to such

providers. Usually, but not necessarily, a Blue Cross plan or private insurance company. See also carrier and fiscal agent, fiscal intermediary.

**intermediary letter (IL)**
A letter from the Bureau of Health Insurance to the intermediaries in the Medicare program which provides them with administrative direction or policy. Thee letters form a numbered series in which the Social Security Administration has made much of the policy for the Medicare program over the last decade.

**intermediate care faclity (ICF)**
An institution recognized under the Medicaid program which is licensed under state law to provide, on a regular basis, health-related care and services to individuals who do not require the degree of care or treatment which a hospital or skilled nursing facility is designed to provide, but who because of their mental or physical condition, require care and services (above the level of room and board) which can be made available to them only through institutional facilities. Public institutions for care of the mentally retarded or people with related conditions are also included. The distinction between "health-related care and services" and "room and board" has often proven difficult to make but is important because ICFs are subject to quite different regulation and coverage than institutions which do not provide health-related care and services. An ICF/MR is an ICF which cares solely or particularly for the mentally retarded.

**intermediate service**
See services, levels of service.

**intermittent**
1. Off and on; periodic; once in a while; occasionally; now and then; comes and goes; stopping and starting again at intervals. 2. A disease which entirely subsides or ceases at certain intervals, as in fever and shivering. 3. Pausing from time to time. 4. Reviews or payments done periodically or at intervals.

**intermittent irrigation**
Same as plain irrigation but done through a closed catheter system at designated intervals.

**intern**
A graduate of a medical, osteopathic or dental school serving a first year period of graduate clinical training.

**internal feedback**
Inside or intrinsic responses one gives back either in writing or verbally.

**internal law**
In conflict of law, it is the laws of jurisdiction other than exception of its choice-of-law rule.

**internal quality audit**
Procedure carried out by staff or internal committees through which health care institutions can determine if their services meet pre-established standards.

**Internal Revenue Code**
The code of the United States Government tax laws.

**International Classification of Disease, Adapted for use in the United States (ICDA)**
A United States Public Health Service official adaptation of a system for classifying diseases and operations for the purpose of indexing hospital records developed by the World Health Organization. Diseases are grouped according to the problems they present. For example, the major infective and parasitic diseases are listed in one section and all malignant neoplasms in another section. A three digit numerical code is used to number the majo disease categories. Subdivisions within categories are numbered with a four digit code. The ICDA is revised every ten years. The eighth version (known as ICDA-8) is now in use and ICDA-9 in preparation. A further revised and expanded version of ICDA-8, known as Hospital-ICDA, was developed by CHPA and is widely used in hospitals and the Professional Activity Study. This version is now in its second edition, H-ICDA-2.

**international law**
Law that applies to the relationships and transactions and interactions between countries. The set of principles that determines which country's courts should hear a complaint or dispute.

**internship**
Any period of on the job training which is part of a larger educational program. In medicine, dentistry, podiatry and some other health professions, a one year program of graduate medical education practically always coming in the year after graduation. Practically all physicians take internships although they are required for licensure in only 39 of the 55 licensing jurisdictions. An internship usually is required for granting of staff privileges. Residencies are increasingly beginning in the first year after graduation, gradually eliminating internships.

**inter-plan bank**
A service provided by the Blue Cross system under which a subscriber receiving care outside his Blue Cross Plan's area will have his bills paid by the local plan.

**interpleader**
A procedure to cause a third person to enter into a lawsuit or risk losing his claim.

**Interpol**
International Criminal Police Organization.

**interpolate**
To insert words or phrases into a completed document.

**interposition**
Where a state may reject an order from the federal government if it believes the federal government has overstepped its authority. The Tenth Amendment provides to the states those powers not delegated to the federal government.

**interpretation**
1. The reading into or deciding of the meaning of a written document. 2. A psychological or psychiatric technique used in some psychological testing and in psychoanalysis, both individual and group. The significance and meaning of behavior, perception and emotions are constructed into a meaningful form.

**interrogatories**
1. Written questions given to the opposing parties in a lawsuit to get written facts and answers given under oath to questions put forth. 2. A part of the discovery process in a lawsuit. 3. Written questions addressed to a witness.

**in terrorum (Lat.)**
In threat.

**inter se (Lat.)**
Among themselves.

**intervening cause**
1. The cause that came in the middle. 2. An indirect cause of an accident or other injury that removes the blame from the person who was the original cause. 3. A cause that comes between the event and the original or proximate cause.

**intervenor**
A person who becomes a party in a lawsuit between two other parties without being legally required to do so.

**intervention**
1. A third party entering in an existing lawsuit between two other parties. 2. Any strategy, procedure, therapy, approach, method or technique that changes, stops, deters or interacts with a problem, disorder, disease or disability of a patient, group or community.

**interview**
A structured communication process for the purpose of obtaining information or to evaluate progress.

**inter vivo (Lat.)**
Between the living.

**inter vivos (Lat.)**
Between the living.

**intestate**
To die without making a will; dying and leaving property that is not disposed of in a will.

**intolerable cruelty**
Same as cruelty, but of a more serious nature.

**in toto (Lat.)**
In whole; complete.

**intra**

**intra-**
Prefix meaning within.
Within.

**intravenous**
Within a vein.

**intra vires (Lat.)**
Within powers.

**intrinsic evidence**
Facts from within a case or evidence gained from a document itself.

**introduction of evidence**
Evidence presented for use or acceptance as facts in a trial.

**introjection**
A mental mechanism, whereby loved or hated objects are used symbolically within oneself.

**intropunitive**
Turning hatred and anger inward or hating oneself, commonly a characteristic of depressed persons.

**introversion**
1. Afraid to interact with others or enter into unfamiliar situations. 2. Turning in to one's self, with no interest in others or the world.

**intrust**
1. To allow another to hold property, money or items of value. 2. To deliver something to another with trust, with an understanding as to what it will be used for and with the understanding that it will be honores. Also, entrust.

**intubation**
The insertion of a tube.

**inure**
To take effect; to result. To come into use.

**inurement**
Use; to a person's benefit.

**invalid**
1. Of no force. 2. Useless. 3. Not binding; lacking legal force; having no authority or value.

**invasion**
The unwarranted or undesired interference in the rights of others; encroachment upon one's rights.

**invasion of privacy**
The unwarranted encroachment upon the personal and private rights of another through the wrongful viewing of private records or information and/or subjecting the person to undesired publicity.

**inventory**
1. Counting all items or goods in stock. 2. A detailed accounting of all items or property.

**in ventre sa mere (French)**
In this mother's womb. Referring to an unborn child.

**investigational new drug (IND)**
A drug available solely for experimental purposes intended to determine its safety and effectiveness and not yet approved by the FDA for marketing to the general public. Prescription of the drug is limited to those experts qualified by training and experience to investigate its safety and effectiveness. Use of the drug in humans requires approval by the FDA of an IND application which provides reports of animal toxicity tests, a description of proposed clinical trials, and a list of the names and qualifications of the investigators. See also new drug application, and new drug.

**invidious**
Offensive.

**invitation**
Inviting someone to come into your building/facility or onto your property. A hospital or nursing home *invites* the public to come in. Under the law of negligence, a hospital must be more careful for the safety of the public invited in than for the safety of a person who is merely allowed in.

**invitee**
A person who by either implied or express invitation goes onto the property of another. A caller, such as a drug salesman, may not be an *invitee*, but a *licensee.*

**invoice**
A list of goods usually giving prices and numbers of each, item by item.

**involuntary manslaughter**
To unintentionally cause the death of another human being. This is still against the law even though unintentional.

**involuntary nonsuit**
Where the plaintiff fails to appear or fails to produce evidence on which a jury could find a verdict.

**involutional melancholia**
Depression that occurs at middle age or the menopausal period, characterized by insomnia, anxiety, and paranoia. There is usually no history of a previous mental illness.

**involutional psychotic reaction**
See involutional melancholia.

**ippissimis verbis (Lat.)**
In the very same words. In the exact words.

**ipse dixit (Lat.)**
He himself said it.

**ipso facto (Lat.)**
By the fact itself.

**I.Q.**
Intelligence quotient. A measure of intelligence, based on a psychological test.

**irradiation**
Expousre to rays that can penetrate the body, such as x-rays, gamma rays, infrared rays, or ultraviolet rays.

**irrational**
Making decisions that appear correct but are not; a state of emotional confusion.

**irregularity**
1. Failure to use proper procedures. 2. Failure to take the usual or proper formal steps. This may invalidate a lawsuit or cause a default judgment.

**irrelevant**
1. Not important or related to the issue. 2. Unimportant to subject or dispute.

**irreparable injury**
1. Harm that cannot be overcome, repaired or properly reinstated by money alone. 2. Harm that is serious enough to justify an injunction.

**irresistible impulse**
Loss of control due to temporary insanity. An impulse or urge that is beyond control so that a person cannot stop from doing an act of committing a crime. A questionable test used to decide how a person will be treated; as a criminal, or as a mental patient.

**irrevocable**
1. Not capable of being undone or revoked. 2. Incapable of being recalled, stopped or changed. 3. Not revocable. 4. Not able to be repealed or annulled.

**irrigation, plain**
The process of introducing a solution into the bladder through a catheter, then emptying the solution out.

**irritant**

An agent or substance that causes unpleasant responses, such as itching, swelling or a reaction by the tissues.

**isolation**

**isolation**

The separation of patients having communicable diseases from
1. To set apart an idea from the attached feeling tone. 2. The segregation of patients with communicable diseases or special others for a specified time. problems. 3. The state of being separated and kept apart for the protection of self or others for health and medical reasons. Three types are common: 1) strict: limiting the movement and social contacts of a patient suffering from or a carrier of a communicable disease to prevent the spread of the disease to others, 2) modified: making an effort to control specified aspects of care in order to prevent cross-infection, 3) reverse: the seclusion of a patient in a near germ-free environment in order to protect the patient from cross-infection.

**isotope**

One or more of several chemical elements in which all atoms have the same atomic number with each separate one having varying atomic weights. Some are radioactive and can be used in radiation treatment procedures.

**issue**

1. Something in contention. 2. An event, action or occurrence entered into. 3. Conflict. 4. To promulgate or give out officially. 5. The fact or law being discussed. 6. A single point of dispute. 7. Descendants, children, grandchildren. 7. Joint submission of a claim for a decision at law.

**-ist**

Suffix meaning specialist.

**itemize**

To list each piece or object item by item; breaking a list down into individual separated parts.

**I.V. piggyback**

The attachment of a second intravenous solution (I.V.) onto the initial I.V. line, making one solution piggybacked onto the original one.

# J

**j.**
Abbreviation for Judge; justice; journal.

**jactitation**
1. A false boastful statement that results in harm to another. 2. Making false claims or untrue boasting.

**jail**
1. A place for holding persons taken into custody and placed under confinement. 2. Used to hold persons who have broken the law or have been convicted of a misdemeanor or those awaiting trial, who cannot get out on bail. 3. To jail is to place into confinement of a prison or jail.

**jailbird**
One who is often in jail because of habitual law breaking activities.

**jail fever**
Slang for typhus fever.

**jape**
To mock, make fun of; one who uses trickery.

**jargon**
The technical or characteristic terminology of a particular group, profession or culture.

**J.C.A.H.**
Joint Commission on Accreditation of Hospitals. See these words.

**J.D.**
Juris Doctor or Doctor of Jurisprudence. The basic law degree which replaced the LL.B. Other law degrees offered include the LL.M., LL.D., B.L., J.C.D., D.C.L., etc.

**Jehovah's Witnesses**
A church and religious group that has certain limited beliefs with regard to health care. They do not believe in blood transfusions yet believe in surgery, presenting legally complex situations in emergency care, as it is almost impossible to perform some surgical procedures without a transfusion of blood.

**jeopardy**
1. Risk; danger; hazard; peril. 2. The risk a defendant has in a criminal trial of being convicted.

**J.N.O.V.**
Judgment non obstant veredicto.

**jobber**
1. A purchaser; one who purchases and sells goods or services for others. 2. A wholesaler or middle man. 3. One who does work by the job. 4. One who carries on official business for his own gain.

**John Doe**
A fictitious name used in lawsuits where no real defendant is yet known. Also placed in legal documents when the actual person is not known at the time the document was written.

**joinder**
1. The bringing together of causes. 2. Uniting together. 3. Accepting an issue as offered.

**joinder of claims**
When a party asserting a claim joins a claim with other claims that he already has against the opposing party.

**joinder of issues**
When a lawsuit is in its advanced states, where one side claims facts to be true and the opposing side denies them.

**joinder of parties**
1. United as parties to an action. 2. All persons against whom rights are claimed, as either co-plaintiffs or co-defendants. 3. A new person joining a lawsuit, on either side of the complaint or suit.

**joint**
1. Combined, shared, united; undivided. 2. A joint effort owned by two or more parties. 3. Slang for a marijuana cigarette.

**joint adventure; joint venture**
1. A business deal or administrative effort between two persons, companies or organizations, i.e., between two hospitals. 2. A one time group business deal.

**joint and several**
1. Where the creditor has the option to sue the debtors either as a group or individually. 2. United together in an obligation either individually or collectively.

**Joint Commission on Accreditation of Hospitals (JCAH)**
A private, non-profit organization whose purpose is to encourage the attainment of uniformly high standards of institutional medical care. Comprised of representatives of the American Hospital Association, American Medical Association, American College of Physicians, and American College of Surgeons, the organization establishes guidelines for the operation of hospitals and other health facilities and conducts survey and accreditation programs. A staff of medical inspectors will visit hospitals by invitation and examine the operation of the hospital, the organization of its medical staff and its patient records. Hospitals with 25 or more beds are eligible for review. On the basis of inspection reports, the hospital may be granted "full accreditation" (for three years), "provisional accreditation" (one year), or none. Accreditation has been

used by, or adopted as a requirement of specific public programs and funding agencies, e.g., hospitals participating in the Medicare program are deemed to have met most conditions of participation if they are accredited by the JCAH.

**joint conference committee**
In a health care facility this is made up of officers of the medical staff and members of the governing board in order to maintain communications between board and medical staff. This committee, though common, is not always found in hospitals and health care facilities.

**joint purchasing agreement**
A formal agreement among two or more health facilities or programs to purchase professional services, equipment or supplies. The agreements simplify purchasing or result in economies of scale intended to lower costs to the programs. The purchased services or supplies may be shared or simply distributed among the programs.

**joint underwriting association (JUA)**
An association consisting of all insurers authorized by a state to write a certain kind of insurance, usually some form of liability insurance such as malpractice insurance. Such associations may be required or voluntarily agree to write malpractice insurance on a self-supporting basis. They may write such insurance on an exclusive basis, which means individual carriers cannot write such insurance, or on a non-exclusive basis. The JUA approach has been used in state legislation to assure the availability of malpractice insurance. Examples of the powers given to such associations are included in the medical malpractice insurance legislation recently enacted in New York. There, the JUA can issue policies, develop rates, employ a service company to handle the insurance (including claims adjustment), assume re-insurance from its members, and cede reinsurance.

**joint venture**
See joint adventure.

**journal**
1. A book or record that is written and kept up on a regular basis. 2. A periodical professional magazine.

**jousting**
This term is commonly referred to in relationship to medical records, when complaining, belittling, blaming others or criticizing others to defend oneself is done in the chart or to others in person or in court when defending the medical record.

**J.P.**
Justice of the Peace. A local lower level judge and court.

**judge**
1. The person placed in judgment and who presides over and runs a courtroom. 2. One who decides all legal questions, and decides cases. 3. To decide or evaluate. 4. A person appointed to make decisions.

**judge advocate**
A military legal officer who acts as a judge or a lawyer.

**judge-made law**
1. Law created by judicial precedent rather than by a statute. 2. Where a judge changes the law to reflect an intent that was never contemplated by the legislature. Also, see law precedent; common law; judicial opinion.

**judgment (also spelled judgement)**
1. The official determination of a judge or court on legal matters heard. 2. A final decision based on the facts of a case. 3. The comparing or evaluation of one's choices within one's own set of values for the purpose of choosing a course of action. Judgment is intact if one's behavior is consistent with reality; judgment is said to be impaired if the chosen course of action is not consistent with reality.

**judgment creditor**
A creditor who has proven a debt is due and has obtained a judgment and uses the court to collect it.

**judgment debtor**
One against whom a judgment has been made, and who is to make payments to the judgment creditor.

**judgment, estopped by**
An estoppel imposed by a valid decision previously handed down by a competent court.

**judgment in personam**
A judgment against a specific person, over whom the court has jurisdiction.

**judgment, interlocutory**
A judgment made during the litigation process to settle a point which must be determined before continuing. Not a final determination of a case.

**judgment non obstante veredicto (Lat.)**
Judgment not withstanding a verdict, judgment n.o.v. When a judge overrules the decision of a jury which is contrary to law.

**judgment note**
The document a debtor gives to a creditor to allow a confession of judgment.

**judicial**
1. Judges, courts, statutes, law and their functions. 2. Related to a court or a judge. 3. Dealing with jurisprudence. 4. The branch of government that interprets law and decides legal issues, as opposed to the legislative branch.

**judicial action**
Any legal or court action.

**judicial comity**
A court in one jurisdiction is to utilize the decisions of equal and superior courts in other jurisdictions to make decisions from as a matter of practice rather than as matter of law.

**judicial confession**
A confession made before a judge or court.

**judicial errors**
Errors of the court that require a reversal or a revision of opinion.

**judicial notice**
A court's recognition of certain facts susceptible to readily available proof, or which are of common knowledge, without the necessity of proof, i.e., the result of a sharp knife drawn over skin.

**judicial opinion**
1. Judge-made laws. 2. Final decisions made by judges on the appellate level which are referred to at a later date and are used to make new decisions on new cases. 3. A precedent is set by a court's decision on previous cases, thus are used to determine future disputes.

**judicial question**
1. A dispute that is heard by a court; those issues decided by the courts.

**judicial review**
The power of a court to review laws, to declare a statute unconstitutional and/or to interpret laws.

**judiciary**
1. Pertaining to a court of justice, judges, courts and their processes. 2. The branch of government that judges, reviews, studies and interprets the law. See judicial.

**jungle rot**
A skin condition, usually a fungus infection, resulting from a long exposure to tropical climates.

**jura eodem modo destituuntur quo constituunter (Lat.)**
Laws are abrogated by the same means by which they are constituted.

**jura fiscalia (Lat.)**
(Great Britain) Fiscal rights.

**jural**
Basic law of rights and obligations. Legal rights and obligations as opposed to moral rights.

**jurat**
A statement on an affidavit swearing to where, when and before whom it was sworn.

**jure uxoris (Lat.)**
The right of a wife.

**juridical**
1. Related to the court system or a judge. 2. Conforming to law and the court. 3. Regular legal procedures.

**jurisdiction**
1. The limitation on the courts, judges, police, etc. 2. The region or geographical area within which a court has the authority, right and power to carry out its prescribed activities. 3. The subject matters which a court has the authority to hear and decide upon and that are legally binding. 4. The extent of authority a court has. 5. The right to decide a question properly presented in court.

**jurisdictional dispute**
A dispute between unions. Dealing with union members and what the members are or are not allowed to do.

**juris doctorate**
Doctor of Laws. The basic law degree, abbreviated J.D.

**jurisprudence**
1. The study of law. 2. Philosophy of law. 3. System of laws.

**jurist**
1. Judge. 2. An expert in the field of law.

**juristic act**
An act having a legal ramification.

**juristic person**
1. Legal aspects of the individual person. 2. For legal purposes, it is natural persons, individuals and corporations.

**juror**
A person who serves on a jury.

**jury**
Several persons randomly selected and put under oath to weigh and review facts of a case and determine fairness, truth and decide guilt or innocence. A grand jury is used to review complaints and accusations about crimes and hear preliminary evidence. Formal accusations or indictments are then made. A trial jury hears evidence and decides guilt or innocence on criminal cases or liability in civil actions.

**jury box**
The closed-off area in the court where the jury sits.

**jury commission**
A special selected group of private citizens with authority to select names of jurors. This can also be done by a jury clerk.

**jury list**
List of prospective jurors, from which a jury is selected.

**jus (Lat.)**
Right; justice; law; a body of law.

**jus disponendi (Lat.)**
The right of disposing.

**jus mariti (Lat.)**
The right of the husband.

**just**
1. True, correct, proper, rightful, equitable. 2. Legal; lawful. 3. Impartial right; fair; upright; honest.

**jus tertii (Lat.)**
1. The right to property by a person not involved in a lawsuit. 2. The right of a third party.

**justice**
1. The use of legal authority and power to uphold that which is right, fair and lawful. 2. Impartiality, fairness and equality in treatment under the law. 3. Dealing uprightly with others. 4. Legal administration. 5. A judge of higher courts.

**justice of the peace**
A judge or court at the local level.

**justiciable**
That which can properly be determined in a judicial proceeding.

**justification**
1. The act of showing that something is right or just. 2. A strong or good enough reason that facts will stand up in court. That which justifies.

**juvenile**
1. Pertaining to youth, adolescence or childhood. 2. Immature; immature behavior.

**juvenile court**
1. A court that tries children under a certain age. 2. The court used to hear cases of either delinquent, neglected children and arrested adolescents.

**juxtaposition**
Side by side; close together.

**J visa**
A special visa category authorized by the U.S. Information and Educational Exchange (Smith-Mundt) Act of 1948. It is a product of the concept of the educational exchange initiated by the Fulbright program. Individuals with J visas may be admitted to the United States for the purpose of pursuing a full-time program of study (such as residency), but must be absent from the United States for two years after their studies have ended before they can reenter as an immigrant. In 1970 legislation was passed which eliminated this requirement for foreign medical graduates coming to the United States on private funds as long as they were not from a country where their special skills were in short supply. However, waivers may be obtained by those physicians who are from

countries where their skills are in short supply if the home country has not objected to their immigration to the United States. Waivers are rarely, if ever, denied, primarily for lack of objection from home countries. See also labor certification and schedule A.

# K

**Kahn test**
A blood test based on assessing and analyzing certain elements in the blood. Cancer and syphilis can be diagnosed with this test.

**kangaroo court**
1. A mock court. 2. An unofficial court with no authority or legal powers, so often uses force or violence for its power.

**keep**
1. To watch, to defend. 2. To carry on. 3. To manage; to tend to. 4. To shelter. 5. To maintain continuously. 6. To store safely. 7. To protect.

**Kefauver-Harris Amendment (1962)**
This amendment requires that effectiveness of new drugs must be demonstrated before they are allowed to be provided to patients and prescribed by physicians. The law was extended in 1976 to include the safety and effectiveness of medical devices. Devices must be demonstrated and proven effective before they are allowed to be used in the treatment of patients.

**Kelly forcep**
A type of small surgical clamp used to stop the flow of blood from blood vessels by clamping off the vessel; a hemostat.

**Kelvin scale**
A scale on which a unit of measure corresponds to the celsius (centigrade) scale. Freezing is 273.15 K degrees. (32°F)

**Kentucky January**
A program designed to teach students about the problems of delivering health care in a rural community and how to work with other disciplines in solving them. The project was supported by the Division of Associated Health Professions and the Area Health Education System of the Kentucky State Council on Public Higher Education. The project provided allied health students with an overview of the totality of health care in a variety of practical situations and was supported by an Allied Health Special Project Grant to the University of Kentucky. This project permitted the students to obtain a better understanding of their chosen professions and incorporate this experience into their existing community health curriculum.

**Keogh Act plan**
A plan, available since 1963, under the Self-Employed Individual's Tax Retirement Act (Keogh Act), which permits a self-employed individual (such as a private physician) to establish a formal retirement plan including himself and to obtain tax advantages similar to those available

for qualified corporate pension plans. Self-employed individuals can annually set aside up to fifteen percent of earned income or $7,500, whichever is less, and take a tax deduction for it.

**Kerr-Mills**
Popular name for the Social Security Amendments of 1960 which expanded and modified the federal government's existing responsibility for assisting the states in paying for medical care for the aged poor. The Act liberalized federal sharing in vendor payments for medical care under the federal/state old-age cash assistance program. It also created a new public assistance category—Medical Assistance for the Aged (MAA). The medically indigent eligible for assistance under this program were persons age 65 or over whose incomes were high enough that they were not eligible for Old Age Assistance but who needed help in meeting the costs of their medical care. The federal share of medical payments ranged between 50 and 80 percent depending on the per capita income of the states with no limitation on the maximum amount of payment. The Social Security Amendments of 1965 established the Medicaid program, which substituted a single program of federal assistance for medical vendor payments under the categorical cash assistance and MAA programs. The concept of medical indigency was extended to needy, disabled, blind, and dependent children and their families. In July, 1970, federal sharing in vendor payments became available only under Medicaid.

**key issues/constraints affecting plan implementation**
In health planning these are the issues and constraints that are deemed by the Health Systems Agency to be influential or deleterious to the implementation of the Health Systems Plan.

**key-man health insurance**
An individual or group insurance policy designed to protect an essential employee or employees of a firm against the loss of income resulting from disability. If desired, it may be written for the benefit of the employer, who usually continues to pay the salary during periods of disability.

**key numbers**
A legal referencing system. It classifies legal subjects by topics and subtopics, with a key number and sign of a key given to each topic. It is used to find cases listed by subject in the American Digest System and the National Reporter System.

**key primary professional**
Health care professional who is first seen for general health care, e.g., general practitioner, family physician, etc.

**Kg.**
Kilogram.

**Kg.-m.**
Kilogram-meter.

**kHz**
Kilohertz.

**kickback**
Money or favors given to a public or corporate official for personal use, for a favor done or for swinging a deal the way of the person paying the kickback.

**kidnapping**
1. Illegally holding a person against his will. 2. To carry off a person by force or fraud.

**kidney dialysis**
See renal dialysis.

**killing by misadventure**
The accidental killing of a person while engaged in a lawful activity.

**kin**
See kindred.

**kind**
1. A group, class or division. 2. Humane treatment. 3. Type; like.

**kindred**
Blood relationships. Family; kinfolk.

**kinematograph**
A device used to show pictures of objects in motion.

**kinesiology**
The study of the motion and biomechanics of the human body.

**kinesthesia**
The awareness one has of the position and the movement of parts of one's body.

**kineticist**
A specialist in kinetics.

**kinetics**
The study of the rate of change of certain factors in the body.

**kinetocardiogram**
The device that records slow vibration of the chest in the area of the heart.

**kinetocardiography**
The recording of vibration (usually slow) of the chest in the area of the heart.

**kinetograph**
A device used to record movements in the muscles or organs.

**kinship**
Those persons who are descendents of a common ancestor.

**kite**
Negotiable instrument that has no value which is written to temporarily maintain credit or to raise money.

**kiting**
1. Writing a check against an account that cannot cover it, often before funds have time to be added to the account. 2. Writing checks on a checking account before putting enough money in to cover them. 3. Increasing the quantity of a drug ordered by a prescription. Either the patient or pharmacist may kite the quantity of the original prescription. When done by a pharmacist, he then provides the patient with the quantity originally prescribed but bills a third party, such as Medicaid, for the larger quantity. When done by a patient, it is usually because the patient is dependent upon the drug in question. See also shorting and fraud.

**kleptomania**
An irresistible compulsion to steal.

**kleptophobia**
The fear of becoming a thief or of being stolen.

**Kline test**
A test used to test for syphilis.

**km.**
Kilometer.

**Knights-move thought**
A thought process disorder seen in some schizophrenic patients characterized by bizarre and tortuous ideas.

**knockout drops**
Chloral hydrate.

**knowingly**
1. With full knowledge, design and intention. 2. Willfully. 3. In a knowing way.

**koro**
A form of anxiety seen in the oriental cultures, where the male patient believes his penis is shrinking into his abdomen and will possibly disappear. A similar disorder has occurred in females, who imagine the breasts are disappearing into the chest.

**Korsakoff's psychosis**
A mental disorder of alcoholism with symptoms of a loss of memory, lying and making up stories to cover up the problems.

**Kosher**
That which is sanctioned by Jewish law.

**kr.**
Kryptor.

**krypton - 81m.**
The shortest-lived radioactive isotope gas used in medical treatment, having a half-life of 13 seconds.

**kv.**
Kilovolt.

**kvp.**
Kilovolt peak.

**K-Y jelly**
A lubricating salve used to lubricate fingers, hands or devices used in a physical examination of a patient.

**kymograph**
A device used to record physiological reactions on a graph placed on a revolving drum.

# L

**labeling**

All labels and other written, printed, or graphic matter upon or accompanying a food, drug, device, or cosmetic, or any of their containers or wrappers (section 201(m) of the Federal Food, Drug, and Cosmetic Act). Labeling for all of these products is regulated by the FDA, while advertising for these products (with the exception of prescription drugs) is regulated by the Federal Trade Commission. Labeling cannot contain any false or misleading statements and must include adequate directions for use, unless exempt by regulation. Courts have taken a broad view of the term labeling in FDA cases: it includes all written material that is associated with a product (including leaflets, books, and reprints of journal articles or materials that explain or are designed to be used with the product) and point-of purchase display material (such as placards and signs). Written material need not have been provided to the purchaser at the same time as the product to be considered labeling. See also package insert, Physician's Desk Reference and compendium.

**labile**

Unstable rapidly changing emotions.

**laboratory animal technician**

Possesses knowledge and skills similar to the animal technician, but training has been exclusively oriented to laboratory animals.

**laboratory assistant**

A person who works under the direct supervision of a medical technologist, pathologist, physician, or qualified scientist, in performing routine laboratory procedures requiring basic technical skills and minimal independent judgment, in chemistry, hematology, and microbiology.

**labor certification**

Certification by the U.S. Department of Labor which certain aliens (such as foreign medical graduates) seeking to immigrate to the United States in order to work must obtain before they may obtain a visa. People in occupations which the Department of Labor feels are in short supply throughout the country (such as physicians and nurses but not dentists) are given such certification after review of the applicant's qualifications (such as ECFMG certification). See also schedule A and J visa.

**labor dispute**

A disagreement between employees who are members of a union and an employer, over job content, work environment, benefits, wages, etc.

**Labor Management Reporting and Disclosure Act of 1959**
See Landrum-Griffin Act.

**labor union**
An organization formally established to represent employees with the goal of improving benefits, wages and working conditions.

**laches**
1. An unjustified or inexcusable delay in filing or asserting a claim which results in the claim being dismissed. 2. Neglect or omission to assert a claim on time.

**laetrile**
A drug substance derived from apricot pits. Some authorities claim that it has therapeutic value in treating various forms of cancer while other authorities claim it has no value and could possibly be harmful, as it contains a cyanide compound.

**laissez faire**
1. As used in business, this refers to little governmental interference so individuals can pursue their own self interests while unfettered competition will maintain prices and wages at normal levels. 2. In management this refers to leaving the employees alone, having trust and confidence in their ability, thus delegating almost total responsibility to them, which allows them to function to the highest level of their innate capacity. 3. Generally, this is letting people alone, non-interference; letting people fix their own conditions.

**lalophobia**
Fear of speaking.

**LaMaze**
The most popular orientation toward natural childbirth. Based on reconditioning the expectant mother from realization of pain to concentration on breathing and relaxation techniques. Expectant mothers are taught different breathing regimens for each stage of labor and are taught to focus on something in the first stage. The coach is taught to help keep the mother in control.

**Landrum-Griffin Act**
A federal act that allows rights to members of a union. It changed the Taft-Hartley Act and regulates the internal affairs of unions. This was enacted due to fiscal abuse and poor administration by some unions. Known as the Labor Management Reporting and Disclosure Act of 1959 (LMRDA).

**Lanham Act**
A federal statute (1964) controlling the laws of trade and service markes and trade names.

**lapse**
1. The termination of a right because of its lack of use within a set time period. 2. Forfeiture of a privilege by failing to meet on obligation. 3. In

insurance, the termination of an insurance policy upon the policyholder's failure to pay the premium within the time required.

**lapsed funds**
In the federal budget, unobligated budget authority that by law has ceased to be available for obligation because of the expiration of the period for which it was available.

**lapsus calmi (Lat.)**
A slip of the pen. See also lapsus linguae.

**lapsus linguae (Lat.)**
A slip of the tongue.

**larceny**
Stealing; felonious thievery; Taking of anothers property without consent and with the intent of depriving the true owner of its ownership.

**laryngoscope**
A visual examining instrument with a light used to visualize the larynx.

**laryngoscopy**
A process of visually examining the larynx.

**lascivious**
To excite lustful desires; immoral.

**laser**
Light amplification by stimulated emission of radiation. An instrument or device that produces an intense energy thin beam of light that is highly controllable and is able to be direct or aimed at will.

**last clear chance**
The legal concept that a person is liable if he has the last clear chance to avoid injury or damage and fails to do so.

**last dollar coverage**
Insurance coverage without upper limits or maximums no matter how great the benefits payable. See also first dollar coverage.

**last resort**
1. Used to identify the court of last resort, which is when there is no higher appeal process remaining. 2. A court from which there is no appeal.

**latent**
1. Remaining hidden or undeveloped; not apparent. 2. Not discovered by ordinary observation. 3. Undeveloped; dormant. Not obvious by appearance, i.e., latent guilt.

**latent defect**
A defect that is hidden and not readily or easily discoverable upon inspection. Opposite of apparent defect.

**latent homosexuality**
Unexpressed homoerotic wishes that are held in check. Many have questioned the validity of the theory of latent homoeroticism. See also bisexuality, homosexuality, overt homosexuality.

**lateral**
A side; away from the midline.

**lateral support**
1. The right to have one's land supported or held up by the surrounding land. 2. Right to not have one's land undermined.

**laundry and linen services**
May be a part of central supply or the materials management department and does such tasks as collecting, sorting, washing, drying, pressing, mending of sheets, gowns, uniforms and other cloth items used in a health care setting.

**law**
1. Any set of rules established to control acts or behavior. 2. A complete set of rules and limitations of a culture or society. 3. An act or bill passed by a legislature. 4. The regulations, principles, standards and rules of a government. 5. The system of justice and courts that uses rules to defend rights, property, fairness, business society and human activity. Synonyms include: common law, act, code, enactment, ordinance, principle, regulation, statute.

**law, French**
The Norman/French language used by William the Conquerer, which was introduced to England after the Norman conquests of 1066.

**lawful**
Allowed by law; legal; authorized by law; legitimate; not against the law; within the law; that which is recognized by the law; that which conforms to the law.

**law merchant**
Generally accepted practices, customs or standards that merchants commonly use, which over the years have become a part of law.

**law of the case**
1. To refuse to reopen a settled case. 2. Acknowledging a previous decision on a specific subject matter.

**law reform**
1. Making a change in a law. 2. Bringing test cases to court.

**law reports**
Published series containing case decisions as decided by a court.

**lawsuit**
1. A suit, in equity or law brought to court. 2. A civil proceeding to enforce a right as opposed to a proceeding to convict a criminal. 3. A case brought before a civil court to have a dispute decided by a judge or jury.

**lawyer**
1. An attorney, legal counselor. 2. One who is trained, schooled and licensed to practice law. 3. One who professionally advises and counsels others on legal matters and represents them in hearings and in court.

**laxative**
A drug that stimulates the bowel and causes bowel movement activity.

**lay**
Laity, or a non-professional; the general public or an average individual. Those not belonging to, or associated with a profession.

**lay advocate**
A legal paraprofessional or non-lawyer who helps in legal matters or who helps represent persons in hearings of public agencies such as public health departments or health system agencies.

**L.E.A.A.**
Law Enforcement Assistance Administration. A federal agency that provides money to states and local governments to deter crime.

**leaching**
1. The removal from the soil of mineral substances by the action of erosion. 2. The passing of surface water over garbage or wastes that have been placed in the ground. The water washes substances out of the waste, including those that are harmful such as pathogens or radioactive material. These harmful substances then work their way underground to eventually pollute water supplies such as wells, rivers, and lakes. In the past, outdoor toilets and cesspools were serious health hazards due to the leaching process.

**leading case**
1. A case that sets a precedent or establishes a principle of law. 2. A landmark decision or case.

**leading question**
1. To ask a question in a way that can suggest the answer sought. 2. A question that leads a witness to the desired answer.

**lead poisoning**
Lead compounds can cause poisoning when swallowed or breathed. Inorganic compounds cause symptoms of lead colic and lead anemia, whereas organic lead compounds affect the nervous system.

**lease**
1. A contract used in the rental of land or buildings. 2. A contractual agreement where one party provides another with an item for its use. 3. The legal document or agreement allowing one to use something for a set payment at fixed intervals.

**leasehold**
An estate in realty held under a lease; an estate for a fixed term of years.

**leave**
1. Permission to not be present; to go away from. 2. A permission granted. 3. A formal farewell.

**LeBoyer**
A French physician who believes that traditional obstetrics cause trauma to the baby during birth. He advocates that the delivery room have soft music, low lights, a warm temperature, and calm voices. The newborn is given a bath immediately following birth to enhance transition into the new environment.

**L.Ed.**
Lawyer's edition of the U.S. Supreme Court Reports.

**ledger**
1. An account book, used in bookkeeping to record monetary transactions. 2. A business accounting book.

**legacy**
1. A gift given by a will. 2. The disposition of personal property by a will.

**legal**
Required or allowed by law; authorized by or permitted by law; not stopped or forbidden by law; concerning the law.

**legal age**
1. Age of majority, which is from age 18 to 21, depending on the state. 2. The age at which one is old enough to enter into a legal contract. 3. Not a minor or a juvenile.

**legal aid**
Free legal help provided to poverty level persons or those who cannot afford a lawyer.

**legal cap**
Legal stationery or paper. It is a long tablet of paper that has a wide left-hand margin and a narrow right-hand margin.

**legal consideration**
Consideration that is lawful; is legally binding as recognized by the courts.

**legal detriment**
1. Taking on liabilities enforceable by law. 2. Changing one's financial position. 3. Subjecting one's self to duties that are enforceable in court.

**legalese**
Legal jargon.

**legal ethics**
The professional behavior and duties owed by lawyers to their clients, to other professionals and to the public.

**legal fiction**
An assumption made by a court used to decide a dispute even though it is not supported by facts.

**legal malpractice**
Consists of failure of an attorney to use such skill, prudence and diligence as lawyers of ordinary skill and capacity commonly possess and exercise in performance of tasks which they undertake, and when such failure proximately causes damage it gives rise to an action in tort. See malpractice, medical malpractice. Neel v. Magana, Olney, Levy, Cathcart and Gelfand, 6 Cal.3d 176, 98 Cal. Rptr. 837, 838, 491 P.2d 421. (Black's Law Dictionary, West Pub. Co.)

**legal proceedings**
1. Any legal actions in a court. 2. The correct process of presenting a legal action and having it heard in court, according to established rules and procedures in law.

**legal realism**
A part of jurisprudence that utilizes psychology, anthropology, business, sociology, economics, etc. to explain or make legal decisions or judgments.

**legal representative**
One who legally represents or handles another's involvement in the law, a court, suit, trial or hearing. See lawyer.

**legal residence**
The place in which a person or persons actually live, domicile.

**legal right**
A right guaranteed by law, or that would hold up in court.

**legal services corporation**
The federal program of legal aid.

**legal tender**
Official medium of exchange, such as money.

**legend**
The statement, "Caution: federal law prohibits dispensing without prescription," required by section 503(b)(4) of the Federal Food, Drug, and Cosmetic Act as a part of the labeling of all prescription drugs (and only such drugs). Legend drug is thus synonymous with prescription drug.

**legend drug**
See legend.

**legislate**
To renew, create, enact and pass laws such as statutes; ordinances in a legislative body.

**legislation**
1. The process or system through which laws are created, enacted passed or removed. 2. The bills that are in the process of being considered to be made into law.

**legislative**
1. The lawmaking part of government. 2. Those activities requiring legislative action in order to expedite the implementation of the Health Systems Plan.

**legislative authority**
Refers to Section 1513 of P.L. 93-641 that outlines Health System Agency Planning and Development functions.

**legislative courts**
Higher level courts that are established by a legislature, such as Congress, state legislatures or the Constitution.

**legislative facts**
Facts that aid administrative agencies in deciding legal questions on statutes in order to make regulations or rules.

**legislative history**
The written record of the writing of an Act of Congress or state legislature. It may be used in writing rules or by courts in interpreting the law, to ascertain or detail the intent of the Congress if the Act is ambiguous or lacking in detail. The legislative history is listed in the slip law and consists of the House, Senate and conference committee reports (if any), and the House and Senate floor debates on the law. The history, particularly the committee reports, often contains the only available complete explanation of the meaning and intent of the law.

**legislative intent**
1. The intent or purpose of enacting a statute which a court analyzes to help interpret a statute which is ambiguous or inconsistent with another statute. 2. The process by which a judge or agency decides what the lawmakers meant when they passed a law. This process utilizes legislative records and hearing reports; a way of interpreting statutes.

**legislative purpose rule**
Also referred to as legislative intent. Interpreting what the law previously was and trying to decide what the law is trying to do or change. A way of interpreting statutes. That is, the judge will look at a vague law, and after researching it, he or she will interpret according to the way it is believed the legislative body meant it or what purpose they had in mind when passing the law.

**legislator**
A Senator, Congressman, a member of city council, or a county commissioner or other public official who is involved with law making.

**length of stay (LOS)**
1. The length of an inpatient's stay in a hospital or other health facility. It is one measure of use of health facilities, reported as an average

number of days spent in a facility per admission or discharge. It is calculated as follows: total number of days in the facility for all discharges and deaths during the same period. In concurrent review, an appropriate length of stay may be assigned each patient upon admission. Average lengths of stay vary and are measured for people with various ages, specific diagnoses, or sources of payment. 2. In PSRO, it is a criterion which defines the expected point at which patients of similar age and diagnoses or condition would be expected to be ready for discharge. This projection is established by the PSRO based upon an analysis of regional norms and, where available, PSRO area norms for lengths-of-stay.

**lesbianism**
Female homosexuality also known as Sapphism.

**Lese majesty (french)**
Treason

**lesion**
1. Damage; injury. A change or deterioration in a part of one's body due to injury or illness. 2. An area of tissue that does not function due to damage from trauma or disease. Ulcers, abscesses and tumors are considered lesions.

**lessee**
1. The one doing the leasing; the person to whom a lease contract is made. 2. One who leases or pays money for the use of something from someone else.

**lesser offense**
A crime that is a lesser crime or a lesser part of a more serious crime. A misdemeanor is a lesser offense of stealing.

**lessor**
One who leases or receives money for the use of something. One who grants a lease.

**let**
1. To give or award one of many bidders a contract. 2. To hire out; to lease. 3. To allow or permit.

**lethal**
Capable of causing death.

**letter**
1. The exact, specific, precise and literal meaning of a law or document, as in the letter of the law. 2. The precise language of a subject or policy rather than the philosophical intent. 3. A formal document as drawn up by someone with legal authority, as a letter of attorney.

**letter of credit**
A formal statement provided by a money lending institution indicating that it will support a financial agreement.

**letters of administration**
A court drawn document specifically identifying and instructing a person to take charge of the distribution of the property of a dead person.

**letters rogatory**
A request from a court of one jurisdiction to a court of another jurisdiction. This is usually a request that a witness be examined by interrogatories.

**letters testamentary**
See letters of administration.

**leukapheresis**
The selective removal of leukocytes from withdrawn blood, which is then transfused into the patient.

**leukocyte**
A white blood cell.

**levels of service**
When providing health care services such as examinations, evaluations, treatment, counseling, conferences with or concerning patients, preventive pediatric and adult health supervision and similar services necessitating the wide variations in skill, effort and time required for the prevention, diagnosis and treatment of illness and the promotion of optimal health, there are seven levels of recognized service or care: minimal, brief, limited, intermediate, extended, comprehensive, unusually complex. See services for detailed descriptons of these seven levels.

**levy**
1. Assess and collect. 2. To impose. To levy a tax is to pass a tax law in the legislature to collect taxes. 3. To seize or collect. 4. To seize property as ordered by a court ordered writ of execution.

**lewd**
Unacceptable in a sexual way; immoral. See lascivious.

**lex (Lat.)**
Law; a collection of laws.

**lex domicilii (Lat.)**
The law of the domicile, law of the court.

**lex fori (Lat.)**
Law of the court. The law of a state or county where a dispute was decided.

**lex loci (Lat.)**
The law of the place; law of the local. The legal jurisdiction of the state or country where the acts of a civil suit occurred or a contract was made.

**lex loci contractus (Lat.)**
The law of the place of a contract.

**lex loci delicti (Lat.)**
The law of the place of the wrong.

**lex non scripta (Lat.)**
Unwritten law.

**lex rei sitae (Lat.)**
The law of the place of a dispute.

**lex salica (Lat.)**
Salic Law. Laws from 5th century France, which said that females could not inherit land, and by extension of this law, succession to the crown of France could only be a male.

**lex scripta (Lat.)**
Written law.

**leze majesty (French)**
Treason.

**liability**
1. Something one is bound to do, or an obligation one is bound to fulfill, by law and justice. A liability may be enforced in court. Liabilities are usually financial or can be expressed in financial terms. Also, the probable cost of meeting such an obligation. 2. Any legal obligation or responsibility. 3. An act one is answerable to. 4. A debt; an amount owed. 5. To be liable. 6. A loss; an incident; an occurrence; obligation or involvement that works to one's disadvantage.

**liability insurance**
An insurance contract to have an insurance company pay for any liability or loss in return for the payment of insurance premiums.

**liable**
1. Legally bound. 2. Legally required to make good any loss, damage or harm done. 3. Being responsible for one's acts, such as harm done to another. 4. A duty or obligation enforceable in court. 5. Responsible; answerable.

**Liaison Committee on Graduate Medical Education (LCGME)**
A subgroup of the Coordinating Council on Medical Education intended to serve as the accrediting agency for graduate medical education; application to be officially designated in this role is expected to be submitted to the U.S. Office of Education. The committee includes representatives of the American Board of Medical Specialists, American Hospital Association, American Medical Association, Association of American Medical Colleges, and Council on Medical Specialty Societies.

**Liaison Committee on Medical Education (LCME)**
A joint committee of the American Medical Association and the Association of American Medical Colleges responsible for accrediting medical schools. Established in 1942, the LCME is recognized for this purpose by the U.S. Commissioner of Education and the National Commission on Accrediting. The committee is made up of six representatives of the AMA Council on Medical Education, six

representatives of the AAMC Executive Council, two representatives of the public, and one representative of the federal government. While all medical schools are now accredited, there are different types and grades of accreditation which are not constant among schools. In addition to accreditation the LCME and the two councils it represents have also been performing advisory functions for the medical schools with respect to their programs. See also LCGME, CCME, and ECFMG.

**libel**
1. A written defamation of character. 2. A common law wrongdoing; False and malicious written statements that cause harm or injury to a person's profession, position or reputation. 3. Statements in writing, or on film that include defamatory remarks. Libel is actionable without proof of actual damage.

**libelant**
The plaintiff.

**libelous**
1. To be defamatory in nature. 2. To cause harm to or injure a person's position, profession or reputation.

**liberty**
1. Freedom; to be free from any unlawful, forceful or illegal personal false imprisonment or restraint. 2. The personal right to be free within established limits.

**Library of Congress system**
A system of storing or shelving books, which is by subject area and by a number which is assigned by time of publication order which is by the Library of Congress.

**license**
1. A permission granted to an individual or organization by competent authority, usually public, to engage in a practice, occupation or activity otherwise unlawful. Since a license is needed to begin lawful practice, it is usually granted on the basis of examination and/or proof of education rather than measures of performance. License when given is usually permanent but may be conditioned on annual payment of a fee, proof of continuing education, or proof of competence. Common grounds for revocation of a license include incompetence, commission of a crime (whether or not related to the licensed practice) or moral turpitude. Possession of a medical license from one state may (reciprocity) or may not suffice to obtain a license from another. There is no national licensure system for health professionals, although requirements are often so nearly standardized as to constitute a national system. 2. Formal permission authorized by law as indicated by a certificate or document to do something specific. 3. Acting without legal restraint; disregarding the law. 4. Permission to practice or deviate from a strict rule of conduct. See national boards, Federation Licensing Examination, accreditation, certification and institutional licensure.

**licensed nursing personnel**
Under Medicare, registered nurses or practical (vocational) nurses licensed by the state in which practicing.

**licensed practical nurse (LPN)**
1. A nurse who has practical experience in the provision of nursing care and/or completed a 9 month to one year education program but is not a graduate of a formal Bachelor degree, Associate degree or diploma school program of nursing education (see e.g., diploma school). The education, required experience, licensure and job responsibilities of LPNs are fairly variable. 2. According to JCAH accreditation of long term care facilities, it is a nurse who is a graduate of an approved school of practical (vocational) nursing and/or is licensed by waiver to practice as a practical (vocational) nurse.

**licensed vocational nurse (LVN)**
See licensed practical nurse.

**licensee**
1. One who holds a license. 2. A person allowed on property with permission but without invitation or enticement. 3. Used in tort law in some situations to identify an invited person guest as a licensee, not an invitee.

**licensure**
The process by which an agency of government grants permission to persons meeting predetermined qualifications to engage in a given occupation and/or to use a particular title, or grants permission to institutions to perform specified functions.

**licensure and certification**
Certification and licensure of home health care services and facilities including shelter care, long-term care and acute care.

**licensure, limited**
Physician licensure that restricts practice to a specific institution (such as a mental hospital) designated by the state. Holders of these licenses are often FMGs.

**licentiousness**
1. Acting with disregard for ethics, law, or rights of others. 2. Lewdness or unacceptable behavior.

**lien**
1. A legal claim against property rather than a claim against a contract. 2. An incumbrance upon a property. 3. A claim for a payment of a debt.

**lienee**
A person who has a lien against him. A person whose property is subject to a lien.

**lienor**
One who holds a lien.

**lieu (French)**
Place.

**life costs**
Mortality, morbidity and suffering associated with a given medical procedure or disease. Life costs of diagnosis and therapy may be contrasted with their financial costs, and the money required for their provision. Life costs of treating a disease can be compared with the mortality, morbidity and suffering (life costs) resulting from the untreated disease, while financial costs are compared with the various monetary costs of not treating the disease. Use of life costs in assessing the costs of medical procedures avoids the need for assigning dollar values to mortality and morbidity.

**life expectancy**
The average span of time an individual born at a certain point in time can reasonably expect to live. The average age one is expected to live.

**life in being**
The time remaining which a person has to live.

**life insurance**
Insurance which pays a specific amount to the beneficiary when the insured dies. Various types of life insurance include: whole-life, term, and straight or ordinary life. The various approaches include: A) Commercial term life: A group insurance paid to survivor(s) upon death of the insured. Provided by an employer for each of his employees. B) Commercial term life: An individual insurance paid to survivor(s) upon death of the insured. Coverage for a single person usually purchased by, or, for that person. C) Commercial whole life: A group insurance in which payment is made to survivor(s) upon death of insured to a certain age, or, if still alive upon reaching that age, paid to the insured. Provided by an employer for each of his employees. D) Commercial whole life: An individual insurance in which payment is made to survivor(s) upon death of insured to a certain age, or, if still alive upon reaching that age, paid to the insured. Coverage for a single person usually purchased by, or for that person.

**life lie**
A belief or conviction based on fantasy around which a person structures his or her philosophy, behavior, attitudes and life pursuits.

**Life Safety Code**
A fire safety code prepared by the National Fire Protection Association. The provisions of this Code (NFPA, 21st edition, 1967) relating to hospitals and nursing facilities must (except in instances where a waiver is granted) be met by facilities certified for participation under Medicare and Medicaid. The Secretary of HHS may accept a State's fire and safety code, in lieu of the 1967 edition of the Life Safety Code, if he finds that it is imposed by law and will provide adequate protection for inpatients of nursing facilities. The code is based on the Southern Standard Building Code which contains optimum, not minimum, standards.

**lifestyle**
The values, beliefs, behaviors and activities utilized in one's daily living as influenced and affected by physiologic, psychosocial, environmental, economic and religious factors.

**life table**
A vital statistics table displaying the conditions of mortality for selected or specified age groups within a population. Based on age-specific mortality rates, the life table predicts the probability of dying at a given age. Used in underwriting to calculate risks.

**lifetime disability benefit**
A payment to a disabled person to help replace lost income as long as he or she is totally disabled, even for a lifetime.

**lifetime reserve**
In the hospital insurance program of Medicare, a reserve of 60 days of inpatient hospital care available over an individual's lifetime that the individual may use after he has used the maximum 90 days allowed in a single benefit period. See also spell of illness.

**L.I.F.O.**
"Last in, first out," method of determining the value of an inventory.

**limitation**
1. A time restriction. 2. To be restricted or limited. 3. A time period fixed by law during which a legal action can be brought or settled. See statute of limitations.

**limited**
1. Narrowed; restricted. 2. Restricting the liability of shareholders of a corporation so they cannot be sued for corporate actions. 3. Can be a limited company; "limited" is the English equivalent of corporation, abbreviated Ltd.

**limited insurance**
A contract which covers only specified diseases or accidents and restricts indemnity payments. Insuring clause of contracts can be either limited or comprehensive.

**limited partnership**
One type of a business owner arrangement where two or three physicians, psychologists or other health care practitioners, act as general partners and are responsible for all acts of the partnership. Other individuals involved or a part of the group may be limited partners and may purchase an interest in the group but have no voice in the management. The limited partnership minimizes liability exposure of partners to the amount of his or her investment. A partnership by law requires at least one general partner, who is subject to the claims of the creditors, while the limited partners may be exposed only to the extent of the investment. The disadvantage of a limited partnership is finding and identifying an entity willing to take on the responsibility of a general partner.

**limited services**
See services, also levels of service.

**limits of liability**
In insurance, limits on dollar coverage contained in an insurance policy. Malpractice insurance generally contains such limits on the amounts payable for an individual claim, or in the policy year, e.g. $100,000 to $200,000, and $300,000 to $600,000, respectively. Excess coverage describes insurance with limits higher than these conventional amounts. It may also be used to refer to limits on professional liability imposed by law. Several states have enacted legislation, for example, which would place a limit of $500,000 on any malpractice award. Such laws are being challenged as to their legality and, in some instances, have been ruled unconstitutional.

**Lindbergh Act**
The federal statute that makes it illegal to transport a kidnapped person across the border of a state.

**lineal**
Made up of lines; in line.

**lineal relationships**
1. A direct line to one's ancestors. 2. Pertaining to a direct descent from an ancestor. 3. A direct line.

**line of credit**
The highest allowable amount of credit given to a customer.

**liniment**
An oily salve, lotion or liquid used on the skin.

**liquidate**
1. To clear up, pay off or settle an account or debt. 2. To make into cash. 3. To settle the affairs of a company, organization or business and distribute the money or goods.

**liquidated**
Paid off or settled up.

**liquidated claim**
1. A claim or debt bound by an agreement or by a court order. 2. Ascertained; established; fixed; settled. 3. A claim that has a specific fixed amount put on it by the court or by a mutual agreement.

**liquidated damages**
1. A money amount established by the parties to a contract which must be paid off. 2. This occurs if a contract is reached by either party. 3. The party breaching the contract would pay damages to the other party. See damages, liquidated.

**liquidation**
1. To liquidate. 2. The ending or closing of a business or company.

**lis pendens (Lat.)**
1. A notice that a lawsuit is pending; a suit awaiting filing. 2. The public announcement of a pending suit against certain property, which gives notice to anybody, especially prospective buyers, that property is subject to a claim.

**listed**
According to JCAH for psychiatric, alcoholism and drug abuse facilities accreditation purposes, this is used to indicate equipment or materials included in a list published by a nationally recognized testing laboratory, inspection agency, or other organization concerned with product evaluation. The organization periodically inspects the production of listed equipment or materials, and the organization's list states that the equipment or material either meets nationally recognized standards or has been tested and found suitable for use in a specified manner.

**listing**
A right to sell offered to more than one agent at a time.

**lithium therapy**
The treatment of manic emotional states with lithium salts.

**litigant**
A party to litigation; a party to a lawsuit or involved in a legal proceeding.

**litigate**
The act of carrying on a lawsuit; to hold a trial; to go through the litigation process.

**litigation**
1. The process of carrying on a lawsuit. 2. The activities of the process of the law. 2. To go through all legal ramifications of a suit or trial.

**litigious**
1. One who likes to create and bring lawsuits; starting many lawsuits. 2. Subject to disagreement, debate or dispute.

**live birth**
The complete expulsion or extraction from its mother of a product of conception, irrespective of the duration of the pregnancy, which, after such separation, breathes or shows any other evidence of life, such as beating of the heart, pulsation of the umbilical cord or definite movement of voluntary muscles, whether or not the umbilical cord has been cut or the placenta is attached; each product of such a birth is considered live born. It should be noted that this definition includes no requirement that the product of conception be viable or capable of independent life and thus includes very early and patently non-viable fetuses. This has meant that the definition is often not strictly applied and suggests the need for the addition of a viability criteria or the use of a different term (e.g. viable birth) which includes such a criteria.

**living trust**

A trust that is in effect while the person creating it is living. "Inter vivos trust."

**living will**

A short document stating that should a circumstance arise where there is no chance to recover from an illness or injury, then the person creating or signing the document would like to be allowed to die without being placed on machines which prolong one's life by artificial means. The legal status of such a document has not yet been established.

**LL.B.**

Bachelor of Laws, the basic law degree, later replaced by J.D.

**LL.M. and LL.D.**

Law degrees of a higher status. LL.M.-Masters, LL.D.-Doctorate.

**L.M.R.D.A.**

Labor Management Reporting and Disclosure Act of 1959. Also known as the Landrum-Griffin Act.

**loading**

In insurance, the amount added to the actuarial value of the coverage (expected or average amounts payable to the insured) to cover the expense to the insurer of securing and maintaining the business, i.e., the amount added to the pure premium needed to meet anticipated liabilities for expenses, contingencies, profits or special situations. Loading costs for group health insurance range from 5 to 25 percent of premiums; for individual health insurance they go as high as 40 to 60 percent.

**loan consent**

In finance, this is interest rates expressed in percentage form of indebtedness which do not change during the term of the loan.

**loan constant**

Interest rates in percentage form representing indebtedness which remains unchanged during the term of the loan.

**loan package**

A financial proposal containing all items and estimates necessary for a money lending agency to decide whether or not to give a loan. These items would include information on the borrower, loan application, credit report, financial statement, employment letters and information and estimates on the property or equipment.

**loan ratio**

In finance this is a percentage of the amount of a loan to the value of property. Usually, the higher the percentage, the greater the interest charged. Maximum percentages for banks, savings and loans, or government insured loans, are set by statute.

**loan shark**

One who illegally lends money at interest rates higher than allowed by law.

**loath**
Unwilling, reluctant, indisposed, averse, disinclined.

**lobbying**
Efforts by the provision of information, argument or other means by anybody, other than a citizen acting in his own behalf, to influence a governmental official in the performance of his duty. Federal legislation governing lobbying activities (title III of the Legislative Reorganization Act of 1946) does not define the terms lobbying or lobbyist. The Act requires registration by any person "who, by himself or through any agent or employee or other persons in any manner whatsoever, directly or indirectly, solicits, collects, or receives money or any other thing of value to be used principally to aid or the principle purpose of which person is to aid . . . the passage or defeat of any legislation by the Congress." Paid lobbyists are required to register with the Clerk of the House and the Secretary of the Senate and to file quarterly financial reports with the House Clerk. The term derives from the frequent presence of lobbyists in the lobbies of Congressional and other governmental chambers.

**lobotomy**
A neurosurgical procedure in which one or more nerve areas in a lobe of the cerebrum of the brain are severed. Prefrontal lobotomy is the disconnecting through surgery of one or more nerve tracts in the prefrontal area of the brain. This treatment is used in certain severe mental disorders that do not respond to other treatments.

**local action**
1. A lawsuit brought in one place or one locale. 2. An action against a locality. 3. Actions that of necessity or due to jurisdiction, must be brought in a specific place.

**local adaptation syndrome (LAS)**
The reaction of one's body or body parts to stress.

**local issues/needs**
Concerns identified by local groups and residents which are considered as being important to them.

**locality**
In Medicare, the geographic area from which a carrier derives prevailing charges for the purpose of making reasonable charge determinations. Usually a locality is a political or economic subdivision of a state and should include a cross-section of the population with respect to economic and other characteristics. See also catchment and health service areas.

**locality rule**
In malpractice, a rule which bases the standard of care a physician owes a patient on the standard of care generally attained in a specific locality. The most restrictive form of the rule is that the measure of a physician's duty of care to a patient is that degree of care, skill, and diligence used by physicians, generally, in the same locality or community. A less restrictive form holds that a physician owes that degree of care to a

patient which is exercised by physicians, generally, in the same or similar localities or communities. The rationale for the more expansive rule, being applied more widely by courts today, is that the earlier emphasis on locality is no longer appropriate in light of better communications, and the standardization of hospital procedures and physician licensure brought about by state statutes and regulations.

**local option**
Local regulation of the sale of alcoholic beverages used in prohibition or restriction of alcohol sales.

**lock hospital**
A facility used to treat venereal disease.

**lock-in**
In finance, this is a loan that does not allow prepayment so that the borrower is "locked in" to the loan for a specified period.

**lockout**
1. Stopping work; refusing to allow employees to work. 2. Locking the employee out so he can't work, a tactic used by unions or employers when a dispute is unsettled.

**loco parentis**
See in loco parentis.

**locus (Lat.)**
1. Place. 2. Anatomical place of origin.

**locus poenitentiae (Lat.)**
1. Place of repentance. 2. A point, place, or opportunity to withdraw from a contemplated agreement. Also, a point at which one may withdraw from committing a crime; renouncing the intention to commit a criminal act.

**locus sigilli (Lat.)**
The place of the seal. The place on a document where a seal is affixed. Abbreviated L.S.

**lodger**
One who stays in a building owned and operated by another. The person staying has no control over the room lived in. For example, a patient admitted to and staying in a hospital. This is a controversial issue with nursing home residents.

**log**
A journal or record that is frequently used to record daily or periodic events or advancements in ones activities or projects.

**logging in**
1. Creating a log. Recording or creating an original record. 2. Writing down the names of persons brought to a police station.

**logic function**
A computer function. The comparing of numbers and testing of data for certain conditions.

**-logy**
Suffix meaning study; study of.

**long-arm statute**
A statute that exists in some states that allows a court to have jurisdiction over items or persons involved in a claim, dispute or crime who are in another state at that time.

**long-range recommended actions**
Those actions which are suggested to satisfy and insure the attainment of the stated goals and objectives.

**long-stay setting (or long-term inpatient setting)**
A setting which provides health care services to patients who stay overnight in the institution but fifty percent or more of whom remain in the institution thirty days or longer. A long-stay setting may be the usual place of residence of some or all its patients. See long-term care, long-term care facilities.

**long-term capital gain**
Income or financial gain on the sale of a capital asset which has been owned for a specified time (usually one year or longer) which is taxed at a special rate and not as ordinary income.

**long-term care**
Health and/or personal care services required by persons who are chronically ill, aged, disabled, or retarded, in an institution or at home, on a long-term basis. The term is often used more narrowly to refer only to long-term institutional care such as that provided in nursing homes, homes for the retarded and mental hospitals. Ambulatory services, like home health care, which also can be provided on a long-term basis, are seen as alternatives to long-term institutional care.

**long-term care administrator**
A person trained in a specialized area of health administration focusing on the operation of long-term care facilities. Directs, plans, and coordinates operations and activities of extended care facilities. Most commonly this refers to nursing home administrators.

**long-term care facilities**
1. Nursing homes that provide continuity of care for the aged or chronically ill patient. Some are skilled nursing care homes or intermediate care and provide rehabilitative programs for the convalescing patient. Recreational therapy, physical and occupational therapies, social services and other special services are provided for the ambulatory and bedridden patients. Long-term care facilities generally offer a comprehensive care program and usually are participants in Medicare and Medicaid programs. 2. Facilities designed, staffed and operated to render comprehensive, long range health services to those in need of such services. See nursing homes.

**long-term disability income insurance**
To pay benefits to a covered or insured disabled person as long as he or she remains disabled. Usually up to a specified time period, exceeding two years.

**long-term financing**
Loans financed for a term of ten years or more.

**long term hospital**
See hospital, long term, long-term care, long-term care facilities, long-stay setting.

**loop**
1. The repeating or going around of a group of computer functions. 2. The repetition of a group of instructions in a routine until certain conditions are reached. 3. Completing a set of functions and then starting them over.

**loose-leaf service**
Books published in loose-leaf binder form that have current reports on various areas of law. As laws are passed or changes are made, new pages are issued to be added to or replace the old ones.

**L.O.S.**
Length of stay. See average length of stay, length of stay.

**loser**
A department or service in a hospital or health care facility that does not generate enough money to support itself, thus a service or department that loses money; a department or service that causes a continued deficit in the budget.

**loss**
Destroyed; wasted away; failure to win. Loss can be at different levels or amounts: i.e., heavy losses, total loss. 2. Technical loss in health care law is when something remains but is rendered useless as in an eye being blinded or a hand that is paralyzed. 3. In insurance, the basis for a claim under the terms of an insurance policy. 4. Any diminution of quantity, quality or value of property, resulting from the occurrence of some peril or hazard.

**loss-of-income benefits**
Payments made to an insured person to help replace income lost through inability to work due to an insured disability.

**lot**
1. A piece of land of predetermined size. 2. Items that are a separate sale, delivery, or purchase. 3. A portion or a parcel. 4. A number of items in a group.

**loth**
Unwilling. See loath.

**lotions**
Liquids or salves which have limited medicinal effect and often have an insoluble powder.

**lower court**
A court which has only limited authority; an inferior court.

**L.S.**
Locus sigilli, the place of the seal. These letters were once used next to a signature to make a contract formal.

**LSD**
Lysergic acid diethylamide. A potent psychotogenic drug discovered in 1942. LSD produces psychotic-like symptoms and behavior changes, hallucinations, delusions and time-space disorientation.

**Ltd.**
Limited. The British equivalent of corporation. See limited.

**lucre**
Profit; gain. Often used with a negative connotation in referring to profit gotten in a somewhat illegal or immoral way.

**lumbar puncture**
The insertion of a needle into the spinal canal in the lumbar region; a spinal tap.

**lump sum settlement**
1. Payment of a debt in a large payment at one time rather than in smaller amounts over time. 2. Payment of a large sum of money to settle a debt as it might have otherwise gone on forever. 3. Payment of benefits of medical insurance in one check to the injured party or beneficiary.

**lunacy**
Insanity; craziness; mental illness.

**lymphatic**
Referring to lymph or the lymph vessels.

**lysergic acid diethylamide**
See LSD.

**lysis of a fever**
The gradual reduction of a high body temperature back to normal.

# M

**macro-**
Prefix meaning large.

**magistrate**
1. A judge, usually in local and regional courts, who is limited in function and power. 2. A public officer. 3. A justice of the peace.

**magna culpa (Lat.)**
Great fault or blame. Gross negligence.

**magnetic tape**
1. Audio recording tape. 2. In computers, it is a storage, input, and output medium in which data are recorded on the surface of a strip of tape in the form of magnetized spots.

**mailbox rule**
An acceptance to an offer is effective when it is posted in the mailbox; at that moment, a contract is formed and the offer cannot thereafter be revoked.

**mail-order insurance**
Health and other disability insurance secured in response to public or personal solicitation by mail and advertising. It usually requires no physical examination, but rather a statement of health completed by the insured, and becomes effective upon return of the application by mail and approval by the mail-order insurer. The scant health information required, the complexities of medical histories, and the relative difficulty of excluding preexisting conditions have contributed to relatively high premiums and loadings, and low rates of claims recovery from mail-order insurance.

**maim**
To harm or cripple; to injure a person.

**maintainor**
1. A third party interfering in a suit in which he has no interest in order to assist one of the parties against the other. 2. One who supports a lawsuit.

**maintenance**
1. The offense committed by a maintainor. 2. Unethical or illegal support of a lawsuit. 3. Unethical financial support of a client by an attorney while a lawsuit is pending.

**maintenance department**
See physical plant.

**maintenance drug therapy**

After a drug has reached its maximal effect, the dosage is reduced and then kept at the minimal therapeutic level in order to prevent a relapse.

**maintenance services**

Services provided to individuals with chronic physical and mental ill-health conditions in order to prevent deterioration in those conditions, as well as services provided to individuals in need of assistance in activities of daily living. The purpose of such services is to enable an individual to participate in the community to the fullest degree to which that individual is capable. Maintenance services do not include habilitative or rehabilitative services, since the primary purpose of the latter services is to restore functional ability rather than maintain an existing level of function.

**major**

1. Most important; greatest. 2. One no longer a minor; a person who is of age.

**majority**

1. Being of age; no longer a minor; of legal age. 2. The age at which one can ideally manage his own affairs. 3. More than half; greatest percentage; the most or greatest amount.

**major medical**

Insurance designed to offset the heavy medical expenses resulting from catastrophic or prolonged illness or injuries. Generally, such policies do not provide first dollar coverage, but do provide benefit payments of 75 to 80 percent of all types of medical expenses above a certain base amount paid by the insured. Most major medical policies contain maximums on the total amount that will be paid (such as $50,000); thus they do not provide last dollar coverage or complete protection against catastrophic costs. However, there is a trend toward $250,000 limits or even unlimited plans. In addition, benefit payments are often 100 percent of expenses after the individual has incurred some large amount ($500 to $2,000) of out-of-pocket expenses. The various financing mechanisms for major medical are: A) Medicare, Part A: government-supplemented health insurance for the aged and totally disabled which helps pay the expenses of a patient in a hospital, skilled nursing (extended care) facility, or at home receiving services from a home health agency. B) Medicare, Part B: supplementary medical insurance benefits for the aged and disabled. A voluntary program (client pays a monthly premium), which helps pay the cost of physicians' services, outpatient hospital services, medical services and supplies, home health services, outpatient physical therapy, and other health services. C) Medicaid: state and federal payment for medical assistance for certain low-income individuals and families (eligible for welfare or medically indigent). D) CHAMPUS: (Civilian Health and Medical Program of the Uniformed Services): health care benefits available to dependents, children and spouses of all uniformed military service personnel, and to retired military service personnel and dependents of retired or deceased retired personnel. Covered services include: inpatient hospital care, outpatient medical care, surgery, treatment for nervous and mental conditions and contagious diseases. F) Veteran's Benefits: Medical and dental services available to any veteran who has been honorably discharged from the armed services. Benefits are most available to those with service connected disabilities. G) Private commercial insurance through one's employment or paid by oneself.

**major medical expense insurance**
Health insurance to finance the expense of major illnesses and injuries. Major medical policies usually include a deductible clause, which means that the individual or another insurer contributes toward the cost of the medical expenses. A policy especially designed to help offset heavy medical expenses, resulting from catastrophic or prolonged illness or injury. See major medical.

**major surgery**
Surgery in which the operative procedure is hazardous. Major surgery is irregularly distinguished from minor surgery according to whether or not it requires a general anesthetic, involves an amputation above the ankle or wrist, or includes entering one of the body cavities (abdomen, chest or head).

**major tranquilizer**
Drugs that have antipsychotic properties. The phenothiazines, thioxanthenes, butyrophenones, and reserpine derivatives are typical major tranquilizers, which are also known as neuroleptics and antipsychotics.

**maker**
One who makes or prepares a legal document. One who signs a negotiable instrument, which binds the signer or maker to pay on it. A check is an example.

**mal-**
Prefix meaning bad.

**mala fides (Lat.)**
Bad faith.

**mala in se (lat.)**
1. Wrong in itself. 2. An act which is morally wrong, independent of any statute that may declare it wrong. 3. Wrongs in and of themselves 4. Natural wrongs, i.e., murder.

**malaise**
A general feeling of being unwell, restless, indisposed and having physical discomfort.

**malefactor**
One who has committed a crime.

**malfeasance**
1. Committing an illegal or evil act. 2. When personnel perform an act which is unlawful.

**malice**
1. Intentionally causing harm or injury without just cause or excuse. 2. Evil intent.

**malice aforethought**
With an evil intention, but not necessarily with an intent to produce a negative result.

**malicious**
1. With malice or negative intent. 2. Intent to harm someone or to commit a serious crime. 3. Done intentionally without excuse.

**malingering**
The willful, deliberate and fraudulent feigning or exaggeration of the symptoms of illness or injury, done for the purpose of a consciously desired end such as collecting insurance or some other benefits.

**malnutrition**
Any nutritional disorder, usually associated with undernourished or poorly nourished; imbalance in the intake of the various nutrients.

**mal ojo (Spanish)**
Evil eye. A disorder that occurs in the Mexican-American culture. This is characterized by a female child experiencing an adult looking at her with lust, thus causing a curse-type disorder to fall upon the child. Also referred to as just "ojo." Founded on emotional and supernatural powers.

**malpractice**
1. Professional misconduct or lack of ordinary skill in the performance of a professional act. A practitioner is liable for damages or injuries caused by malpractice. Such liability, for some professions like medicine, can be covered by malpractice insurance against the costs of defending suits instituted against the professional and/or any damages assessed by the court, usually up to a maximum limit. 2. Malpractice requires that the patient demonstrate some injury and that the injury be caused by negligence. 3. The professional misconduct or unreasonable lack of skill, improper discharge of duties, or failure to take necessary precautions and to meet the standards of care which results in harm or injury to another. 4. Professional misconduct due to unreasonable incompetence primarily applicable to the medical and legal professions. 5. Professional misconduct or unreasonable lack of skill. This term is usually applied to such conduct by doctors, lawyers and accountants. Failure of one rendering professional services to exercise that degree of skill and learning commonly applied under all the circumstances in the community by the average prudent reputable member of the profession with the result of injury, loss or damage to the recipient of those services or to those entitled to rely upon them. It is any professional misconduct, unreasonable lack of skill or fidelity in professional or fiduciary duties, evil practice, or illegal or immoral conduct. Matthews v. Walker, 34 Ohio App. 2d 128, 296 N.E.2d 569, 571, 63 0.0.2d 208. See also discovery rule, standard of care, claims incurred policy, claims made policy. (Black's Law Dictionary, West Pub. Co.)

**malpractice insurance**
Insurance against the risk of suffering financial damage because of malpractice. See malpractice.

**mal puesto (Spanish)**
Bad or evil place. A disorder related to sorcery that occurs in the Mexican-American culture. It is believed that an illness or disorder is caused by passing, going in, or having an association with a place or spot that is evil. Based on emotional, supernatural powers.

**maltreatment**
Improper or unskillful treatment of a patient by a health care provider which is due to his or her willfulness, neglect or lack of knowledge or skill. This principle does not imply that this conduct by the health care provider is either willful or grossly careless in his or her treatment of the patient.

**malum prohibitum (Lat.)**
Singular-mala prohibita. 1. Any wrong that is prohibited. 2. An act made wrong because it is prohibited by a statute. 3. Conventional wrongs; things thought to be harmful or wrong. 4. Breaking manmade rules, i.e., breaking the speed limit.

**management**
The process of allocating an organization's inputs (human and economic resources) by planning, organizing, directing, and controlling for the purpose of producing outputs (goods and services) desired by its customers so that organization objectives are accomplished. In the process, work is performed with and through organization personnel in an ever-changing environment.

**management audit**
Assessment of financial statements and status and management by a certified public accountant or other knowledgeable professionals. They review the adherence to governing policy, profit capability, controls, operating procedures, and relations with employees, customers, patients, clients and the general public.

**management information system**
A system (frequently automated or computer based) which produces the necessary information in proper form and at appropriate intervals for the management of a program or other activity. The system should measure program progress toward objectives and report costs and problems needing attention. Special efforts have been made in the Medicaid program to develop information systems for each State program.

**management team**
Individuals who plan, coordinate, evaluate, direct and apply the principles and practices of management and administration to an organization's operation, such as a hospital, through a coordinated effort.

**manager**
1. A person who is in charge of and administers a business or company.
2. A member of the House of Representatives who conducts an

impeachment hearing in the Senate. 3. One who conducts the affairs of a business or department. See health services administrator.

**mandamus ((Lat.)**

1. We command. 2. An order issued by a court to a public official, commanding him to perform an act that it is his duty to do. 3. A writ that tells a governmental department to do something.

**mandate**

1. A directive or an order from a high official or higher court. 2. A command; an order. 3. Authorization or power to do certain acts.

**mandatory**

1. Obligatory; required; commanded by formal power or authority; must be followed or obeyed. 2. Imperative; that which must be completed as requested.

**mandatory licensure**

State laws that require all persons who practice in a particular profession, such as nursing or medicine, to be licensed. See licensing.

**mania**

A state of excitability, agitation, and hyperactivity. Excessive symptoms are seen in the manic phase of manic-depressive illness.

**manic-depressive illness**

A mental disorder characterized by severe changes of mood with a tendency to reoccur. In the manic state, the patient is elated and hyperactive; in the depressed state the patient suffers from a depressed mood, anxiety, and possible physical slowing down that can lead to stupor. In the cyclic form of the disorder, the affected person has at least one of each kind of episode.

**manifest**

Evident; obvious; unmistakable.

**Mann Act**

The White Slave Traffic Act of 1910. An act making it unlawful for anybody to transport females across state lines for the purpose of prostitution or debauchery, or any immoral purpose.

**manpower**

The type, level, number and distribution of the personnel needed to accomplish the goals and objectives of an institution, organization, program or a region, i.e., as outlined in a health systems plan.

**manslaughter**

1. The unpremeditated killing of another person. 2. Illegally killing a person without malice, either expressed or implied. 3. The taking of another's life upon a sudden heat of anger. This is unlawful and may be voluntary.

**manual arts therapist**

This person utilizes industrial arts such as woodworking and graphic arts to rehabilitate disabled patients. Under the direction of a physician, he plans and administers rehabilitation programs. A 4 year bachelor's degree in manual arts therapy, industrial arts or industrial education supplemented by a minimum 2 month clinical training program is required. Clinical training is offered by hospitals and rehabilitation centers.

**marathon**
An extended group therapy session that usually lasts from 8 to 72 hours or more.

**marginal cost**
In health economics, the change in the total cost of producing services which results from a small or unit change in the quantity of services being produced. Marginal cost is the appropriate cost concept to consider when contemplating program expansion or contraction. Economies of scale will result from the expansion of a program when marginal cost is less than average or unit cost.

**marginal tax rate**
The tax rate, or percentage, which is applied on the last increment of income for purposes of computing federal or other income taxes.

**marijuana**
Dried leaves and flowers of Cannabis sative (Indian hemp). It causes physical and mental or emotional changes when smoked or ingested in sufficient quantity. The physical changes include increased heart rate, rise in blood pressure, dryness of the mouth, increased appetite and occasional nausea, vomiting and diarrhea. The mental or emotional changes include dreamy state level of consciousness, disruptive chain of thoughts, disturbances of time and space, and alterations of mood. In strong doses, marijuana can produce hallucinations and, at times, paranoid ideas and suspiciousness. It is also known as pot, grass, weed, tea, and Mary Jane.

**marital**
Concerned with marriage. Pertaining to a husband and wife or matrimonial matters, such as marital counseling.

**marital counseling**
Marriage counseling. A trained counselor assists married couples to resolve problems that arise and trouble them in their marital relationship.

**marked-sensed punching method**
In computers, it is a technique for detecting special pencil marks entered in specific positions on a card and the computer then automatically translates the marks into punched holes.

**market value approach**
In finance this is one method for appraising the value of a property or equipment. It is comparing the price of similar properties (comparables) recently sold and the circumstances of the sales.

**mark-up**
In Congress, a meeting of a Congressional committee at which the committee itself writes law to recommend to the full Congress, makes

decisions on appropriations, or otherwise makes policy. Usually takes place after public hearing on the subject matter. See also executive session.

**marshal**
A federal police officer appointed to the federal courts to enforce the law and keep order. Similar to a state sheriff.

**marshaling**
1. The act of ordering, arranging or ranking. 2. Arranging and ranking of capital assets when planning to pay off debts.

**Martindale-Hubbell**
Books that list lawyers by location and area of practice.

**masochism**
Asexual deviation, where sexual gratification is achieved from being maltreated by the partner or by oneself; self-punishment. See also sadism, sadomasochistic relationshiop.

**mastectomy**
The surgical removal of the breast.

**master**
1. The agent or responsible one. 2. An employer or principal person who is responsible for the acts of employees. 3. The person who is responsible for acts of those working under him or her; the physician/nurse relationship. The physician is the master and the nurse is legally the servant.

**master lease**
The major or main lease which controls subsequent leases or subleases which covers more property than subsequent leases.

**master, special**
A court official empowered to represent the court in special transactions.

**masticate**
To chew; to chew food.

**MAST suit**
Military Anti-Shock Trousers. Used in emergency care to treat hypovolemic or cardiogenic shock. The pants are pulled on the legs up to and over the abdomen and then inflated. The pressure compresses the veins, thus increasng venous return to the heart.

**masturbation**
See autoerotism.

**matching (funds)**
Money, equipment, vehicles, buildings, office space and sometimes personnel, which is provided by local Health and Human Service agencies to be used as a contribution to a project for which the federal government is providing a grant, demonstration contract or other contract. The federal government usually provides three-fourths of the

money the first year of funding, with one-fourth being "matched" or provided by the state or local agency in the form of matching funds or equivalent amounts through in-kind support, which is any other items other than actual money. Some grants are provided on a diminishing federal contribution and an increased match by the state or local agency, e.g., three-fourths by the federal government and one-fourth by the agency the first year, half by each the second year and one-fourth by the federal government and three-fourths by the agency the third year, with the idea that the state or county would be able to come up with the remainder of the money. This notion created by the federal government has not been effective for the most part, as the state and local governments usually cannot generate the extra money to compensate for the withdrawn federal funds.

**material**
1. Essential; necessary; pertinent; getting to the basic issue. 2. Facts or evidence important enough to sway the final decision of a case.

**material allegation**
An allegation that is a part of a claim or a defense.

**material evidence**
Evidence that proves or disproves substantial matters of a dispute.

**material fact**
1. A fact that is central and basic to the final decision of a case. 2. In insurance, a fact that could influence the type and nature of an insurance policy.

**material issue**
An issue that is disputed and is subject to the process of a trial.

**materials management department**
This department has also been called purchasing and stores. It is responsible for ordering supplies, materials, furniture, equipment, both medical and administrative. It purchases, receives, maintains and stores an inventory and delivers these items to the units, departments or services of the health care facility where they are used.

**material witness**
A person who knows specific facts and who can provide relevant evidence and testimony at trial.

**maternal**
Related to being a mother; belonging to or coming from a mother.

**maternal and child health services (MCH)**
Organized health and social services for mothers (particularly) as they need family planning and pregnancy related services), their children, and (rarely) fathers. Mothers and children are often considered particularly vulnerable populations with special health needs; their health to be a matter of high public priority; and particularly benefited by preventive medicine. Therefore such services are sometimes separately organized and funded from other health services. One example is the Maternal and

Child Health Program operated by the Federal Government under the authority of title V of the Social Security Act.

**maternal mortality rate**
The number of deaths attributed to the birth processes per 1,000, 10,000 or 100,000 live births.

**maternity benefits**
Coverage under insurance for the costs of pregnancy, labor and delivery, and in some cases, family planning, post-partum care and complications of pregnancy. Health insurance policies take different approaches and apply different conditions to maternity benefits. See also exclusions, and flat, swap and switch maternity.

**matriarchal order**
The mother as head of the house or family.

**matrilineal**
Descending through the female side of the family.

**matter**
1. A subject or issue worthy of dispute or discussion; an important fact. 2. An event, deal, or transaction. 3. An issue of a lawsuit.

**matter in pais**
Facts that are not a matter of record.

**matter of fact**
An issue or concern that is solved by obvious facts and evidence or the testimony of the witnesses.

**matter of law**
Any question that is solved through the process of testing the issues through applying the law to the matters and facts of the case.

**matter of record**
1. The official recording of an issue or statement of the court as it is stated. 2. Any matter or issue that is recorded and can be proven by the record of the court. 3. Any issue that can be proved by checking any official record of the court.

**maturation**
The process of growth, physically, emotionally, and socially, to full development.

**maturity**
1. When a debt, obligation, or insurance becomes due. 2. Date or time when a document is in full force or fully developed.

**maxim**
1. Specific and concise statement about the law. 2. A principle or rule of conduct that works when applied to most cases. 3. A general statement of truth; a law or rule.

**Maximum Allowable Cost Program (MAC)**
A federal program which will limit reimbursement for prescription drugs under the Medicare and Medicaid programs, and Public Health Service projects to the lowest cost at which the drug is generally available. Specifically, the program limits reimbursement for drugs under programs administered by HHS to the lowest of the maximum allowable cost (MAC) of the drug, if any, plus a reasonable dispensing fee, the acquisition cost of the drug plus a dispensing fee, or the providers' usual and customary charge to the general public for the drug. The MAC is the lowest unit price at which a drug available from several sources or manufacturers can be purchased on a national basis.

**maximum security unit**
That part of a mental institution used for those who have committed crimes or who are considered dangerous to others.

**may**
Used in JCAH accreditation as a term in the interpretation of a standard to reflect an acceptable method that is recognized but not necessarily preferred. See shall or must and should.

**mayhem**
1. To maim another person. 2. To intentionally maim or mutilate or injure a person's body. 3. Violently causing a serious wound. 4. To limit or deprive a person's bodily function which he would need for self-defense.

**McCarran-Ferguson Act.**
The act of March 9, 1945, (15 U.S.C. 1011-15) which declares a general policy that federal laws which regulate or affect business and commerce are not to be interpreted as affecting the insurance business unless specifically provided for. Also known as the McCarran-Wiler Bill (S. 1508) and Public Law 15. Prior to a Supreme Court decision in 1944 insurance was not considered a matter of commerce and thus not subject to federal law. When the Supreme Court found insurance to be a matter of commerce it became necessary to clarify the effect of existing federal law on it. The Act has the effect of leaving regulation of insurance to the states unless specifically undertaken in federal law.

**M.C.E.**
Medical Care Evauations. See these words.

**mean**
Average, a statistical measurement; the adding of a set of scores and then dividing by the number of scores. See also average.

**mean deviation**
Average variation, a statistical measure of variation. It is derived by dividing the sum of deviations in a set of variables by the number of cases involved. See also deviation.

**medex**
Physician assistant programs developed specifically for former military medical corpsmen with independent duty experience. They train as

physician assistants, especially for general practitioners in rural areas. Most Medex, as graduates of the programs are called, have been trained to work with specific physicians. The first such program was begun in 1969 by Richard A. Smith at the University of Washington, in cooperation with the Wasington State Medical Association. The programs generally consist of three months of university training and twelve months of preceptorship.

**median**
The middle number or value of a set of numbers. See also average.

**media nox (Lat.)**
Midnight.

**mediate data**
Data from which facts can, with a reasonable amount of certainty, be inferred.

**mediate testimony**
Secondary evidence.

**mediation**
1. Friendly intercession. 2. An invited intervention in a dispute. 3. Caling in of an intermediary. 4. A third party who is used to decide issues and provide solutions to disputes. The decision has no legal backing, differing from arbitration, which can have the backing of the court.

**medic**
1. A physcian, doctor or surgeon. 2. A medical student, intern or resident. 3. A military medical corpsman who gives first aid and medical care in the field or in combat.

**medicable**
That which can be cured, healed or medically treated.

**Medicaid (Title XIX)**
A federaly-aided, state operated and administered program which provides medical benefits for certain low-income persons in need of health and medical care. The program, authorized by title XIX of the Social Security Act, is basically for the poor. It does not cover all of the poor, however, but only persons who are members of one of the categories of people who can be covered under the welfare cash payment programs--the aged, the blind, the disabled, and members of families with dependent children where one parent is absent, incapacitated or unemployed. Under certain circumstances states may provide Medicaid coverage for children under 21 who are not categorically related. Subject to broad federal guidelines, states determine the benefits covered, program eligibility, rates of payment for providers, and methods of administering the program. Medicaid is estimated to provide services to sme 25 million people, with federal-state expenditures of approximately $12.5 billion in fiscal year 1975. As of 1981, Arizona is the only state without a Medicaid program in operation. See eligibility, extended care facility.

**Medicaid mill**

A health program which serves, solely or primarily, Medicaid beneficiaries, typically on an ambulatory basis. The mills originated in the ghettos of New York City and are still found primarily in urban slums with few other medical services. They are usually organized on a for-profit basis, characterized by their great productivity, and frequently accused of a variety of abuses (such as ping-ponging and family ganging).

**medical**

**Medi-Cal**

California's version of Medicaid.

1. In JCAH accreditation, this is of, pertaining to, or dealing with the healing arts and the science of medicine. 2. Pertaining to the science, study, or practice of medicine, the art of healing diseases or providing treatment and cures for illness and disease.

**Medical Assistance Program**

The health care program for the poor authorized by title XIX of the Social Security Act, known as Medicaid.

**medical associations**

There are many kinds of medical associations; some are legal, formal associations such as cooperatives, corporations and chartered institutions. There are partnerships of three or more practitioners that fit the broader definition of association. There are also practitioners who share practice or resources with others under a single name, however, these are associations only in a very loose or broad sense.

**medical audit**

Detailed retrospective review and evaluation of selected medical records by qualified professional staff. Medical audits are used in some hospitals, group practices and occasionally in private, independent practices for evaluating professional performance by comparing it with accepted criteria, standards and current professional judgment. A medical audit is usually concerned with the care of a given illness and is undertaken to identify deficiencies in that care in anticipation of educational programs to improve it. See also concurrent review and medical care evaluation studies.

**Medical Audit Program (MAP)**

An extension of the Professional Activities Study (PAS), in which data are displayed in comprehensive quarterly reports by hospital department. The reports are for use by hospital clinical departments in conducting a comprehensive medical audit and in retrospective utilization review. See also Commission on Professional and Hospital Activities.

**medical care evaluation studies (MCE STUDIES)**

1. Retrospective medical care review in which an in-depth assessment of the quality and/or nature of the use of selected health services or programs is made. Restudy of a MCE study assesses the effectiveness of corrective actions taken to correct deficiencies identified in the original study, but does not necessarily repeat or replicate the original study.

Utilization review requirements under Medicare and Medicaid require utilization review committees in hospitals and skilled nursing facilities to have at least one such study in progress at all times. Such studies are also required by the PSRO program. 2. In-depth assessment of the delivery and organization of health care services designed to assure that said services are appropriate, of optimum quality and provided in a timely fashion. Other terms that are commonly associated with MEE are medical audit, patient care audit, patient care evaluation, patient care assessment.

**Medical College Admission Test (MCAT)**
A nationally standardized test generally required or strongly recommended by nearly all medical schools in the United States as part of their admission process. The results of the test are evaluated along with other evidence of student ability to handle medical school course work by admissions committees. The test, administered by the Psychological Corporation, is designed to provide objective measures of academic ability and achievement through tests of verbal ability, quantitative ability, science knowledge and general information. It cannot and does not claim to measure motivation, the nature or sincerity of interest in the study of medicine, or the personal characteristics that are of basic importance to the practitioner or teacher of medicine.

**medical communications specialist**
Knows the properties and capabilities of communications media and applies this knowledge to the design and improvement of communication processes in the health field.

**medical computer language**
See MUMPS, CAPER.

**medical computer specialist**
combines a knowledge of computer science and health science to provide systems and programming support in the medical field.

**Medical Consumer Price Index (MCPI)**
Medical component of CPI, giving the trends in medical care charges based on specific indicators of hospital, dental, medical, and drug prices.

**medical deduction**
The federal income tax deduction for expenditures on health insurance (one half of such expenditures up to a maximum of $150) and other medical expenses in excess of three percent of income.

**medical/dental secretary**
Assists physicians and/or dentists through the use of medical shorthand, typing, filing, accounting, appointment scheduling, receptionist duties, and office management.

**medical device**
See device, Kefauver-Harris Amendment.

**medical director**

A physician who is in charge of medical matters of a health facility or organization and is usually appointed by the governing body to function in a leadership capacity. The scope of responsibilities varies with each position and generally includes patient/doctor relationships, doctor/doctor or doctor/administrator relationships; it may or may not include business or non-medical administrative duties.

**medical eligibility**

Eligibility for Medicare Part A Hospital Insurance benefits applies to individuals age 65 or over who are entitled to monthly social security benefits; qualified railroad retirement beneficiaries age 65 or over; and uninsured persons age 65 or over who meet the requirements of a special transitional provision. Those persons permanently disabled were given eligibility in 1972 by Public Law 92-603 (H.R.-1). Supplementary medical insurance Part B is also available effective July 1973. A person eligible for hospital insurance is enrolled automatically.

**medical emergency**

The sudden and unexpected onset of an illness or condition, manifesting symptoms such as severe chest pains, convulsive seizure, hemorrhage, or unconsciousness. Not to be confused with accidental injury.

**medical examiner**

1. A coroner or related public health officer. 2. A physician who examines applicants for insurance purposes.

**medical expense insurance**

A health insurance that provides benefits for medical care on an outpatient basis. The company may limit the amount it will pay per call or the total amount for all calls. It may also exclude the first few calls made by the physician at the beginning of an illness.

**medical foundation**

An organization of physicians, generally sponsored by a state or local medical association. Sometimes called a foundation for medical care. It is a separate and autonomous corporation with its own board of directors. Every physician member of the medical society may apply for membership in the foundation and, upon acceptance, participate in all its activities. A foundation is concerned with the delivery of medical services at reasonable cost. It believes in the free choice of a physician and hospital by the patient, fee-for-service reimbursement and local peer review. Many foundations operate as prepaid group practices or as an individual practice association for an HMO. While these are prepaid on a capitation basis for services to some or all of their patients, they still pay their individual members on a fee-for-service basis for the services they give. Some foundations are organized only for peer review purposes or other specific functions.

**medical graduate, foreign (FMG)**

A graduate of a medical school outside the United States, Puerto Rico or Canada who was not a U.S. or Canadian citizen at the time of graduation.

**medical graduate, United States (USMG)**
Any graduate of a U.S., Puerto Rican, or Canadian medical school, irrespective of citizenship.

**medical graduate, United States foreign (USFMG)**
A graduate of a medical school outside the United States, Puerto Rico, or Canada who was a U.S. citizen at the time of graduation.

**Medical Group Management Association (MGMA)**
The official professional organization for administrators and managers of medical groups, clinics, group practices and related organizations. See Medical Group Management Information Services (MGMIS)

**Medical Group Management Information Service (MGMIS)**
Activity of the Medical Group Management Association located in Denver, Colorado. Formerly known as the Library Reference Service. The purpose of the Information Service is to assist persons involved in or desiring to learn more about the management of medical group practices, health maintenance organizations, and evolving forms of medical care in which group practice is an essential organizational component. The MGMA Information Service provides opportunities for continuing education for MGMA members and others in medical group business management by collecting, classifying, storing, and disseminating information on medical group business management and by stimulating the creation of new information. The Information Service was the first such service covering medical group practice management on a national scale.

**medical habilitation and rehabilitation services**
The medical evaluation of the needs of the ill or disabled individual, and the design, management and evaluation of a habilitation or rehabilitation program to meet those needs.

**medical illustrator**
Demonstrates medical facts by the creation of illustrations, models and teaching films; serves as a consultant, advisor, and administrator in the field of medical illustration.

**Medical Impairment Bureau (MIB)**
A clearinghouse of information on people who have applied for life insurance in the past. Any adverse medical findings on previous medical examinations are recorded in code and sent to companies subscribing to the service. This service raises interesting legal and confidentiality questions, especially with respect to information produced by medical examinations.

**Medical Indemnity of America, Inc. (MIA)**
A stock insurance company organized in Ohio in 1950 by Blue Shield plans to serve as national enrollment agency, to assist individual plans in negotiating contracts, and to serve large national accounts in which two or more plans are involved. See also Health Service, Inc.

**medical indigency**
Having enough money for the basics of life, but not enough money for health insurance or to pay medical bills. The condition of having insufficient income to pay for adequate medical care without depriving oneself or dependents of food, clothing, shelter, and other essentials of living. Medical indigency may occur when a self-supporting individual able under ordinary conditions to provide basic maintenance for himself and his family, is, in time of catastrophic illness, unable to finance the total cost of medical care. See also medically indigent, spend down, and medically needy.

**medical jurisprudence**
Forensic medicine. Health care law, medical law. See forensic.

**medical laboratory scientist**
Performs clinical analysis procedures and research in the medical/clinical laboratories utilizing disciplines such as chemistry, biochemistry, bacteriology, and microbiology. Traning at the graduate level is required for job entry.

**medical laboratory technician**
Medical laboratory technicians perform routine clinical laboratory tests which require minimal exercise of independent judgment. Under the supervision of a medical technologist or pathologist, they perform laboratory tests in chemistry (qualitative and quantitative analyses of body constituents), hematology (blood counts, blood cell identification), urinalysis, blood banking (routine typing and cross-matching, immunological tests for the detection of antibodies), microbiology (antibiotic susceptibility testing), and parasitology (organism identification). As a part of their work, medical laboratory technicians utilize laboratory instruments ranging from microscopes to highly sophisticated instruments such as automated blood analyzers and electronic cell counters. Certification is awarded by the Board of Registry following succesful completion of an examination. The requirements for taking the certifying examination include a high school diploma or equivalent, either graduation from an AMA- approved school or completion of a basic military laboratory course, and a year of experience.

**medical librarian**
Combines a degree in library science with specialized knowledge of medical librarianship and bibliography, to acquire, organize, catalog, retrieve and disseminate medical information.

**medically**
A medical concern; according to the rules of medicine; for the purpose of curing and healing.

**medically indigent**
A person who is capable of sustaining himself financially and is able to pay for the basics in life but too poor to have enough money to meet his medical expenses or buy health insurance. It may refer to either persons whose income is low enough so that they can pay for their basic living costs but not their routine medical care, or alternately, to persons

with generally adequate income who suddenly face catastrophically large medical bills. See also medical indigency, medically needy and spend down.

**medically needy**

In the Medicaid program, persons who have enough income and resources to pay for their basic living expenses (and so do not need welfare) but not enough to pay for their medical care. Medicaid law requires that the standard for income used by a state to determine if someone is medically needy cannot exceed 133 percent of the maximum amount paid to a family of similar size under the welfare program for families with dependent children (AFDC). In order to be eligible as medically needy, people must fall into one of the categories of people who are covered under the welfare cash assistance programs; i.e., be aged, blind, disabled, or members of families with dependent children where one parent is absent, incapacitated or unemployed. They receive benefits if their income after deducting medical expenses (see spend down) is low enough to meet the eligibility standard.

**medically underserved area**

1. A geographic location (i.e., an urban or rural area) which has insufficient health resources (manpower and/or facilities) to meet the medical needs of the resident population. Physician shortage area applies to a medically underserved area which is particularly short of physicians. Such areas are also sometimes defined by measuring the health status of the resident population rather than the supply of resources, an area with an unhealthy population being considered underserved. The term is defined and used several places in the PHS Act in order to give priority to such areas for federal assistance. 2. A comprehensive federal designation of a geographic area. The designation is designed to measure the extent of personal health care services and needs in a particular area. It is based upon a set of four weighted tables, each of which is designed to measure an important aspect of the health resources or needs of the area. The variables considered are: 1) percentage of the population below poverty level; 2) percentage of the population over 65 years old; 3) infant mortality rate; 4) primary care physicians per 1,000 population.

**medically underserved population**

The population of an urban or rural area with a shortage of personal health services or another population group having a shortage of such services. A medically underserved population may not reside in a particular medically underserved area, or be defined by its place of residence. Thus migrants, Native Americans or the inmates of a prison or mental hospital may constitute such a population. The term is defined and used several places in the PHS Act in order to give such populations priority for federal assistance, e.g., in the HMO and NHSC programs.

**medical malpractice**

In medical malpractice litigation, negligent is the predominant theory of liability. In order to recover for negligent malpractice, the plaintiff must establish the following elements: 1) the existence of the physician's duty to the plaintiff, usually based upon the existence of the physician-patient relationship; 2) the applicable standard of care and its violation; 3) a compensable injury; and, 4) a casual connection between the violation of the standard of care and the harm complained of. Kosberg v. Washington Hospital Center Inc., 129 U.S. App. D.C. 322, 394 F. 2d 947, 949. See also Captain of ship, malpractice, discovery rule, maltreatment.(Black's Law Dictionary, West Pub. Co.)

**medical necessity**
In determining eligibilty for home health care under Medicare, it means that it must be medically contraindicated for the patient to leave home. The following examples will differentiate between Medicare covered status and noncovered status. Patient requires aid of supportive devices; covered: wheelchair-confined patient who requires wheelchair cab for any transportation (in other words, he requires special transportation to obtain medical services). See eligibility, home health care.

**medical office assistant**
Medical office assistants help physicians examine and treat patients and perform the administrative tasks required to maintain an efficient medical practice. For example, they may prepare patients for examination or treatment, take temperatures, measure height and weight, sterilize instruments, and assist in certain examinations or treatments. They also may act as secretary, receptionist, and bookkeeper for the physician.

**medical radiation dosimetrist**
Involved in treatment planning and radiation dosage calculation, usually under a physician's or radiologist's supervision. Calculates radiation dosage in the treatment of malignant disease and plans the direction of radiation to its target in the safest way. Minimum education required is a baccalaureate degree; graduate training is preferable.

**medical radiographer**

**medical radiographer**
Another term for x-ray technician or radiologic technologist.
A technician educated in x-ray diagnostic radiology, thera- peutic radiology and/or nuclear medicine. See radiographer.

**medical radiography**
The current terminology for radiologic technology or x-ray technology.

**medical record**
1. A record kept on patients which properly contains sufficient information to identify the patient clearly, to justify his diagnosis and treatment, and to document the results accurately. The purposes of the record are to serve as the basis for planning and continuity of patient care; provide a means of communication among physicians and any professional contributing to the patient's care; furnish documentary evidence of the patient's course of illness and treatment; serve as a basis for review, study, and evaluation; serve in protecting the legal interests of the patient, hospital, and responsible practitioner; and provide data for use in research and education. Medical records and their contents are not

usually available to the patient himself. The content of the record is usually confidential. Each different provider in a community caring for a given patient usually keeps an independent record of that care.
2. In JCAH long-term care facility accreditation, this is clinical documentation of an individual's health care, including, but not limited to, the medical, nursing, social, and rehabilitative care provided to a patient/resident. See also problem-oriented medical record.

**medical record administrator**
An individual who plans, designs, and manages systems of patient administrative and clinical data, and patient medical records, in all types of health care institutions. The minimum educational requirements for professional registration as a medical record administrator is a baccalaureate degree in medical record science or medical record administration in a program accredited by the American Medical Association in collaboration with the American Medical Record Association. The AMRA maintains a list of persons who have successfully completed the national registration examination that qualified them to use the professional designation of registered record administrator. Recent graduates must meet a continuing education requirement five years after initial registration. The administrator is the most highly trained of several types of medical records personnel, including the medical record technician, See qualified medical record administrator.

**medical record committee**
A committee of hospital personnel who utilize medical records. The committee is to assist in upgrading the records and make them more efficient to use. The handling and storage of medical records may also be a task for this committee.

**medical record practitioner (Medicare).**
A person who 1) is eligible for certification as a registered record administrator (RRA), or an accredited record technician (ART), by the Amercian Medical Record Association under its requirements in effect on the publication of this provision; or 2) is a graduate of a school of medical record science that is accredited jointly by the Council on Medical Education of the American Medical Association and the American Medical Record Association. See qualified medical record practitioner, medical record technician.

**medical records department**
This department manages, maintains, stores, and retrieves both old and new patient records and related patient care statistics.

**medical record technician (or accredited records technician— ART).**
Medical record technicians provide records assistance to medical record administrators by performing many essential technical activities in the medical record department of a health care institution or agency. Their duties are varied and dependent on the size of the facility in which they work. In a small facility they are likely to work independently with only occasional consultation with a medical record administrator. In some cases they may be employed as directors of medical record departments.

In general, medical record technicians compile and maintain medical records and review them for completeness and accuracy. They code symptoms, diseases, operations, procedures, and other therapies according to standard classification systems and post codes on medical records to facilitate information retrieval. Technicians maintain and use a variety of health record indexes and compile medical care and census data for public health and other statistical reports. They assist the medical staff by tabulating data from records for research purposes and for use in evaluating and planning health care services programs. Other responsibilities include transcription, directing the routine operation of a medical record department, and either filing or directing filing by medical clerks. See qualified medical record technician.

**medical review**
Review, required by Medicaid, by a team composed of physicians and other appropiate health and social service personnel of the condition and need for care, including a medical evaluation, of each inpatient in a long-term care facility. By law, the team must review the: care being provided in the facilities; adequacy of the services available in the facilities to meet the current health needs and promote the maximum physical well-being of the patients; necessity and desirability of the continued placement of such patients in the facilities; and feasibility of meeting their health care needs through alternate institutional or noninstitutional services. Medical review differs from utilization review in that it requires evaluation of each individual patient and an analysis of the appropriateness of his specific treatment in a given institution, whereas utilization review is often done on a sample basis, with special attention to certain procedures, conditions or lengths of stay. See also continued stay review.

**medical self-help**
A concept that involves basic emergency care, but is expanded to cover situations where there are no doctors available.

**medical service plan**
An organization for the billing, collection, distribution and/or use of all specifically identified portions of the professional fees covered by participating physicians.

**medical services**
In health insurance, these services are provided by the primary physician who refers the patient to another physician.

**Medical Services Administration (MSA)**
The bureau which administers the Medicaid program at the federal level. It is part of the Social and Rehabilitation Service, which administers most of the welfare programs within the Department of Health and Human Services. Direct administration of Medicaid programs is carried out by the states.

**medical social worker**
Provides link between organized social services and those who need the services to solve medical problems. Prepared to identify and understand the social and emotional factors underlying patients' illness and to

communicate these factors to the health team; to assist patients and their families in understanding and accepting the treatment necessary to maximize medical benefits and their adjustment to permanent and temporary effects of illness; to utilize resources, such as family and community agencies, in assisting patients to recovery. See qualified medical social worker.

**medical staff**

Collectively, the physicians, dentists, and other professionals responsible for medical care in a health facility, typically a hospital. Such staff may be full-time or part-time, employed by the hospital or not, and include all professionals who wish to be included (open staff) or just those who meet various standards of competence (closed staff). Staff privileges may or may not be permanent or conditioned on continued evidence of competence.

**medical staff equivalent**

In JCAH long-term care facility accreditation, this is an organized medical staff which provides services to one or more facilities or serves a group of facilities.

**medical technologist**

A specially trained individual who performs a wide range of complex and specialized procedures in all general areas of the clinical laboratory. The minimum educational requirement for one of several certification programs in medical technology is a baccalaureate degree with appropriate science course requirements plus a 12-month structered AMA approved medical technology program and an examination; or a baccalaureate degree with appropriate science course requirements and experience. The medical technologist is the most highly trained of several types of clinical laboratory personnel, including the medical laboratory technician, and medical laboratory assistant. As highly skilled laboratory scientists with a strong generalist orientation, medical technologists have an ability to perform or supervise tests and procedures in hematology, bacteriology, serology, immunology, clinical chemistry, blood banking, urinalysis, mycology, and parasitology. They perform complex analyses requiring the exercise of independent judgement, correlate test results, and must be able to interpret their findings with respect to disease or normality. They must have knowledge of physiological conditions affecting test results and must produce reliable and valid results that can be confirmed by statistical measurements of precision and accuracy. See medical laboratory technician. See qualified medical technologist.

**medical trade area**

An area from which one or more specified providers draw their patients; similar to catchment area except that it is defined by the patients rather than the provider.

**medical transcriptionist**

Skilled in typing, medical spelling, medical terminology, and the proper format of medical records and reports; prepared to transcribe medical dictation using mechanical dictating equipment.

**medicament**

A drug or herb used for healing, treating, curing or relieving pain; a medicine.

**Medicare(Title XVIII)**

A nationwide health insurance program for people aged 65 and over, for persons eligible for social security disability payments for over two years, and for certain workers and their dependents who need kidney transplantation or dialysis. Health insurance protection is available to insured persons without regard to income. Monies from payroll taxes and premiums from beneficiaries are deposited in special trust funds for use in meeting the expenses incurred by the insured. The program was enacted July 30,1965, as title XVIII—Health Insurance for the Aged—of the Social Security Act, and became effective on July 1,1966. It consists of two separate but coordinated programs: hospital insurance (Part A), and supplementary medical insurance (Part B).

**Medicare benefits**

As outlined in the Social Security Handbook, a person under hospital insurance protection means that the individual may have benefits paid on his behalf or, in certain cases, paid to him for the covered hospital and related health care services. The Medical Insurance plan adds to the protection provided by the basic hospital insurance plan and covers a substantial part of physicians' services, surgery and a number of other health items and services. The benefit period includes 90 days of hospital care plus a lifetime reserve of 60 days. A benefit period begins when a person is admitted to a hospital and terminates if a person has not been a patient for 60 consecutive days in the hospital or in a skilled nursing home. The original act used 'spell of illness' and allowed skilled nursing care even if it was not in a 'skilled' nursing home. Now, benefits are limited and are paid to participating hospitals and 'skilled' nursing facilities. The hospital insurance covers the cost of general hospital care, room and board, operations, drugs, medical supplies, diagnostic tests, laboratory fees, and physical therapy. Some services are not allowed, i.e., telephone, television, private room (except as a medical necessity), and personal items. The cost to the patient includes the initial hospital deductible, which is changed every year.

**Medicare/Medicaid (Medi-Cal)**

This program, also known as Medi-Medi, covers those persons protected under both the Medicare plan and the Medicaid (or Medi-Cal) plan.

**medicaster**

A medical charlatan or medical quack.

**medicate**

1. To give anything medicinal. 2. To treat with medicine or drugs.

**medication**

In JCAH long-term care facility accreditation, this is any substance, whether legend or over-the-counter drug, that is taken orally or injected, inserted, topically applied, or otherwise administered to a patient/resident.

**medication, administration**

The route or process by which drugs are taken or administered. Four methods are usually used. 1) Oral administration: the process of taking drugs either in liquid or solid form (tablet, capsule), for absorption into the body and the gastrointestinal tract. 2) Inhalation administration: the process of administering drugs through a gas or vapor form, so the drug will be absorbed through the respiratory tract. 3) Topical administration: the administration of drugs in liquid form (lotion, liniment), semi-solids (ointment, cream), or solid form (Lozenges, suppositories), for absorption through the skin or mucous membranes. 4) Parenteral administration: the administration of drugs in a solution or in suspension by injection or intravenously. There are several methods of parenteral administration. They are A) intradernal (I.D.): injecting a small amount of a solution (usually O.1 cc.) just below the surface of the skin, forming a wheal. This method is used for a local effect, rather than a systemic effect, e.g., local anesthetic, Tb skin test. B) Intravenously (I.V.): injecting varying amounts of soluble solutions directly into a vein for immediate absorption. C) Subcutaneous (S.C.) or hypodermic (H): the injecting of a small amount (0.5 to 2.0 cc.) of highly soluble medication into the tissue directly under the skin. D) Intramuscularly (I.M.): Injecting a large amount (up to 5 cc.) of a solution into the muscle.

**medication aide**

In JCAH long-term care facility accreditation, this is any unlicensed personnal who have successfully completed a state- approved training program in medication administration.

**medicinal**

Having the ability to heal or relieve disease.

**medicine**

The art and science of promoting, maintaining and restoring individual health, and of diagnosing and treating disease.

**medico (Spanish)**

Physician or an equivalent health care practitioner.

**medico, ca (Spanish)**

Medical; medicinal personal construct. See construct.

**medico-legal**

Pertaining to medicine and law.

**Medicredit**

One of several proposed national health insurance plans which are designed to encourage the voluntary purchase of qualified private health insurance policies by granting tax credits against personal income taxes to finance, in part or in whole, the premium cost of such plans. In addition, the proposal would provide for the federal payment of premiums for qualified policies for poor individuals or families with no tax liability.

**Medigap insurance**
Supplemental insurance designed to fill in some of the gaps in Medicare's coverage or the gaps between private insurance and Medicare's coverage.

**M.E.D.I.H.C.**
Military Experience Directed Into Health Careers. A program that recruits qualified veterans with military health care experience and attempts to place them in health care jobs in areas of shortages of health personnel.

**medi medi**
See Medicare/Medicaid (medical).

**meeting of minds**
A contract; a clear understanding of a contract by both parties, with no secret purpose or intention.

**melancholia**
An old term for depression. Involutional melancholia refers to a debilitating state of depression.

**melancholia agitata**
Agitated depression, common to senile psychosis.

**member**
1. Belonging to an organized group or effort. 2. A part of the body, usually a limb. 3. A person who is eligible to receive, or is receiving, benefits from a health maintenance organization (usually) or insurance policy (occasionally; see beneficiary). Usually includes both people who have themselves enrolled or subscribed for benefits and their eligible dependents. See also subscriber, and insured.

**member co-payment**
One type of cost sharing whereby the insured pays a specified amount per unit of service, such as $1.00 per visit or one-half of prescription drug cost, with the insurer paying the remainder of the cost. Unlike coinsurance, the amount of co-payment does not vary with cost of services.

**membership corporation**
A corporation created for social, charitable, political purposes that is an organization which is not-for-profit or non-stock.

**memorandum**
1. A written record of events; an informal written communication. 2. A written summary of a meeting. 3. A written proposed agreement. 4. A message from one member of an organization to another. 5. A document establishing that a contract exists. 6. A brief submitted to a judge. 7. A brief written summary of the terms of a contract, promise or transaction.

**memorandum decision**
An appellate court's decision that determines which party prevails, but gives no reason for the decision.

**memorandum of understanding (MOU)**
An agreement, usually between an PSRO and a hospital, fiscal intermediary, or state agency, identifying the respective responsibilities of each party for various activities and costs.

**memory**
1. Ability to retrieve past impressions, experiences and learned ideas. 2. Storage in a computer. That part of the computer that stores and holds data.

**menarche**
The onset of menstruation.

**menopause**
Cessation of menstruation that occurs usually around the age of 45 to 50 years.

**menses**
Menstrual flow.

**mens rea (Lat.)**
Guilty mind; wrongful intent; with a harmful purpose.

**mental adaptive mechanisms**
See mental mechanisms.

**mental age**
A measure of mental ability as determined by standard psychological testing. See also I.Q.

**mental anguish**
Mental or emotional feelings that occurred during or after an injury, harm or grief, fear, shame, humiliation, despair. Used in deciding damages in a lawsuit. Also referred to as mental suffering.

**mental cruelty**
Cruelty on the part of one spouse to another which is not physically harmful but causes mental distress or anguish to such a degree so as to make the marriage intolerable.

**mental disorder**
Either mental illness or disease, or mental retardation, a general term for abnormal functioning or capacity of the mind or emotions; the absence of mental health.

**mental health**
The capacity in an individual to form harmonious relations with others; to participate in, or contribute constructively to, changes in his social and physical environment; and to achieve a harmonious and balanced satisfaction of his own potentially conflicting instinctive drives—harmonious in that it reaches an integrated synthesis rather than the denial of satisfaction to certain instinctive tendencies as a means of avoiding the thwarting of others. This attempt at a definition should be compared with that of health. Mental health is a concept influenced by both biological and cultural factors and highly variable in definition, time

and place. It is often operatively defined as the absence of any identifiable or significant mental disorder, and sometimes perversely used as a synonym for mental illness (for instance in speaking of coverage of 'mental health benefits' under NHI) apparently because it is thought to be a more genteel term. See also CMHC and clinical psychologist.

**mental health plan**
Plan of an entity of the state that addresses the provision of services designed to prevent emotional and behavioral dysfunctions in the residents.

**mental health services**
The diagnosis and treatment of emotional and mental diseases and conditions or their symptoms through the administration of medication and specialized therapy.

**mental health technologist**
See human services/mental health technologist.

**mental illness**
All forms of illness in which psychological, intellectual, emotional or behavioral disturbances are the dominating feature. The term is relative and variable in different cultures, schools of thought and definitions. It includes a wide range of types (such as psychic and physical, neurotic and psychotic), and severities. It would be useful to distinguish mental diseases (those with an identifiable physical cause) and mental illnesses (those with no known cause and those with emotional, familial, social or other causes) but this is not regularly done. See also mental health and mental disorders.

**mental mechanisms**
Coping and defensive behavior adjustments which occur with or without the person being aware of them; an inner desire may arise from the unconscious mind, while the conscious mind realizes that satisfaction of the desire is not acceptable. Mental mechanisms are used to compensate for an emotional, social or environmental lack, to cope with and to overcome insecurity, defend one's pride, shift the blame, provide a self-alibi, deny a problem while saving face, or justify actions in some way or another.

**mental retardation**
The absence of normal mental development, usually measured by the intelligence quotient and considered to be present in individuals scoring less than 70 on the Stanford-Binet scale. Many synonyms are used: mental deficiency, subnormality, handicap and disability. Various types (intellectual, emotional) and degrees (borderline—68-85 on the Stanford-Binet, mild—57 to 67, moderate—36 to 51, severe—20 to 35, and profound—under 20) are described. Mental retardation is one type of developmental disability and mental disorder.

**mental retardation aide**
Works under the supervision of a professional staff in attending to the physical needs and well-being of mentally retarded patients and in assisting with teaching and recreation processes.

**mental status**
The results of a psychiatric examination in which a patient's general health, speech patterns, perception, general mood and other such characteristics are assessed or renewed.

**mental suffering**
See mental anguish.

**mental well-being**
A feeling of contentment, emotional stability, peace of mind, and a satisfaction with life. See mental health.

**mercantile**
Pertaining to trade; the buying, selling, and trading goods or services; dealing with commerce.

**Merck Manual**
One of the most widely used of all medical books on diagnosis and therapy. The contents of this book include diseases, disorders, genetics, poisoning, physical agents that cause illness, prescriptions as set forth by the pharmacologic therapeutic classification system of the American Hospital Formulary Service. Each disease and disorder covered is presented in a standardized way, discussing etiology, epidemiology, pathology, symptoms and signs, diagnosis and prognosis, prophylaxis, treatment, complications, etc.

**mescaline**
A hallucinogenic drug obtained from the peyote cactus.

**mesmerism**
Hypnotism.

**messenger and transport service**
This service provides for the delivery of mail, supplies and the moving and transportation of patients.

**metabolic disease screening**
Preventive procedures for detecting disease in respiration, circulation, peristalsis, muscle tone, body temperature, glandular activity and other vegetative functions of the body.

**-meter**
Suffix meaning measure.

**methadone**
A drug used mostly in treatment of heroin addicts, methadone hydrochloride is a long acting synthetic narcotic drug developed in Germany as a substitute for morphine. It is used in detoxification and maintenance of opiate addicts.

**'me too' drug**
A drug that is identical, similar, or closely related to a drug product for which a new drug application has been approved. Many 'me too' drugs on the market are essentially copies of approved new drugs but were introduced by the manufacturers without Food and Drug Administration approval on the theory that the NDA holder, or pioneer drug, had become generally recognized as safe and effective. Other 'me too' products are being marketed with abbreviated new drug applications (ANDAs), which require the submission of manufacturing, bioavailability and labeling information, but not data relating to safety and effectiveness, which are assumed to be established. See also GRAS and GRAE.

**metrazol shock treatment**
A rarely used form of shock treatment. A convulsive seizure is induced by the injection of the drug Metrazol.

**M.G.M.A.**
Medical Group Management Association.

**Mickey Mouse**
1. Any act, procedure, rule, policy or related phenomenon that is simple-minded, elementary or ineffective. 2. Ridiculous, childish or foolish. 3. Purposeless, inefficient and lacking efficacy.

**microbiology technologist**
Works with a minimum of supervision by a pathologist, physician, or laboratory director, in performing bacteriological, viral, parasitological, immunologic, and serologic procedures in a clinical laboratory setting. Generally not a medical technologist by degree; education in microbiology is required. See medical technologist.

**microfilm**
An information storage method where positive films are used to store information reduced without altering or changing the information content or the original document. This process allows reduced storage requirements, reduced mailing costs as well as use of paper products. Microfilm is processed on rolls, cartridges and on film cards called microfiche.

**microorganism**
1. Bacteria, fungi, and viruses. 2. Organisms too small to be seen with the naked eye. Also called microbes.

**midnight census**
See average daily census.

**midwife**
See nurse-midwife.

**miedo (Spanish)**
Fear, dread or apprehension. An early form of mal puesto, where the victim is usually so frightened that he or she imagines seeing frightful things that do not exist. These are based on natural, emotional and supernatural forces. See mal puesto, demencia.

**migraine**
A severe headache affecting one side of the brain. This disorder is manifested by nausea and disturbed vision and may be associated with emotional conflicts.

**milieu therapy**
A method of therapy that emphasizes a positive socio-environmental situation for the benefit of the patient.

**milliequivalent**
The numbers of grams of a solute in one milliliter of a normal solution, abbreviated mEq.

**milliliter**
A unit of volume in the metric system equal to one cubic centimeter; abbreviated ml.

**minim**
A unit of liquid measure equal to 0.0616 ml.

**minimal brain damage or dysfunction**
A behavior pattern of childhood characterized by learning problems, hyperactivity, irritability, and short attention span.

**minimal services**
See services, also levels of service.

**Minnesota Multiphasic Personality Inventory (MMPI)**
Questionnaire type of psychological test for ages 16 and over, with 550 true-false statements that are coded in 14 scales, ranging from a social to a schizophrenia scale.

**minor surgery**
Surgery in which the operative procedure is not hazardous: e.g., repair of lacerations, treatment of fractures, and biopsies. See also major surgery.

**minor tranquilizer**
Drug used to diminish stress, restlessness, and pathological anxiety without producing any antipsychotic effect. Meprobamate and diazapoxides are commonly used minor tranquilizers.

**minutes**
In JCAH accreditation, this is a record of business introduced, transactions and reports made, conclusions reached, and recommendations made. Reports of officers and committees may be summarized briefly or mentioned as having been presented. In either case, a copy of the report is filed in the committee report book and the page number is included in the minutes.

**M.I.S.**
A set of formalized computer procedures, used to provide information for management, planning and control.

**miscellaneous expenses**
In connection with hospital insurance, hospital charges other than for room and board, such as X-ray, drug, laboratory, or whatever ancillary charges are not separately itemized.

**misdemeanor**
An unlawful act or crime of a less serious nature than a felony and punishable by a fine or short-term imprisonment, usually less than one year, or both fine and imprisonment.

**misfeasance**
1. Occurs when a person performs a legal act, but in an improper or negligent manner. 2. Doing an illegal or improper act. 3. The doing of an improper act otherwise considered proper. 4. Doing something wrong.

**misjoinder**
The improper joinder of claims or parties involved in a lawsuit.

**mislaid property**
Property put in place by its rightful owner, and then forgotten. Such property is not considered lost.

**misnomer**
1. A mistake. 2. An error in an explanation. 3. A name wrongly used for an individual or a corporation. When the correct party can be identified, a misnomer will not void a contract.

**misprision**
1. Misconduct in or failure in a public duty. 2. Negligence in one's duty. 3. Negligence, malpractice, failing to carry out the responsibility of a high public office. 4. Failing to report a crime.

**misprision of felony**
Concealing a felony one is not an accessory to.

**misprision of office**
Incompetent or contempt administration of one's official office; misconduct in public office.

**misrepresentation**
A false or misleading presentation of oneself. A statement that is not known to be false as made, is an innocent misrepresentation. Knowingly making a false or untrue statement is a fraudulent misrepresentation.

**mistrial**
1. A trial that has been stopped and invalidated because some fundamental procedure has not been followed. 2. A trial that has not been carried through to the finish. 3. A trial that the judge dismisses because of a major defect in procedure.

**mists**
Liquid droplets suspended in the air, caused by or generated by condensation from a gaseous to a liquid state or by breaking up and dispersing a liquid by atomizing. Mist is a finely divided liquid suspended in the air.

**mitered corner**
The way of tucking in the sheets on a hospital bed so that the corners are well-anchored. See hospital corner.

**mitigate**
1. To alleviate; to diminish or reduce. 2. Lower the extent of a decision.

**mitigating circumstances**
Facts that justify a reduction in the charge against a person; providing a more lenient sentence or reducing the damages in a civil suit.

**mitigation**
Reduction; lowering the severity of a penalty or punishment.

**mitigation of damages**
Facts or evidence that demonstrate the amount of a claim for damages is too high, unjustified or unrealistic.

**mittimus**
The court order used to send a convicted person to prison. A writ that transfers records from one court to another.

**mixoscopia**
A sexual deviation where a person achieves an orgasm by watching one's partner have sex with another person.

**M.M.P.I.**
See Minnesota Multiphasic Personality Inventory.

**M'Naghten's Rule**
1. A test of criminal responsibility. 2. If a person is not aware of the nature and extent of his acts due to mental incompetence, he cannot be held responsible for those acts.

**m.o. (Lat.)**
Modus operandi. In English, manner or mode of operation. See Modus operandi.

**mobile intensive care (MIC)**
Personnel trained at various levels and aspects of emergency care to provide efficient emergency care to the ill or injured at the scene of the accident and also during the transportation of the victim to the emergency care center or emergency room. The care provided in a MIC system is provided by advanced life support teams, also referred to as mobile intensive care paramedics.

**mobile setting**
A movable structure or specially equipped vehicle used to provide continuing or periodic health care services in a location selected to assure geographic accessibility to an identified target population; or a vehicle used to provide health care services during transportation of patients. See mobile intensive care unit.

**mode**
The number or value which occurs most frequently in a series of numbers or observations that are ordered from least to most.

**model A**
A national Blue Cross association automated, computerized system for processing Medicare admissions and paying claims.

**modernization**
Remodeling, renovation or, sometimes, replacement of health facilities and equipment to bring them up to current construction standards, into compliance with fire and safety codes, or to meet contemporary health delivery needs and capabilities. Usually implies no increase in facility capacity, e.g., in the case of a hospital the total number of available beds would not be increased. Defined and supported under the Hill-Burton program (title XVI of the PHS Act).

**modification**
A reduction, change or alteration. A slight change or revision. A limitation or qualification.

**modifiers**
In health insurance, modifiers of service description are allowed and are provided in the procedure coding manual. The use of modifiers permits the physician to indicate those circumstances in which his usual procedure is altered (increased or decreased) and/or the service itself is changed from that described by its five-digit code. The modifier code system is used by the majority of physicians in only a small portion of services, since relatively few of the modifiers will be applicable to their practices. Properly used, the modifiers obviate the necessity for more extensive reporting of the modifying circumstances. Specific modifiers are listed at the beginning of each section in the procedure coding manual.

**modus (Lat.)**
Method, manner or way. The means or system used.

**modus operandi (Lat.)**
Method of operation. A specific technique, a set of circumstances, specific characteristics or methods of a person's actions; the usual methods employed by a specific criminal.

**moiety**
Half. One of two equal parts.

**monitor**
1. Closely checking out and observing contaminated areas to determine whether they are safe for workers. 2. To keep watch on the condition of a patient.

**monomania**
A mental illness characterized by preoccupation with one thing. A partial insanity.

**monopoly**
One organization only controlling the manufacture, sale or distribution of money, goods or services.

**Montgomery straps**
Ties used to hold dressings in place.

**mood**
Feelings or the emotional tone that is experienced by a person.

**moot**
1. A pretend subject for argument; not genuine, undecided, unsettled. 2. Abstract; not a real dispute. 3. For the sake of argument; a practice situation.

**moot court**
A mock court, held for the arguing of abstract cases which do not involve real persons' participation. A moot court is usually a part of legal education.

**moral turpitude**
Lewd or immoral behavior; a crime that is more than just breaking of the law, which could include bizarre acts, acts of baseness, vileness, or being contrary.

**moratorium**
A delay; an authorized and enforced delay; to prevent an occurrence or act.

**morbidity**
1. The extent of illness, injury, or disability in a defined population. It is usually expressed in general or specific rates of incidence or prevalence. Sometimes used to refer to any episode of disease. 2. Sickness rates. The morbidity rate is the ratio of the number of persons ill in a certain population. See mortality.

**morbidity incidence rate**
The number or reported cases of a specific or any given disease during a period of a year per 100,000 population. An estimate is usually made in the middle of the year.

**morbidity prevalence rate**
1. The number of cases of a given disease at a particular time per 100,000 population at that same time. 2. A picture of a specific disease at a given period of time per 1,000, 10,000 or 100,000 population. See prevalence.

**morphology**
The branch of science that studies the structure and form of living organisms.

**mortality**
Death. Used to describe the relation of deaths to the population in which they occur. The mortality rate (death rate) expresses the number of deaths in a unit of population within a prescribed time and may be

expressed as crude death rates (e.g., total deaths in relation to total population during a year) or as rates specific for diseases and, sometimes, for age, sex, or other attributes (e.g., number of deaths from cancer in white males in relation to the white male population during a year). See perinatal mortality.

**mortgage**
Property offered as security for payment of a debt with the borrower retaining the possession and full use of the property. The legal document by which real estate is offered as security for the repayment of a loan.

**mortgage banker**
A bank or other business organization which provides mortgage financing with its own monies rather than serving as only a mortgage broker. Following borrowing, the bank may sell the mortgages to investors.

**mortgage broker**
A business entity that has the purpose of bringing together a borrower and a lender to obtain a loan against real property by providing a mortgage or deed of trust as security. Also called a loan broker, this person puts together loan applications and charges a fee for his services.

**mortgage company**
A business entity that is authorized to service real estate loans for a fee.

**mortgage warehousing**
One finance method whereby a mortgage company holds loans which are usually sold, in order to sell them later at a better price and/or use them as collateral to borrow new money to loan.

**morto-**
Prefix meaning death.

**mother surrogate**
Mother substitute.

**motion**
1. Requesting a court to rule on an issue or provide an order directing some act to be done. 2. A formal procedure used in a meeting to propose an action. 3. To request that the court dismiss the case.

**movant**
1. One who makes a motion. 2. One who initiates a motion before a court.

**move**
The act of putting a motion into discussion.

**M.U.G.**
MUMPS users group. An organization of medical computer specialists who use and work with the MUMPS program. See MUMPS.

**multidisciplinary team**
According to JCAH for psychiatric, alcoholism and drug abuse facilities accreditation purposes, this is a group of clinical staff composed of representatives from different professions, disciplines or service areas.

**multilateral**
Many sided; on many sides.

**multiphasic screening**
The combined use of a group or battery of screening tests as a preventive measure to attempt to identify any of the several diseases being screened for in an apparently healthy population.

**multiple personality**
Psychiatric term for a dissociative reaction in which a person has two or more distinctive personalities, each one knowing nothing of the others.

**multiplicity of actions**
Improperly starting several lawsuits on the same issue.

**multi-source drug**
A drug that is available from more than one manufacturer or distributor, often under different brand names. Limits on reimbursement are more likely to be feasible for multi-source drugs than drugs available from only a single source. A drug may not be available from more than one source because it is protected by a patent; only one company has obtained FDA marketing approval; or the demand for it is such that only one supplier has entered the market. See also Maximum Allowable Cost Program.

**multispecialty group**
A medical group composed of three or more physicians representing two or more fields of medicine.

**multitial**
Legal relations in rem.

**M.U.M.P.S.**
Massachusetts General Hospital's multi-programming system. A medical computer language developed and demonstrated through grants from the National Center for Health Service Research (NCHSR), put into practical use between 1970 and 1980. Prior to the development of MUMPS, no such computer language existed. FORTRAN and COBOL did not adapt well to medical use as they require a lengthy process. MUMPS handles a broad range of medical data and is easily updated. The language is flexible and easy to learn, inexpensive to use, and improves the quality and efficiency of health care. Some of its features include: time and database sharing and hierarchical and file structure. See CAPER.

**mun.**
Abbreviation for municipal.

**municipal**
Local governments. Usually city government and its laws.

**municipal corporation**
A city government, a municipality.

**municipal law**
City laws, usually called ordinances.

**muniments**
Deeds or documents showing evidence of land ownership; a title to land.

**murder**
The unlawful killing of another human being with malice aforethought. Manslaughter is an unplanned murder with no premeditation or malice aforethought. Second degree murder lacks the premeditation aspect, but is still an unlawful act.

**music therapist**
These therapists use individual and group musical activities with physically and mentally ill patients to accomplish therapeutic aims, to create an environment conducive to therapy, and to influence behavior.

**mutatis mutandis (Lat.)**
With necessary detailed changes. A part of a document may remain the same but names can be changed.

**mutilate**
1. To mangle or maim. 2. To damage or injure; to cut off a limb.

**mutilation**
1. The act of cutting, shredding, tearing, or otherwise destroying a document. 2. To destroy its legal effect. 3. The act of injuring or mutilating.

**mutual**
Joint; done together; reciprocal; shared in common. See mutual insurance company.

**mutual benefit associations**
Fraternal or social organizations or corporations for the relief of members of the organization from specified perils or costs such as the costs of illness. Such associations pay losses with assessments on their members intended to liquidate specific losses rather than by fixed premiums payable in advance.

**mutual company**
A company or business in which the consumers are the owners and also receive profits from the company.

**mutual fund**
1. A business or company established as an investors pool. 2. A group that jointly invests money and buys stock in other companies.

**mutual insurance company**
Insurance companies with no capital stock, owned by the policyholders. Earnings over and above payment of losses, operating expenses, and reserves are the property of the policyholders and returned to them in

some way such as dividends or reduced premiums. See also stock insurance company.

**mutuality of contract**
1. Reciprocity of obligation of making a contract binding. 2. A binding obligation of performance. 3. Each side of an agreement must keep a promise to do an act to make a contract binding.

**mutual mistake**
A misunderstanding on the same important issue by both parties to a contract sufficient to negate or void the contract.

**myelogram**
An x-ray of the spinal cord.

**myocardial infarction**
Heart attack; cardiac arrest; obstruction of the blood flow to an area of cardiac tissue.

**myopia**
Near-sightedness.

**mysophobia**
Fear of germs and dirt.

# N

**naked**
1. Incomplete. 2. Lacking authority. 3. Without force. 4. Outfront.

**named insured**
1. The person whose name appears on an insurance policy for health, life, or property. 2. The policyholder of an insurance policy.

**narcissism**
Self-love. The word is derived from Narcissus, a Greek mythology figure who fell in love with his own image.

**narcolespy**
Uncontrollable and irresistible desire to sleep.

**narcosis**
Drug-induced stupor.

**narcosynthesis**
Psychoanalysis with the patient sedated.

**narcotic**
A drug which causes insensibility and stupor while at the same time relieves pain.

**narcotic blockade**
The use of specific drugs to inhibit the effects of other drugs like heroin, and thus is used to aid in the treatment of opiate addicts.

**narcotic drug**
As set out in the Comprehensive Drug Abuse Prevention and Control Act of 1970, any of the following drugs, whether produced directly or indirectly by extraction from substances of vegetable origin, or independently by means of chemical synthesis, or by a combination of extraction and chemical synthesis: opium, coca leaves, and opiates; a compound, manufacture, salt, derivative or preparation of opium, coca leaves, or opiates; and a substance (and any compound, manufacture, salt, derivative, or preparation thereof which is chemically identical with any of the substances referred to above. The term is very irregularly used, sometimes being any drug which dulls the senses and reduces pain, sometimes being any drug whose use is subject to special governmental control. Narcotics include heroin, morphine, demerol, and methadone. They do not, by the first definition, include marijuana, hallucinogens, amphetamines or barbiturates. The narcotics are among the most common causes of drug dependence. See Schedule of drugs.

**nati-**
Prefix meaning birth.

**national accounts**
In health insurance, a national group with employees in two or more plan areas, which designates one location as the control plan for all enrollment and coverage history for members of that group. Claims received in a local plan are wired to the control plan for payment approval.

**National Association for Practical Nurse Education and Service (NAPNES)**
This organization is concerned only with practical nurse education and services at the practical nurse level. The NAPNES provides accrediting and consulting services for schools involved in practical nurse training as well as educational services.

**National Association of Dental Service Plans (N.A.D.S.P.) (Delta Dental Plans).**
A dental prepayment plan developed with the cooperation of the American Dental Association (ADA), which was underwritten by ADA and now is an autonomous agency supported by state dental service plans and dental societies. See Delta Dental plans.

**national board examinations**
Standard national examinations developed and administered by the National Board of Medical Examiners. They are given in three parts which are generally taken during the second and final years of medical school and the internship year. Successful completion of the national boards is a requirement for licensure as a physician in some states and an acceptable alternative to the state's own medical examinations in other states. See also Federation Licensing Examination.

**National Board of Medical Examiners (NBME)**
An organization founded in 1915, which includes among its members representatives from the Federation of State Medical Boards of the United States, Council on Medical Education of the American Medical Association, Association of American Medical Colleges, American Hospital Association, Armed Services, United States Public Health Service, and Veterans Administration. Members at large are elected from among leaders in medicine throughout the United States. The purposes of the Board are: to prepare and administer qualifying examinations of such high quality that legal agencies governing the practice of medicine within each state may, at their discretion, grant successful candidates a license without further examination (see FLEX and national board examinations); to consult and cooperate with the examining boards of the states; to consult and cooperate with medical schools and other organizations or institutions concerned with maintaining the advancing quality of medical education; to assist medical specialty boards and societies in establishing measurement of clinical knowledge and competence for purposes of certification and assessment; and to study and develop methods of testing and evaluating medical knowledge and competence.

**National Federation of Licensed Practical Nurses (NFLPN)**
The official national organization for licensed practical/vocational nurses (LPN) founded in 1949 to establish policy and become the official voice for LPNs. The federation conducts workshops and holds an annual convention. The NFLPN also represents LPNs in all affairs of the profession relating to its welfare and its role in nursing. Its official publication is the journal *Nursing Care.*

**National Formulary (NF)**
A compendium of standards for certain drugs and preparations that are not included in the United States Pharmacopeia (USP). It is revised every five years, and recognized as a book of official standards by the Pure Food and Drug Act of 1906. See formulary, compendium.

**national health insurance (NHI)**
1. A term not yet defined in the United States. 2. A proposed prepaid comprehensive insurance program that would be mandatory and be funded by payroll deductions for all U.S. citizens. See also medical deduction, national health service, social insurance, and socialized medicine.

**national health priorities**
The health priorities specified by the 93rd U.S. Congress and listed in Section 1502 of P.L. 93-541. See health systems priorities.

**national health service**
Often used synonymously with national health insurance. They are sometimes usefully distinguished by applying the former to health programs in which the national government directly operates a health system which serves some or all of its citizens and the latter to programs in which the government insures or otherwise arranges financing for health care without arranging for, owning or operating it (although NHI proposals usually include some measure of regulation of the financed services). See also social insurance and socialized medicine.

**National Health Service Corps (NHSC)**
A program which places U.S. Public Health Service personnel in areas with a critical shortage of health manpower (see medically underserved population) for the purpose of improving the delivery of health care and services to persons residing in such areas. The Corps was established by the Emergency Health Personnel Act of 1970, P.L. 91-623, as amended by the Emergency Health Personnel Act Amendments of 1972, P.L. 92-585 (section 329 of the PHS Act). The first Corps members were assigned in January, 1972.

**National Health Service Corps programs**
Programs operated by the federal government pursuant to Section 329(b) of the Public Health Service Act, the Manpower Training Act of 1971 (P.L. 92-157), and Section 74(F) of the Public Health Service Act as amended.

**National Health Survey**
A continuing health survey by the National Center for Health Statistics of the Dept. of Health and Human Services, which includes studies to determine the extent of illness and disability in the population of the United States, describe the use of health services by Americans, and gather related information. It conducts a continuing household interview survey of a sample of the population, surveys certain medical records, surveys a sample of the population through health examinations, and conducts related developmental and evaluative studies.

**National Institute of Health**
One of the major institutes under the Department of Health and Human Services, which has several subunits including the National Library of Medicine, the Fogarty International Center for the Advanced Study of Health Sciences, and eleven research institutes which carry out and support programs of basic and clinical research. They are: National Institute on Aging; National Cancer Institute; National Heart and Lung Institute; National Institute of Dental Research; National Institute of Neurological Disease and Stroke; National Institute of Arthritis, Metabolism and Digestive Diseases; National Institute of Allergy and Infectious Diseases; National Institute of Child Health and Human Development; National Institute of General Medical Sciences; National Eye Institute; National Institute of Environmental Health Sciences.

**National Institute of Occupational Safety and Health (NIOSH)**
Under the Center for Disease Control, NIOSH conducts research and studies and develops standards related to work environment, health and safety.

**National Interns and Residents Matching Program (NIRMP)**
The official cooperative plan for first-year appointments in graduate medical education of the American Hospital Association, American Protestant Hospital Association, Association of American Medical Colleges, Catholic Hospital Association, American Medical Association, American Student Medical Association, and American Board of Medical Specialties. The program operates as a clearinghouse for matching preferences of medical students for internships and residencies with available positions in accord with hospital lists of preferences among graduating students. In order to participate in the program, hospital program directors sign the program's hospital agreement, which commits the institution to participate in the NIRMP as a corporate entity, and list with the NIRMP all programs and positions being made available to students.

**National League of Nursing (NLN)**
The official nursing organization that has taken on a national role of improving nursing education and services. The NLN has two major divisions—one for individual members and one for agency and institutional members. The NLN is open on the individual level to anyone providing nursing care, from the RN down to nursing assistants. Among the many roles of the NLN, it is the official accrediting body for schools of nursing. Its official journal is *Nursing Outlook*.

**National Reporter System**
Court cases, in book form, which cover decisions of appellate courts. They are reported by region. For example, the North Eastern Reporter (Illinois, Indiana, Massachusetts, New York, and Ohio) is abbreviated "N.E." and in more recent books, N.E.2d (second). The Reporter System includes all federal cases and those state court cases decided by the court of last resort.

**native American**
One whose ancestry originates on the North American continent; the American Indians.

**natural childbirth**
A very general orientation where the mother is awake and aware at birth of her child. She has gone through some preparation to decrease and minimize use of pain-reduction drugs. It does not mean a painless birth.

**Natural Death Act**
The act of removing life-sustaining equipment and procedures from patients with a terminal illness. The patient usually has written a "living will" requesting such actions.

**natural law**
1. Wrongs that are considered immoral, dangerous or harmful by most societies. 2. Rules of conduct that are the same everywhere. 3. The rules that are basic to society and human behavior. 4. Moral law. See mala in se.

**natural person**
A human being; as differing from an artificial creation such as a corporation.

**naturopath**
A nonmedical health practitioner who practices therapy utilizing natural things such as light, heat, water, nutrition, etc. but uses no drugs in treatment.

**naturopathy**
A drugless system of therapy, making use of physical forces such as air, light, water, diet, heat and massage.

**nausea**
The sensation or feeling that one has to vomit.

**N.B. (Lat.) Nota Bene**
1. Mark well. 2. Note well. 3. Observe; used for emphasis. 4. Emphasizes one thing.

**near poor**
Those people who make enough money to meet daily needs but who cannot meet poverty guidelines or quality for any type of county, state or federal government assistance when an emergency arises. This group of people make too much money to receive aid and too little money to pay for medical bills, automobile bills or other emergencies. They usually have no insurance to help pay for these emergencies either. The elderly,

some racial minorities and students often fall into this income area. (Some suggest it is the income bracket somewhere between $5,000 and $15,000, depending on certain factors such as location and inflation.)

**nebulize**
Change a liquid, medication or other substance into a mist or spray.

**nebulizer**
An atomizer or sprayer; a mist maker.

**necessary**
See need.

**necessary cause**
A condition or factor which must be present or which is necessary for a specific disease to occur.

**necro-**
Prefix meaning death.

**necromania**
Unhealthy preoccupation with dead bodies. Also called necrophilia.

**necrosis**
Dead tissue.

**need**
Some thing or action which is essential, indispensable, required or cannot be done or lived without; a condition marked by the lack or want of some such thing or action. The presence or absence of a need can and should be measured by an objective criterion or standard. Needs may or may not be perceived or expressed by the person in need and must be distinguished from demands, expressed desires whether or not needed. Like appropriateness, need is frequently and irregularly used in health care with respect to health facilities and services (see certificate-of-need) and people (see medically needy). It is thus important to specify what thing or action's need is being considered, by what criteria the need is to be established, by whom (provider, consumer, or third party), and with what effect (since payment for services by insurance is, for instance, sometimes conditioned upon the necessity of their provision).

**need assessment**
Portion of the plan development process which involves assessment of health status and health system and goal setting but is prior to objective and priority setting.

**need for a specific allied health occupation**
An adequate minimum quantity and quality of persons in that allied health occupation which the consensus of a wide variety of persons believes ought to be available to the citizens of the U.S. for the purpose of remaining or becoming reasonably healthy.

**ne exeat (Lat.)**
A writ forbidding a person from leaving a local city or area.

**nefas (Lat.)**
Wrong, unjust.

**negative averment**
1. A negative declaration. 2. A positive declaration in which some negative is used. 3. A statement in the negative.

**negative covenant**
A party agrees and is obliged to refrain from committing an act, usually having to do with the use of real property.

**negative pregnant**
In a testimony, a denial that implies an affirmation of the truth or a fact.

**neglect**
1. Carelessness. 2. Failure to do that which normally is expected to be done. 3. Lack of due care. 4. Failure to properly care for a child. 5. Habitual lack of attention.

**negligence**
1. The failure to exercise reasonable, usual, ordinary or expected care, resulting in harm or injury. 2. Doing something carelessly or failing to do something that should have been done. 3. The omission of doing what a reasonable man would do, using ordinary considerations which commonly regulate human behavior. 4. The doing of some act, behavior or activity that a reasonable and prudent man would not do. Negligence is characterized by inattention, recklessness, thoughtlessness, wantonness, and inadvertence. The law of negligence is based on reasonable care under all circumstances. Negligence is often referred to in degrees of care or degrees of failure to exercise the proper degree of care. These degrees are "gross," "ordinary," and "slight." These degrees indicate only that certain levels of care or caution are required, but failure to exercise care at a demanded or expected level is negligence. (38 Del. Laws, c. 26. Gallegher v. Davis, 7 W.W. Harr. 380, 183 A. 620) See also comparative negligence, contributory negligence, gross negligence, ordinary negligence, passive negligence, slight negligence, subsequent negligence, wanton negligence, willful negligence, reasonable man, standard of care, foreseeability.

**negligent**
1. Not exercising due care. 2. Careless. 3. The commission of an act or the failure to perform an act that a "reasonable man" would not do under the same circumstance.

**negotiable instrument**
1. A document which has been signed and which contains a promise to pay a specific sum upon demand or at a specific time. 2. It must have printed on it "pay to the order of" (a specific person) or "pay to bearer." Negotiable instruments include checks, notes, drafts and bills of exchange.

**negotiate**

1. To bring about a compromise by negotiation. 2. To discuss, arrange or bargain. 3. Do business. 4. To place into circulation. 5. To tender a negotiable instrument for payment.

**negotiation**

1. Conferring, bargaining or discussing a matter. 2. Carrying on a discussion to reach an agreement or compromise. 3. The process by which a negotiable instrument is presented for payment.

**neighborhood health center**

Developed in the 1960's era with funds from the Office of Economic Opportunity and the old Department of Health, Education and Welfare. They provided comprehensive ambulatory services for special populations consisting mostly of the poor and elderly. The neighborhood health centers were developed to overcome the demeaning, impersonal, crowded, and long waiting conditions while trying to receive health care in county hospitals, or state medical school teaching hospitals' outpatient services. A broad range of primary and secondary ambulatory care services are provided by salaried physicians and other health care providers, with an emphasis being placed on preventive health care with some nonmedical support services also provided. Consumers were to have a major role in the governing of the facility. These programs are now on the down turn.

**nemine contradicente (Lat.)**

No one dissenting or contradicting.

**nemine dissentiente (Lat.)**

Unanimous non-dissent, no one dissenting.

**nemo (Lat.)**

No one; no one person; no person.

**nemo dat quod non habet (Lat.)**

No one can give what he does not have.

**nemo est supra leges (Lat.)**

No one is above the law.

**nemo potest plus juris ad alium transferre quam ipse habet (Lat.)**

No one can transfer a greater right to another than he himself has.

**neonatal mortality**

The death (mortality) of live born children who have not reached 4 weeks or 1 month of age, usually measured as a rate: number of neonatal deaths per 1,000 live births in a given area or program and time period. Early neonatal deaths (those occurring in the first week of life) are sometimes also reported. See also mortality, infant and perinatal mortality.

**neoplasm**

A new growth; a tumor.

**nepotism**
Hiring one's relative; providing favors to one's relatives by providing them employment or a position.

**net**
1. Actual items remaining. 2. Free from charges, expenses, commissions and fees. 3. What is left after all expenses or debts have been paid. 4. Actual weight excluding the weight of the container. 5. What is left after everything is deducted.

**net income**
The difference between a health facility's adjusted gross income and its operating expenses. This may or may not include depreciation figures.

**net lease**
A lease requiring payment of not only rent but also taxes, insurance, utilities and maintenance. The terms net net, net net net, or triple net are also used.

**net worth**
Difference between total assets and liabilities of an individual, hospital, nursing home, corporation, etc.

**neuroleptic**
A major tranquilizer. See Antipsychotic drug.

**neurologic**
Pertaining to the nervous system.

**neurologist**
A physician who specializes in disorders and diseases of the nervous system.

**neurology**
The medical specialty that deals with disorders and diseases of the nervous system.

**neuropsychiatry**
The medical specialty that incorporates psychiatry and neurology.

**neurosis**
A mental disorder. A form of mental illness that is characterized by anxiety. Although neuroses do not overtly distort reality, it can be severe enough to impair one's effectiveness and functioning. The following are types of neurosis: anxiety, hysterical, phobic, obsessive-compulsive, depressive, neurasthenic, depersonalization, and hypochondriacal. Due to the vagueness of this term it now has only limited use.

**new drug**
A drug for which pre-marketing approval is required by the Federal Food, Drug, and Cosmetic Act. A new drug is any drug which is not generally recognized, among experts qualified by scientific training and experience to evaluate the safety and effectiveness of drugs, as safe and effective for use under its prescribed conditions of use. Since 1962, most new prescription drugs have been subject to the new drug application and

premarket approval process for new drugs. The vast majority of drugs marketed over-the-counter, however, have not been through the new drug approval process. See also GRAS and GRAE, not new and 'me too' drugs.

**new drug application (NDA)**
An application which must be approved by the FDA before any new drug is marketed to the general public which provides information designed to demonstrate safety and effectiveness. Once the application is approved, the drug may be prescribed by any physician or other health professional authorized to prescribe under state law. The NDA must include: reports of animal and clinical investigations; a list of ingredients including the active drug and any vehicle, excipient, binder, filler, flavoring, and coloring; a description of manufacturing methods and quality control procedures: samples of the drug; and the proposed labelling. Approval of an NDA must be based on valid scientific evidence that the drug is safe, and adequate and well-controlled clinical studies (such as random controlled trials) demonstrating that it is effective for its intended, i.e., labeled, uses. NDA also commonly refers to the FDA's approval of an application, i.e., the manufacturer's license to market the drug. See also investigational new drug.

**new illness**
In health insurance, for the purpose of determining payment of office visits, a new illness is one which begins with a series of office visits separated by 120 days from the date of the last visit.

**New Jersey rule**
A ruling by the Supreme Court of New Jersey which held that contingency fees must be scheduled according to the size of the award, with the percentage of the award going to the claimant's lawyer declining as the size of the award increases. For example, in New Jersey, lawyers may receive 50 percent of a $1,000 settlement, but only 10 percent of any amount recovered over $100,000. A number of states have adopted variations of the New Jersey rule.

**new matter**
New issues or facts that have not previously been alleged in a pleading.

**new patient**
One new to the physician, office, or facility. The initial comprehensive history and examination need not be done at the time of the first visit.

**newspaper policy**
One type of life or health insurance sold in newspapers.

**next cause**
The closest or most related cause of harm or injury; the proximate cause. See proximate cause.

**next friend**
A person not formally appointed who acts on behalf or represents one who is legally incapable or is disabled, such as an infant or someone who is retarded.

**next of kin**
Family or those closely related to a dead person. Usually the dead person's spouse, children or brothers and sisters.

**nexus (Lat.)**
A connection; a link in a series; a joining.

**NFPA**
National Fire Protection Association.

**N.H.R.D.**
National Health Planning and Resource Development Act (P.L. 93-641). See these words.

**night hospital**
1. A halfway house type facility. 2. A part time hospital in which psychiatric patients are allowed to work and function in the outside community during the day and work hours and then return to the hospital at night.

**night terror**
A relatively new term used to describe a sleep disturbance characterized by a person sweating, talking incoherently, crying, sleepwalking and often showing fear or talking about fearful situations. This is not a nightmare, as the person does not remember any part of the night terror, whereas nightmares cause no physical reaction and are remembered.

**nihil (Lat.)**
Nothing.

**nil (Lat.)**
Nothing.

**N.I.O.S.H.**
National Institute of Occupational Safety and Health.

**nisi (Lat.)**
Unless. A court order that will be enforced unless the person named in it appears in court to show cause why it should not be enforced.

**nisi prius (Lat.)**
Unless before; a trial court.

**nisi prius court (Lat.)**
A court that conducts a trial with a judge and a jury. This court is distinguished from an appellate court.

**N.L.A.D.A.**
National Legal Aid and Defender Association.

**N.L.R.A.**
National Labor Relations Act.

**N.L.R.B.**
National Labor Relations Board.

**no contest**
Not challenged. See nolo contendere.

**nocti-**
Prefix, meaning night.

**nocturnal enuresis**
Uncontrolled urination at night; bedwetting.

**no-fault insurance**
Automobile insurance that provides coverage against injury or other loss without the need to determine responsibility for an accident. Coverage and benefits vary widely; this insurance or law exists in only a few states.

**noise**
Any unwanted sound.

**nolle prosequi (Lat.)**
A plaintiff or a prosecutor deciding and announcing that he will not further prosecute a pending case. When a case ends, it is nolled or nolled prossed.

**nolo contendere (Lat.)**
I will not contest it. In a criminal action, admitting guilt indirectly without admitting guilt.

**nominal**
1. Slight, small, token amount. 2. Not real or substantial; in name only.

**nominal damages**
Compensation given to the plaintiff when his case is proven, but the actual injury or loss was not proven.

**non (Lat.)**
Not.

**non age**
Not yet of legal age; still a minor.

**nonassertion**
As used in assertiveness training, it is to violate one's own rights by not expressing honest feelings, thoughts and beliefs and permitting others to walk over oneself. Expression of one's thoughts and feelings in an apologetic, diffident, self-effacing manner so others can easily disregard them; to appease others to avoid conflict.

**non-assigned**
Health care providers who will not accept patients or programs under certain health care programs administered by the Federal government.

**noncancellable, or noncancellable and guaranteed renewable policy**
An insurance policy that the insured has the right to continue in force to a specified age, by the timely payment of premiums. During the specified period that the policy is in force, the insurer has no right to make any unilateral change in any provision of the policy.

**non compos mentis (Lat.)**
1. Not of sound mind. 2. Insane; suffering a mental illness. See insanity.

**nonconfining sickness**
An illness which prevents the insured person from working but which does not result in confinement to a hospital or to one's home.

**noncontributory**
One type of health insurance that is done on a group basis, for which the employer pays the entire premium.

**nondelegated hospital**
A hospital for which all PSRO program health care review activities are performed by a PSRO.

**nondisabling injury**
An injury or illness which may require medical care but does not produce loss of working time or income.

**nondisclosure**
1. Failure to disclose. 2. Not telling all the facts.

**nonduplication of benefits**
When a patient is covered under more than one group of medical or dental programs. The carrier with a nonduplication provision—as distinguished from a coordination of benefits provision—assumes no liability, frequently leaving the patient with out-of-pocket expenses.

**nonfeasance**
1. Nonperformance of an act that one is duty-bound to perform. 2. Failure to perform a required duty. 3. The failure to perform a duty or act that a professional is required to perform.

**non obstante veredicto (Lat.)**
Notwithstanding the verdict. When a judge overrules a jury by rendering the judgment in a lawsuit to one suit when the jury gave the verdict to the other side.

**nonoccupational policy**
A contract that insures a person against off-the-job accident or sickness. It does not cover disability resulting from injury or sickness covered by Workers' Compensation. Group accident and sickness policies are frequently nonoccupational.

**non-participating hospital**
A hospital which has not contracted with a reciprocating Blue Cross plan.

**nonparticipating insurance company**
See stock insurance company.

**non-pathogen**
A microorganism that is not disease producing.

**nonprofit**
Any school, agency, organization, or institution which is a corporation or association, or is owned and operated by one or more corporations or associations, no part of the net earnings of which inures, or may lawfully inure, to the benefit of any private shareholder or individual.

**non-profit hospital**
A hospital which is a corporation which turns its profits back into the hospital and has a non-taxable status. It is usually community own or owned by a church or society or other services minded organization. See proprietary hospital.

**nonprofit school**
1. A school owned and operated by one or more occupations or associations, no part of the net earnings which inures, or may lawfully inure, to the benefit of any private shareholder or individual. 2. As applied to any training center for allied health professions means such a training center which is an entity, or is owned and operated by an entity, no part of the net earnings of which inures or may lawfully inure, to the benefit of any private shareholder or individual; and as applied to any entity means an entity no part of the net earnings of which inures or may lawfully inure to the benefit of any private shareholder or individual.

**non prosequitur (Lat.)**
1. He does not follow up. 2. A judgment given to a defendant because the plaintiff has failed to follow up on a lawsuit or claim that has been filed. 3. A default judgment.

**non repet (Lat.)**
Do not repeat.

**non-service-connected disability**
In the Veterans' Administration health care program, a disability which was not incurred or aggravated in the line of duty during active military service. Care is available from the program for such disabilities on a bed-available basis after service-connected disabilities are cared for.

**nonsuit**
1. A judgment against a plaintiff when he fails to prove his case or fails to appear in court. 2. A judgment not fully on the merits but on the failure to present a prima facie case. See directed verdict.

**nonurgent**
Any health care emergency not requiring the resources of an emergency service, with the disorder being minor or nonacute.

**nonverbal communication**
Communication through facial expression, gestures and posture; body language.

**norm(s)**
1. Numerical or statistical measure(s) of usual observed performance. For example, a norm for care of appendicitis would be the usual percentage

of appendices removed in cases diagnosed as appendicitis which are shown by pathology to be diseased. A norm can be used as a standard but does not necessarily serve as one. Both norm and standard imply single, proper values rather than a range. 2. The average, normal, usual expected behavior, action, ability or level of achievement.

**normal saline**
An isotonic concentration of salt (NaCl) in water.

**normo-**
Prefix meaning rule; order; average; normal.

**Norris-Laguardia Act**
A federal act (1932) established to prevent certain injunctions against strikers or unions and prohibits "yellow dog" contracts.

**nosocomial**
Pertaining to or originating from a hospital.

**nosology**
The science of the classification of diseases.

**no-strike clause**
A clause put into a labor contract by management, whereby a union relinquishes its rights to strike.

**notary public**
A minor public official who witnesses signatures on documents, administers oaths, certifies the validity of legal documents, and performs witnessing duties for the business and legal community.

**notation voting**
Boards or legislature casting votes without any meeting. This is not ethical or legal in most situations.

**notch**
A sudden and sharp discontinuity in health or financial benefits for individuals with slightly different income. In certain public and medical assistance programs, an additional dollar of income can mean a total loss of benefits. For example, in Medicaid, families just below the income eligibility standard receive fully subsidized coverage while families with only slightly more income and just above eligibility standards receive no benefits. Substantial incentives for families to restrict their incomes in order to remain eligible may result. Spend down provisions are used to compensate for notches. A notch may also occur when, without change in eligibility, cost-sharing requirements increase suddenly with a small change in income.

**note**
1. A legal document that may be exchanged for money. Whoever signs the note promises to pay a specific amount of money by a certain time. 2. A record of a legal proceeding or ruling in a court.

**not-for-profit carriers**
Insurance programs, service corporations or prepayment plans organized under state not-for-profit statutes for the purpose of providing health care insurance coverage (for example, Delta Dental Plans, Blue Cross and Blue Shield Plans).

**not-for-profit hospital**
See proprietary hospital, non-profit.

**notice**
1. To become aware of. 2. To pay attention to. 3. To give a formal warning. 4. A formal action which can be part of a legal agreement. 5. The act of delivering legal documents.

**notice of lis pendens**
See lis pendens notice.

**notice to produce**
A lawful notice requiring a party or witness to bring certain documents for inspection by a party or to trial.

**notifiable**
A disease which providers are required (usually by law) to report to federal, state or local public health officials when diagnosed (such as tuberculosis, diphtheria and syphilis). Notifiable diseases are those of public interest by reason of their infectiousness, severity or frequency. See also registration and quarantine.

**notification of changes in patient status (Medicare)**
The facility has appropriate written policies and procedures relating to notification of the patient's attending physician and other responsible persons in the event of an accident involving the patient, or other significant change in the patient's physical, mental, or emotional status, or patient charges, billings, and related administrative matters. Except in a medical emergency, a patient is not transferred or discharged, nor is treatment altered radically, without consultation with the patient or, if he is incompetent, without prior notification of next of kin or guardian.

**not new**
A drug for which premarketing approval by the Food and Drug Administration is not, or no longer, required. A drug may become "not new" upon a ruling by the FDA that the safeguards applicable to approved new drugs, e.g., maintenance of records and submission of reports, are no longer required. See also 'me too' drug.

**notorious**
Common knowledge; known to all.

**N.O.V. (Lat.)**
Non obstante veredicto. See these words.

**novation**
1. The substitution of a new contract for an earlier one, which ends the old agreement or promise. 2. A new formal contract which ends all related previous agreements. 3. Placing a new professional in a

responsible position held previously by a person under a contractual agreement.

**N.S.A.**
National Security Agency.

**N.S.F.**
1. National Science Foundation. 2. Not sufficient funds.

**nuclear family**
1. Immediate members of a family, including the parents and the children. 2. As used in JCAH accreditation it is the conjugal family composed of parents and children living under one roof. Assumed to be the predominant form of family life today, as compared to the extended family in the past in which the conjugal family plus blood relatives from two or more generations live under one roof. Modified extended families are still very much in evidence where two or more generations live in close proximity and maintain close contact, but not under one roof.

**nuclear medicine**
For JCAH accreditation purposes this is the scientific and clinical discipline concerned with diagnostic, therapeutic (exclusive of sealed radium sources), and investigative use of radionuclides.

**nuclear medicine technologist**
Nuclear medicine technologists are involved in both diagnostic and therapeutic procedures, preparing and using radioactive nucleides in laboratory procedures, scanning-imaging, and function studies. Under the guidance of a nuclear medicine physician, the technologist receives, positions, and attends to patients, makes dose calculations for in vivo studies, performs a wide variety of diagnostic tests on human beings or on body fluids, and applies radioactive materials in treatment procedures. Nuclear medicine technologists are responsible for the safe disposal or storage of radioactive materials and for the inventory and control of radiopharmaceuticals. Nearly all nuclear medicine technologists are employed in hospitals or clinics.

**nuclear radiation**
A process that accompanies the transformation of atoms from unstable to stable states by the release of excess energy in the form of electromagnetic waves or atomic particles.

**nude pact**
See nudum pactum.

**nudum pactum (Lat.)**
A bare agreement; a promise not supported by consideration, and therefore not enforceable and is completed only by honesty and good will.

**nugatory**
A wasted effort. Ineffectual; futile.

**nuisance**

1. Anything that unnecessarily or unreasonably annoys or disturbs. 2. Violating the public's health, safety, or decency. A nuisance may be stopped by a civil lawsuit or enforcing public law.

**null**

Having no legal effect or validity; void.

**null hypothesis**

In research, the expected outcome is stated in a way that says nothing will happen in hopes of rejecting this position once results have been found.

**nullify**

1. To void. 2. To render invalid.

**nullity**

1. Nothing. 2. Having no legal force. 3. Ineffectual.

**nunc dimittis (Lat.)**

1. Now you let depart. 2. A departure or farewell, usually from life. 3. A dismissal.

**nunc pro tunc (Lat.)**

1. Now for then. 2. Acts performed with a retroactive effect. 3. Legal authority which clears the health care provider for giving treatment which has already been done.

**nuncupative will**

An oral declaration intended to serve as a will, made shortly before death and later put in writing by one of the witnesses.

**nurse (R.N.)**

A professional person qualified by education and authorized by state law to practice nursing. There are many different types, specialties and levels of nurses whose names are generally descriptive of their special responsibilities (such as charge or head, hospital, private or private duty, public health, and school nurses). See also nurse anesthetist, midwife and practitioner.

**nurse aide/orderly**

These individuals may be called hospital attendants, nurse aides, nurse assistants, nurse attendants, orderlies, or some variation of these titles. However, they all perform tasks delegated or assigned by the professional nursing staff, including assisting in direct patient care of a routine nature, making beds, escorting patients to other hospital departments, setting up and moving equipment, delivering messages, counting linens, etc. May also include, where hospital policy permits, the taking of vital signs, and in the case of orderlies, includes performing heavier work in the nursing unit and maintaining equipment and may include setting up of traction and performing male catheterization. See nurse assistant, nurse aide, orderly, hospital attendant, nurse attendant.

**nurse anesthetist**

A registered nurse who has had special training in anesthesia so that she is prepared to work under supervision of an anesthesiologist or physician in administering anesthetic agents to patients before and during surgical and obstetrical procedures and operations. See certified registered nurse anesthetist.

**nurse midwife**

A registered nurse who, by virtue of added knowledge and skill gained through an organized program of study and clinical experience recognized by the American College of Nurse-Midwives, has extended the lawful limits of her practice into the management and care of mothers and babies throughout the maternity cycle, so long as progress meets criteria accepted as normal.

**nurse-midwifery practice**

Nurse-midwifery practice is the independent management of care of essentially normal newborns and women, antepartally, intrapartally, postpartally and/or gynecologically, occurring within a health care system which provides for medical consultation, collaborative management, or referral and is in accord with the *Functions, Standards and Qualifications for Nurse-Midwifery Practice* as defined by the American College of Nurse-Midwives.

**nurse practitioner**

A registered nurse qualified and specially trained to provide primary care, including primary health care in homes and in ambulatory care facilities, long-term care facilities and other health care institutions. Nurse practitioners generally function under supervision of a physician but not necessarily in his presence. They are usually salaried rather than being reimbursed on a fee-for-service basis, although the supervising physician may receive fee-for-service reimbursement for their services. See also physician assistant and Medex.

**nurse, psychiatric**

A member of the mental health care team. She works with patients in the psychiatric hospital milieu, and conducts individual, family, and group psychotherapy.

**nurses fees**

A provision often found in a medical expense reimbursement policy that allows for payment of nursing services provided to a patient. In most cases, the services are provided by a visiting nurse or a home care agency nurse in the home.

**nursing**

1. The unique function of the nurse is to assist an individual, sick or well, in the performance of those activities contributing to health or its recovery (or to peaceful death) that he would perform unaided if he had the necessary strength, will or knowledge. (From International Council of Nurses) This includes assisting patients in carrying out therapeutic plans initiated by physicians and other health professionals and assisting other members of the medical team in performing the nursing function and

understanding health needs of patients. The specific content of nursing care varies in different countries and situations, and it is important to note that, as defined, it is not given solely by nurses but also by many other lay persons, paraprofessionals and advanced specialty trained nurses such as nurse practitioners, i.e., pediatric nurse practitioners, geriatric nurse practitioners, etc. 2. According to the American Nursing Association in Standards of Nursing practice, nursing practice is defined as a direct service that is goal oriented, and is adaptable to the needs of the individual, the family and community during health and illness.

**nursing assistant**

A term which is currently starting to replace "nurse's aide" and "orderly," as it provides more prestige to the position and has no gender related connotation. This person usually performs an increasing number of duties, such as bedmaking, feeding, bathing, taking temperature, elevation, and assisting the patient and the nursing staff.

**nursing audit**

Reviewing a patient's charts by peers (nurses) to determine the competency of nursing care.

**nursing care**

Nursing care is provided on four different levels: 1) promotion of health, 2) prevention of disease or injury 3) restoration of health and 4) consolation of the dying. Professional nursing care activities can include the following: assisting patients with basic needs, administering drugs, medications and treatments, patient observation with regard to response and adaptation, patient observation with regard to response to treatment, teaching self care, counseling on health matters, directing rehabilitation activities, patient aftercare, planning, and providing mental, social and emotional support for the patient. See nursing, nursing process.

**nursing differential**

A differential (8½ percent of routine inpatient nursing salary costs) added to the costs of such services to reflect the supposedly above average costs of providing routine inpatient nursing care to Medicare beneficiaries. Medicare reimburses hospitals more by this amount for nursing services than do other insurance programs which cover the general population. There has been much recent controversy over the need for the differential.

**nursing home administration**

The performance of any act or the making of any decision involved in the planning, organizing, directing and control of the operation of a nursing home or its equivalent. (American College of Nursing Home Administrators)

**nursing homes**

1. Generally, a wide range of institutions, other than hospitals, which provide various levels of maintenance and personal or nursing care to people who are unable to care for themselves and who may have health problems which range from minimal to very serious. The term includes free standing institutions, or identifiable components of other health

facilities which provide nursing care and related services, personal care, and residential care. Nursing homes include skilled nursing facilities, intermediate care facilities, and extended care facilities but not boarding homes. 2. Any institution caring for the elderly and/or patients in need of skilled nursing care. Usually it is expected that a certain level of nursing care be given. Nursing homes offer custodial and personal care, nursing care as well as social and rehabilitative services. The home should be a well-equipped, clean and pleasant facility with a courteous, cheerful, well-trained staff. 3. A long term care facility having 50 percent or more of its residents receiving one or more nursing services and having at least one registered nurse or licensed practical nurse for 35 or more hours of employment per week. See long term care facility, skilled nursing care facility.

**nursing process**
Describes the methods and steps that a nurse uses when planning and implementing patient care. It is based on the scientific method of problem solving and includes 4 basic components 1) assessment, 2) planning, 3) implementation, and 4) evaluation.

**nursing service**
1. In JCAH hospital accreditation, this is patient care services pertaining to the curative, restorative, and preventive aspects of nursing that are performed and/or supervised by a registered nurse pursuant to the medical care plan of the practitioner and the nursing care plan. 2. In JCAH long-term care facility accreditation, this is patient/resident care services that pertain to the curative, restorative, and preventive aspects of nursing and that are under the supervision of a registered nurse pursuant to the multidisciplinary patient/resident plan of care.

**nursing unit**
1. A geographic division of a hospital determined by medical specialty or service provided, including medical, surgical, recovery, coronary care, intensive care, obstetrical, pediatric and psychiatric units, etc. A supervisor or charge nurse of a unit manages several professional staff and other support personnel, such as aides, orderlies, ward clerks and unit managers. 2. In JCAH accreditation, this is an organized jurisdiction of nursing service in which nursing services are provided on a continuous basis.

**nutrient**
Substances found in food which are digested and absorbed by the body and used as food and energy needed to sustain life.

**nutrition**
The science of food, the nutrients and other substances therein, their action, interaction, and balance in relation to health and disease, and the processes by which the organism ingests, digests, absorbs, transports, utilizes, and excretes food substances. In addition, nutrition must be concerned with social, economic, cultural, and psychological implications of food and eating. (Council on Foods and Nutrition, American Medical Association, 1963.)

**nutritional care**

The application of the science and art of human nutrition in helping people select and obtain food for the primary purpose of nourishing their bodies in health or disease throughout the life cycle. This participation may be in single or combined functions; in foodservice systems management to groups; in extending knowledge of food and nutrition principles; in teaching these principles for application according to particular situations; and in dietary counseling.

**nutritional deficiency disease**

A disease such as rickets which is caused by an insufficient quantity of necessary vitamins and minerals in the body due to the lack of proper food.

**nutritionist**

Adapts and applies food and nutrient information to the solution of food problems, the control of disease, and the promotion of health. Performs nutrition research, instructs groups and individuals about nutritional requirements, and helps people develop meal patterns to meet their nutritional needs.

**nymphomania**

An unhealthy and somewhat compulsive need in women for sexual intercourse. See also satyriasis.

# O

**oath**
1. The giving of a solemn declaration of truth, fact, or giving evidence in a court of law. 2. Swearing to tell the truth. There are two basic types of oaths: 1) assertory oath—asserting something is true; 2) promissory oath—making a promise to do something.

**obese**
Excessively fat; having a high amount of fatty tissue over normal body weight; being more than 20% over your normal body weight, which is sometimes measured by how much you weighed at age 20.

**obiter**
In passing; incidentally.

**obiter dictum (Lat.)**
Something said in passing. Words in a judicial opinion, not a part of the decision. A general comment of a judge.

**object**
1. To oppose an action or statement of the opposing party in court or a lawsuit as being incorrect, biased, improper, unfair, or failing to follow procedure. 2. To assert that a decision or action made by a judge is incorrect or wrong. 3. To express opposition. 4. To formally oppose.

**objection**
1. Having grounds to object. 2. Presenting an adverse argument. 3. Disapproval. 4. Disagreement. 5. An expression of disapproval.

**objective**
1. Something that is determinable, known, external to one's mind; actual or real. 2. Features and characteristics of an object. 3. Being without judgment, prejudice, bias or a demeaning position. 4. A sign, symptom or condition that is easily observed by others besides the patient. 5. A lens in a microscope. 6. In health planning, management or administration, it is any short term, measurable, specific activity having a specific time limit or time line for completion. It is usually a quantified statement of a desired outcome in the near future. Objectives are used to reach goals (goals being generalized aims of an organization, project or plan). Objectives include specifying who, to what extent, under what conditions, by what standards and within a specific time period certain activities are to be performed and completed. 7. According to JCAH for psychiatric, alcoholism and drug abuse facilities accreditation purposes, this is an expected result or condition that takes less time to achieve than a goal, is stated in measurable terms, has a specified time for achievement, and is related to the attainment of a goal.

**obligation**
1. A legal duty. 2. An expectation created by a contract. 3. An official written promise; a duty to perform a written promise. 4. A duty to perform or act. 5. An agreement or promise bound by a legal penalty.

**obligations**
1. In the federal budget, amounts of orders placed, contracts awarded, services rendered, or other commitments of federal budget authority made by federal agencies during a given period which will require outlays of federal funds during the same or some future period. 2. Debts owed or agreements yet to be completed or fulfilled.

**obligatory**
Legally or morally bound.

**obligee**
1. One to whom a duty is owed. 2. A person to whom another party is bound by a contract. 3. One on whose behalf an obligation exists.

**obligor**
1. One who is obligated. 2. One who binds himself to another party by a contract. 3. One who owes another a duty. 4. One bound to perform an obligation.

**obliterate**
1. To destroy. 2. To erase. 3. To cross out written words or phrases. 4. To remove all traces of something.

**obloquy**
1. To cause shame or disgrace. 2. To blame. 3. To censure. 4. To reproach. 5. Verbal abuse or reproach.

**obscene**
1. Immoral. 2. Foul. 3. Indecent. 4. Lewd. 5. Filthy.

**obscenity**
1. An obscene act or presentation. 2. The state of being morally and socially unacceptable.

**obsession**
Dwelling on something to excess. A persistent impulse that cannot be eliminated from consciousness by logical effort. See also compulsion.

**obsessive-compulsive personality**
A personality disorder in which a person is a perfectionist with overattention to detail, excessively conscientious, demanding and usually overinhibited.

**obstante (Lat.)**
Withstanding.

**obstetrical technician**
Under the supervision of the nursing and medical staff, the obstetrical technician assists in the care of women in labor and in delivery rooms before, during, and after delivery. They may perform various hygienic

procedures, routine laboratory procedures, sterilize and maintain equipment, and maintain supplies in the delivery rooms. This is a fairly small occupational group.

**obstetrics**

The branch of medicine concerned with and treating the birth process and related conditions, disorders and events which are medically associated which precede and follow birth.

**obstetric services**

The diagnosis and treatment of any abnormalities during pregnancy, and services for the promotion and maintenance of optimum mental and physical well-being of the individual woman and her child from the onset of labor until the end of the perinatal period.

**obstructing justice**

1. Stopping or interfering with the functioning of the courts or the litigation process, or court officials. 2. Keeping a witness from appearing in court. 3. Withholding evidence.

**occult**

1. Concealed; hidden; secret. 2. The acts or occurrences that are mysterious, supernatural and beyond human understanding. 3. Mystic arts and studies related to magic, witchcraft, astrology and folk beliefs.

**occupancy**

The ratio of inpatient census to number of available beds. This is usually calculated and presented as a percentage of beds in use. See occupancy rate.

**occupancy rate**

A measure of inpatient health facility use, determined by dividing available bed days by patient days. It measures the average percentage of a hospital's beds occupied and may be institution-wide, or specific for one department or service.

**occupational health and safety**

Actions taken to assure the recognition, prevention and control of occupational health hazards and illnesses, and to promote the physical and mental well-being of employed persons.

**occupational health services**

Health services concerned with the physical, mental and social well-being of man in relation to his work and working environment, and with the adjustment of man to his work and work to man. The concern is thus wider than the safety of the workplace, and includes health and job satisfaction. In the United States the principal federal statute concerned with occupational health is the Occupational Safety and Health Act administered by the Occupational Safety and Health Administration (OSHA) and the National Institute of Occupational Safety and Health (NIOSH).

**occupational medicine**
A specialty of medicine that is involved with the treatment and prevention of occupationally related injuries and illnesses arising out of the course of employment.

**Occupational Safety and Health Act of 1970 (OSHA)**
A Federal level law enacted to assure that every working man and woman in the United States has a safe and healthful working environment. The Act authorizes the Secretary of Labor to set mandatory standards for safety and health, provide for research and development in industrial health, encourage the institution of new industrial health programs, and provide for enforcements of established standards.

**Occupational Safety and Health Administration**
An agency under the Department of Labor that was created by Section 6(a) of the Williams-Steiger Occupational Safety and Health Act of 1970 (84 Stat. 1593). This act provides for the promulgation as an occupational safety or health standard any national consensus standard, and any established federal standard, unless determined that the promulgation of such a standard would not result in improved safety or health for specifically designated employees. The legislative purpose of this provision is to establish standards with which industries are generally familiar, and on whose adoption interested and affected persons have already had an opportunity to express their views. Such standards are either 1) national consensus standards on whose adoption affected persons have reached substantial agreement, or 2) federal standards already established by federal statutes or regulations.

**occupational therapist**
A specially trained individual who evaluates the self-care, work and leisure performance skills of well and disabled clients of all age ranges; and plans and implements programs, and social and interpersonal activities designed to restore, develop and/or maintain the client's ability to satisfactorily accomplish those daily living tasks required of his specific age and necessary to his particular occupational role. Formal educational preparation of an occupational therapist requires at least four academic years of college or university work, leading to a baccalaureate degree, plus a minimum of 6 months' field work experience. Those persons already having a baccalaureate degree in a field other than occupational therapy may enroll in a post-baccalaureate program leading to a master's degree in occupational therapy or a certificate of proficiency in occupational therapy. See qualified occupational therapist.

**occupational therapist, qualified**
According to JCAH for psychiatric, alcoholism and drug abuse facilities accreditation purposes, this is an individual who is a graduate of an occupational therapy program approved by a nationally recognized accrediting body, or who currently holds certification by the American Occupational Therapy Association as an occupational therapist, registered, or who has the documented equivalent in education, training, and/or experience; who meets any current legal requirements of licensure or registration; and who is currently competent in the field.

**occupational therapy**

Any activity in which one engages for evaluation, diagnosis and treatment of problems interfering with functional performance in persons impaired by physical illness or injury, emotional disorder, congenital or developmental disability, or the aging process in order to achieve optimum functioning and for prevention and health maintenance. Specific occupational therapy services include, but are not limited to, activities of daily living (ADL); the design, fabrication, and application of splints; sensorimotor activities; the use of specifically designed crafts; guidance in the selection and use of adaptive equipment; therapeutic activities to enhance functional performance; pre-vocational evaluation and training; and consultation concerning the adaptation of physical environments for the handicapped. These services are provided to individuals or groups through medical, health, educational, and social systems and for the maintenance of health through these systems.

**occupational therapy assistant (Medicare)**

A person who: 1) is eligible for certification as a certified occupational therapy assistant (COTA) by the American Occupational Therapy Association under its requirements in effect on the publication of this provision; or 2) has 2 years of appropriate experience as an occupational therapy assistant, and has achieved a satisfactory grade on a proficiency examination approved by the Secretary, except that such determination of proficiency shall not apply with respect to persons initially licensed by a state or seeking initial qualification as an occupational therapy assistant after December 21, 1977.

**O.D.**

Optometrist. See this word.

**odium**

Hatred; general ill-feeling against someone.

**Oedipus complex**

An unconscious tendency or sexual orientation of a child toward the parent of the opposite sex.

**O.E.O.**

Office of Economic Opportunity.

**of counsel**

1. Employed as a lawyer. 2. One who assists a lawyer.

**off**

1. Postponed. 2. Ended. 3. Terminated.

**offense**

1. Commission of a crime. 2. The breaking of laws.

**offer**

1. To present a proposal. 2. To make a proposition. 3. To attempt to have evidence admitted into a trial. 4. In contract law, an offer is a proposal to make a deal.

**offeree**
One to whom an offer is extended.

**offeror**
One who makes an offer.

**office call**
See visit.

**officers of the court**
All personnel who work in or assist the court.

**office visits**
Those services performed by a physician in his own office, or in an out-patient facility of a hospital, such as an out-patient clinic, examining or treatment room, etc.

**official**
1. One holding a position of authority. 2. Directives from one of authority. 3. In pharmacy, pharmaceuticals authorized for medical use. 4. Authoritative.

**official notice**
Notice coming from a source of authority, usually an administrative agency.

**offset**
A counterclaim; a set-off.

**of record**
Officially recorded.

**ointment**
A semisolid salve or lotion that is rubbed on parts of the body.

**Old-Age, Survivors, Disability and Health Insurance Program (OASHDI)**
A program administered by the Social Security Administration which provided monthly cash benefits to retired and disabled workers and their dependents and to survivors of insured workers; it also provides health insurance benefits for persons aged 65 and over, and for the disabled under age 65. The health insurance component of OASHDI was initiated in 1965 and is generally known as Medicare. Commonly known as social security, the legislative authority for the program is found in the Social Security Act, originally enacted in 1935. The program is an example of social insurance.

**old Bailey**
Criminal court utilized in London.

**old country**
The nation or country from which a person originated or immigrated. Often refers to European countries.

**old guard**
Any group of persons with long tenure with an organization, who are conservative and defenders of the old way of doing things and are resistant to organizational change.

**olfactory**
Referring to the sense of smell.

**oligophrenia**
Mental retardation.

**olograph**
See holograph.

**-ology**
Suffix meaning study of.

**-oma**
Suffix meaning morbid growth; tumor.

**ombudsman (Swedish)**
A special person or public official who acts as an advocate for a special group with power to investigate illicit acts, misconduct and provide legal help in wrongdoings, such as a nursing home ombudsman.

**omen**
An event, experience or occurrence that is believed by some to predict good or evil or the occurrence of future events; a prognostication of future events; a sign.

**omission**
Being omitted, not included or neglected. An act of omission is failing to do what is expected or what is a part of one's duty. See act of omission; negligence.

**omit**
1. To purposefully leave out; failure to include; to not give or provide; to not mention. 2. To neglect, fail to do or to use.

**omnibus (Lat.)**
1. Containing two or more separate items. 2. Concerning two or more different and independent subjects.

**Onanism**
Coitus interruptus or masturbation.

**once-over**
To take a quick and comprehensive check for the last time; a swift examination; an appraisal in a rapid, yet complete fashion.

**oncology**
The branch of medicine that studies tumors.

**oncometer**
An instrument of medicine that is used to measure variations in size of the viscera.

**oncost**
Overhead or overhead expenses.

**on demand**
1. Immediately payable. 2. Something must be presented or given up upon the presentation of an official document or note.

**one party coverage**
In health insurance, one person coverage; that is, coverage for the subscriber only.

**onerous**
Burdensome. In contract law, when one party's obligations far exceed his advantages, the agreement is said to be onerous.

**on-line**
In computers or data processing, it is when the equipment that provides direct interface with the central processing unit of a computer is fully installed and functioning.

**on-line data processing**
A method of processing medical records or business data in which input and output are under the control of a central processing unit. Current information is introduced into the processing system as soon as it occurs.

**on or about**
Close to; approximate.

**onus**
Burden; encumbrance.

**onus probandi (Lat.)**
Burden of proof.

**O.P.D.**
Outpatient department. See these words.

**open**
1. To begin. 2. Making available. 3. To be visible. 4. To have no time limitation. 5. To be frank and honest with nothing hidden.

**open and shut**
An issue or case that is easily, clearly, and obviously determined and ended.

**open door**
An unrestricted or unlimited admission or allowance, such as open door policy.

**open-end credit**
Revolving charge plans that can be paid off in small payments. Credit cards are an example.

**open-ended programs**
In the federal budget, entitlement programs for which eligibility requirements are determined by law, e.g. Medicaid. Actual obligations and

resultant outlays are limited only by the number of eligible persons who apply for benefits and the actual benefits received. See also entitlement authority.

**open enrollment**
A period when new subscribers may elect to enroll in a health insurance plan or prepaid group practice. Open enrollment periods may be used in the sale of either group or individual insurance and be the only period of a year when insurance is available. Individuals perceived as high-risk (perhaps because of a preexisting condition) may be subjected to high premiums or exclusions during open enrollment periods. In the Health Maintenance Organization Act of 1973 (P.L. 93-222) the term refers to periodic opportunities for the general public, on a first come, first served, basis, to join an HMO. The law presently requires that HMOs have at least one annual open enrollment period during which an HMO accepts, "up to its capacity, individuals in the order that they apply" unless the HMO can demonstrate to HHS that open enrollment would threaten its economic viability. In such cases, HHS can waive the open enrollment requirement for a period of up to three years.

**opening statement**
1. The first remarks to a jury at the start of a trial. 2. At the beginning of a trial when each side explains the facts and how they will be proven.

**open-minded**
1. being open to progress, both sides of an issue or new ideas without prejudgments, preevaluations or bias. 2. Free from prejudice.

**openness**
Being frank and forthright, not hiding or withholding information or secrets; having trust in one's communication with another; a willingness to disclose.

**open panel group practice**
A dental care plan characterized by the beneficiary choosing among all the dentists participating or with dentists accepting or refusing clients/beneficiaries.

**open shop**
1. A hospital or other facility where non-union persons may work. 2. Where both union and non-union workers can be employed.

**open staff**
Where any licensed physician may admit his own private patient to a hospital and care for him there. This used to be widespread in practice, but is now very rare.

**open wound**
An injury or wound where the skin or mucous membrane has been cut open to expose underlying tissue.

**operant conditioning**
The term was created by psychologist B.F. Skinner to describe behavioral change taking place as a result of reinforcing behavior. A behavior

therapy theory and process by which environmental or social events called reinforcers are given following an individual's behavior, depending on whether it is negative or positive, so the behavior is likely to occur more or occur less in the future.

**operating cost**
The financial requirements necessary to operate an activity which provides health services. These costs include all costs incurred after the date the activities commenced. They normally include the costs of personnel, material, overhead, depreciation, and interest.

**operating expenses**
(Related to investments) The cost of running a business or services, such as management, utilities, and day to day expenses, as well as taxes, insurance and employee related expenses, plus a reserve of money for replacement items.

**operating room technician**
This individual works as a general technical assistant on the surgical team under the direct supervision of the operating room nurse and the medical staff. They prepare patients for surgery, maintain antiseptic conditions, arrange supplies and instruments, and assist the surgeon during operations. This is a fairly small occupational group.

**operation**
Any medical procedure or act performed on the body with instruments or by the hands of a physician or surgeon. See also major, minor and cosmetic surgery.

**operational control**
In health care administration, it is the process of assuring that specific tasks are carried out effectively and efficiently.

**operational mode**
In clinic management it is a way of classifying medical groups. Most medical group practices have been free standing; fee-for-service organizations and have not been linked contractually or organizationally to another organization or entity such as a hospital or medical school. The following classifications are listed, but not limited, under operational mode: free standing, hospital affiliated, university affiliated, industry affiliated, university hospital affiliated.

**operational performance in health care organizations**
Indicators of operational performance are the comparison with actual desired levels of inventory, occupancy rates in hospitals, and waiting times in physicians' offices, etc.

**operation of law**
The process by which rights or liabilities are given to or are owned by a person automatically, without his or her act or cooperation.

**opinion**
1. A decision or statement given by a judge about the outcome or final decision of a case. 2. A statement by a lawyer for a client, giving a belief about how the law applies to his case.

**opinion evidence**
What a witness believes about facts, rather than what the witness saw or heard. Opinion evidence is usually admissible only when it comes from an expert witness such as a physician.

**opinion of the court**
The decision given by an appellate court. One judge writing the opinion for the court. Judges who agree, but for different reasons, may write their opinions explaining their reasons. Judges who disagree with the majority may write dissenting opinions.

**opportunity cost**
In health economics, the value that resources, used in a particular way, would have if used in the best possible or another specified alternative way. When opportunity costs exceed the value the resources have in the way they are being used, they represent lost opportunities to get value from the resources. One opportunity cost of devoting physician time to tertiary care is the lost value of devoting the same time to primary care. Opportunity costs are the appropriate cost concept to consider when making resource allocation decisions. Actual costs often, but not always, can be assumed to represent (be proportional to) opportunity costs. See also marginal cost.

**opprobrious**
Infamous; not worthy of respect. Disgraceful, abusive.

**opprobrium**
Disgrace or reproach as a result of a wrongdoing, shame.

**-opsy**
Suffix meaning view.

**opthalmic dispenser**
Adapts and fits corrective eyewear as prescribed by the opthalmologist or optometrist.

**opthalmic laboratory technician**
Operates machines to grind lenses and fabricate eyewear to prescription.

**opthalmic medical assistants**
Under the direction and supervision of the opthalmologist, they perform a variety of tasks, including technical laboratory duties and office assistance, which allows physicians more time for decision making and other activities which require professional judgment and expertise. Opthalmic assistants take medical histories, administer diagnostic tests using precision instruments, make anatomical and functional ocular measurements, and test eye functions including visual acuity, visual fields, and sensorimotor functions. They often carry out very technical measuring and testing procedures and, in some cases, even provide technical assistance to the

opthalmologist in opthalmic surgery. They change eye dressings, administer eye drops or oral medications, and instruct patients in inserting, removing, and caring for contact lenses. Other duties include caring for and maintaining optical and surgical instruments.

**opthalmic photographer**
One who does opthalmic photography. See these words.

**opthalmic photographic technologist**
One who does opthalmic photography. See these words.

**opthalmic photography**
A specialized field dealing solely with the eye and related problems. There are two major divisions of opthalmic photography: 1) Slit lamp photography, which deals with photography of the anterior segment of the eye. The camera has an independent variable width beam of illuminating light (thus, slit lamp), which can be rotated through a 180° arc in front of the eye. This method gives illumination of etiologies that may otherwise be obscured in normal flood-lamp type photography. Corneal endothelial cells may be illuminated and counted by this method, as well as iris and crystalline lens disease entities. 2) Posterior or fundus photography is the second major area and involves two areas of study in the posterior segment of the eye. In the first area, fundus photography is a static color documentation of the interior of the eye using a specially prepared optical system allowing the photographer to view and photograph the retina and vitreous through a dilated pupil with 35mm film. A technique known as stereophotography reveals elevation differences in the retina, and abnormalities in the vitreous. The other aspect of fundus photography is called fluorescein angiography. It involves a photographic technique formulated by Novotney and Alvis in 1961, of injecting an intravenous bolus of sodium fluorescein, then taking rapid sequential photographs of the vasculature of the retinal areas as the dye enters the vascular system.

**opthalmic photography technician**
An allied health profession that utilizes the photographing of the inner parts of the eye for diagnostic or research purposes. No specialized training has yet been established.

**opthalmologist**
A physician specializing in the diagnosis and treatment of all eye diseases and abnormal conditions including refractive errors. They may prescribe drugs and lenses, and perform surgery or other treatment. Opthalmologists represented about 12 percent of all surgical specialists among non-federal physicians in the United States during 1970. A state Medicaid plan must provide that there will be an examination by a physician skilled in diseases of the eye, or an optometrist, when a decision is to be made whether an individual is blind according to the state's definition. A state supervising opthalmologist must review each eye examination report in making the state agency's decision that the applicant does or does not meet the state's definition of blindness, and determining if and when reexaminations are necessary. See also optician.

**opthalmoscope**
A hand held instrument used to examine the interior of the eye, utilizing a high-powered focused light.

**optical scanner**
A computer-type device that photoelectrically speed-reads data from a page and puts it directly into a computer.

**optical scanning**
A method utilizing an optical scanner for reading symbols and converting them to data into a computer through the use of magnetic ink or optical marks.

**opticians**
Health workers who fit, supply, and adjust eye glasses according to prescriptions written by opthalmologists or optometrists in order to correct a patient's optical or muscular vision defect. In some states, opticians also fit contact lenses. They do not examine the eyes or prescribe treatment. Qualification for initial licensure usually includes successful completion of written, oral, and practical examinations. Apprenticeships are required in most licensing states, with an alternative being the completion of a one- or two-year training program.

**option**
As used in law, it is when a person is allowed to pay money for the right to buy or sell something at a certain place and within a certain time.

**optional services**
Services which may be provided or covered by a health program or provider, and, if provided, will be paid for in addition to any required services which must be offered. In addition to the required services under Medicaid, if states elect to include any of the optional services in their programs, matching funds under title XIX are available. The optional services states may offer are the following: prescribed drugs, clinic services, dental services, eyeglasses, private duty nursing, skilled nursing facility services for individuals under 21, care for patients under 21 in psychiatric hospitals, intermediate care facility services, prosthetic devices, physical therapy and related services, other diagnostic, screening, preventive and rehabilitation services, optometrists' services, podiatrists' services, chiropractors' services, care for persons 65 or older in institutions for mental diseases and care for patients 65 and older in tuberculosis institutions. States may also offer any "medical care, or any other type of remedial care recognized under state law, furnished by licensed practitioners within the scope of their practice as defined by state law" that is not specifically excluded from coverage by title XIX (the exclusions are: care or services for inmates of public nonmedical institutions; inpatient services in a mental institution for individuals over 20 and under 65, and services for persons under 65 in a tuberculosis institution.) See also basic and supplemental health services.

**option contract**

A contract supported by consideration which allows the right to buy on the terms stated and for a specific period of time. The offeror may not withdraw or revise the terms of the offer.

**optometric assistants**

Perform a variety of tasks which are generally less complex than those of the optometric technician. They keep records, act as receptionists, assist patients with frame selection, and order prescribed lenses. They may do visual-acuity testing, color-vision screening, as well as visual-field testing. In addition, assistants may also provide patients with instructions on the use and care of different types of lenses. The specific duties are determined by the employing optometrist. In large practices, they may specialize in any of the following functions: laboratory, contact lens, visual training, chairside assistance, or office administration. Those in smaller practices may assume all of these duties. Most optometric assistants work for optometrists engaged in private practices of varying sizes. Others are employed by clinics, government agencies, optical-instrument manufacturers, health maintenance organizations, and various branches of the Armed Forces.

**optometric technicians**

Optometric technicians assist the optometrist with vision care services. They measure the curvature of the cornea, test the ability of the patient to see numbers or letters of a specific size at a specified distance, and record eye pressures or tensions. They determine the power of lenses in old and new prescriptions, assist the patient in frame selection, and take facial and frame measurements. They may also perform opthalmic laboratory work, modify conventional glasses or contact lenses, keep an inventory of optometric materials, and clean and care for instruments. Other duties may include bookkeeping, secretarial, and office management responsibilities. In all cases, their duties are performed under the supervision and guidance of an optometrist.

**optometrist**

A practitioner concerned with problems of vision. Optometrists examine the eyes and related structures to determine the presence of any abnormality, and prescribe and adapt lenses or other optical aids. They do not prescribe drugs, make definitive diagnosis of or treat eye diseases, or perform surgery. An accredited doctor of optometry degree requires a minimum of two years of pre-optometry college education and four years of professional training in a school of optometry. The degree and an optometry board examination are required by all states for licensure for the practice of optometry. Effective October 30, 1972, a state which previously covered optometric services under Medicaid, and which, in its Medicaid formal plan, specifically provides coverage for eye care under physicians' services which an optometrist is licensed to perform, must reimburse such care whether provided by a physician or an optometrist. Optometrists thus may not be excluded as potential providers in these states. See also opthalmologist and optician.

**optometry**
A profession concerned with the problems of human vision. Optometrists examine the eyes and related structures to determine the presence of any visual, muscular, neurological, or other abnormality. They prescribe and adapt lenses or other optical aids and may use visual training aids (orthoptics) when indicated to preserve or restore maximum efficiency of vision. Most optometrists fit and supply the eyeglasses they prescribe. Some states have passed legislation that allows optometrists to prescribe drugs in their treatment of patients.

**-or**
Suffix meaning one who.

**oral**
Referring to the mouth.

**oral contract**
1. A contract that is spoken and is not in writing. 2. A verbally expressed contract. 3. An expressed agreement as opposed to an implied agreement.

**oral hygiene**
The cleaning and freshening of a patient's teeth, gums and mouth on a constant and regular basis.

**order**
1. A written directive from a judge. 2. A directive of a court to appear at a trial or hearing. 3. A command given by a public official. 4. A direction to pay something.

**orderly**
A hospital attendant with no professional training or schooling, most often a male, who does non-nursing general chores, especially attending to the needs of male patients.

**order to show cause**
A court order made ex parte requiring a party to appear in court to show cause as to why a claim or decision should not be made final. See rule nisi, rule to show cause.

**ordinance**
1. A law passed by a municipal legislative body. 2. A statute at the local or city level. 3. A rule or regulation of a local government.

**ordinary negligence**
The lack of or omission of care which an ordinary, prudent and reasonable person would usually take for his or her own concerns or care. The failure to exercise care of an ordinarily reasonable and prudent person in the same situation. Under normal circumstances, a person is expected to know and understand the results of his or her acts. See Negligence.

**ordinary person**
Any person of ordinary diligence, reasonableness, prudence and care in relation to acts, behaviors, duties or any other particular thing.

**organ bank**
A service provided in some major hospitals through which a supply of human tissue, organs and bone is acquired and maintained for use or replacement in other patients.

**organic brain syndrome (OBS)**
A psychotic or nonpsychotic disorder caused by impaired organic functioning of the brain.

**organic disease**
Any illness caused by damage or change in an organ or tissue.

**organic law**
1. Basic. 2. The most fundamental of governmental law.

**organic matter**
Compounds containing carbon.

**organism**
Any living thing, such as a human being, an animal, germ, etc., particularly one having several parts, each specializing in a particular bodily function.

**organizational performance**
The ability of a health care organization to properly articulate and coordinate its various components necessary for the delivery of efficient, effective and quality hospital care to patients.

**organization performance processes**
-Vertical differentiation: this establishes the hierarchy and levels in a health care organization. -Horizontal differentiation: This helps separate activities so that health care management may be performed more effectively and efficiently. This is done through the formation of departments and sections.

**organized**
Administratively and functionally structured.

**organized medical staff**
In JCAH accreditation, this is a formal organization of practitioners, with the delegated responsibility and authority to maintain proper standards of patient/resident care and to plan for continued betterment of that care.

**orgasm**
The height of sexual excitement, accompanied by a feeling of physiologic and psychologic release, with uncontrollable rhythmic contractions of the genitals.

**orgasmic dysfunction**
The inability to achieve orgasm

**orientation**
Awareness of time, place, and person

**orifice**
Any opening that serves as an entrance and/or outlet to a body cavity or organ.

**original jurisdiction**
The authority of a court initially to try a case or to hear an appeal.

**ortho-**
Prefix meaning straight.

**orthopsychiatry**
A therapy method that psychiatry, psychology and other sciences use to promote healthy emotional development and growth.

**orthoptics**
A technique of eye exercises designed to correct the visual axes of eyes not properly coordinated for binocular vision. See also orthoptist.

**orthoptist**
A specially traned individual who works under the supervision of an opthalmologist in testing for certain eye muscle imbalances and teaching the patient exercises to correct eye coordination defects. The majority work in the private offices of opthalmologists, while others are employed in hospitals and clinics. The American Orthoptic Council is the regulating board for orthoptists. The council administers the national board examination, a person needs a minimum of 2 years of college, and 15 months of training in a training center or 24 months preceptorship training.

**orthostatism**
Erect posture of the body in standing position.

**orthotic/prosthetic assistant**
Assists the orthotist/prosthetist in caring for patients by making cases, measurements, and model specifications and fitting supportive appliances and/or artificial limbs.

**orthotist**
See prosthetist.

**orthotist/prosthetist**
Writes specifications for, makes, fits, and repairs braces and appliances and/or artificial limbs following the prescription of physicians.

**O.S.H.A.**
Occupational Safety and Health Administration. See these words.

**-osis**
Suffix, meaning abnormal condition.

**Osler, Sir William (1849-1919)**
A Canadian-born physician, successively professor of medicine at McGill University, the University of Pennsylvania, Johns Hopkins University and the University of Oxford. Considered one of the greatest American physicians and one of the founders of modern academic medicine.

**osmotic pressure**
The amount of atmospheric pressure required to oppose osmosis.

**ostensible**
1. That which is intended to be obvious. 2. That which is apparent or visible. 3. The power a principal gives to an agent. 4. The authority a physician gives to a nurse or medical technologist.

**osteopathy**
A school of healing based on the theory, originally propounded in 1874 by Dr. Andrew Taylor Still, that the normal body, when in correct adjustment, is a vital mechanical organism naturally capable of making its own responses to and defense against disease, infections and other toxic conditions. The body is seen as structurally and functionally coordinate and interdependent, abnormality of either structure or function constituting disease. The physician of this school searches for, and if possible corrects any peculiar position of the joints or tissues, or peculiarity of diet or environment which is a factor in destroying the natural resistance. The measures he may use are physical, hygienic, medicinal, and surgical. He is now distinguished from the allopathic physician mainly, if at all, by his greater reliance on manipulation. Osteopaths are licensed to perform medicine and surgery in all states, eligible for graduate medical education in either osteopathic or allopathic programs, reimbursed by Medicare and Medicaid for their services, supported under health manpower legislation, and generally treated identically with allopathic physicians. See also homeopathy and naturopathy.

**ostomy**
Suffix meaning make a new opening.

**otologist**
A physician who specializes in surgery and diseases of the ear.

**otomy**
Suffix, meaning cut into; incision.

**outcome measure**
A measure of the quality of medical care in which the standard of judgment is the attainment of a specified end result, or outcome. The outcome of medical care is measured with such parameters as improved health, lowered mortality and morbidity, and improvement in abnormal states (such as elevated blood pressure). Any disease has a "natural history" which medical care seeks to alter. To measure the effectiveness of a particular medical action in altering a disease's natural history is to carry out an outcome measure. Such measures are a way to measure the effectiveness of medical care, and a way to measure the quality of medical care. To carry out cost-benefit analyses of medical care such measures are not necessary. However, they are difficult to devise, and have not often been done in comparing medical settings. It is possible to carry out a random controlled trial using outcome measures to compare the therapeutic effect of any drug or medical procedure on a disease to its "natural history" without treatment, or with a treatment already in

use. Some argue that this should be done before any new medical procedure is put into use. See also input, process and output measures.

**outlays**
In the federal budget, actual expenditures of federal funds, including checks issued, interest accrued on the public debt, or other payments (minus refunds and reimbursements). Total budget outlays consist of the sum of the outlays from appropriations and other funds included in the budget universe, less offsetting receipts. Off-budget federal agencies are not included in the budget universe and their outlays are excluded from total budget outlays. While budget authority is usually obligated in the fiscal year for which it is appropriated, it may be outlaid, once obligated, over several years.

**out-of-pocket payments or costs**
Those borne directly by a patient without benefit of insurance, sometimes called direct costs. Unless insured, these include patient payments under cost-sharing provisions.

**outpatient**
A patient who is receiving ambulatory care at a hospital or other health facility without being admitted to the facility. Usually does not mean people receiving services from a physician's office or other program which does not also give inpatient care. Outpatient care refers to care given outpatients, often in organized programs. Outpatients are also called ambulatory patients or clinic patients.

**outpatient department (OPD)**
This department provides nonemergency ambulatory care, as contrasted with formal admission to the hospital and inpatient care. The department may have several specialty clinics and may be staffed by full-time doctors, nurses, clerks and technicians.

**outpatient medical facility**
A facility designed to provide a limited or full spectrum of health and medical services (including health education and maintenance, preventive services, diagnosis, treatment, and rehabilitation) to individuals wo do not require hospitalization or institutionalization (outpatients).

**outpatient programs**
According to JCAH for psychiatric, alcoholism and drug abuse facilities accreditation purposes, these are programs that provide services to persons who generally do not need the level of care associated with the more restrictive environments of inpatient or residential programs. Such programs are usually located in facilities classified as business occupancies in Chapter 13 of the 1973 edition of the Life Safety Code (NFPA 101).

**output**
1. The data that comes out of a computer after it has been processed. 2. The process of transferring data from an internal storage to an external storage area of a computer. 3. The end product of any activity. It is often associated with communication processes, information systems, production tasks and management activities.

**output contract**
A contract in which a buyer agrees to purchase the entire production or output of a particular item. See requirements contract.

**output measures**
Used synonymously with measures of the productivity of health programs and manpower, process measures or outcome measures.

**output media**
The forms, tapes, printouts or devices on which processed information appears.

**Outrageous Conduct, Doctrine of**
Any act or behavior which is beyond all decency and is regarded as unacceptable and intolerable.

**outreach**
According to JCAH for psychiatric, alcoholism and drug abuse facilities accreditation purposes, this is the process of systematically interacting with the community to identify persons in need of services, alert persons and their families to the availability of services, locate needed services, and enable persons to enter the service delivery system.

**outreach worker**
A professional or paraprofessional worker who is usually in the social service areas. This worker goes into the community to visit individuals in need, or thought to be in need of social or health care. The worker tries to establish a level of need and types of services needed to fill their social or health care needs.

**ovary**
Female gonad.

**over**
1. Having higher authority or position. 2. More than or above. 3. Duration. The sickness was over a period of one year. 4. Covering or complete. The wound healed over. 5. To release or give up, as in to hand over.

**overbed cradle**
A specialized frame set over a patient while lying in bed. Used to protect the body from contact with the bed covers.

**overcharge**
To charge too much.

**overcome**
1. To prevail over. 2. To master.

**overcompensation**
Real or imagined physical or psychological deficit or insufficiency which one has that causes or inspires exaggerated efforts to overcome any lacks.

**overdraft**
Taking out more than you have in.

**overdraw**
See overdraft.

**overhead**
The general costs of operating an entity which are distributed to all the revenue producing operations of the entity, but which are not directly attributable to a single activity.

**overnutrition**
The over-supply of calories, vitamins, minerals, or other nutrients.

**overreach**
In contract law, an overreach is when a party in a superior position makes unfair demands or requires concessions from the party in an inferior bargaining position.

**overrule**
1. To have authority over. 2. To supercede; a higher court rejecting the legal principles on which the case was based. 3. A superior court voiding a lower court's opinion.

**overt**
1. An act outwardly done. 2. Any action done with no attempt to conceal it. 3. Open; clear. 4. Extremely obvious.

**over-the-counter drug (OTC drug).**
A drug which is advertised and sold directly to the public without prescription (e.g., aspirin).

**overt homosexuality**
The actual physical involvement in homoeroticism. See also homosexuality, latent homosexuality.

**overtime**
Any amount of time worked beyond the expected, set or standard workday or workweek. Some personnel may require payment of overtime wages as set forth by federal or state wage/hour laws. For exempt employees (professional staff), payment for extra hours worked such as for weekends is built into the basic salary, income distribution, or bonus plans. Certain statutes require that certain nonphysician and nonprofessional personnel be paid overtime for extra hours of work. Provisions should be made in personnel handbooks to clearly indicate which employees must be paid overtime according to law.

**ovulation**
The discharge of a mature egg from the ovary of the female.

**ovum**
The female reproductive egg cell.

**ownership disclosure**
Disclosure by a health program of all ownersip interests in the program. By law, each skilled nursing facility participating in Medicare and Medicaid must supply ownership information to the state survey agency and each intermediate care facility must supply such information to the

state licensing agency. Full and complete information must be supplied on the identity of: each person having (directly or indirectly) an ownership interest of ten percent or more in such facility; in the case of a facility organized as a corporation, each officer and director of the corporation; and in case the facility is organized as a partnership, each partner. Any changes which affect the accuracy of this information must be promptly reported.

**oxo-**
Prefix meaning oxygen.

**oyer and terminer (french)**
Hear and decide; some higher criminal courts carry this title.

**oyez**
"hear ye"; cried out in some courtrooms at the beginning of a court session.

# P

**P.A.**
1. Professional Association. 2. Physician's Assistant.

**package insert**
Labeling approved by the Food and Drug Administration for a prescription drug product, which accompanies the product when shipped by the manufacturer to the pharmacist, but usually does not accompany a dispensed prescription. The package insert is directed at the prescribing professional, principally the physician, and states the appropriate uses of a drug, the mode of administration, dosage information, contraindications, and warnings. The legal effect of prescribing the drug in ways not described in the package is unclear. See also compendium and Physicians' Desk Reference.

**packing**
1. Attempting to sway a legal decision your way through improperly placing persons on a jury, a court or an agency hearing. 2. Improperly placing specific persons on a jury. 3. The process of filling an open wound with an absorbent material such as gauze.

**pact**
An agreement.

**pactum (Lat.)**
1. A pact. 2. A bargain.

**pain**
Any unpleasant feeling or sensation or suffering experienced by the stimulation of certain nerve endings: may be caused by threat or be a fantasy, disease, injury or mental perception.

**pain-pleasure principle**
A psychological concept stating that man tends to seek pleasure and avoid pain.

**pain threshhold**
The amount of stimulation required for pain to be felt.

**pairing**
1. Two or more persons not voting on a certain bill in a legislature. 2. Agreeing to refrain from.

**pais (French)**
Outside the court.

**palliative**
Providing relief but not a cure.

**palpable**
1. That which is tangible. 2. Plain. 3. Easily seen. 4. Obviously evident. 5. Clear to the mind. 6. Notorious. Usually in reference to an error or an abuse of authority.

**palpation**
Feeling with the hands and the fingers.

**pandemic**
When a disease is widespread or worldwide or affects large numbers of people at the same time and crosses over community or country boundaries.

**pander**
1. To procure. 2. To pimp. 3. To solicit prostitution. 4. To provide a means to help one satisfy vices or ambitions.

**panel**
1. A jury list. 2. The group of jurors as a whole. 3. A group of judges or arbitrators used to decide an issue. See registry.

**panel group practice**
See closed-panel group practice, open-panel group practice.

**panic**
An intense state of anxiety, associated with mental, emotional and personality disorganization.

**panphobia**
Fear of everything.

**pantomime**
Gesticulation; psychodrama without the use of words.

**paper of a lawsuit**
1. All documents; short for "commercial paper"; a negotiable instrument. 2. A document or legal instrument that is written.

**par**
1. At face value. 2. Equal to a pre-established value.

**paralegal**
A non-lawyer who works to assist a lawyer.

**parallel citation**
A court's decision which is published in more than one publication.

**paralogia**
see evasion.

**paralysis**
The loss of all or part of one's motor function of a part of the body.

**paralysis agitans**
See Parkinsonism.

**paramedic**
Having completed a more advanced level of training than the emergency medical technician, the paramedic responds to medical emergencies, evaluates the nature of the emergency, and carries out specified diagnostic and treatment procedures under standing orders or in communication with professional medical personnel. Paramedics may provide advanced life support services such as intravenous drug administration and cardiac arrhythmia control. See emergency medical technician.

**paramedical**
Having indirect or peripheral association with the practice of medicine.

**para-medical personnel**
Those health personnel who are not doctors. It includes medical technicians, health aides, record keepers, family health workers, nutritionists, dental hygienists, physician assistants, and health associates, but there seems to be no agreed upon list of included occupations. See also allied health personnel.

**paramnesia**
Memory confusion in which reality and fantasy are confused. It is observed in certain types of schizophrenia and organic brain syndromes.

**paramount title**
1. A holder of a legal instrument who has superior right to real property. 2. Any title that will prevail over another title. 3. A title that is better than a previously held title. 4. A title of seniority.

**paramour**
An illicit lover. A person who substitutes for or replaces a husband or wife but without any legal right or obligations attached to the marriage.

**paranoid**
A mental state marked by symptoms of systematized delusions, with signs of disorganization. Common symptoms are fear and excessive distrust.

**paranoid delusion**
See delusion.

**paraplegia**
Paralyzed from the waist down; paralysis of both legs, usually caused by destruction of the spinal cord as a reslt of injury or disease. Sensation may or may not be lost, depending on the level and extent of destruction.

**parapraxis**
Slips of the tongue caused by unconscious thoughts.

**para-professional**
A person who assists a professional or does some of the basic duties of a professional. In health care, this person is usually referred to as an allied health professional.

**parasitic disease**
A disease which is caused by a plant or animal living within or on another living organism at whose expense it obtains some advantage.

**parasympathetic nervous system**
The segment of the autonomic nervous system that controls the life-sustaining organs of the body.

**parcener**
A joint heir.

**pardon**
A power given to a president or governor to exempt a person from punishment.

**parens patriae (Lat.)**
1. Father of the country. 2. The power and right of government, to take over treatment or care for minors or others who cannot legally care for themselves.

**parental rejection**
Withholding of love, affection and attention from a child by one or both parents. The child develops great emotional needs and hostility, which can be directed outwardly in the form of tantrums, or inwardly against himself in the form of psychosomatic disorders, self-hate and self-pity.

**parenteral product**
According to JCAH for psychiatric, alcoholism and drug abuse facilities accreditation purposes, this is a sterile, pharmaceutical preparation ingested by the body through a route other than the alimentary canal.

**pares (Lat.) Equals.**

**paresthesia**
Strange feelings or sensations felt on the skin, including burning, tickling and tingling.

**pari delicto (lat.)**
Equal fault.

**pari materia (lat.)**
On the same subject: interdependent.

**pari passu (Lat.)**
Equally; without preference or discrimination.

**parity**
1. Equality. 2. In epidemiology, the classification of women by their number of live-born children (e.g., a woman of parity 4 has had four live-born children). In medical usuage, the classification of women by the total number of births they have had, including both live births and stillbirths; or the total number of times a woman has been pregnant minus the number of abortions and/or miscarriages occurring up to 28 weeks of gestation.

**Parkinsonism**
A chronic disease that is shown by rhythmical muscular tremors known as pill rolling, accompanied by spasticity and rigidity of movement, propulsive gait, droopy posture, and mask-like facies. It is usually seen in later life as a result of arteriosclerotic changes in the basal ganglia.

**Parkinsonism-like effect**
A common side effect of antipsychotic drugs. Typical symptoms include motor retardation, physical rigidity, changes in posture, tremor, and autonomic nervous system disturbances.

**parliamentary law.**
Rules policy and procedures used by legislatures to conduct business.

**parol**
1. Oral. 2. Oral evidence. 3. Evidence a witness gives verbally. 4. Not appearing in the written contract.

**parole**
Being allowed to leave prison prior to a sentence being completed.

**parol evidence**
Evidence given verbally rather than in writing.

**parol evidence rule**
In substantive law, a rule that declares that when the terms of a contract have been written in which an agreement with both parties is reached, oral evidence will not supercede the written contract.

**parol promise**
A simple contract; a verbal promise.

**partial-day programs**
According to JCAH for psychiatric, alcoholism and drug abuse facilities accreditation purposes, these are programs that provide services to persons who generally do not require the level of care provided in the more restrictive environments of residential or inpatient programs. Partial-day programs are designed for patients who spend only part of a 24-hour period in the facility. Partial-day programs that provide sleeping accomodations are usually located in facilities classified as residential occupancies in Chapter 11 of the 1973 edition of the Life Safety Code (NFPA 101). Partial-day programs that provide treatment and care services only during the day are usually located in facilities classified as business occupancies in Chapter 13 of the 1973 edition of the Life Safety Code.

**partial disability**
In insurance this term describes any illness or injury that prevents a person from performing some of the functions of his regular job.

**partial hospitalization**
Formal programs of care in a hospital or other institution for periods of less than 24 hours a day, typically involving services usually provided to inpatients. There are two principal types: night hospitalization for patients who need hospitalization but can work or attend school outside the

hospital during the day; and day hospitalization for people who require in-hospital diagnostic or treatment services but can safely spend nights and weekends at home.

**partial hospitalization, psychiatric**
A method of part-time therapy and the treating of mental illness in which the patient goes to a hospital on a part-time basis. See also day, night, and weekend hospital.

**partial insanity**
Monomania. See this word.

**partially delegated hospital**
A hospital to which the PSRO has assigned either concurrent review or MCE study functions. May also indicate that within the concurrent review process the hospital assumes the responsibility for either the physician advisor or the review coordinator function. The PSRO retains final responsibility for the effective performance of all review conducted by the hospital review committee. See medical care evaluations, PSRO.

**participating hospital**
A hospital which has an agreement with an insurance company like a Blue Cross plan to provide hospital services to its enrolled members.

**participating insurance company**
See mutual insurance company

**participating physician (member physician)**
A doctor who has joined an insurance group or enrolled with the insurance company and agreed to accept its contracts.

**participating special facility**
A non-hospital health care facility which has a written agreement with an insurance company like Blue Cross and provides a specialized type of care.

**participation**
A physician participates in an insurance plan when he agrees to accept the plan's preestablished fee or reasonable charge as the maximum amount which can be collected for services rendered. A non-participating physician may charge more than the insurance program's maximum allowable amount for a particular service. The patient is then liable for the excess above the allowed amount. This system was developed in the private sector as a method of providing the insured with specific health care services at no out-of-pocket costs. The term is used more loosely in Medicare and Medicaid to mean any physician who accepts reimbursement from either program. Approximately half of Medicare claims are paid to physicians who participate by accepting assignment. Any physician accepting Medicaid payments must accept them as payment in full. A hospital or other health program is called a participating provider when it meets the various requirements of, and accepts reimbursement from, a public or private health insurance program. See also conditions of participation and penetration.

**particulars**
1. The specific details of a complaint. 2. Items listed on a bill or ledger.

**particulars, bill of**
1. An itemized written account of the issues of a claim. 2. An informal statement by a plaintiff as to a cause of action, or a defendant's set-off.

**parties**
Several persons or groups of persons involved in a lawsuit; all persons or organizations involved in a legal proceeding.

**partner**
1. An individual in a partnership. 2. A "silent" partner is one not publicly known as a partner. 3. A "special" or "limited" partner puts in a fixed amount of money, gets a fixed amount of profit, and is usually not liable for anything beyond the initial investment.

**partnership**

**partnership**
Two or more persons in a contractual agreement to carry on a business. A business agreement between two or more persons, often physicians, who agree to share profits and losses in an unincorporated business arrangement. Each partner is a legal agent of the other and can be legally held responsible for the acts of the other, including malpractice, torts, or negligence, and each is legally bound by the acts of the other just as if they were performed by both or the other partners. In a partnership each partner has a vested interest and incentive in the business, decision and policy making, and profit. The disadvantages of a partnership are that the partners share responsibility for the professional and business mistakes of one another, tax benefits are limited, and a partnership can be dissolved with the withdrawal of a single partner. See limited partnership.

**Partnership for Health**
A synonym for the old comprehensive health planning program. The first set of amendments to the program were made in 1967 by P.L. 90-174 which was given the short title, Partnership for Health Amendments of 1967, hence the name.

**-partum**
Suffix, meaning birth; labor.

**party**
1. A person taking part in or involved in a transaction, lawsuit or any legal claim. 2. Those persons taking part in a transaction or proceeding. 3. A plaintiff or a defendant in a lawsuit. 4. One who takes direct part in a legal proceeding.

**party of the first part**
A phrase used instead of the name of a party in a document.

**pass**
1. To pronounce. 2. To pass judgment. 3. Enacted successfully.

**passim (Lat.)**
1. Here and there. 2. In various places. 3. Throughout. 4. General reference to a work.

**passive**
1. Inactive. 2. Not involved. 3. Apathetic.

**passive-dependent personality**
A personality disorder marked by indecisiveness, emotional dependency and lack of self-confidence.

**passive exercise**
Therapeutic exercise in which the movement is not provided by the patient but by a machine or therapist.

**passive negligence**
Those defects, obstacles or problems on premises that are allowed to exist and which cause danger to arise from the mere physical condition of the property, building or physical plant itself.

**passivity**
Lethargic; lacking energy or will.

**patency**
Open, not shut or clogged up.

**patent**
1. Apparent, evident, plainly visible. 2. Open; obvious. 3. a right to control the manufacture and sale of a discovery or invention. 4. A grant of privilege or property by the government.

**paternal**
Belonging to or coming from the father.

**paternity suit.**
A lawsuit used to prove a person is the real father of an illegitimate child. This is usually done to enforce his obligations to provide child support.

**patho-**
Prefix, meaning disease.

**pathological**
Abnormal or diseased.

**pathology**
The study of disease processes.

**pathology department**
A clinical department and service in most major health care facilities. In hospitals, laboratories are provided to examine and analyze tests on human tissue, bone, and excretions, which assist in the diagnosis and treatment of patients. This department is under the supervision of a physician, and, in a large health care facility and large hospital, may include many sub-departments and allied health personnel such as medical technologists who do special analysis and related research.

**-pathy**
Suffix, meaning disease process.

**patient**
One who is receiving health services; sometimes used synonymously with consmer. See also inpatient, outpatient, and private and service patient.

**patient activities coordinator**
See qualified patient activities coordinator.

**patient advocate**
A person who works for a patient and can speak or act on the patient's behalf. See patient representative.

**patient bed days**
See patient days.

**patient/client bill of rights**
Documents made available to patients/clients describing their rights under treatment by or through a health care provider or facility. See Appendix, bill of patients rights.

**patient compliance**
1. When a patient follows the doctor's orders. 2. When a patient sticks to the treatment plan; follows through, and completes the proper taking of drugs, showing up for therapy and follows prescribed orders when away from the health care provider and/or health care facilities.

**patient consent**
See informed consent.

**patient days**
A measure of institutional use, usually measured as the number of inpatients at a specified time (e.g., midnight). The total number of inpatient days of care provided in a specified or set time period. For example, if there were 60 inpatients in a health facility for each day for 10 days, this would be 600 patient days for this set time period. See occupancy rate.

**patient education**
1. Those health experiences designed to influence learning which occur as a person receives preventive, diagnostic, therapeutic, and/or rehabilitative services, including experiences which arise from coping with symptoms, referral to sources of information, prevention, diagnosis, and care, and contacts with health institutions, health personnel, family, and other patients. 2. A specially designed or planned combination of learning and motivation activities used to assist people who have an illness, disease or disorder, in order to change their behavior and beliefs towards a life style conducive to good health.

**patient educator**
This is an individual with advanced education and specialized training in communication and interpersonal relations skills and educational methods who also has an expertise in medicine, diseases and health and wellness facts. This individual has additional knowledge and skills in new medical

technologies, belief structures, motivation, patient counseling, educational media, and behavior modification, so that when assisting a patient in a combination of learning belief modification, behavior change, value clarification activities, the patient can activate and adopt behaviors conducive to wellness and a healthful lifestyle.

**patient mix**

1. The numbers and types of patients served by a hospital or other health program. Patients may be classified according to their homes (see patient origin study), socioeconomic characteristics, diagnoses, or severity of illness. Knowledge of a program's patient mix is important for planning and comparative purposes. See also scope of services. 2. This term is also used to identify the different types or sources of payment.

**patient origin study**

A study, usually undertaken by an individual health program or health planning agency, to determine the geographic distribution of the homes of the patients served by one or more health programs. Such studies help define catchment and medical trade areas, and are useful in locating and planning the development of new services.

**patient representative**

The patient representative has the responsibility to meet the personal, social and comfort needs of the patient, and in health services to respond to patient's inquiries and concerns about his/her care such as hospital services, procedures, treatment, etc. He or she is also to help with problems and concerns the patient and/or family may have as well as serving as a part of the health care institution's complaint mechanism and to act as a support factor in the institution's risk management program.

**patient service representative**

A person who has a varied background who works in a hospital assisting with Medicare, Medicaid and private insurance company forms by filling them out and assisting with the money collection process. This is opposed to the patient representative, who is a social service worker and an advocate of the patient. See patient representative.

**patient's right to privacy**

No unauthorized persons are allowed to view the patient's medical record or his person without consent. The right to privacy applies to any communications made to the physician and entered in the medical record and on matters related to medical treatment. Some states have passed statutes that allow personal information to be released to governmental agencies or pharmaceutical companies as long as the patient's privacy and anonymity is preserved.

**patriarchal**

A family system in which the father is the head of the house or family.

**patrilineal**

Descending through the male line.

**paucital**
Legal relations in personam.

**pavor nocturnus**
Nightmare

**pawn**
To allow personal property to be held by another as security for money.

**payable**
1. Owing. 2. To be paid now or in the future; that which is due.

**payback period**
A finance and budgeting method that determines the length of time needed to recover the initial investment of money in a project. Often discounted cash flow analysis is not used in determining the payback period and therefore is not as effective in making long term decisions, as is adjusted rate of return or net present value.

**payee**
1. To whom a negotiable instrument is made out. 2. To whom something has been paid, or is about to be paid.

**payment, cost-based**
One method of payment of medical care programs by third parties, typically Blue Cross plans or government agencies, for services delivered to patients. In cost-related systems, the amount of payment is based on the costs to the provider of delivering the service. The actual payment may be based on any one of several different formulae, such as full cost, full cost plus an additional percentage, allowable costs, or a fraction of costs. Under Medicare, Part A services—including those provided by interns and residents in approved training programs—are reimbursed on a cost basis. Also reimbursable to the hospital under Part A are the teaching, administrative, and supervising activities of physicians not in training.

**payment, fee-for-service**
Payment by the patient of a fee to a physician for the performance of a specific service or procedure.

**payment, lump sum**
Payment for professional patient care services based on a negotiated agreement between the payor and individual physicians, physician groups, or institutions. The agreement establishes the services to be provided, the amount of payment, who will provide the services, and describes the client group without necessarily specifying the population of the group or the services to be provided its members. This payment method is used by the Maternal and Child Health Program (Title V) and by many state and local governments to provide physician services to specified client groups.

**payment, unified**
Payment for services of teaching physicians and house officers in cases where the latter are employees of a physician organization rather than a

hospital. As recognized by Medicare in a modified form, payment is made wholly from Part B (The Supplemental Medical Insurance Program) for cost reimbursement of house officer salaries and Part B for direct patient care services of physicians.

**payroll**
Those employees entitled to monetary compensation for work or personal services rendered. Payments are also made for payroll-associated costs such as insurance, income tax, retirement and Social Security withholdings.

**payroll deduction**
A specified amount taken out of pay to finance a benefit. Payroll deductions may be either a set payroll tax, such as the social security tax, or a required payment for a benefit, for example, a group health insurance premium. A payroll deduction generally refers to any amount withheld from the earnings of an employee.

**payroll tax**
A tax liability imposed on an employer, or employee, related to the amount of the company payroll or individual pay, the revenues from which are used to finance a specific benefit. In the health field, payroll tax is often used synonymously with the social security tax. That tax, it is important to note, is not applied on total payroll, but rather on the wages of each employee up to a set maximum. The ceiling on wages to which tax is applied means that the tax rate varies with income in a regressive manner. A government requirement that a employer pay a set portion of the premium on group health insurance benefits for his employees is in reality a payroll tax on the employer, although it is not often recognized as such. Since the amount paid by the employer would be a set amount per employee not related to the amount of an individual's earnings, its impact as a tax would be regressive.

**P.C.**
1. These letters often appear after a physician's name and mean professonal corporation. 2. Corporation set up by doctors, or other professionals who share facilities, professions or who work together.

**P.D.R.**
Physician's Desk Reference. See these words.

**peace bond**
A sum of money held to assure good behavior by a certain person for a specific period of time.

**peculation**
Embezzlement. See this word.

**pecuniary**
Pertaining to or related to money. Having a monetary concern.

**pederasty**
Anal intercourse between males. A criminal offense in many states.

**pediculosis**
Infestation with lice.

**pedophilia**
A sexual deviation where a child is used for sexual purposes; sexual acts with children.

**peer review**
The evaluation by practicing physicians or other professionals To assess the effectiveness and efficiency of services ordered. Evaluation is performed by other practicing physicians or other members of the profession whose work is reviewed (peers). Frequently refers to the activities of the Professional Standards Review Organizations (PSRO) which in 1972 were required by P.L. 92-603 to review services provided under the Medicare, Medicaid, and Maternal And Child Health programs. Local PSROs which receive federal guidance and funding from HHS, are staffed by local physicians, osteopaths, and non-physicians. Their duties include the establishment of criteria, norms and standards for diagnosis and treatment of diseases encountered in the local PSRO jurisdiction, and review of services that are inconsistent with the established norms, e.g., hospital stays longer than the normal length of stay. The norms may be input, process, or outcome measures. Peer review has been advocated as the only possible form of quality control for medical services because it is said that only a physician's professional peers can judge his work. Peer review has been criticized as having inherent conflict of interest since, a physician will not properly judge those who will judge him, and also as not adequately reflecting patient objectives and points of view. See PSRO or professional standards review committee.

**peers**
Equals. Those of the same rank or status; those average persons of a community or profession.

**pejoration**
A worsening.

**pelf, pelfe**
Ill-gotten gains; booty.

**penal**
Punishment or punishable; concerning a penalty. Pertaining to criminal law.

**penalty**
A punishment imposed by law. Paying for a breach of a contract.

**pendency**
After beginning and prior to terminating.

**pendente lite (lat.)**
1. Pending the suit. 2. During the period of time a lawsuit is being heard.

**pendent jurisdiction**
The authority given to federal courts to hear and decide all issues against a defendant, even if the issues are not involved with federal law.

**pending**
Not yet decided; not finished or completed. Awaiting completion or approval.

**penetration**
1. In marketing insurance or HMOs, the percentage of possible subscribers who have in fact contracted for benefits (subscribed). Participation is sometimes used synonymously (see saturation). 2. In sexuality, this is when the penis enters the vagina.

**penis envy**
A Freudian concept that maintains that the woman envies the man for having a penis. It is sometimes used to refer to the woman's generalized envy of the man.

**penrose drain**
A flexible, rubber tube used to drain secretions from a wound or incision.

**Pension Reform Act of 1974**
Public Law P.L. 93-406, "Employee Retirement Income Security Act of 1974." This act established mandatory rules for retirement plan participation. The vesting of participants' rights by means of a three-way option plan with minimum funding standards and more stringent fiduciary laws is also required. Financial statements are to be audited. A pension benefit guaranty corporation is to be established to insure plans against failure. The law does not require an employer to establish plans nor does it apply to all retirement plans.

**people**
1. All persons in a nation or state. 2. All persons as a whole.

**per (Lat.)**
By; through; by means of; during.

**per autre vie (Lat.)**
1. For another life. 2. For as long as another, specified person is alive.

**per capita (Lat.)**
1. "By heads" or by the head. 2. Individual person sharing equally.

**percentage participation**
One stipulation in a health insurance contract which states that the insurer will share losses in an agreed proportion with the insured person. An 80-20 participation is often used, where the insured person pays 20% of his losses and the insurance company pays the remaining 80%. This is a typical arrangement with the policyholder paying the 20% like a deductible.

**perception**
The meaningful organization of man's intellectual, sensory and emotional capacities. Through perception man makes sense out of the many stimuli of his world; the understanding an experience or knowledge; an awareness of a person, thing, or situation.

**percipient**
Perceiving; one who perceives, or sees something.

**per curiam (Lat.)**
1. By the court. 2. By the entire court, as opposed to by a single judge.

**per diem (Lat.)**
By the day. Through the course of the day. This term is used in reference to compensation for meals, lodging, expenses etc. incurred in a day of work or services. Travel allowances are provided on a "per diem" basis.

**per diem charge**
The amount of money charged for services, care or treatment through the period of one day. See hospital service charge, per diem cost.

**per diem cost**
Literally, cost per day. Refers, in general, to hospital or other inpatient institutional costs per day or for a day of care. Hospitals occasionally charge for their services on the basis of a per diem rate derived by dividng their total costs by the number of inpatient days of care given. Per diem costs are averages and do not reflect true cost for each patient. With this approach, patients who use few hospital services (typically those at the end of a long stay) subsidize those who need much care (those just admitted). Thus the per diem approach is said to give hospitals an incentive to prolong hospital stays. See cost per patient day.

**peremptory**
1. Barring further action. 2. Absolute; conclusive; final. 3. Not requiring an explanation. 4. Cause not need to be shown. 5. Arbitrary; decisive. 6. That which cannot be denied, opposed or changed.

**peremptory challenge**
Used in jury selection; a challenge to a prospective juror used to disqualify him from being empaneled for no given reason. Peremptory challenges vary and are established by statute.

**peremptory ruling**
A judge's decision that overrules the final decision of a jury.

**perfect**
1. To leave nothing wanting. 2. Complete; enforceable; exact. 3. Without defect. Totally correct.

**perfidy**
1. The deliberate violation of an agreement. 2. The violation of trust and faith. 3. Breach of faith or trust.

**performance**
1. Carrying out a deal, promise or contract. 2. Completing an obligation according to present terms. 3. The fulfillment of a contract or a promise.

**performance appraisal (evaluation)**
A criterion measurement that is used in the work setting to pinpoint strengths and weaknesses of individuals, groups and organizations. It is used as an information source for reward, promotion, change, personal and staff development, organizational modification and job description refinement. Information gained from evaluation and appraisal of job performance is useful in planning, organizing, controlling and directing work performance.

**performance budget**
A budgeting method where it is prepared at the end of the accounting period, which shows what income and what costs should have been in the actual operations of the facility.

**performance, specific**
1. Carrying out a contract according to specific terms agreed-upon. 2. To seek a remedy. One may sue for specific performance, rather than suing for damages for nonperformance.

**peril**
Cause of a possible loss; such as an accident, death, sickness, fire, flood, or burglary. See also insurance and hazard.

**perinatal mortality**
Death (mortality) during the late prenatal period (variously defined, conventionally occurring after the 28th week of gestation or with a fetus weighing over 1,000 grams, including stillbirths), birth process and the early neonatal period, and usually measured as a rate: number of perinatal deaths per 1,000 live births in a given area or program and time period. See also health status, and infant and neonatal mortality.

**periodic table**
The systemic classification of elements according to atomic numbers, and by physical and chemical properties.

**perjury**
1. Lying under oath. 2. To give false testimony or swear falsely to a document; evidence or facts in a legal proceeding.

**perm. (abbrev.)**
Permanent.

**permanent disability**
An illness or injury that prevents an insured person from performing all the functions of his or her regular job.

**permissive**
1. Allowed. 2. Tolerated.

**permissive licensure**
A legal rule that allows practitioners who are not licensed to practice, but does not offer them protection from the licensing agency or organization.

**perpetrator**
1. One who commits a crime. 2. By whose agency or direction an illicit act occurs.

**perpetual inventory**
A stock control system where the counting of units of goods at any time may be obtained directly from the records without doing an actual physical count of the goods. A record is kept in units and/or values for stocked items or goods. It is a running record of items or goods ordered, received, and used, and the balance left on hand.

**perpetuating testimony**
A method of gathering and preserving testimony. A deposition taken from a prson who is in ill, or a person about to leave the state.

**perpetuation of evidence**
Assuring that evidence is available for a trial that may occur at a later date.

**perquisites**
Extra benefits provided in a job that are supplemental to one's salary. Benefits incidental to a job or a position, other than salary.

**per quod (Lat.)**
Whereby.

**per se (Lat.)**
By himself, herself, itself. In itself; alone. In and of itself; taken along; inherent.

**persistency**
In insurance, the rate at which policies written in a given line of insurance or for members of a given group are maintained in force until the completion of the terms of the policies.

**person**
A human being or individual or incorporated group having certain legal rights or responsibilities; a natural person, as opposed to a corporation which is called an artificial person.

**personal**
1. Private, individual, not public. 2. Having to do with movable property as opposed to affixed property. 3. Belonging to a person.

**personal care**
In nursing home care, it usually consists of assistance in walking, buttoning clothes, getting in and out of bed, bathing, dressing and eating, taking drugs and preparation of special diets prescribed by a physician.

**personal health care**

A major subsystem of the overall health system which includes those services delivered to individuals in order to improve or maintain their health status. Major service categories within personal health care include: prevention and detection, diagnosis and treatment, habilitation and rehabilitation, maintenance, and person health care support.

**personal health care support services**

Services which do not involve direct medical care, but which assist in the prevention, diagnosis and treatment of diseases or ill-health conditions, or in the habilitation, rehabilitation or maintenance of ill or disabled individuals.

**personal health services**

All those health services provided to specific individuals. Contrasted with environmental and community health, public health, consultation and education services and health education, which are all usually directed at populations, not individuals, and are undertaken to promote healthful environments, behavior or lifestyles.

**personal health status**

Level of health of the individuals of a group population.

**personal injury**

Harm done to a person's body. The harm or injury a person suffers.

**personality**

1. Personal property. 2. The constant configuration and behavior of a person, showing his physical, emotional, mental status as well as attitudes, beliefs and interests, which are the sum total of adjustment to life.

**personal physician**

The physician who assumes responsibility for the comprehensive medical care of an individual on a continuing basis. The physician obtains professional assistance when needed for services he is not qualified to provide, and coordinates the care provided by other professional personnel in light of his knowledge and understanding of the patient as whole. While personal physicians will have an interest in the patient's family as they affect his patient, the personal physician may not serve the entire family directly, e.g., a pediatrician may serve as a personal physician for children, while an internist or other specialist may serve in this capacity for adults. Personal physician is sometimes more simply defined for any given patient as the one the patient designates as his personal or principal physician. See also family physician and private patient.

**persona non grata (Lat.)**

An unwelcome person. A person who is unacceptable.

**personnel department**

This administrative department recruits, interviews, and screens applicants for health care facilities positions, provides benefits and maintains salary scales. The department keeps records of present and past employees and provides orientation for new employees. The director of personnel maintains a control system over positions of employment so that jobs cannot be increased without approval of the administration. Personnel departments also get involved with labor relations and risk appraisal.

**personnel record**
According to JCAH for psychiatric, alcoholism and drug abuse facilities accreditation purposes, this is the complete employment record of a staff member or an employee, including job application, education and employment history, performance evaluation, and, when applicable, evidence of current licensure, certification, or registration.

**per stirpes (Lat.)**
1. By roots. 2. Through or by roots or stocks, by representations. A method of dividing by estates, "by representation" or by groups, whereby the children share equally in their deceased parents' share.

**persuasive authority**
All law that a judge might use in making a decision. A persuasive decision often is given by a famous judge, or comes from a powerful court.

**perversion**
Deviation from the expected norm. A psychological term that often refers to sexual deviation. See also sexual deviation.

**pesticides**
A group of chemicals used to control or kill pests such as rats, insects, fungi, bacteria, etc. that affect man or agricultural products. Included are insecticides, herbicides, fungicides, rodenticides, miticides, fumigants and repellents.

**PET**
See Positron Emission Tonography.

**petition**
1. A written prayer or request for certain things or that a court take a particular action on. 2. A written application for redress. 3. "Petition" is used in some states in place of "complaint." 4. A request made to a public official. 5. An official plea on an issue or complaint; sometimes petition is synonymous with complaint.

**petitioner**
1. A plaintiff; one who initiates a petition. 2. One initiating an appeal to a higher court. 3. An appellant. 4. One who petitions the court.

**petition in bankruptcy**
1. A written plea to a court for bankruptcy. 2. Debtor requesting relief from debts.

**petit jury (petty jury)**
A small or lower level jury. A trial jury.

**petit larceny**
A misdemeanor; theft of property of little value, usually below fifty dollars.

**petty theft**
Stealing that involves items of lesser worth. Petty larceny. Theft of something of little value.

**pH.**
The acidity or alkalinity of a solution with neutral being as 7. Acidity is less than 7 and alkalinity being more than 7 up to the strongest being 14.

**P.H.A.**
Public Housing Administration.

**phantasy**
See fantasy.

**phantom limb**
A sensation that an arm, leg, finger, etc. is still there even though it has been amputated. Pain and feeling seem to still exist when in reality the part is not attached. This is due to the severed nerves providing a sensation to the nervous system.

**phantom pain**
A pain that continues to exist after the source of it has been removed, such as pain perceived to be in a foot after it has been amputated.

**pharmaceuticals**
Drugs and related chemicals used by the public, including not only such medicinals as aspirin and antibiotics but also such nutrients as vitamins and amino acids for both human and animal use. See drug.

**pharmacist**
1. A professional person qualified by education and authorized by law (usually by obtaining a license) to practice pharmacy. 2. Under Medicare, he or she is licensed as a pharmacist by the state in which practicing and has training or experience in the specialized functions of institutional pharmacy, such as residencies in hospital pharmacy, seminars on institutional pharmacy, and related training programs. See qualified pharmacist. 3. According to JCAH for psychiatric, alcoholism and drug abuse facilities accreditation purposes, this is an individual who has a degree in pharmacy and is licensed and registered to prepare, preserve, compound, and dispense drugs and chemicals in the state in which he or she practices.

**pharmaco-**
Prefix, meaning drug or chemical.

**pharmacology**
A science which studies the action or interaction of drugs upon animals and humans.

**pharmacopoeia**
A list of products, substances, or drugs used in medicine, including their description and formulas.

**pharmacy**
1. The science, art and practice of preparing, preserving, compounding, dispensing and giving appropriate instruction in the use of drugs. 2. A place where pharmacology is practiced. 3. Usually this department or service purchases drugs and medications, maintains a supply, fills requisitions for medical care services and nursing units. It also may fill prescriptions for individual patients. The department is run by the chief pharmacist; a special drug and therapeutics committee provides communication and interaction with the medical staff. The pharmacy maintains the formulary, a list of drugs that the medical staff finds acceptable for use in the hospital. (See formulary). Generic names are listed and the pharmacist may substitute clinically similar drugs. This reduces drug inventories and helps contain the cost of drugs as it allows bulk purchasing and the use of low-cost generic name drugs.

**pharmacy assistant**
Works under the supervision of a pharmacist; assists the pharmacist in selected activities including medication profile reviews for drug incompatibilities, prescription packaging, handling of purchase records, and inventory control. Where state law permits, may administer drugs to patients under the supervision of a registered pharmacist.

**pharmacy services**
Assist the pharmacist in selected activities in pharmacy departments to provide pharmaceutical services to patients, nurses, and physicians.

**phenothiazine**
A drug known for its antipsychotic property. As a class, the phenothiazine derivatives are among the most widely used drugs in medical practice, particularly in psychiatry.

**Philadelphia lawyer**
Formerly used to praise a lawyer's skill, this word has come to mean a lawyer who is unpredictable, sly, tricky or untrustworthy.

**philo-**
Prefix, meaning attracted to; like; love.

**phobia**

**-phobia**
Pathological and restraining fear associated with some specific object Suffix, meaning fear. or situation. See also acrophobia, agoraphobia, alurophobia, algophobia, claustrophobia, erytophobia, mysophobia, panphobia, xenophobia, zoophobia.

**phobo-**
Prefix, meaning fear.

**-phoria**
Suffix, meaning emotions; feeling; or mental state.

**photo scan**

A two-dimensional picture of the gamma rays emitted by a radioisotope showing a varying concentration of bones and tissues of the body with a printout from the light source of the exposure on the film.

**photo therapy**

A treatment usually used on babies suffering from hyperbilirubinemia and jaundice. A specialized type of light is shown on the patient which reduces the condition to normal.

**-phylaxis**

Suffix, meaning protection.

**physiatrics**

Rehabilitation, physical therapy and physical medicine. See physical medicine.

**physiatrist**

See qualified physiatrist.

**physical examination**

Inspecting, examining and assessing the body by a health care provider qualified to do so, utilizing special tools and instruments such as the stethoscope, blood pressure cuff, fluoroscope, lab tests, x-rays, etc. to determine health status and levels of wellness or signs and symptoms of illness and disease.

**physical fact**

1. A fact that is obvious and indisputable. 2. An unquestionable fact; law of nature.

**physical medicine**

This department can include specialty areas such as physiatry, physical and rehabilitative medicine. Physical medicine is involved with the diagnosis and treatment of the disabled, convalescent, and physically handicapped patient, by using heat, cold, exercise, water, etc., as treatment and therapy. Physical therapists assist the physiatrist and provide much of the therapy. Occupational therapy and speech therapy may also be included in this department.

**physical medicine services**

According to JCAH accreditation it is those services such as physical therapy, occupational therapy, or other physical restorative and maintenance services that are provided in the specialty of physical medicine.

**physical plant and maintenance department**

The deparment of a health care facility that is responsible for upkeep, repair and maintenance of the facility such as painting, carpentry and maintenance. It also provides and maintains the steam and heating plant, electricity, air conditioning, emergency power, fire alarm systems, elevators, etc., as well as the grounds and parking lots.

**physical therapist**

A specially trained and licensed individual who uses physical agents, biomechanical, and neurophysiological principles, and assistive devices in relieving pain, restoring maximum function, and preventing disability following disease, injury or loss of a bodily part. Physical therapists are employed by rehabilitation centers, schools, or societies for crippled children, and public health agencies. A license is required to practice physical therapy in the 50 states, the District of Columbia, Puerto Rico, and the Virgin Islands. To obtain a license, an applicant physical must have a baccalaureate degree or certificate from an approved school of physical therapy and pass a state board examination. See qualified physical therapist.

**physical therapist (qualified consultant) (Medicare)**

A person who is licensed as a physical therapist by the state in which practicing, and 1) has graduated from a physical therapy curriculum approved by the American Physical Therapy Association, or by the Council on Medical Education and Hospitals of the American Medical Association, or jointly by the Council on Medical Education of the American Medical Association and American Physical Therapy Association; or 2) Prior to January 1, 1966, was admitted to membership by the American Physical Therapy Association, or was admitted to registration by the American Registry of Physical Therapists, or has graduated from a physical therapy curriculum in a 4-year college or university approved by a state department of education; or 3) has 2 years of appropriate experience as a physical therapist, and has achieved a satisfactory grade on a proficiency examination approved by the Secretary, except that such determinations of proficiency shall not apply with respect to persons initially licensed by a state or seeking qualification as aphysical therapist after December 21, 1977; or 4) was licensed or registered prior to January 1, 1966, and prior to January 1, 1970, had 15 years of full-time experience in the treatment of illness or injury through the practice of physical therapy in which services were rendered under the order and direction of attending and referring physicians; or 5) if trained outside the United States, was graduated since 1928 from a physical therapy curriculum approved in the country in which the curriculum was located and in which there is a member organization of the World Confederation for Physical Therapy, has 1 year of experience under the supervision of an active member of the American Physical Therapy Association, and has successfully completed a qualifying examination as prescribed by the American Physical Therapy Association.

**physician**

1. A professional person qualified by education and authorized by law (usually by having obtained a license) to practice medicine. 2. A doctor with the degree of M.D., D.O. and board certified. 3. According to JCAH, this is an individual who has received a Doctor of Medicine or Doctor of Osteopathy degree and is currently fully licensed to practice medicine. See teaching physician.

**physician assistant (PA)**

A specially trained, and licensed (when necessary) or otherwise credentialled, individual who performs tsks, which might otherwise be performed by physicians themselves, under the direction of a supervising physician. Also known as physician extenders and by many other synonymous terms. Many were paramedics initially trained by the military (e.g. corpsmen and pharmacists' mates) and later further trained medical schools to assist physicians in civilian health services (see Medex). Other examples of similar occupations are dentists' assistants, nurse practitioners, nurse midwives, psychiatric therapy assistants and rehabilitative personnel. Physician assistants are usually salaried rather than reimbursed on a fee-for-service basis, although the supervising physicians may receive fee-for-service for their services.

**physician assistant-primary care**

These individuals, who represent the majority of physician's assistants, perform physician-delegated functions in the areas of family practice, general internal medicine, general practice, pediatrics, emergency medicine, and obstetrics. They take medical histories, perform detailed physical examinations, conduct visual and auditory tests, and otherwise assist the physician in patient care responsibilities.

**physician assistant-specialty**

Specialty-trained physician's assistants perform physician- delegated functions in such areas as orthopedics, surgery, urology, pathology, allergy, and dermatology. These individuals take case histories, perform physical examinations, conduct routine tests appropriate to the medical specialty, perform routine laboratory tests, and otherwise assist physicians in specialty-oriented patient care responsibilities.

**physician assistants training program**

An educational program which has as its objective the education of individuals who will, upon completion of their studies in the program, be qualified to effectively provide health care under the supervision of a physician.

**physician, attending**

The physician legally responsible for the care given a patient in a hospital or other health program. Usually the private physician of a private patient who is also responsible for the patient's outpatient care. An attending physician can be assigned to a patient if the patient does not have his own physician when admitted to the hospital.P

**physician, contact**

General and family practitioners, general internistis, and general pediatricians who make up the majority of physicians of first contact in the medical care system. Other physicians also engage in primary care.

**physician extender**

See physician assistant.

**physician, hospital based**
A physician who spends the predominant part of his practice time within one or more hospitals instead of in an office setting, or providing services to one or more hospitals or their patients. Such physicians sometimes have a special financial arrangement with the hospital (salary or percentage of fees collected), and include directors of medical education, pathologists, anesthesiol- ogists, and radiologists as well as physicians who staff emergency rooms and outpatient departments.

**physicians' and surgeons' professional liability insurance**
Malpractice insurance. See this word.

**Physician's Desk Reference (PDR)**
An annual compendium of information concerning drugs, primarily prescription, and diagnostic products published primarily for physicians and widely used as a reference document by physicians, other health manpower and patients. The information is primarily that included in the labeling or package insert, for the drug required by the Food and Drug Administration and covers indications, effects, dosages, administration, and any relevant warnings, hazards, contraindications, side effects and precautions. The PDR is distributed free or at reduced cost to many physicians and other providers through the patronage of the drug manufacturers which have paid by column-inch for having information on their products included. It is the only readily available source of identifying photographs of drugs. The drugs are listed by brand name for each manufacturer, and are indexed by manufacturer, brand name, drug classification, and generic and chemical name.

**physician shortage area**
An area with an inadequate supply of physicians, usually defined as an area having a physician to population ratio less than some standard, such as 1 to 4,000. See also medically underserved area.

**physician's profile**
A compilation of each doctor's charges and the payments made to him through the years for each specific professional service rendered to a patient. As charges are increased, so are payments, and the profile is then updated through the use of computer data.

**physician, teaching**
Any fully-trained physician (M.D., D.O., or Oral Surgeon D.D.S.) not enrolled in a graduate training program who is responsible for or directly engaged in any patient care activities performed by a physician; and is responsible for the instruction, supervision or both, of interns, residents, or fellows.

**physio-**
Prefix, meaning nature.

**physiology**
The study of the function of living organisms and their parts.

**physiotherapist**
A member of the health care team who assists patients with problems related to musculoskeletal system. See physical therapy.

**physiotherapy**
Therapy, treatment and rehabilitation techniques utilizing physical agents, such as hydrotherapy, heat, light rays, etc.

**pica**
A hunger for something not fit to eat.

**Pick's disease**
A presenile degenerative brain disease. See also Alzheimer's disease.

**piercing the corporate veil**
A court refusal to recognize a corporation as a legal entity, making those individuals who run the corporations personally responsible for its activity.

**pig**
A container made out of lead used to ship or store radioactive materials.

**ping-ponging**
The practice of passing a patient from one physician to another in a health program for unnecessary cursory examinations so that the program can charge the patient's third-party for a physician visit to each physician. The practice and term originated and is most common in Medicaid mills.

**PKU (phenylketonuria)**
A congenital protein-related metabolic disease that, if untreated in infancy, leads to mental retardation.

**P.L.**
Public Law, as in P.L. 93-641, or public law number 93-641.

**placebo**
An inactive or inert substance, preparation or procedure (such as an injection of sugar water) used in random controlled trials to determine the efficacy of the substance, treatment or preparation being tried (and usually indistinguishable from it), or given to please or gratify a patient or physician. In many controlled trials of pain medicines (such as of Darvon) the placebo gives much, and as much, relief from pain perceived by the patient as does the pain medicine. See also Hawthorne effect.

**plagiarism**
Illegally using literary compositions of another and passing it off as one's own work. See copyright.

**plain error rule**
This rule allows an appeals court to reverse a decision because of an error in the proceedings; even if no objection was given during the proceeding.

**plain meaning rule**
Using the obvious, plain and simplest meaning of the words of the law. One way of interpreting statutes.

**plaintiff**
1. The person initiating a lawsuit against another person or party. The person initiating a petition. 2. The party who has been harmed or injured and has brought a lawsuit to seek damages. 3. The person or persons who bring a civil action against the defendant.

**plaintiff in error**
The appellant who seeks a review of a decision. An appellant.

**plan 1. A set of decisions on what short- or long-range actions should be taken to produce future changes in order to attain explicitly stated desired results. 2. May be used to refer to an insurance company or to describe each of the not-for-profit Blue Cross organizations throughout the country.**

**plan development process**
A cyclical process of expressing community values and long-range aspirations for health status and health system performance, projecting and evaluating the capabilities of current health services to address them, and designing and choosing among actions which will close the gaps between projected and desired levels of community health and health system performance.

**plan, implementation**
See plan, annual, implementation plan.

**planning**
The conscious design of desired future states (described in a plan by its goals and objectives, and description and selection among alternative means of achieving the goals and objectives), and the conduct of the activities necessary to the designing (such as data gathering and analysis) and the activities necessary to assure that the plan is achieved. There are many different definitions of planning and descriptions of different types, including: long-range or perspective (covering 15 or more years); mid-range or strategic (5-15 years); short-term or tactical (1-3 years, see budget); health facilities or manpower; community or program; categorical or comprehensive health; normative (based on norms or standards with legal basis); and inductive or deductive (used when the planning is done locally and consolidated and used at state and federal levels (bubbled up), or vice versa (trickled down), respectively). The extent to which planning is responsible by definition for implementation of the plans is controversial, as is its relation to management. See also health planning and policy.

**planning cycle**
The scheduled sequence of a set of formal steps and procedures to be performed over a predetermined period of time. The planning cycle is repeated for each successive planning period and ends with the selection and dissemination of a plan or plans.

**planning system**
A formal set of rational procedures--involving steps in data collection and analysis for projections of the future, setting of goals and objectives, generation of alternative actions and selection among them--to guide the process of decision-making during the development of a plan.

**plan selection**
This fourth phase of plan development involves an analysis of the cost-benefits and cost-effectiveness of implementing each of the available alternative plans. The alternatives are compared with respect to their overall effect on all priority objectives, their respective feasibility, public acceptability, and comparative cost. Plan selection ends with a selection of the preferred alternative plan.

**plasma**
The fluid portion of the blood.

**plea**
1. A defendant's official answer to a complaint. 2. A pleading in a legal action. 3. Motion or pleading to a court. 4. In equity, an answer as to why a suit should not be heard or entered.

**plea bargaining**
The process of making a deal between a prosecutor and the defendant's lawyer, used to reduce sentencing or the charges against the denfendant.

**plead**
1. To make a pleading. 2. To present a motion to a court. 3. To argue a case in a hearing or trial.

**pleading**
1. The making of an official written statement to a court. 2. The first document filed is a complaint; the response to the complaint is the answer. Motions and all documents given to a court are usually called pleadings.

**plea in abatement**
A plea that does not challenge the complaint but challenges the manner, place or time a dispute is brought.

**plea in bar**
A plea that defeats a plaintiff's entire action.

**pledge**
Allowing possession of personal property to be given to another person until the completion of the promise, or pay that person the debt owed to him.

**plenary**
1. Full; whole; complete. 2. Concerning every person or every thing.

**pleonexia**
A psychiatric disorder where the patient has excessive desires to acquire wealth or objects.

**P.L.I.**
Practicing Law Institute; a non-profit publishing and legal continuing education organization.

**pluralism**
In psychiatry, the idea that a multitude of factors may affect one's behavior.

**plurality**
The greatest number; more than half.

**P.L. 1122**
The number of the section of the federal Social Security Act dealing with capital expenditures for medical care facilities. 'Section 1122 Review' of proposed facility construction; changes in services and/or equipment is authorized by this portion of the act.

**P.L. 93-641**
The National Health Planning and Resource Development Act of 1974. Replaces: 'Hill-Burton', 'Regional Medical Programs', and 'Conprehensive Health Planning Agencies.' See HSA and Health Systems Agency.

**pneumoencephalogram**
An x-ray of the cerebrospinal spaces after they are filled with air.

**pneumonia**
Inflammation of the lungs with exudation and consolidation.

**pneumoventriculogram**
An x-ray of the ventricles of the brain after oxygen is put into them.

**pocket part**
An addition to lawbooks that updates them; a pocket with leaflets is found inside the back cover.

**podiatric assistant**
Supports the podiatrist in his service to patients by preparing patients for treatment, sterilizing the instruments, performing general office duties, and assisting the podiatrist in preparing dressings, administering treatments, and developing x-rays.

**podiatrist**
1. A health professional responsible for the examination, diagnosis, prevention, treatment, and care of conditions and function- ing of the human foot. A podiatrist performs surgical and other operative procedures, prescribes corrective devices, and prescribes and administers drugs and physical therapy. 2. Medicare regulations state that the doctor of podiatry is considered a 'physician,' but only with respect to functions he is legally authorized to perform as such by the state in which he performs them. However, certain types of foot treatment or care are excluded, whether performed by a doctor of medicine or a doctor of podiatry. 3. According to JCAH, this is an individual who has received a Doctor of Podiatric Medicine degree and is currently fully licensed to practice podiatry.

**point**

1. An important issue that is the focus of concern or attention. 2. A legal issue or argument. 3. Money charged for lending money.

**points and authorities**

A memorandum used to support a legal position.

**police power**

A government's power to create, carry out and enforce laws or restrict rights for the health, safety and welfare of the public; the power to license occupations such as physicians.

**policies**

Guidelines, rules and directives established in companies and health care institutions which employees must operate and perform their work duties within.

**policy**

1. A course of action adopted and pursued by a government, party statesman, or other individual or organization; any course of action adopted as proper, advantageous or expedient. The Congress makes policy by writing legislation and conducting oversight activities. The term is sometimes used less actively, to describe any stated position on matters at issue. In insurance, a written contract of insurance between an insurer and the insured. In the executive branch of the federal government, policies are documents which interpret or enlarge upon rules, and are sometimes referred to as guidelines. Policies bear the same relationship to rules (regulations) as rules do to law, except that, unlike regulations, they do not have the force of law. 2. General rules and procedures of an organization. See personnel policies and procedures.

**policy, public**

General rules and expectations used in controlling a society or representative of that society.

**policy term**

The period for which an insurance policy provides coverage or is in force.

**polio-(poliomyelitis)**

An acute viral disease marked clinically by fever, sore throat, headache, vomiting, and often stiffness of the neck and back. Severe forms may result in paralysis.

**political question**

An issue that courts can not and will not hear because it is a decision to be made by the executive branch of government.

**polling the jury**

1. Asking each individual jury member for his or her decision. 2. To question jurors one at a time in open court. 3. To require a jury to voice its verdict.

**pollution**
Contamination of water, atmosphere or soil beyond that which is natural or normal.

**poly-**
Prefix, meaning many.

**polydipsia**
Excessive thirst.

**polydrug**
A medicinal substance, usually narcotic, which contains many different drugs.

**polygamy**
Illegally having more than one husband or wife at the same time.

**polyphagia**
Pathological overeating.

**POMR**
Problem-Oriented Medical Record. See these words.

**pool**
See insurance pool.

**poor**
See poverty.

**popular name tables**
Legal reference charts used to find laws and statutes by their popular names.

**population and family planning specialist**
Serves in an administrative and planning role specifically oriented toward the use of demography, demographic techniques, and reproductive physiology to plan, conduct, and evaluate family planning programs. See family planning.

**population density**
The number or concentration of people of a given area.

**population segment**
The quantifiable number of persons who share similar health care service needs which can be translated into a relatively predictable pattern of health services utilization.

**portent of embarrassment**
The fear of being demeaned or belittled for inferior or inadequate performance in one's duty or profession.

**positive evidence**
Direct and final proof of an issue.

**positive law**
Law enacted by a legislature.

**Positron Emission Tomography (PET scanner)**
Invented in 1973. PET can peer into the skull to learn how brain cells react to a radioactive substance that is almost painlessly injected into the body. It allows one to look at the brain and not only localize brain disturbances, but measure how bad they are.

**posse commitatus (Lat.)**
1. The power of the state. 2. Citizens used by law officers to help enforce the law, usually only in emergency.

**possession**
1. To have ownership and control. 2. Rightful occupancy of land or buildings. 3. Holding or possessing something. 4. To have or hold drugs illegally is illegal possession of drugs.

**possessory action**
A legal action used to gain and control property, but with no attempt to get legal ownership.

**post-**
Prefix, meaning after; past.

**post-date**
To date a document later than the date it is signed.

**postea**
In common law, a record of nisi prius proceedings. It is endorsed by the judge and delivered to the winning party following final disposition of a case.

**posterior frame**
A frame on which the patient lies when in a supine position.

**(postero)**
Prefix, meaning back; behind.

**post mortem (Lat.)**
1. After death. 2. Examining a dead body in order to determine the actual cause of death. 3. An autopsy.

**postmortem care**
The preparation of the deceased by health care providers for transportation to the mortuary, funeral home or morgue.

**postnatal**
Following the birth of a child.

**postoperative care**
A series of activities aimed at meeting the patient's psychological and physical needs directly after surgery, which begins when the patient is removed from surgery.

**postpartum**
Following childbirth.

**postpartum care**
Includes hospital and office visits following the birth of a baby.

**postprandial**
After a meal.

**potency**
A male's ability to achieve an erection in order to have sexual intercourse.

**poverty**
The condition of having an inadequate supply of money, resources, goods, or means of subsistence. A difficult concept to define in practice, there is no single national definition of poverty. Three of the most commonly cited measures are the low income level developed by the Bureau of the Census, income poverty guidelines published by the Community Services Administration of HHS (formerly the OEO guidelines) and the lower budget developed by the Bureau of Labor Statistics. Each of these uses a different method to measure poverty and arrives at a different dollar result. The Census low-income level is the measure accepted by the Office of Management and Budget for official data on low income persons. Eligibility for food stamps is based on a formula which uses low income thresholds. The Community Services Administration (CSA) poverty guidelines are essentially the Census low income levels rounded off to the nearest $10 for easy application, and are primarily used in determining eligibility for participation in programs initiated under the Economic Opportunity Act. The Bureau of Labor Statistics income levels for an urban family and retired couple are based on a budget for a "modest but adequate" standard of living. In essence, the budget represents a detailed listing of items to meet the normal needs of a family or retired couple as judged adequate by the experts drawing up this hypothetical budget. These items are indexed to the Consumer Price Index. Income eligibility for welfare programs provides a different definition of poverty. Under the Aid for Families with Dependent Children (AFDC) program the poverty levels vary significantly by state. Under the Supplemental Security Income (SSI) program a nationwide standard has been established. Medicaid income levels are based on, but are not necessarily equivalent to, the levels established under AFDC and SSI. Since all of these vary and are raised with inflation, they are not provided here.

**poverty area**
An urban or rural geographic area with a high proportion of low income families. Normally, average income is used to define a poverty area, but other indicators, such as housing conditions, illegitimate birth rates and incidence of juvenile delinquency are sometimes added to define geographic areas with poverty conditions. The term is defined precisely, albeit confusingly, in P.L. 93-641 (section 1633(15) of the PHS Act).

**power**
1. The right to control or do something. 2. The ability to control something. 3. Authority given to carry out tasks or insure rules or laws are upheld.

**power of appointment**
A document that gives someone the power to decide who receives money or property from an estate and how it will be used.

**power of attorney**
A document authorizing a person to act as an attorney or agent.

**practical nurse**
See licensed practical nurse.

**practice**
1. The use of one's knowledge in a particular profession. The practice of medicine is the exercise of one's knowledge in the promotion of health and the treatment of disease. 2. A usual way of doing things, custom. 3. The common way, customary, regular, repetition. 4. Procedures used in pleading and in court. 5. To repeat a behavior over and over until it is an easily done act.

**practice plan**
See medical service plan.

**practice privileges**
1. In JCAH long-term care facility accreditation, this is permission to render care within well-defined limits based upon the individual's professional license and his or her training, experience, competence, ability and judgment. 2. In a facility permission is given to licensed physicians to render medical care within well-defined limits. Physicians must meet the requirements of the facility for medical staff membership to be accepted on the medical staff.

**practitioner**
1. One who practices a profession; a physician or other health care professional who provides health care services. 2. According to JCAH long-term care accreditation, this is any appropriately licensed individual who may be granted clinical privileges in the hospital, specifically physicians (M.D. or D.O.), dentists, and podiatrists.

**praecipe**
A motion of official request that does not need the courts or a judge's approval, as it can be completed by the clerk of the court.

**prayer**
1. A request hoped for or desired as a part of a legal pleading. 2. Asking for relief, help, action or damages from the other party.

**preadmission certification**
Review of the need for proposed inpatient service(s) prior to time of admission to an institution. See also concurrent review and prior authorization.

**pre-admission testing (PAT)**
Tests and examinations performed in the hospital on an outpatient basis prior to admission for care as an inpatient.

**preamble**
The introduction to a document, such as a summary of why it was written.

**precatory**
1. A recommendation that is advisory only. 2. Counseling that is not legally binding. 3. Expression of a desire of something wanted.

**PRECEDE**
This is an acronym for Predisposing, Reinforcing and Enabling Causes in Educational Diagnosis and Evaluation. This is a 7-phase health education planning model which directs a health educator's efforts to results rather than inputs. The seven phases include 1 & 2) epidemiological and social diagnosis, 3) behavioral diagnosis, 4 & 5) educational diagnosis, 6) administrative diagnosis.

**precedent**
1. A judicial interpretation of a legal issue which will be followed in the future. 2. A court decision and understanding that gives authority and direction on how to decide a future similar issue of law. 3. Something that must occur before something else may be accomplished or take place.

**precept**
A directive given by a person having authority to give such a command.

**precinct**
A police district or an election district.

**precipe**
See praecipe.

**precognition**
1. Interviewing and questioning of a witness before a hearing or a trial begins. 2. In psychology, this refers to thoughts or emotional states that are at a lower conscious level and have not yet reached the thinking or conscious level.

**predisposing factor**
Any characteristic, condition or circumstance that affects a patient or community to be motivated toward a certain health behavior.

**pre-emption**
1. The first right or chance to be in line to purchase or receive something. 2. The act of doing or the right to do something before somebody else does it.

**pre-emptive**
A right to the exclusion of others.

**pre-existing condition**
1. A physical condition that existed before the insured's policy was issued. Some companies will not cover these conditions and others will pay only after a certain waiting period. 3. An injury occurring, disease contracted, or physical condition which existed prior to the issuance of a

health insurance policy. Usually results in an exclusion from coverage under the policy for costs resulting from the condition.

**preference**
1. The paying of a debt by an insolvent debtor. 2. Right to be paid first before other creditors. 3. A broke person paying off a creditor more than a fair share of what he has left.

**preferential debts**
1. Those debts in bankruptcy that have a priority. 2. Debts that can be satisfied before others.

**prefrontal lobotomy**
See lobotomy.

**prejudice**
1. Bias. 2. A strong belief in something or against someone. 3. Opinionated. 4. Favoring one side in a dispute. 5. Harmful to one's rights. 6. As in prejudicial error which is serious enough error to be appealed. 7. Negative evaluations, beliefs, judgments or opinions formed without factual knowledge. 8. Irrational suspicion or hatred.

**prejudice, without**
1. Negotiations, decisions, agreements, offers, admissions and judgments that are carried out at no risk to the parties involved 2. "With prejudice" refers to a final judgment adverse to the plaintiff, just as if the action had been tried to the end.

**premeditation**
1. A predetermined act. 2. Planning in advance about how to do something. 3. Deliberation. 4. Prior consideration.

**premium**
1. Money paid to an insurance company for insurance coverage. 2. Payment made periodically to keep an insurance policy in force. 3. The amount of money or consideration which is paid by an insured person or policyholder (or on his behalf) to an insurer or third party for insurance coverage under an insurance policy. The premium is generally paid in periodic amounts. It is related to the actuarial value of the benefits provided by the policy, plus a loading to cover administrative costs, profit, etc. Premium amounts for employment related insurance are often split between employers and employees (see contributory insurance). Premiums paid by the employer are non-taxable income for the employee. Premiums are paid for coverage whether benefits are actually used or not; they should not be confused with cost-sharing, like copayments and deductibles which are paid only if benefits are actually used.

**preoperative care**
The period prior to undergoing surgery when psychological and physical preparations are made according to the special needs of the individual patient. Preparation for surgery starts from the time the patient is admitted to the hospital to the actual time of the surgical operation.

**prepaid expenses**
An accrual accounting method which pays for goods or services in advance which provides savings to the organization in the next operating and budget cycle.

**prepaid group practice**
An arrangement where a formal association of three or more physicians provides a defined set of services to persons over a specified time period in return for a fixed periodic prepayment made in advance of the use of service. See also group practice, medical foundation and health maintenance organization.

**prepaid group practice plan**
A health insurance plan under which specified health services are provided by participating physicians to a pre-enrolled group of persons, who pay fixed periodic payments in advance, on behalf of each person or family. If a health insurance carrier is involved, it contracts to pay in advance for the full range of health services to which the insured is entitled under the terms of the health insurance contract. One approach to such a plan is a health maintenance organization. See health maintenance organization.

**prepaid health plan (PHP)**
Generically, a contract between an insurer and a subscriber or group of subscribers whereby the PHP provides a specified set of health benefits in return for a periodic premium. The term now usually means organizational entities in California which provide services to Medi-Cal (the name for California's Medicaid program) beneficiaries under contract with the State of California.

**prepared childbirth**
General terminology to describe courses which prepare expectant parents for pregnancy and childbirth. These courses include information, hospital tours, and often several methods of managing labor.

**prepayment penalty**
Money charged for the privilege of paying off a debt in advance.

**prepayment premiums**
Medical insurance benefits paid for in advance, generally through monthly premiums. Synonymous with insurance, sometimes refers to any payment ahead of time to a provider for anticipated services (such as an expectant mother paying in advance for maternity care), sometimes distinguished from insurance as referring to payment to organizations, (such as HMOs, prepaid group practices and medical foundations) which, unlike an insurance company, take responsibility for arranging for and providing needed services as well as paying for them.

**preponderance of evidence**
Evidence of greater weight which is adequate to overcome doubt and to dispel speculation.

**prerogative**
1. A special authority or privilege. 2. A special choice of a person. 3. Official power. 4. Special allowance of an action. 5. An exclusive privilege, advantage or power.

**prerogative writs**
A special action of a court taken only under special circumstances, such as a mandamus or habeas corpus.

**presbyopia**
Presby means old. A vision disorder that occurs in old age because the lens of the eye tends to solidify in a certain shape and the person loses his or her ability to focus.

**prescription**
1. A document allowing open possession and limited to a specific time period set by law. 2. The acquisition of rights to property by long-term uninterrupted use. 3. An order signed by a physician to a pharmacist to provide a specific amount of a drug or medicine. 4. A written order or direction for the preparation and administration of a drug or other remedy by a physician, dentist or other practitioner licensed by law to administer such a drug. Prescriptions may be written as orders in hospitals and other institutions for drugs to be given inpatients, or given to outpatients to be filled by a pharmacist. The prescription properly specifies the drug to be given, the amount of the drug to be dispensed, and the directions necessary for the patient to use the drug.

**prescription drug**
A drug available to the public only upon prescription. The availability of such drugs is thus limited because the drug is considered dangerous if used without a physician's supervision. See also ethical and over-the-counter drugs.

**present**
1. In the here and now. 2. Immediate. 3. The one at hand. See presentment.

**presentation**
See presentment.

**presentence investigation**
1. An investigation carried out by court-appointed physicians, psychologists, social workers, psychiatrists, to learn of a person's background. This is done to ascertain his potential for rehabilitation or integration back into society.

**presentment**
1. Presenting a negotiable instrument, and expecting payment on it. 2. A statement from a grand jury to a court stating that it believes that a crime has been committed and that the named person is responsible.

**presents**
1. This document. 2. A guess without facts to back it up. 3. An inference based on usual occurrences.

**present value**
The current value of cash flows that will be received or paid later. The value of money is adjusted for inflation for the time value of money and is discounted at the same interest rate.

**President's budget**
In the federal budget, the budget for a particular fiscal year specifying proposed budget authority, obligations and outlays transmitted to the Congress by the President in accordance with the Budget and Accounting Act of 1921, as amended. Some elements of the budget, such as the estimates for the legislative branch and the judiciary, are included without review by the Office of Management and Budget or approval by the President. The budget is presently submitted in January for the fiscal year beginning during the calendar year.

**pressure sore**
Referred to as a decubitus ulcer or bedsore. A skin disorder commonly occurring in persons confined to lying or sitting positions, such as long-term care patients. It is caused by continuous pressure in a localized area, interfering with circulation, resulting in an open sore.

**presumption**
1. To assume a fact is true by reviewing the factual occurrence of other events. 2. A conclusion. 3. A presumption of fact is an assumption that because one thing is true another thing is also true.

**presumption of innocence**
Assuming that a person is innocent of any wrong doing until fault or guilt is established by evidence and proven by the due process of law.

**presumptive**
1. Founded on presumption; assumed. 2. It may be concluded or inferred. See presumption.

**preterlegal**
Beyond the law; illegal, illicit, not legal.

**pretermit**
To neglect.

**prevailing charge**
A charge which falls within the range of charges most frequently used in a locality for a particular medical service or procedure. The top of this range establishes an over-all limitation on the charges which a carrier, which considers prevailing charges in reimbursement, will accept as reasonable for a given service, without adequate special justification. Current Medicare rules state that the limit of an area's prevailing charge is to be the 75th percentile of the customary charges for a given service by the physicians in a given area. For example, if customary charges for an appendectomy in a locality were distributed so that 10 percent of the services were rendered by physicians whose customary charge was $150, 40 percent by physicians who charged $200, 40 percent who charged $250, and 10 percent who charged $300 or more, then the prevailing charge would be $250, since this is the level that, under Medicare

regulations, would cover at least 75 percent of the cases. See also actual charges & fractionation.

**prevalence**
The number of cases of disease, infected persons, or persons with some other attribute, present at a particular time and in relation to the size of the population from which drawn. It is a measurement of morbidity at a moment in time, for example, the number of cases of hemophilia in the country as of the first of the year. The prevalence of arthritis is high relative to its incidence. Prevalence equals incidence times average case duration.

**prevention and detection services**
Services delivered to individuals in order to promote optimum physical and mental well-being, including protection from the development of disease and ill-health, or to identify disease or ill-health at the presymptomatic or unrecognized symptomatic stage to permit early intervention.

**preventive detention**
Holding a person against his will assuming that he may commit an illegal act. This is unconstitutional in almost all cases.

**preventive law**
Helping a person to avoid legal problems.

**preventive medicine**
Care and health education aimed at preventing disease or its consequences. It includes health care programs aimed at warding off illnesses (e.g., immunizations), early detection of disease (e.g., Pap smears), and inhibiting further deterioration of the body (e.g., exercise or prophylactic surgery). Preventive medicine developed subsequent to bacteriology, and was concerned in its early history with specific medical control measures taken against the agents of infectious diseases. With increasing knowledge of nutritional, malignant and other chronic diseases, the scope of preventive medicine has been extended. It is now operatively assumed that most if not all problems are preventable at some stage of their development. Preventive medicine now includes health education as a major concern with general aims of improving the healthfulness of our environment and our relations with it through such things as avoidance of hazardous substances, modified diet, and family planning. In particular, the promotion of health through altering behavior, especially by health education, is gaining prominence as a component of preventive care. See also public health, consultation and education services, community medicine, health education.

**preventive psychiatry**
See community psychology/psychiatry.

**price variance**
The assessment of how actual prices agree with budgeted prices, the difference between the actual prices and the budgeted prices are

multiplied by the actual quantity of goods or services purchased. Also called rate variance.

**prima facie (Lat.)**
1. At first sight; on the face of it; as it appears on the face of it; on the first appearance. 2. Presumably; a fact considered to be true unless proven otherwise.

**prima facie case**
A case based on evidence that appears to be sufficient enough to determine a negative outcome for the defendant.

**primary authority**
The first and basic binding authority.

**primary care**
Basic or general health care which emphasizes the point when the patient first seeks assistance from the medical care system and the care of the simpler and more common illnesses. The primary care provider usually also assumes ongoing responsibility for the patient in both health maintenance and therapy of illness. It is comprehensive in the sense that it takes responsibility for the overall coordination of the care of the patient's health problems, be they biological, behavioral or social. The appropriate use of consultants and community resources is an important part of effective primary care. Such care is generally provided by physicians, but is increasingly provided by other personnel such as physician assistants and family nurse practitioners. See also family and personal physician, secondary and tertiary care, general practice, care primary.

**primary care facilities**
Those facilities, regardless of location or structure, that offer services on a need/demand basis to the public. Those entities designed, equipped, staffed, organized and operated as an integral part of a comprehensive health care system and which offer health services in an available, personalized and continuous fashion on an outpatient basis.

**primary evidence**
The best and surest evidence.

**primary gain**
The reduction of tension, anxieties, symptoms or conflict of neurotic disorders.

**primary payer**
Denotes insurer obligated to pay losses prior to any liability of other, secondary insurers. Under current law, Medicare is a primary payer with respect to Medicaid; for a person eligible under both programs, Medicaid pays only for benefits not covered under Medicare, or after Medicare benefits are exhausted. See also duplication and coordination of benefits.

**primary psychological prevention**
Those measures needed to prevent an emotional or mental disorder such as nutrition education or substitute parents.

**primary reserve**
That part of an insurance company's reserves set aside for losses incurred but not reported (IBNR).

**prime**
First; high quality; major; original; most important; the best.

**primogeniture**
First child born. An old rule that the first son inherits everything.

**primus inter pares (Lat.)**
First among equals.

**principal**
1. Head, director, main, major, chief, most important, primary. 2. The most legally responsible person in a relationship. 3. A basic sum of money. 4. A person acting in his own behalf. 5. One in a position of authority. 6. An employer, a physician, or anyone else who as another person (an agent) do things for him. 7. The main person committing a crime.

**principle**
1. A doctrime. 2. A rule or belief used to determine an issue. 3. A legal truth. 4. A basic legal expectation or doctrine.

**prior authorization**
1. An administrative procedure where a doctor or dentist submits a treatment plan to the insurance carrier before treatment is initiated. This procedure is common in dental contracts, the Medicaid program, and the Medi-Cal program. 2. Also referred to as preauthorization, precertification, predetermination, pre-estimate of cost and pretreatment estimate. 3. In health care, a requirement imposed by a third party, under some systems of utilization review, that a provider must justify before a peer review committee, insurance company representative, or state agent the need for delivering a particular service to a patient before actually providing the service in order to receive reimbursement. Generally, prior authorization is required for non-emergency services which are expensive (involving a hospital stay, preadmission certification, for example) or particularly likely to be overused or abused (many state Medicaid programs require prior authorization of all dental services, for instance).

**prior determination**
Similar to prior authorization but less restrictive in that payment will be made if prior authorization is not sought, provided that it would have approved the service as needed.

**prior hearing**
A previously held hearing of an administrative agency which is required to occur before any action can be taken.

**priorities**
The relative importance and emphasis attached to various goals, objectives and, by extension, the actions designed to achieve them.

**priority**
Lists, problems, concerns, ramifications and alternatives ranked according to desirability, preference, importance, value and effectiveness.

**priority levels(planning)**
In health or institutional planning: there are four steps or levels that have to be addressed. They are:

Level 1 - The goal will be developed with objectives and with long-range recommended actions and resource requirements to meet those actions and will receive first priority in the agency's Annual Implementation Plan (AIP).

Level 2 - The goal will be developed with objectives and with long-range recommended actions and resource requirements to meet those actions and will be considered for the Annual Implementation Plan (AIP) with the understanding the goal is a second priority.

Level 3 - The goal, together with any objectives and long-range recommended actions and resource requirements that are given by the community will be included in the overall plan but there will not be provision in the first year Annual Implementation Plan.

Level 4 - The goal should be included in the HSP and notation should be made of consideration given it, together with objectives that were considered, but will not be included in the Annual Implementation plan nor will recommended actions be developed for it. See Annual Implementation Plan.

**prisoner**
Anyone deprived of liberty.

**privacy**
1. The right to have one's personal life and activities kept to himself, to be left alone, and not be presented to the public. 2. Respect for confidential information of a person.

**private**
Individual and personal; not for use by the general public or government.

**private duty nurse**
A registered nurse who works on her own by offering skilled nursing services in a person's home to care for a sick, injured or disabled family member or individual who pays her directly for her services.

**private health agency**
A nongovernmental agency concerned with health, organized as one of three types: 1) nonprofit incorporated (voluntary), 2) nonprofit unincorporated (voluntary) or 3) proprietary (commercial). Also called a voluntary health agency. Many deal with a disease or disability or body part that can be diseased or injured, i.e., The American Heart Association.

**private law**
1. Law dealing with private individuals or a group. 2. The law controlling the relationships among and between persons and groups. 3.

Opposite public law. 4. Laws that deal with the private sector and/or its relationship to society and between private parties.

**private patient**

A patient whose care is the responsibility of an identifiable, individual health professional (usually a physician) who is paid directly (by the patient or a third-party) for his service to the patient. The physician is called a personal physician and the patient is his private patient. Private patients are contrasted with public, service or ward patients whose care is the responsibility of a health program or institution. Public patients are often cared for by an individual practitioner paid by the program (such as a member of the house staff) but the program, rather than the individual, is paid for the care. The distinction is important to third-party payers (including Medicare) because situations arise in which payment is made to both a program and an individual practitioner for the same services. The term occasionally refers to a patient occupying a room in an institution by himself (a private room). See also private practice.

**private practice**

Medical practice in which the practitioner and his practice are independent of any external policy control. It usually requires that the practitioner be self-employed, except when he is salaried by a partnership in which he is a partner with similar practitioners. It is sometimes wrongly used synonymously with either fee-for-service practice (the practitioner may sell his services by another method; i.e., capitation); or solo practice (group practice may be private). Note that physicians practice in many different settings and there is no agreement as to which of these does or does not constitute private practice. Regulation, which does exert external control, is not generally felt to make all practice public. The opposite of private practice is not necessarily public, in the sense of employment by government. Practitioners salaried by private hospitals are not usually thought to be in private practice.

**privilege**

1. Being allowed to do something you usually are not allowed to do. 2. A special right to be preferred. 3. Exempt from regular duty; getting preferential treatment.

**privileged communication**

Any statement, paper, document or communication made in confidence or trust to a counselor, psychologist, physician, lawyer or spouse. The law protects such a fiduciary from revealing confidential information, even in a trial.

**privileged relations**

A special or confidential relationship between two persons of such a nature that would exempt them from being forced to testify against themselves based on any communication they might have had with another, such as physician/patient, or psychologist/client. See fiduciary.

**privileges and immunities**

1. A principle provided by the constitution in that no state may treat a person from another state unfairly. 2. No state shall make or enforce any

law which shall abridge the privileges or immunities of citizens of the United States.

**privity**
1. Private information. 2. Having inside information. 3. Having a direct financial relationship. 4. Rights and duties of a contract. 5. Mutual relationships to the same right or property. 6. Two or more persons with an interest in something that if one of them has a legal involvement it would be representative of the other or both.

**privy**
One who is privity of a contract or with another person. Private.

**pro (Lat.)**
1. For. 2. For probable cause. 3. Having a fairly sound suspicion, that is provable by facts, that a crime has been committed. 4. It is not what the law enforcement official finds out after an arrest or search but what was known before the action was taken. Cause as supported by circumstances.

**probable cause for arrest**
Arrest for strong circumstances that are more than a suspicion, but less than proven facts that a crime has been committed.

**probate**
The court that handles the distribution of an estate or will. It may also handle such matters as mental illness commitments.

**probation**
1. Allowing a convicted person to stay out of jail based on expected good behavior and the condition that he or she will commit no further illegal acts or have no encounters with the law. 2. A trial period sometimes given to new employees to see if they are capable of doing the work or if they will fit into the job. In governmental jobs, it is usually a period of 6 months.

**probationary period**
A specified number of days after the date of the issuance of the policy during which coverage is not afforded for sickness. See waiting period.

**probationer**
A person free on probation based on expected future good behavior or supervised behavior.

**probative**
1. Tending to prove a fact. 2. Providing actual proof.

**probative facts**
Facts that prove other needed facts of an issue in a lawsuit.

**probity**
Honesty.

**Problem-Oriented Medical Information System (PROMIS)**
A computerized medical record system. Medical data base and source tapes, along with functional specification and documentation of PROMIS,

were developed by the Medical Center Hospital of Vermont with the support of the National Center for Health Services Research (NCHSR). PROMIS categorizes patient data according to relevant medical problems, recording the reasons for each medical service provided and how it relates to the total regimen of care. PROMIS also provides a guide to basic medical practices for each phase of care and warns of inadvisable therapy and drugs.

**problem oriented medical record (POMR)**
A medical record in which the information and conclusions contained in the record are organized to describe each of the patient's problems. The description properly includes subjective, objective and significant negative information, discussion and conclusions, and diagnostic and treatment plans with respect to each problem. The record, which was developed by Lawrence Weed, M.D., has gained increasing acceptance and can be contrasted with the traditional medical record which is differently and less formally organized, usually recording all information from each source (history, physical exam and laboratory) together without regard to the problems which the information describes.

**pro bono (Lat.)**
Free or charitable legal services for a community or public organization.

**pro bono publico (Lat.)**
For the good of the public.

**procedural law**
1. The process of carrying out the procedures necessary for a lawsuit. 2. Law governing procedure or practice.

**procedure**
1. The process and step by step method used in carrying out a lawsuit. 2. A technical predetermined system and method of carrying out legal actions. 3. A method or technique used in therapy or treatment. 4. A step by step outline of the mode used by a hospital or other institution to accomplish a specific objective or task.

**procedure coding manual**
A booklet produced by the medical and health insurance companies with the intent of helping the health care provider to file an insurance claim so to express precisely and concisely each service provided or rendered. A code and narrative description is provided for services, treatments and procedures in the areas of medicine, surgery, radiology, nuclear medicine, pathology and for special services.

**proceeding**
1. The process and procedure of hearing a case in court. 2. The orderly process of a lawsuit or hearing. 3. A record of a hearing or court.

**process**
1. A court order for a defendant to appear in court or risk losing the lawsuit. 2. A summons. 3. A court order that takes jurisdiction over person or property. 4. Carrying out the method of doing things. 5. Regular procedures moving forth step by step. 6. The manner in which

planning for the health systems plan or institutional plan is to take place. It details the areas of responsibilities among the planning entities in the development of the plan.

**process measure**
An indicator of the quality of medical care used to assess the activities of health manpower and programs in the management of patients. Process measures document the process of care used for various populations or diagnoses; for example, the fraction of people with hypertension who receive an intravenous pyelogram or the percentage of cases of strep throat which are cultured before treatment. They do not necessarily measure the results of care although they measure the use of diagnostic and treatment methods which are thought or proven to be effective. Generally, such measures indicate the degree of conformity with standards established by peer groups or with expectations formulated by leaders in the profession. See also input, outcome and output measures.

**process server**
A court official who delivers a summons.

**prochein ami (French)**
Next friend.

**pro confesso (Lat.)**
As confessed.

**proctor**
Someone given authority to oversee or to manage another person's activity.

**proctoscope**
A lighted optical instrument used to visually examine the interior of the rectum.

**proctoscopy**
The act of viewing the interior of the rectum with a lighted optical instrument.

**procure**
1. To acquire or gain something for someone. 2. Obtain, solicit.

**produce**
1. To bring forward; to show. 2. To yield up. 3. To provide. 4. To exhibit.

**producing cause**
See proximate cause.

**productivity**
How much output can be obtained from a unit of input by utilizing production measures. Physician productivity generally is measured by number of physician hours spent, number of patient visits, expenditure of supplies; and a unit of output is measured by the number of patiets seen, number of office visits, dollar amount of income generated.

**professio juris (Lat.)**
In contract law this is to have one state or country decide all legal issues of a contractual agreement.

**profession**
The act of professing, a group of persons with a common interest united together for advancement of the common interest.

**professional**
Formal education and examination are required for membership in a profession; certification or licensure is required for membership, reflecting community sanction or approval, there exists regional or national professional associations; there is a code of ethics governing the activities of individuals in a profession. Usually for a person to be a professional there is a body of systematic scientific knowledge and technical skill required; and the members function with a degree of autonomy and authority, under the assumption that they alone have the expertise to make decisions in their area of competence. Medicine is often considered the occupation which most closely approaches the prototype of a profession.

**Professional Activity Study (PAS)**
A shared-computer medical record information system purchased by hospitals from the Commission on Professional and Hospital Activities (CPHA) in Ann Arbor, Michigan, a nonprofit computer center. Information flows into the system through a discharge abstract completed by the hospital medical record department on every discharged patient. The patient information is displayed back to the hospital in a series of monthly, semi-annual, and annual reports which compare its average lengths of stay, number and types of tests used, and autopsy rates for given diagnostic conditions with those of other hospitals of similar size and scope of services (good examples of process measures). See also ICDA.

**professional component**
In health insurance, under certain circumstances, the physician may wish to submit a charge for the professional component of a procedure rather than for a technical component. Under these circumstances the professional component charge is identified by adding a modifier number to the usual procedure number, found in the procedure coding manual when filing his insurance forms. See procedure coding manual.

**professional corporation (PC)**
A legal entity established to function in the business world distinct from its several members. A PC is created and operates under authority from a state through the articles of incorporation. This legal entity may be for-profit, not-for-profit, as a personal holding company or for tax shelter purposes under Subchapter S of the Internal Revenue Code. Also referred to as a professional association, a PC requires shareholders to be licensed in the same profession (medicine, dentistry, architecture, and the like), with sole incorporators acting as members of the board of directors. The advantages of a PC are limited liability for the professional stockholder(s), centralized administration, continuity of corporate life, free

transferability of stock; and tax shelters. The disadvantages are loss of a degree of stockholder autonomy in decision policy making, scrutiny from state and federal governments, substantial legal service requirements, and the possibility of double taxation.

**professional liability**
Obligation of providers or their professional liability insurers to pay for damages resulting from the providers, acts of omission or commission in treating patients. The term is sometimes preferred by providers to medical malpractice because it does not necessarily imply negligence. It is also a term which more adequately describes the obligations of all types of professionals, e.g. lawyers, architects and other health providers, as well as physicians.

**professional liability insurance**
See malpractice insurance.

**Professional Standards Review Organization (PSRO)**
1. A group of physicians working with the government to review cases for hospital admission and discharge under government guidelines. 2. A physician-sponsored organization charged with comprehensive and ongoing review of services provided under the Medicare, Medicaid and Maternal and Child Health programs. The purpose of this review is to determine for purposes of reimbursement under these programs whether services are: medically necessary; provided in accordance with professional criteria, norms and standards; and, in the case of institutional services, rendered in an appropriate setting. The requirement for the establishment of PSROs was added by the Social Security Amendments of 1972, P.L. 92-603, to the Social Security Act as part B of title XI. PSRO areas have been designated throughout the country and organizations in many of these areas are at various stages of implementing the required review functions. See also peer and medical review, PSRO, standards.

**proffer**
1. To offer. 2. To present for acceptance. 3. Avowal. 4. To offer services.

**proficiency testing**
Assesses technical knowledge and skills related to the performance requirements of a specific job, whether such knowledge and skills were acquired through formal or informal means. Section 241 of the Social Security Amendments of 1972, P.L. 92-603, requires the Secretary of HHS, in carrying out his functions relating to qualifications for health manpower, to develop and conduct a program to determine the proficiency of individuals in performing the duties and functions of practical nurses, therapists, medical technologists and cytotechnologists, radiologic technologists, psychiatric technicians, or other health care technicians and technologists. The program is to use formal testing of the proficiency of individuals, and is not to deny any individual, who otherwise meets the proficiency requirements for any health care specialty, a satisfactory proficiency rating solely because of his failure to meet formal educational or professional membership requirements. Proficiency examinations are to determine the necessary work qualifications of health personnel (therapists, technologists, technicians and others) who do not

otherwise meet the formal educational, professional membership, or other specified criteria established under Medicare regulations so that services provided by these individuals will be eligible for payment. See also equivalency testing.

**profile**

A longitudinal or cross-sectional aggregation of medical care data. Patient profiles list all of the services provided to a particular patient during a specified period of time. Physician, hospital, or population profiles are statistical summaries of the pattern of practice of an individual physician, a specific hospital, or the medical experience of a specific population. Diagnostic profiles are a subcategory of physician, hospital, or population profiles with regard to a specific condition or diagnosis.

**profit**

The gain made by the sale of goods or services after deducting the value of the labor, materials, rents, interest on capital and other expenses involved in the production of the good or service. Economists define profit as return to (or on) capital investment, and distinguish normal (competitive) and excessive (more than competitive) profit. Profit in the sense of a profit-making or proprietary institution is present when any of the net earnings of the institution inure to the benefit of any individual. The concept of profit is very hard to define operationally or in detail, and unreasonable or excessive profit even more so. It is important to recognize that reasonable profit on investment must vary with the risks involved in the investment. Profit bears a close relationship to the balance of supply and demand, being a measure of unmet demand.

**pro forma (Lat.)**

As a matter of form; a formality.

**prognosis**

The prediction or opinion of the outcome of a disease, condition or disorder.

**program**

1. In computerized medical records, medical insurance, business records or medical research, it is a group of related routines that solve a given problem or command the computer. A plan or routine for solving a problem on a computer. 2. Another term for agency or department. 3. A set of planned activities designed to achieve specified objectives in a given period of time. 4. A group of projects providing related services which together address a common purpose (e.g., a maternal and child health program). 5. According to JCAH for psychiatric, alcoholism and drug abuse facilities accreditation purposes, it is a general term for an organized system of services designed to address the treatment needs of patients.

**program effectiveness**

The extent or level of quality and quantity which a program has attained in meeting objectives as a result of planned activity.

**program efficiency**
The resourceful use of time, materials and personnel in the attainment of a program's objectives as compared to total resources expended.

**program evaluation**
According to JCAH for psychiatric, alcoholism and drug abuse facilities accreditation purposes, this is an assessment component of a facility that determines the degree to which a program is meeting its stated goals and objectives.

**programming**
The process of planning the procedural steps and the order to be taken in order to produce a given report, document or to command a computer to perform certain functions.

**program objective**
A statement of activity directed towards a desired outcome specifying who is to do what, how much, at what point in time, according to the implementation of a plan. See objective.

**progressive patient care (PPC)**
A system under which patients are grouped together in units depending on their need for care as determined by their degree of illness rather than by consideration of medical specialty. There are three conventional levels or stages of progressive patient care: intensive care, that needed for critically ill patients; intermediate care, that intermediate between intensive and minimal; and minimal care or self-care, which seems self-explanatory. Except for the development of intensive care units, the concept of progressive patient care does not appear to have had much impact on the organization of hospitals and other health programs.

**progressive tax**
A tax which takes an increasing proportion of income as income rises, such as the federal personal income tax. Incremental increases in taxable income are subject to an increased marginal tax rate. See also regressive and proportional tax.

**progress notes**
The hour by hour or day by day notation in the medical record by the physician that indicates the assessment and activities related to the therapy and treatment program and the prescribed care of the patient. The patient's medical record contains information concerning the patient's diseases, disorders or conditions, needs, recovery, improvements and results of tests and examinations. As the patient's conditions changes, so does the treatment plan and these factors are progressively noted in the medical record by the physician.

**pro hac vice (Lat.)**
For one particular occasion only; for this occasion.

**prohibition**
A legal order to stop or not engage in certain acts.

**prohibition, writ of**
1. A court order. 2. A writ directing a person not to do something which the court has been made aware of. 3. A writ from a higher court to a lower court directing it to cease certain activities.

**project**
A set of activities to be carried out by a provider organization. Projects include development and demonstration of manpower, budgets, operations and operating policies (e.g., a project to establish and operate a family planning center).

**project grant**
A grant of federal funds to a public or private agency or organization for a specified purpose authorized by law, such as development of an emergency medical services system, or conduct of a continuing education program.

**projection**
A mental mechanism or defense mechanism that blames or places responsibility on another for one's own failures, inadequacies, shortcomings or mistakes; not being responsible for one's own behavior.

**projective test**
A psychological test that helps a subject reveal his own feelings, intelligence level, personality, or psychopathology. Examples include the Rorschach and Thematic Apperception Test.

**prolix**
Verbose, drawn out; wordy, tedious, tiresome, prolonged.

**prolixity**
Being verbose, using drawn out superfluous statements. Being prolix.

**PROMIS**
Problem-Oriented Medical Information System. See these words.

**promise**
1. An agreement that legally, or otherwise commits the person who made it to keep the agreement or do an act. 2. An orally expressed or written statement by one person to another. 3. An agreement usually involving something of value to be given in return for services performed.

**promisee**
One to whom a promise is made.

**promisor**
One who makes a promise.

**promissory estoppel**
A binding promise that expects some action to be taken by a promisee. Such a promise is legally binding and has the effect of a contract if it would be unfair or cause an injustice not to have it binding.

**promissory note**
A written promise to pay, as agreed, a sum of money at a certain time, place, and/or circumstance.

**promulgate**
1. To publish. 2. To formally announce. 3. To make public. 4. To officially and formally present to the public.

**prone**
Lying face downward.

**proof**
1. Convincing evidence. 2. Enough evidence is shown so that there is no doubt that the facts are true, or that an argument about it shows that the facts are true.

**proof of loss**
A contractual right of an insurance carrier or service corporation to request verification of services rendered through the submission of claim forms, radiographs, dental study models, and/or other diagnostic material.

**proper**
1. Acceptable actions. 2. Having a substantial interest. 3. Suitable or appropriate.

**property**
1. A solid tangible item that may be owned. 2. Any item or object that belongs to someone.

**prophylaxis**
Preventive treatment; prevention of disease.

**proponent**
1. One who makes an offer. 2. A person who puts forward an item, object or suggestion. 3. One who makes a proposal.

**proportional tax**
A tax which takes a constant proportion of income as income changes. The social security payroll tax is proportional up to the $14,000 limit on income to which it applies. See also progressive and regressive tax.

**propound**
1. To offer. 2. To make a proposal. 3. To put forward; to make a proposition.

**proprietary**
1. Holding property. 2. Profit making. 3. Operated for the purpose of gaining a profit. 4. Having to do with ownership. 5. Legal right to ownership.

**proprietary function**
The performance of a function by the board of directors that generally does not fall under general duties imposed upon the board by virtue of its governmental duties; dealing with rights of ownership.

**proprietary hospital**
A hospital operated for the purpose of making a profit for its owners. Proprietary hospitals are often owned by physicians for the care of their own and others' patients. There is also a growing number of investor-owned hospitals, usually operated by a parent corporation which operates a chain of such hospitals.

**pro rata (Lat.)**
Proportionately; by a percentage, fixed rate or share.

**prorate**
1. Break down or divide in sections. 2. Lots, pieces or by items portioned in downward increments.

**prorating**
In budgeting, it is the allocation of an expenditure to two or more different accounts. The allocation is made in proportion to the gain which the expenditure provides in relationship to the programs for which the accounts were established.

**proration**
An adjustment of insurance benefits paid due to a mistake in the premiums paid or the existence of other insurance covering the same accident or disability.

**prorogation**
1. A delay or putting off. 2. A continuance.

**pro se (Lat.)**
For himself in his own behalf.

**prosecute**
To begin and carry out, including follow-up, on a civil lawsuit. To bring a person charged with a crime to trial.

**prosecutor**
A lawyer who works for a county, city, or state as a public official who is a representative of that government who presents the cases against an accused person and asks the court to convict that person of a crime which he has committed.

**prosecutorial discretion**
1. Discretion or decision of a prosecutor. 2. The power of the prosecutor to decide whether or not to prosecute or to decide how serious a charge to present, or whether to go through plea bargaining.

**prospective**
1. Forward in time; events or occurrences of the future. 2. Laws which are preventive in nature.

**prospective budget**
A detailed plan of the projected services, revenues, costs and volume for the next fiscal year.

**prospective reimbursement**
Any method of paying hospitals or other health programs in which amounts or rates of payment are established in advance for the coming year and the programs are paid these amounts regardless of the costs they actually incur. These systems of reimbursement are designed to introduce a degree of constraint on charge or cost increases by setting limits on amounts paid during a future period. In some cases, such systems provide incentives for improved efficiency by sharing savings with institutions that perform at lower than anticipated costs. Prospective reimbursement contrasts with the method of payment presently used under Medicare and Medicaid where institutions are reimbursed for actual expenses incurred, i.e., on a retrospective basis. See also section 222.

**prospective study**
An inquiry planned to observe events that have not yet occurred; compare with a retrospective study which is planned to examine events which have already occurred.

**prospectus**
1. A document of future events. 2. A document of a planned future financial deal. 3. A statement about a corporation or company's stocks, and securities issued as an invitation for investment.

**prosthesis**
Any device, instrument, or object that is an artificial body part used to replace an amputated body limb or part.

**prosthetic/orthotic assistant or technician**
These individuals assist the prosthetist/orthotist in caring for patients by making casts, taking measurements or model specifications, and fitting supportive appliances or artificial limbs.

**prosthetist**
Following the prescription of physicians, usually a specialist in physical medicine, these individuals write specifications for, make, fit, and repair braces, appliances and artificial limbs. Also referred to as orthotist.

**prostitution**
Selling one's body for sexual purposes.

**pro tanto (Lat.)**
For so much; to that extent.

**protective order**
A temporary court order that allows one side of a legal proceeding to not show documents or evidence that were officially requested by the opposing party.

**pro tem (Lat.)**
Short for "pro tempore".

**pro tempore (Lat.)**
For the time being.

**prothonotary**
1. Clerk of the court. 2. Head clerk of a court.

**proto-**
Prefix, meaning first.

**provider**
1. Supplier. 2. Physician. 3. One providing service to a patient. 4. An individual or institution which gives medical care. 5. In Medicare, an institutional provider is a hospital, skilled nursing facility, home health agency, or certain providers of outpatient physical therapy services. These providers receive cost-related reimbursement. Other Medicare providers, paid on a charge basis, are called suppliers. Individual providers include individuals who practice independently of institutional providers. The term must sometimes be distinguished from consumer, for instance when requiring consumer representation in a health program. For these purposes P.L. 93-641 defines the term for individuals as follows (section 1531(3) of the PHS Act): A) who is a direct provider of health care (including a physician, dentist, nurse, podiatrist, or physician assistant) in that the individual's primary current activity is the provision of health care to individuals or the administration of facilities or institutions (including hospitals, long-term care facilities, outpatient facilities and health maintenance organizations) in which such care is provided and, when required by state law, the individual has received professional training in the provision of such care or in such administration and is licensed or certified for such provision or administration.

**provider of health care**
See provider.

**providers of service**
An individual or institution which gives medical care. In Medicare, an institutional provider is a hospital, skilled nursing facility, home health agency, or certain providers of outpatient physical therapy services. These providers receive cost-related reimbursement.

**province**
1. An area of responsibility. 2. An expected duty.

**provisional**
1. Temporarily applied. 2. Applicable. 3. To temporarily enforce a law. 4. A provisional nursing home administrator's license is often called a provisional license as it is issued on a temporary basis and is in effect only until testing or other licensing procedures are passed and completed.

**provisional remedy**
A legal but temporary remedy for an immediate condition or circumstance; an injunction; a temporary enforcement of the law.

**proviso (Lat.)**
1. A condition that is set. 2. A qualification that is made or a limitation placed in a legal paper. 3. A provision. 4. Being provided.

**provocation**
1. Inciting hostility or anger. 2. An act by another that provokes a reaction of rage; something that provokes or causes upset, resentment or irritation.

**proximate**
In immediate relation to or with something else.

**proximate cause**
1. The direct or actual cause that led to an accident, damage, harm or injury. 2. The single most important cause of the damages. The last act prior to injury without which the injury would not have resulted. 4. The act of omission of an act that is complained about which is actually or directly related to the cause of harm or injury. The cause does not have to be the closest cause as far as time, location or space in relationship to the injury. The cause is not always the event that set the incident in motion.

**proximo (Lat.)**
Next.

**proxy**
1. A person who stands in for another person. 2. One appointed to represent another.

**prudent buyer principle**
The principle that Medicare should not reimburse a provider for a cost that is not a reasonable cost because it is in excess of the amount that a prudent and cost-conscious buyer would be expected to pay. For example, an organization that does not seek the customary discount on bulk purchases could, through the operation of this principle, be reimbursed for less than the full purchase price.

**pseudo-**
Prefix, meaning fake or false.

**P.S.R.O. (Professional Standards Review Organization)**
The creation of the Professional Standards Review Organizations (PSROs) was mandated in 1972 by Congress in the 1972 Amendments to the Social Security Act (Public Law 92-603). It was created to assure that health care services and items utilized in health care for which payments are made under Titles V, XVIII, and XIX of the Social Security Act conform to the appropriate and expected high professional standards of health care and are delivered in the most effective, efficient, and economical manner possible, while insuring quality of care. It is based on two fundamental review concepts used in health care settings: 1) that physicians are the most appropriate individuals to assess the quality of medical care, and 2) that local peer review is the most effective means for ensuring health care resources and facilities are appropriately utilized. Four major goals of the PSRO program are: 1) To assure that health care services are of acceptable professional quality; 2) To assure appropriate utilization of health care facilities at the most economical level while being consistent with professional standards; 3) To identify

lack of quality care and overutilization problems in health care practices while working toward improvement; 4) To attempt to obtain voluntary correction of inappropriate or unnecessary practitioner and facility practices and, where unable to do so, recommending sanctions against such practitioners and facilities. See advisory group, Professional Standards Review Organization.

**PSRO Management Information System (PMIS)**
A management information system designed to transmit, process, and analyze information about the PSRO program and project operations so that sound decisions about program operation and policy can be made. At present, PMIS is composed of three interrelated components: the Deliverable Monitoring System, the Federal Reports Manual, and the Contract Management Manual.

**psyche**
Greek work for the mind.

**psychiatric technician**
Works under the supervision of professional and/or technical personnel in caring for mentally ill patients in a psychiatric medical care facility; assists in carrying out the prescribed treatment plan for the patient; maintains consistent attitudes in communicating with the patient in keeping with the treatment plan, and carries out assigned individual and group activities with patients. Also called psychiatric aide.

**psychiatrist**
A physician whose specialty is in the study, diagnosis and treatment of mental disorders. After receiving the M.D. degree, the physician in training to become a psychiatrist spends three years of training as a resident in a psychiatric hospital setting.

**psychiatrist, qualified**
According to JCAH for psychiatric, alcoholism and drug abuse facilities accreditation purposes, this is a doctor of medicine who specializes in the assessment and treatment of individuals having psychiatric disorders and who is fully licensed to practice medicine in the state in which he or she practices.

**psychiatry**
The branch of medicine which deals with behavioral, emotional or mental disorders and related physiological or neurological involvement.

**psycho-**
Prefix, meaning mind.

**psychoactive drug**
Drug that alters one's mind, emotions, i.e., thoughts, feelings or perceptions. Such a drug may help a person to overcome depression, anxiety, or rigidity of thought and behavior. This drug may be used in or in conjunction with psychotherapy.

**psychoanalysis**
Sigmund Freud's system of mental investigation and form of psychotherapy. A technique for determining and understanding the mental processes. Psychoanalysis includes the use of free association, catharsis and the analysis and interpretation of dreams, resistances, and transferences.

**psychologist**
A specially trained professional, usually with an advanced degree (M.A., Ph.D.), and clinical training, who specializes in the study of mental processes and the treatment of mental disorders through testing and psychotherapy. See qualified psychologist.

**psychologist, qualified**
According to JCAH for psychiatric, alcoholism and drug abuse facilities accreditation purposes, this is an individual who meets current legal requirements of licensure, registration, or certification in the state in which the services are rendered, who is currently competent in the field, and who either possesses a doctoral degree in psychology and at least two years of clinical experience in a recognized health care setting or has the documented equivalent in education, training, and/or experience and is currently competent in the field.

**psychology**
The study of the mind and mental and emotional processes.

**psychometry**
The science of measuring mental and psychological functioning and capacity through the use of psychological tests.

**psychomotor**
Body activity or skills related to cerebral or psychic activity.

**psychopathic personality**
One who behaves in unacceptable ways. See antisocial personality.

**psychopathology**
1. The branch of psychology or psychiatry study that deals with mental illness. 2. The existence of emotional or mental illness.

**psychopharmacology**
The study of drugs and their effects on mental and behavioral processes.

**psychophysiological disorder**
Any emotional or mental disorder characterized by physical symptoms related to mental processes. Also known as psychosomatic illness. See these words.

**psychoprophylaxis**
A general term signifying psychological preparation to prevent pain.

**psychosis**
Mental illness where a person's mental awareness, emotional response, recognition of reality, communication and ability to relate to others are impaired enough to interfere with his capacity to deal with the ordinary

demands of life. The psychoses are subdivided into two major types: psychoses associated with organic brain syndromes and functional psychoses.

**psychosomatic illness**
Disease that shows a physical dysfunction or lesion in which psychological and other non-physical factors play a causative role, e.g., asthma, vasomotor rhinitis, peptic ulcer, colonic disorders, arterial hypertension, chronic urticaria, coronary disease and hyperthyroidism. Psychosomatic disorders should be distinguished from mental disorders and from the psychic effects of diseases which are not psychically caused. See psychophysiological.

**psychosurgery**
A surgical treatment procedure that causes the destruction of some region of the brain in order to alleviate severe and otherwise intractable mental disorders. The early and crude lobotomy has been replaced by advanced knowledge and techniques so that this type of psychiatric surgery is now replaced by psychosurgery. Psychosurgery is differentiated from brain surgery in that brain surgery is directed at repairing damaged brain tissue or alleviating symptoms resulting from tumors, accidents, infections or any other disorder where the cause of brain impairment is clear. Whereas psychosurgery includes the destruction of what appears to be normal and healthy brain tissue. This is done in order to eliminate or "cure" serious behavioral and emotional symptoms that other treatment modalities such as drug therapy and psychotherapy have been ineffectual in treating.

**psychotherapy**
A planned and organized treatment for mental illness and behavioral disturbances by a trained person through therapeutic intervention, both verbal and nonverbal, with attempts to remove emotional disturbance, change patterns of behavior, and encourage personality growth and development. Psychotherapy is distinguished from other forms of psychiatric treatment such as drugs, psychosurgery, electric shock treatment, and insulin coma treatment.

**psychotropic drug**
1. Any drug which affects psychic function, behavior or experience. These include, but are not limited to, those which produce drug dependence.

**public**
1. All persons of a society, community, state or nation. 2. A state, nation, or the community as a whole. 3. Affecting all persons.

**public (community) health educator**
A person with professional perparation in health sciences and education including training in the application of selected content from relevant medical, social and behavioral sciences used to educate and influence individuals and group behavior change, learning, mobilization of community health action, and the planning, implementation and evaluation of health education programs. The specific educational methods in which the public health educator is trained include communith organization, health content, communications, group work, and

consultation. Also included in his preparation are the public health sciences of epidemiology, biostatistics, environmental health, microbiology, and public health administration.

**public accountability**
See accountable.

**publication**
1. To make public. 2. A book or other published item provided to the public. 3. Communicating information to another person or party.

**publication of service**
A method of serving a summons by having it printed in a newspaper in an acceptable way.

**public deaths**
Those deaths which accidentally occur on property other than that of the victim.

**public defender**
A lawyer provided by the government to represent persons accused of a crime, who cannot afford a lawyer yet have a right to an attorney. See prosecutor.

**public domain**
1. Owned by the government. 2. Free for anyone's use. 3. Items that are not protected by a patent or a copyright.

**public health**
The science dealing with the protection and improvement of community health by organized community effort. Public health activities are generally those which are less amenable to being undertaken or less effective when undertaken on an individual basis, and do not typically include direct personal health services. Immunizations, sanitation, preventive medicine, quarantine and other disease control activities, occupational health and safety programs, assurance of the healthfulness of air, water and food, health education, and epidemiology are recognized public health activities.

**public health agency**
A governmental tax-supported organization mandated by law for the protection and promotion of the health of the public.

**public health education**
1. A term that is often used synonymously with community health education and refers to five basic phases or types of activities which include community analysis, sensitization, publicity, education and motivation conducted through a process involving health knowledge, awareness, prevention, promotion and motivation aimed at attitude and health behavior change. 2. A process designed to help improve and maintain health status of the general population.

**public health plan**

A plan of the public health department at the state and local levels that addresses the provision of health care services and public and environmental health to the residents of the state or area.

**Public Health Service Act (PHS Act)**

One of the principal Acts of Congress providing legislative authority for Federal health activities (42 U.S.C. 201-300). Originally enacted July 1, 1944 (and sometimes referred to as the Act of July 1), the PHS Act was, when enacted, a complete codification of all the accumulated federal public health laws. Since that time many of the Acts written in the health area, particularly by the Committee on Interstate and Foreign Commerce, have actually been amendments to the PHS Act; revising, extending or adding new authority to it (such as the HMO Act of 1973, P.L. 93-222, which added a new title XIII, and the Health Revenue Sharing and Health Services Amendments of 1975, P.L. 94-63, which revised many existing sections of the Act). A compilation of the PHS Act, as amended, and related Acts is published for public use by the Committee on Interstate and Foreign Commerce. Generally, the Act contains authority for public health programs, biomedical research, health manpower training, family planning, emergency medical services systems, HMOs, regulation of drinking water supplies, and health planning and resources development. See also quotes.

**publici juris (Lat.)**

1. Of public right. 2. Rights that are universal.

**public interest**

Anything that can have an effect on the general public.

**public law**

The area or class of law that deals with the government or the relationship between the government and individual or organizations; laws that deal with the government and public domain. Public law also deals with relationships between private parties and government. Law of the government as opposed to private law. Also it is referred to as administrative law.

**public patient**

See service and private patient.

**public policy**

Laws and general rules to determine public behavior or expectations; for the good of the public.

**publish**

To produce a publication. See publication.

**puffing**

1. Creating a belief or image to a patient or consumer that something is better than it actually is. 2. Intentional giving of misleading information.

**puisne**
A lower-level associated person. Associate subordinate; not a chief or superior.

**pulse**
The rhythmic, recurrent wave of blood in the arteries caused by the contraction of the left ventricle of the heart; used to measure the activity of the heart.

**pulse pressure**
The difference between the systolic and diastolic blood pressures.

**pulse rate**
The number of pulse beats per minute.

**pulse volume**
The force of the blood with each pulse beat.

**punitive damages**
1. Award made by a court to a person who has been harmed. 2. A large award given to serve as a punishment; the award often is not related to the actual cost of the injury or harm suffered, but its purpose is to prevent a similar act from happening again in the future. The money is given to the injured party as a warning to the party who caused the harm. See exemplary damages, recovery.

**purchase**
1. To legally buy or acquire by the giving of money. 2. A transaction creating an agreement to acquire property.

**purchase order**
1. A memo or paper authorizing a person to buy or deliver goods or perform services. 2. A promise to pay for goods or services in written form.

**purchasing and stores**
See materials management.

**purge**
1. To clean. 2. To clear from a charge. 3. To remove guilt. 4. To clear from a contract. 5. To eliminate; to clear a name.

**purport**
1. To act as if it is real. 2. To imply. 3. To profess. 4. To give an impression. 5. To present a false impression.

**pursuant**
1. According to; in accordance with. 2. The carrying out of an act with authority to do so; within the scope of responsibility of authority.

**purview**
1. The meaning, design or reason for a statute or other law. Range, scope or extent.

**putative**
1. To be alleged. 2. To be commonly known as. 3. A supposed occurrence or status.

**pyelogram**
A roentgenogram of the kidney and ureter, showing the pelvis of the kidney.

**pyromania**
A compulsion to set fires.

# Q

**Q-spoiled**
See Q-switched laser.

**Q-switched laser**
A pulsating laser capable of extremely high peak powers for very short durations.

**qua (Lat.)**
1. As. 2. In the capacity of. 3. Considered as. 4. In and of itself.

**quadrangular therapy**
Marital therapy that involves four people: the married couple and a therapist for each spouse.

**quadriplegia**
The paralysis of all four limbs of the body.

**quaere (Lat.)**
1. To query, doubt, question. 2. That which follows is open to question or doubt.

**qualification**
1. To be eligible. 2. Meeting certain requirements. 3. A restriction. 4. Putting limitations on something. 5. In health services, it is meeting standards for program eligibility, licensure, reimbursement or other benefits. Thus a qualified educational program meets accreditation standards, a qualified HMO (for the benefit of mandated dual-choice under section 1310 of the PHS Act) meets the standards imposed by the HMO Act, and a qualified provider for reimbursement by an insurance program meets its condition of participation.

**qualified acceptance**
An acceptance of an agreement or a deal which is limited or conditional.

**qualified administrator**
In JCAH long-term care facility accreditation, this is an individual who is currently licensed by the state in which practicing, if applicable, and is qualified by training and experience for the proper discharge of his or her delegated responsibilities. See health administration, health services administrator.

**qualified audiologist**
For JCAH accreditation of long term care facilities, this is an individual who is certified by the American Speech-Language-Hearing Association as clinically competent in the area of audiology, or who has documented equivalent training and/or experience.

**qualified dietetic service supervisor**
For JCAH accreditation of long term care facilities, this is an individual who is a qualified dietitian, or a graduate of either an approved dietetic technician or dietetic assistant training program or a state-approved course in food service supervision; or an individual who has documented equivalent training and/or experience.

**qualified dietitian**
1. According to JCAH for accreditation purposes, this is an individual who is registered by the Commission on Dietetic Registration of the American Dietetic Association, or has the documented equivalent in education, training, and experience, with evidence of relevant continuing education. 2. For JCAH accreditation of long-term care facilities, this is an individual who has at least a baccalaureate degree with major studies in food and nutrition, dietetics, or food service management; who has one year of internship/experience in the dietetic service of a health care institution; who participates annually in continuing education programs; and who is registered or eligible for registration by the American Dietetic Association; or an individual who has the documented equivalent in education, training, and experience.

**qualified impairment insurance**
A form of substandard or special class of insurance restricting benefits to a particular condition or injury.

**qualified medical radiation physicist**
According to JCAH for accreditation purposes, this is an individual who is certified by the American Board of Radiology in the appropriate disciplines of radiological physics, including diagnostic, therapeutic, and/or medical nuclear physics; or an individual who demonstrates equivalent competency in the disciplines.

**qualified medical record administrator**
1. According to JCAH for accreditation, this is a registered record administrator who has successfully passed an appropriate examination conducted by the American Medical Record Association, or who has the documented equivalent in education and training. 2. For JCAH accreditation of long term care facilities this is an individual who is eligible for certification as a registered record administrator (RRA) or an accredited record technician (ART) by the American Medical Record Association, or who is a graduate of a school of medical record science accredited jointly by the Committee on Allied Health Education and Accreditation (CAHEA) and the American Medical Record Association; or an individual who has documented equivalent training and/or experience.

**qualified medical record technician**
According to JCAH for accreditation this is an accredited record technician who has successfully passed the appropriate accreditation examination conducted by the American Medical Record Association, or who has the documented equivalent in education and training.

**qualified medical technologist**
According to JCAH for accreditation, this is an individual who is a graduate of a medical technology program approved by a nationally recognized body, or who has the documented equivalent in education, training, and/or experience; and who meets current legal requirements of licensure or registration; and who is currently competent in the field.

**qualified nurse anesthetist**
According to JCAH for accreditation, this is a registered nurse who has graduated from a school of nurse anesthesia accredited by the Council on Accreditation of Educational Programs of Nurse Anesthesia or its predecessor and has been certified or is eligible for certification as a nurse anesthetist by the Council on Certification of Nurse Anesthetists, or who has the documented equivalent in training and/or experience; and who meets any current legal requirements of licensure or registration; and who is currently competent in the field.

**qualified occupational therapist**
According to JCAH for accreditation, this is an individual who is a graduate of an occupational therapy program approved by a nationally recognized accrediting body, or who currently holds certification by the American Occupational Therapy Association as an Occupational Therapist, Registered, or who has the documented equivalent in training and/or experience; and who meets any current legal requirements of licensure or registration; and who is currently competent in the field.

**qualified patient activities coordinator**
For JCAH accreditation of long term care facilities this is an individual who is licensed or registered, if applicable, in the state in which practicing and is eligible for registration as a therapeutic recreation specialist by the National Therapeutic Recreation Society; or an individual who has had at least two years of experience in a social or recreational program within the last five years, one year of which was full-time in a patient/resident activities program in a health care setting; or an individual who is a qualified occupational therapist or occupational therapy assistant; or an individual who has the equivalent training and/or experience.

**qualified pharmacist**
For JCAH accreditation of long term care facilities this is an individual who is currently licensed to practice pharmacy by the state in which he or she is practicing and who has formal training or one year of experience in the specialized functions necessary in a long term care facility pharmaceutical service.

**qualified physiatrist**
For JCAH accreditation of long-term care facilities, this is a licensed physician who is certified or eligible for examination either by the American Board of Physical Medicine and Rehabilitation or by a specialty related to rehabilitation, or who has the documented equivalent in training and/or experience.

**qualified physical therapist**
According to JCAH for accreditation, this is an individual who is a graduate of a physical therapy program approved by a nationally recognized accrediting body, or who has the documented equivalent in training and/or experience; and who meets any current legal requirements of licensure or registration; and who is currently competent in the field.

**qualified psychologist**
For JCAH accreditation of long-term care facilities, this is an individual who has a master's or doctoral degree from a program in clinical psychology and has been licensed or certified by the examining board of the state in which practicing, or an individual with equivalent education and/or demonstrated experience.

**qualified radiologic technologist**
According to JCAH for accreditation, this is an individual who is a graduate of a program in radiologic technology approved by the Council on Medical Education of the American Medical Association, or who has the documented equivalent in education and training.

**qualified right**
Gives a person a right to do certain things for certain purposes and under certain circumstances.

**qualified social worker**
According to JCAH for accreditation, this is an individual who has met the requirements of a graduate curriculum in a school of social work, leading to a Master's degree, that is accredited by the Council on Social Work Education; or has the documented equivalent in education, training, and/or experience.

**qualified speech-language pathologist**
For JCAH accreditation of long-term facilities, this is an individual who is licensed by the state, if applicable, and has a Certificate of Clinical Competence in Speech Pathology or a Statement of Equivalence awarded by the American Speech-Language-Hearing Association; or an individual who has documented equivalent training and/or experience.

**qualify**
To become eligible.

**qualitative analysis**
Used to determine the quality or nature of the elements of a problem, compound or substance.

**quality**
1. A measure of the degree to which health services delivered to a patient, regardless of by whom or in what setting provided, resemble satisfactory delivery of services as determined by health professionals. Quality is frequently described as having three dimensions; quality of input resources, (e.g., certification and/or training of providers—both manpower and facility factors); quality of the process of service delivery (e.g., use of appropriate procedure for a given condition); and quality of outcome of service use (actual improvement in condition or reduction of

harmful effects). 2. The nature, kind or character of someone or something; hence, the degree or grade of excellence possessed by the person or thing. Quality may be measured: with respect to individual medical services, the various services received by individual or groups of patients, individual or groups of providers, or health programs or facilities; in terms of technical competence, humanity, need acceptability, appropriateness, inputs structure, process, or outcomes; using standards, criteria, norms or direct quantitative or qualitative measures. See also efficacy, effectiveness, PSRO, QAP, and tissue, medical, peer and utilization review.

**quality assessment**
Measuring or comparing the method or practice used with an accepted standard commonly used to determine the expected level or degree of excellence.

**quality assurance**
Activities and programs intended to assure the quality of care in a defined medical setting or program. Such programs must include educational or other components intended to remedy identified deficiencies in quality, as well as the components necessary to identify such deficiencies (such as peer or utilization review components) and assess the program's own effectiveness. A program which identifies quality deficiencies and responds only with negative sanctions, such as denial of reimbursement, is not usually considered as a quality assurance program, although the latter may include use of such sanctions. Such programs are required of HMOs and other health programs assisted under authority of the PHS Act (e.g., section 1301(c)(8)).

**Quality Assurance Program (QAP)**
A program developed by the American Hospital Association for use by hospital administrations and medical staffs in the development of a hospital program to assure the quality of the care given in the hospital.

**quality food**
Food which has been selected, prepared, and served in such a manner as to retain or enhance natural flavor and identity; to conserve nutrients; and to be acceptable, attractive, and microbiologically and chemically safe.

**quality of care**
As a measure or indication of the health care system, this is usually the degree of excellence or conformation to standards that the various components of the health care system adhere to. Quality of care in the health care setting usually is determined by the level of performance or abilities in efficiency of care, efficacy of care, access to care, satisfaction of care. Availability and acceptability of care may also be considered.

**quality of life**
The perception, belief or expectancy of individuals or groups that their health and personal needs are being satisfied without denying opportunities to achieve personal growth, well-being, happiness and fulfillment.

**quality of services**
The nature and grade of the services being provided to the residents of a particular area at a given point in time.

**quantify**
To measure or express in numbers.

**quantitative analysis**
Used to determine the quantity and nature of elements in a problem, substance or compound.

**quantity**
A goal and/or measure of any organization or of the health care system. That aspect of an organization or system to which measures apply and according to which, part of an organization or system can be compared one to another.

**quantity variance**
A method of determining how well the quantity of a resource was used or controlled; the difference between the actual quantities used and the budgeted quantities for production, multiplied by a standard price. Also called usage variance.

**quantum meruit (Lat.)**
1. As much as he merits or deserves. 2. Bringing suit based on an implied promise or an assumed contract.

**quantum valebat (Lat.)**
1. As much as they were worth. 2. A claim started in order to recover the cost of goods delivered based on an implied promise to pay.

**quarantine**
The limitation of freedom of movement of susceptible persons or animals that have been exposed to a communicable disease, in order to prevent spread of the disease; the place of detention of such persons or animals; or the act of detaining vessels or travelers suspected of having communicable diseases at ports or places for inspection or disinfection. See also public health.

**quare (Lat.)**
Wherefore.

**quare clausum fregit (Lat.)**
Wherefore he broke the close. A legal action against a trespass. This is used to recover damages by an unlawful entry or trespass.

**quash**
1. To make void. 2. To overthrow. 3. To annul. 4. To suppress. 5. To completely do away with.

**quasi (Lat.)**
1. To a certain degree. 2. Analogous to. 3. Almost. 4. As if. 5. Similar. 6. Kind of.

**quasi-contract**
1. An implied contract. 2. A promise with no expressed agreement. 3. A legal obligation imposed by law with the force and legal consequences of a contract. Used to prevent unfair personal gain at the unfair advantage or expense of others.

**quasi-judicial**
1. A semi-judicial case. 2. Deciding function of an administrative agency.

**query (Lat. quaere)**
Question; to question or ask; to inquire.

**queue**
To form into a line while waiting to be treated or served; a line or file of people or things to be served or brought into service.

**qui (Lat.)**
1. He or she. 2. He or she who. 3. One who commits an act.

**quia timet (Lat.)**
1. Because of fears. 2. A request from a court that is similar to an injunction. 3. To protect a person who fears he is in jeopardy.

**quick assets**
Anything that can be directly and immediately turned into cash.

**quid pro quo (Lat.)**
1. Something for something. 2. One thing of value given for another. 3. Consideration. 4. An exchange of items of similar value. 5. Something for something else; in exchange for. 6. Something required in return for another thing of like value. Used in the consideration of health manpower legislation to refer to requirements of health professional schools set as conditions of their receiving federal capitation payments.

**quiescent**
Silent; dormant; inactive, as in a letter or document being silent or inactive.

**quiet**
1. Inactive. 2. Having no interference. 3. Undisturbed.

**quit**
1. To leave a position of employment. 2. To give up possession of a place or position. 3. To end a relationship. 4. To discontinue or stop something.

**quo ad hoc (Lat.)**
1. To this extent. 2. With respect to the following.

**quo animo (Lat.)**
With what intention or motive. See animus.

**quod (Lat.)**
1. That. 2. That which.

**quod bene notandum (Lat.)**
Which may be especially noticed.

**quod erat demonstrandum (Lat.)**
That which was to be proven or demonstrated.

**quod vide (Lat.)**
1. Look at. 2. Which see. 3. Used to refer the reader to something. Abbreviated q.v. Most legal references on law books use the letters Q.V., which means "see that word."

**quorum**
The required number of persons needed or who must be present at a meeting to take action or function legally as a group and for business that was taken care of to be valid. The number required is often a majority of over half of the Board of Directors, governing body, etc.

**quo warranto (Lat.)**
1. To show by what right one has the authority to do an act. 2. With what authority. 3. Legally questioning of the right of a person to undertake an act or to hold an office.

**Q.V. (Lat.)**
Quod vide. "See that word."

# R

**rabbi**
A Jewish person ordained to conduct professional religious activity and provide leadership in Jewish religious ceremonies.

**race statute**
The one who first files a claim on or interest in real property and has prior legal right to that claim. See recording statute.

**rad**
The standard unit or measure of radioactive dose. It supersedes the roentgen. The Atomic Energy Commission has established conservative limits of exposure for the protection of workers around radiation.

**radiation (radioactivity)**
The emission of very fast atomic particles, or rays. Some elements are naturally radioactive while others become radioactive after bombardment with a radioactive material.

**radiation safety**
Actions taken to protect the community from unnecessary exposure to ionizing and non-ionizing radiation from controllable industrial and nuclear sources, and to minimize exposure of patients and medical personnel to clinical radiation.

**radiation therapy technologist**
Working from the prescription and instructions of a physician, radiation therapy technologists use x-ray and electron beam equipment in the therapeutic treatment of disease. They expose specific areas of the body to prescribed doses of ionizing radiations, observe and report patient reactions, and assist in tumor localization and dosimetric procedures. They assist in maintaining the proper operation of controlling devices and equipment, observe safety measures for patients and clinical personnel, and may keep or share in keeping patient records, as well as assisting in the preparation and handling of radioactive materials used in treatment procedures. Nearly all radiation therapy technologists are employed in hospitals or clinics.

**radio-**
Prefix, meaning rays; x-rays; radius.

**radioactivity**
Emission of energy in the form of alpha, beta, or gamma radiation. A few elements, such as radium, are naturally radioactive. Other radioactive forms are induced.

**radiochemical**
Any compound, substance or mixture containing a sufficient amount of radioactivity to be detected by a Geiger counter.

**radiodiagnosis**
A diagnostic procedure which involves x-ray examination.

**radiographer**
Formerly called x-ray technicians and often called radiologic technologists, specialize in the use of x-radiation and other ionizing radiations in order to assist the physician in the diagnosis of disease or injury. Under the general direction of a physician, usually a radiologist, radiographers are primarily responsible for the operation of x-ray equipment and preparation of patients for various types of diagnostic procedures. Radiographers prepare radio-opaque mixtures administered to patients so that internal organs may be observed and identified on film, position patients, adjust x-ray equipment to correct settings, and determine proper voltage, current, and exposure time for the production of radiographs. They assist the radiologist in fluoroscopic procedures and are responsible for maintaining equipment in proper working order, processing film, and keeping patient records. Although examinations are normally conducted in the hospital or a physician's office, radiographers are also capable of operating mobile x-ray equipment at the patient's bedside or in the hospital operating room. The extent of the services provided by the radiographer varies with employment setting and other circumstances. In some states the range of duties of the radiographer is limited by law, e.g., they are prohibited from injecting contrast media into patients. In most locations, however, the range of duties is determined by the hospital, clinic, or other place of employment. In still other situations, the range of duties is determined by the physician responsible for radiographic diagnosis. See qualified radiologic technologists.

**radioimmunoassay**
Antibody reaction based on the use of a radioactively labeled substance which reacts with the substance being tested (e.g., hepatitis antigen).

**radiological warfare**
The purposeful use of radioactively contaminated materials as a weapon of offense in a nuclear war.

**radiologic technologist or technician**
An individual who maintains and safely uses equipment and supplies necessary to demonstrate portions of the human body on x-ray film or fluoroscopic screen for diagnostic purposes, and may supervise and/or teach other radiologic personnel. Approximately one-third of these persons work for hospitals, while the remainder work for independent x-ray laboratories, multi-specialty clinics, in physician's offices, and in government agencies. American Medical Association Council on Medical Education approved radiologic technology programs are conducted by hospitals and medical schools and by community colleges with hospital affiliation. Programs are open to high school graduates, although a few require 1 or 2 years of college or graduation from a school of nursing. The length of training varies from a minimum of 2 years in a hospital

radiology department, or a junior college in affiliation with one or more hospitals offering an associate degree, to a 4-year university course. See qualified radiologic technologist.

**radiology**
A branch of the medical profession which uses ionizing radiation for radiodiagnosis and therapy.

**radiology department**
This clinical department found in health care facilities is under the direct administration of a radiologist who is a physician. Also employed in the radiology department are radiologic technologists, who take x-rays, and could also include nuclear medicine and radiation therapy.

**radio-opaque**
Being visible to x-ray. Substances that make body structures visible or opaque are iodine and barium salts.

**radiotherapy**
Treatment of human disease or disorders with the application of relatively high dosages of radiation.

**radium $^{226}_{88}$ Ra**
The most common of 11 isotopes with a half life of 1602 to 1622 years. A metallic radioactive element found in pitchblende, which exists in a continuous state of disintegration; this makes it useful in treating disease, because it kills cells, especially young, immature, actively growing, abnormal cells such as cancer cells, leukemia cells, etc. (226 is the atomic weight and 88 is the atomic number.)

**radon $^{222}_{86}$ Rn**
One of 23 isotopes with a half life of 3.8 days. It is a radioactive gas, which results as a by-product of radium disintegration. (222 is the atomic weight and 86 is the atomic number.)

**rad. tech.**
See radiographer.

**raise an issue**
To present a concern or an issue. The presentation of a claim in a pleading, the trial proceeding or litigation process.

**raison d'etre (French)**
Reason for being.

**rale**
An abnormal sound heard in a patient's breathing, resembling a rattling or bubbling sound, usually heard on inspiration.

**random**
A statistical term that means that a subject was selected by chance or without any selection or planning.

**random controlled trial (RCT)**

An experimental prospective study for assessing the effects of a particular drug or medical procedure in which subjects (human or animal) are assigned on a random basis to either of two groups, experimental and control. The experimental group receives the drug or procedure while the control group does not. A series of laboratory tests and clinical examinations are performed on both groups in an attempt to detect any difference, usually using the double blind technique. The goals of these studies for drugs are to determine: how the drug is absorbed, metabolized and eliminated; levels of the drug that are tolerated; any obvious toxic effects; long-run toxic and carcinogenic effects; the effectiveness of the drug in prevention or control of a disease or symptom; and the safe and appropriate dosage of the drug for the various patients in whom it will be used.

**range**

1. In statistics, a measure of variation determined by the end values. 2. The distance between the highest and lowest number or values in a series of numbers or observations.

**range of motion (R.O.M.)**

The extent of movement within a given joint, and motion in a joint is achieved through the action of muscles or groups of muscles. Each joint has a normal range. A range of motion of particular importance in rehabilitation is the functional range. This is the range which is less than normal but which enables the limited joint or combination of joints to be functional for performing activities of daily living.

**rape**

1. To take by force. 2. Forceful sexual intercourse with an unwilling woman. A serious crime.

**rapport**

A harmonious accord that shows good relationship between two persons. In a group, it is the mutual responsiveness, as shown by spontaneous and sympathetic understanding of each other's needs.

**raspatory**

A surgical instrument that is a file-like device used to scrape bone surface; a rasp.

**rate**

1. A fixed amount, usually based on a formula or adjustable fee based on a set standard. 2. A regular or usual fee that is charged to all persons for the same service or care. 3. That figure expressed as a ratio that indicates the number of incidents of any given occurrence as they relate to the population of an area, e.g., 20 deaths:1,000 live births.

**rate fixing**

The power to control fees, set charges or control the rate or exchanges that a hospital, health care facility or company may get for its services.

**rates, adjusted or standardized**
Used in vital statistics, these rates are used to compare two population groups in which the age distribution differs.

**ratification**
1. The formal approval of a document. 2. Confirmation of an act. 3. Adoption by proper authority of a proposed action.

**rating**
In insurance, the process of determining rates, or the cost of insurance, for individuals, groups or classes of risks.

**ratio decidendi (Lat.)**
1. The basic and essential issue used in deciding a case. 2. The major reason for or the determining factor in a decision.

**rational behavior therapy (training) (RBT)**
A highly directive form of psychotherapy embracing the cognitive-behavioral areas of psychology used to teach people to have better skill in reasoning, thus having less emotional upset and are better able to cope with problems and stressors of life. Rational and logical thinking enables people to keep their emotions under control. Therefore, through the use of the scientific approach to problem solving, one can see problems more clearly and solve them more effectively. RBT is derived from learning theory and behavior therapy, but goes beyond the mechanical conditioning of reflexes. See rational self-counseling.

**rational emotive therapy (RET)**
This form of psychotherapy contrasts with psychoanalysis, behavior therapy and other related theories. It utilizes an A-B-C theory of personality disturbance (A = activating event, B = belief system, C = disturbed emotional consequences) which helps a person with emotional problems to overcome inappropriate feelings and behaviors in a relatively brief period of time. It employs several methods in the cognitive, emotional and behavioral areas while creating a philosophical view of life. It has also been referred to as a cognitive-behavioral therapy. (Developed by Albert Ellis, Ph.D. psychologist.)

**rationalization**
A mental or defense mechanism in which a person justifies feelings, behavior, and motives that would otherwise be intolerable.

**rational self analysis**
This is the homework behavioral therapy aspect of rational behavioral therapy and rational self counseling that gets the patient/client actively involved in his or her own therapy/treatment program. RSAs help the patient/client to engage in calm, objective self analysis as opposed to emotionally charged, distorted decisions. RSAs help separate feelings from thoughts, thus being able to have an objective view of events. RSAs rely on an A-B-C-D approach to events or upsetting situations, where self talk, emotions and facts are separated out. A = facts and are compared to B, which is the self-talk about the event, C = feelings and emotions,

D = irrational self-talk is compared to "B". Emotions are compared to the facts.

**rational self counseling (RSC)**
Rational self counseling is a personal approach to rational behavioral therapy, which is a constant and continual process that the patient or client does in everyday living to overcome mental, emotional and behavioral problems. A rational self analysis is done to help the patient or client learn to be a more rational person, thus having less emotional upset and fewer self-defeating behaviors.

**ravish**
To rape. To hold or take a person into the care of another person by illicit means. (The latter is an outdated usage.)

**raw data**
Facts that are processed by a computer in order to produce new data or information.

**R.D.**
Registered dietician. See these words.

**re (Lat.)**
Concerning. See also in re.

**reaction formation**
A mental or defense mechanism wherein attitudes and behavior are adopted that are the opposites of beliefs or impulses the individual has.

**readiness**
The state of being ready; maturation and growth needed to be able to perform some activities, such as learning, referred to as readiness to learn.

**ready and willing**
Suggests not only one's ability and capacity to do certain acts or behaviors, but also having a disposition to do them.

**real**
1. Pertaining to land and things on land. 2. Denoting a tangible item rather than a person.

**real evidence**
Actual objects used to prove fact, used for evidence and shown to a judge or jury, such as x-rays, medical records, items or objects used in a crime, wounds, fingerprints, etc.

**reality**
Having an objective view of things and factual events.

**reality-orientation**
A form of therapy used on withdrawn persons or those who have given up. James C. Folsom first organized a "reality-orientation program" in Winter Veterans Administration Hospital in Topeka, Kansas, in 1958. The bulk of the work was done by nursing assistants who spend the

most time with the patients. Folsom believes patients are not ready for remotivation until they have gone through the reality-orientation classes. The program is ideally suited for patients who have been institutionalized for long periods of time or have moderate to severe organic brain impairment. The treatment involves having patients presented with basic personal and current information over and over to each patient, beginning with the patient's name, where he is, and the date. Only when he has relearned these basic facts is the patient presented with other facts such as his age, home town, and former occupation, family, etc.

**reality principle**
In psychoanalytic theory, the construct that pleasure represents the instinctual wishes of a person and is normally modified by the demands, expectations and requirements of society.

**reality testing**
To constantly evaluate the world around you so as to differentiate adequately between reality and the appearance of reality of one's internal world; between self and non-self.

**reality therapy**
A form of psychotherapy based somewhat on psychiatric theory. It leads patients toward reality and toward grappling successfully with the tangible and intangible aspects of the real world; a therapy toward reality. Developed by William Glasser, M.D., a psychiatrist.

**realize**
1. To make real. 2. To convert into monetary form. 3. To cash in.

**realized**
The act of having something come to you either by an understanding or to receive money or property.

**realized profit**
The actual possession of money gained or profits earned and available.

**real time**
The actual time used by a computer. The actual time taken to perform a computation on a computer.

**reasonable**
1. Denoting a decision based on the facts of a situation or case rather than on an abstract legal principle. 2. Possessing the ability to think clearly. 3. Being able to reach sound and competent conclusions. 4. Acting in a sound or sensible manner.

**reasonable act**
Any act that may fairly, justly, and reasonably be expected or required of a party or person.

**reasonable assistance**
Aid and care given in emergencies by one capable of providing basic emergency care.

**reasonable care**

That amount of knowledge and skill ordinarily used by a competent health care provider with equal experience and education in treating and caring for the sick and injured. See reasonable man, standard of care.

**reasonable charge**

For any specific service covered under Medicare, the lower of the customary charge by a particular physician for that service and the prevailing charge by physicians in the geographic area for that service. Reimbursement is based on the lower of the reasonable and actual charges. The term is used for any charge payable by an insurance program which is determined in a similar, but not necessarily identical fashion. See also comparability provision and section 224.

**reasonable cost**

Generally the amount which a third party using cost-related reimbursement will actually reimburse. Under Medicare reasonable costs are costs actually incurred in delivering health services excluding any part of such incurred costs found to be unnecessary for the efficient delivery of needed health services (see section 1861 of the Social Security Act). The law stipulates that, except for certain deductible and coinsurance amounts that must be paid by beneficiaries, payments to hospitals shall be made on the basis of the reasonable cost of covered care. The regulations require that costs be apportioned between Medicare beneficiaries and other hospital patients so that neither group subsidizes the costs of the other. The items or elements of cost, both direct and indirect, which the regulations specify as reimbursable are known as allowable costs. Such costs are reimbursable on the basis of a hospital's actual costs to the extent that they are reasonable and are related to patient care. Under certain conditions the following items may be included as allowable costs: capital depreciation; interest expenses; educational activities; research costs related to patient care; unrestricted grants, gifts and income from endowments; value of services of non-paid workers, compensation of owners; payments to related organizations; return on equity capital of proprietary providers; and the inpatient routine nursing differential. Bad debts may only be included to the extent institutions fail in good faith efforts to collect the debts. See also section 223.

**reasonable doubt**

Knowledge of facts which induces doubt in the mind of an ordinary and prudent person.

**reasonable man (person)**

1. A theoretical ordinary person who possesses the same physical characteristics of the defendant, who possesses foreseeability and who is of good judgment. 2. An expected standard of behavior. 3. An ideal person possessing the same characteristics and physical makeup of any average person with emotional status making no difference. See ordinary person, foreseeability, standard of care.

**reasonableness doctrine**

See reasonable man.

**reasonably prudent man doctrine**
A person who uses ordinary care and skill. See reasonable man.

**rebate**
Money given back at the end of a transaction; a discount.

**rebus sic stantibus (Lat.)**
At this point of affairs. In international law, a phrase often used to terminate an agreement due to a change of circumstances; if an agreement continues, the results would not be of the agreeing parties.

**rebut**
1. To dispute. 2. To defeat the effect. 3. To oppose. 4. To answer to. 5. To take away the effect of the evidence of an argument.

**rebuttable**
Disputable; debatable.

**rebuttal**
The act of refuting through argumentation, by evidence or proof.

**rebutting evidence**
Evidence used to disprove evidence introduced by the opposing party.

**recall**
The process of recollecting thoughts, words, and actions of a past event in an attempt to remember what actually happened.

**recall judgment**
To revoke or reverse a judgment.

**recaption**
1. To recover that which was removed. 2. To take back that which was given away or taken.

**receipt**
1. A printed or written acknowledgment of payment for an object, item or good that has been received. 2. The act of getting or receiving.

**receive evidence**
To admit evidence.

**receiver**
1. One who takes or holds property or items of value. 2. A person appointed by a court to hold and manage money or property. 3. One who accepts stolen goods.

**receiver pendiente lite**
A non-involved or impartial person appointed by the court during litigation to manage, oversee or hold money and accounts or in bankruptcy or foreclosure.

**receivership**
1. Being in the hands of a receiver. 2. Having business affairs taken over by a receiver appointed by a court. A court placing money or property into the hands of a receiver to preserve it for those entitled to it.

**receiving stolen goods**
To purchase or possess any property know to be stolen; a crime.

**recess**
The stopping of a court proceeding for a short period of time. A break in legal proceedings.

**recidivism**
To continually back or support criminal or antisocial behavior, habits, or activities.

**recidivist**
1. A repeating offender. 2. A habitual or continued lawbreaker.

**reciprocal**
An offer made by each side or by each other; a mutual action.

**reciprocate**
To give and take in exchange; to interchange or give something in return.

**reciprocity**
1. In licensure of health manpower, the recognition by one state of the licenses of a second state when the latter state extends the same recognition to licenses of the former state. Licensing requirements in the two states must usually be equivalent before formal or informal reciprocal agreements are made. Reciprocity is often used interchangeably with the term endorsement. 2. The act, process or principles of law where a state allows the same or similar privileges to citizens from another state. 3. An agreement where states exchange privileges or penalties. 4. A mutual and reciprocal agreement.

**recission**
1. In the federal budget, enacted legislation cancelling budget authority previously provided by Congress. Recissions proposed by the President must be transitted in a special message to the Congress. Under section 1012 of the Congressional Budget and Impoundment Control Act of 1974, unless Congress approves a recission bill within forty-five days of continuous session, the budget authority in question must be made available for obligation. 2. In insurance, cancellation, with repayment of premiums of a policy.

**recission of contract**
The rescinding or annulment of a contract. See rescind.

**recital**
An official written statement explaining the purpose and meaning of a document or the reason for the transaction that the document covers.

**recite**
1. To tell in detail. 2. To relate facts of a case. 3. To repeat from memory.

**reckless**
Negligent; careless; not heeding the consequences of one's actions.

**recognition**
1. The identification of facts, evidence, or a object previously known or seen. 2. Formal approval. 3. Items or acts that come under the scrutiny of the law. 4. An item or incident that is recognized by law.

**recognizance**
1. A legal agreement to do a particular act. 2. A type of bail bond used so a person will be obligated to appear in court at a later date. 3. An obligation that is a part of a court record.

**recommended actions and implementation strategies**
The methods and/or techniques to be utilized by health planning in the accomplishment of the stated goals.

**reconcile**
1. To restore a relationship. 2. To adjust or settle differences. 3. To make consistent.

**reconciliation**
1. The restoration of a broken or disrupted relationship. A settlement or adjustment of differences or disagreements.

**reconsideration (Medicare)**
A review of an unfavorable claims adjudication for institutional care (Part A) upon request of beneficiary, his representatives or the provider. Request for reconsideration is made to the intermediary.

**record (noun)**
1. An official report of public acts that is written, printed or published, such as a court record or legislative record. 2. A body of facts that is known and preserved. 3. A formal written account of a case including a written history of actions taken, evidence shown, documents filed, decisions made and opinions written.

**record (verb)**
1. To officially write out in permanent form. 2. To register. To mark or make an indication in written form.

**record linkage**
The method or technique of gathering and the pulling together of information about health care services and other related health events for one patient from many different sources, such as hospital stays, immunizations and visits to physicians. This scattered information is brought together in a common file or record, usually through the use of a computer.

**recoup**
1. To recover or regain. 2. To make a note or agreement good. 3. To repay or reimburse.

**recoupment**
A deduction from a sum owed to a plantiff which deduction grows out of the same transaction between the parties and is based on the plaintiff's failure to fully perform on a contract.

**recourse**
1. The right to receive payment on a negotiable instrument from anyone who has endorsed it if the person who created it fails to make payment. 2. An appeal for aid or protection. 3. Legal avenues that can be used to recover damages.

**recover**
1. To receive compensation for damages through the judgment of a court. 2. To win a lawsuit. 3. To get back or make up for Losses or damage through legal means. 4. Money being paid for damages.

**recovery**
1. The act of regaining a loss. 2. When a lawsuit is decided in your favor it is the amount of money or award given in a judgment upon winning a lawsuit.

**recreational therapist**
1. A person who directs recreational activities in long-term care facilities or recreation centers for special populations such as the elderly, retarded or mentally ill. The activities provide a means of therapy and socialization. Some states refer to this person as an activity director, which is somewhat of a misnomer. 2. A professional person who plans, organizes, and directs medically approved recreation programs such as sports, trips, dramatics, arts or crafts inorder to assist patients in recovering from physical or mental illness and in coping with temporary or permanent disability.

**recreational therapy**
A new type of therapeutic modality that activates social interactions, leisure, crafts, arts and enjoyment in a therapeutic sense. The recreational therapist is concerned with all dimensions of the total person with the aim of providing rehabilitation. The recreational therapist helps patients in nursing homes, state hospitals or other long-term care facilities.

**recreational therapy technician**
This technician assists the recreational therapist in conducting medically approved recreational programs, such as exercise programs dramatics, arts, and crafts.

**recrimination**
The act of answering an accusation or a charge brought by another person; a counter claim.

**rectal digital examination**
An examination procedure where the health care provider uses a gloved finger to examine the innermost areas of the rectum for diagnostic purposes.

**rectal tube**
A tube inserted into a patient's rectum and/or colon to help in the expelling of gas.

**recuperate**
1. To regain. 2. To recover.

**recurring clause**
A provision in some health insurance policies which specifies a period of time during which the recurrence of a condition is considered a continuation of a prior period of disability or hospital confinement rather than a separate spell of illness.

**recusation**
The procedure of disqualifying a judge from a lawsuit because of personal vested interest or bias.

**redeem**
1. To repurchase. 2. To reclaim property. 3. To make good. 4. To turn in for cash. 5. To rescue.

**redemption**
1. To turn in for cash. 2. A seller's right to buy back from the buyer an item sold, at an agreed-upon price.

**redress**
1. To receive reparation or indemnity. 2. To receive satisfaction or compensation from injury or harm done. 3. Payment provided for harm done.

**reductio ad absurdum (Lat.)**
1. Reduce to the absurd. 2. Showing issue or argument that leads to an unfounded and absurd conclusion.

**redundancy**
1. The use of excessive and extraneous material in a pleading or document. 2. To be redundant. 3. Exceeding what is needed; too wordy.

**redundant**
1. Excessive; more than enough. 2. Overabundant, repetitious.

**refer**
1. To direct attention to. 2. Turning a case over to another lawyer. 3. To direct a patient to a professional who has specialized qualifications or has been appointed to, or has more knowledge of the problem or disorder; to direct to.

**referee**
1. An official appointed to hear arguments or arbitrate disputes. 2. An arbitrator.

**referee in bankruptcy**
A federal level judge appointed to hear and judge bankruptcy cases.

**reference**
1. The act of submitting a matter for settlement. 2. Any promise written into a contract where a party will agree to submit certan disputes to arbitration; sending a case to a referee for a decision. 3. To provide information about one's character, credit or qualifications.

**reference projection**
Forecasts of expected future levels, on various types of health planning data, if no actions are taken to alter current activities and commitments. Reference projections include data such as indicators, related demographic and environmental factors, resources, financial factors and health service utilization. The health status health systems, services and resources presented by the reference projection is sometimes termed the Base Case for a particular population.

**referendum**
Placing a proposed law, or repeal of a law, to the vote of the people rather than enacting it through the legislative process.

**referent**
That which is referred to.

**referral**
The practice of sending a patient to another practitioner or to another program for services or consultation. The referring source is not prepared or qualified to provide. In contrast to referral for consultation, referral for services involves a delegation of responsibility for patient care to another practitioner or program, and the referring source may or may not follow up to ensure that services are received. As a physician sends a patient to another physician or health care provider who is a specialist, the referring physician turns over primary responsibility for health care of the patient from one physician to another; in insurance, is not considered a consultation.

**referral protocols**
Those procedures that are followed when referring patients from one service or health care professional to another.

**referred pain**
Pain which is felt in one area but the source of pain is from another area, such as a kidney pain may be referred to the back muscles.

**reflex**
An involuntary activity as a response to a stimulus.

**reformation**
1. The process used by a court for the changing of a written agreement which is usually done for the legal betterment of all involved. 2. To reform or change a written agreement for the better.

**refreshing memory**
1. Used to help a witness remember. 2. The use of documents or items to help remind a witness of details.

**refund**
To give back, to repay.

**refunding**
1. To refinance a debt. 2. The act of returning money for an unacceptable or damaged item or goods.

**refute**
To use argument, discussion or evidence to disprove statements or facts.

**regeneration**
Renewal of damaged or lost cells or tissues.

**regimen**
A regulated pattern of activity; a planned treatment or therapy program.

**regional issues**
Concerns identified by regional groups (subareas) which are considered as being important to them.

**Regional Medical Program (RMP)**
An old and former program of federal support for regional organizations, called regional medical programs, created to improve the care for heart disease, cancer, strokes and related diseases. Created by P.L. 89-239, which is found in title IX of the PHS Act. The programs were heavily oriented towards initiating and improving continuing education, nursing services, and intensive care units. Some features of the RMP program were combined into the health planning program authorized by P.L. 93-641 (see health systems agencies).

**register**
1. A record of vital statistics and public facts such as births, deaths and marriages. 2. The public official who keeps vital records. 3. To record information.

**registered**
1. Facts or information recorded in an official record. 2. To have one's name recorded in a public record or with a legally created office that shows one's legal approval to practice a profession, such as a registered nurse. See licensing, certification and registration.

**registered dietitian (R.D.)**
An A.D.A. dietitian who has successfully completed the examination for registration and maintains registration by meeting continuing education requirements. In providing nutritional care, the R.D. applies the science and art of human nutrition in helping people select and obtain food for the primary purpose of nourishing their bodies in health or disease throughout the life cycle. This participation may be in single or combined functions; in food service systems management; in extending knowledge of food and nutrition principles; in teaching these principles for application according to particular situations; or in dietary counseling. See clinical dietitian.

**registered nurse (RN)**
1. A nurse who has graduated from a formal program of nursing education (see diploma school, associate degree and baccalaureate programs) and been licensed by appropriate state authority. Registered nurses are the most highly educated of nurses with the widest scope of responsibility, including, all aspects of nursing care. 2. According to JCAH for accreditation, this is a nurse who is a graduate of an approved school of nursing and who is licensed to practice as a

registered nurse. See nurse, licensed practical nurse, nurse practitioner and nurse anesthetist.

**registered physical therapist (RPT)**
A person trained, and licensed in physical therapy, to treat disability, injury and disease by external physical means, such as massage, exercise, heat, light, etc. See qualified physical Therapist

**registered records administrator**
Registered records administrators plan, develop, and administer medical record systems for public, private, and military health care facilities. They collect and analyze patient and institutional data, as well as creating and implementing policies and procedures for the collection, storage, retrieval, and release of data for medical, administrative, legal, and research purposes. In smaller facilities a medical record administrator might be hired on a consultant basis to oversee the facility's own staff. In some agencies or institutions, tasks described as those of the administrator might be performed by technicians. In large hospitals, chief medical records administrators direct and coordinate all medical records staff activities, including supervision, training, systems planning, administration, and data analyses. In larger settings, the medical records administrator functions in a more complex professional and administrative role, responsible for planning and developing records systems that meet the standards of a variety of accrediting and regulatory agencies. The administrator designs health record abstracting systems used by staff and researchers and directs the preparation of indexes as well as the collection and analysis of data. Frequently the administrator manages, supervises, and trains the staff to perform subtasks ranging from transcription to analysis. He or she joins hospital management staff in the developement of patient information systems, departmental budgets, and institutional policies, and participates in utilization reviews and the evaluation of patient care services. Employment settings beyond the large hospital include outpatient clinics, ambulatory care centers, health maintenance organizations, nursing homes, professional standards review organizations, government and insurance agencies, universities, colleges, and research centers. See R.R.A., qualified Medical records administrated

**registered respiratory therapist**
According to JCAH for accreditation purposes, this is an individual who has been registered by the National Board for Respiratory Therapy, Inc., after successfully completing all education, experience, and examination requirements.

**registrar**
An official with authority to keep official records.

**registration**
1. The act of recording. 2. The act of creating a special list of people's names. 3. The act of entering names or facts on a list. 4. The process by which qualified individuals are listed on an official roster maintained by a governmental or non-governmental agency. Standards for registration may include such things as successful completion of a written examination given by a registry, membership in a professional association mantaining

the registry, and education and experience such as graduation from an approved program or equivalent experience. Registration is a form of credentialing, similar to certification. Registration is also used to describe the recording of notifiable diseases, or the listing and follow-up of patients with such diseases.

**registry**
A list of individuals who have given explicit indication (for instance by contracting for membership) that they use or rely upon a given health professional or program (whose registry it is) for the services that the professional or program is able to provide. Panel is sometimes used in preference to registry with respect to individual practitioners. The nature of the actual financial and other relationships between a program and the people on its registry are quite variable. Registry also refers to an organization which conducts a registration program for health manpower or the list of individuals such an organization has registered. See also catchment area, enrollment, roster and register.

**regression**
A defense mechanism in which a person mentally returns to earlier thoughts or behaviors.

**regressive tax**
A tax which takes a decreasng proportion of income as income rises, such as sales taxes and the social security payroll tax on earnings above the maximum to which the tax applies. This tax is a constant percentage of income up to the maximum level (wage base) or a proportional tax up to that level. See also progressive tax and marginal tax rate.

**regular**
1. By established rule or order. 2. A usual custom. 3. Steady; uniform; with no unusual deviation or variations. 4. Lawfully conforming to usual practice.

**regular medical expense insurance**
Insurance coverage which provides benefits through payment towards the cost of health services such as doctor fees for non-surgical care that can be in the hospital, at home, or in a physician's office. This also includes x-rays or laboratory tests performed outside of the hospital or other health care facility.

**regulate**
1. To control. 2. To adjust to a standard. 3. To govern according to predetermined rules to keep in proper order.

**regulation**
1. A rule that is created by a branch of government, usually an administrative agency. 2. A rule or a law created by an administrative agency to put forth the specific rules of a statute. 3. The fine details of a statute in health care, which are usually made by a specific health agency and mandated by the proper official lawmaking body. 4. The intervention of government or accreditation associations in the health system by means of rules and regulations which typically influence, control or set standards

relative to the services provided within the health system, which involves the settings, the resources, The services provided, and the manner in which providers of service are reimbursed. 5. The intervention of government in the health care or health insurance market to control entry into or change the behavior of participants in that marketplace through specification of rules for the participants, but does not usually include programs which seek to change behavior through financing mechanisms or incentives. Which regulation does not include private accreditation programs. They may be relied upon by government regulatory programs, as is the Joint Commission on Accreditation of Hospitals and Medicare. Regulatory programs include some certification, some registration, licensure, certificate of need, and the ESP, MAC and PSRO programs. Also, a synonym for a rule published by the executive branch of the federal government implementing a law.

**regulatory agency**
Any agency or subagency of the government which creates regulations and enforces them to control any health or other related activity in a particular area; for example, the federal Food and Drug Administration, county health departments.

**rehabilitate**
1. To restore to a former state, rank or privilege. 2. To restore health and physical strength to a patient.

**rehabilitation**
1. To restore rights, powers, privileges or authority. 2. To clear the character or reputation of a person. 3. Restoration of form and function following an illness or injury. 4. The combined and coordinated use of medical, social, educational and vocational measures for training or re-training individuals disabled by disease or injury to the highest possible level of functional ability. Several different types of rehabilitation are distinguished (vocational, social, medical and educational). Habilitation is used for similar activities undertaken for individuals born with limited functional ability as compared with people who have lost abilities because of disease or injury (see developmental disability). A rehabilitation center is a health program specializing in rehabilitation. 5. The procedures, treatment, therapies and techniques used to achieve maximal function and optimal adjustment for a patient in order to prevent relapses or recurrences of his condition or disability. Rehabilitation is to activate the patient's abilities, self-belief and recoverable functions, which includes individual and group psychotherapy, directed socialization, vocational retraining, education, physical therapy, occupational therapy and recreational therapy.

**rehabilitation counselor**
The rehabilitation counselor works with disabled persons and assists them in locating and securing rehabilitation services designed to equip them for employment, and follows up on job satisfaction after placement.

**rehabilitation counselor aide**
Under the supervision of the rehabilitation counselor, this individual assists in developing and implementing a rehabilitation plan for clients.

Specifically, the aide may conduct interviews, locate employment opportunities, match clients with available jobs, and locate individuals in need of counseling or rehabilitation services.

**rehabilitative services**
Services provided to restore and/or improve lost function following illness, injury or disease.

**rehearing**
To hold a second hearing on a matter previously decided. This is done to allow evidence previously omitted to be presented, or to correct errors.

**reimbursement**
The paying back of monies expended to provide health care services.

**reinstate**
To return to a place, state or condition that has been lost or revoked. To restore to a former position.

**reinstatement**
1. The returning or starting up again of insurance coverage under an insurance policy that has lapsed. 2. To allow insurance coverage to be returned once revoked or discontinued.

**reinsurance**
The practice of one insurance company buying insurance from a second company for the purpose of protecting itself against part or all of the losses it might incur in the process of honoring the claims of its policyholders. The original company is called the ceding company; the second is the assuming compay or reinsurer. Reinsurance may be sought by the ceding company for several reasons: to protect itself against losses in individual cases beyond a certain amount, where competition requires it to offer policies providing coverage in excess of these amounts; to offer protection against catastrophic losses in a certain line of insurance, such as aviation accident or polio insurance; or to protect against mistakes in rating and underwriting in entering a new line of insurance such as major medical.

**relapsing fever**
When a high temperature returns to normal for one or more days and then returns to a feverish state.

**related factor**
Any factor judged to have an impact on the quality of a population's health or the ability of the health system to perform as desired. Trends in population density, ethnicity, occupation and poverty are presumed to affect mortality, morbidity and dysfunctions. Polluting effects of industry and man-made systems also affect health status.

**related system**
Any system which exists for a primary purpose other than improving and maintaining health, but which may also affect the state of health of residents and the performance of the health system (e.g., education, welfare, economic development, etc.).

**relation**

1. A connection between two or more items, persons or things. 2. The act of telling with a retroactive effect.

**relative value scale**

A system of listing medical services where each service or unit of care is given a numerical value that indicates the relative time and complexity of the service or task. A formula is then used to multiply the numerical value against a dollar amount which then is the appropriate fee to be charged.

**relative value scale (or schedule) (RVS)**

A coded listing of physicians or other professional services using a unit system to indicate the relative value of the various services they perform: taking into account the time, skill and overhead cost required for each service, but not usually considering the relative cost-effectiveness of the services, the relative need or demand for them, or their importance to people's health. The units in this scale are based on median charges by physicians. Appropriate conversion factors are used to translate the abstract units in the scale to dollar fees for each service. Given individual and local variations in practice, the relative value scale can be used voluntarily as a guide to physicians in establishing fees for services, and as a guide for insurance carriers and government agencies in determining appropriate reimbursement (e.g., use of relative value scales under Medicare where there is no customary or prevailing charge for a covered service). An example is the scale prepared and revised periodically by the California Medical Association which includes independent scales for medicine, anesthesia, surgery, radiology and pathology. Relative value scales can contain biases favoring certain specialities (such as surgery) or types of services (highly technical or specialized) over others. See also fractionation.

**relator**

1. The name of one against whom a legal action is brought. 2. The name placed on an action or claim.

**release**

1. To set free. 2. To be free from an obligation or from a penalty as in a contract. To be release from a contract. 3. To give up a claim back to the person who owes the claim.

**release form**

A statement signed by a patient, releasing a health care facility or health care provider from responsibility or liability due to the patient refusing treatment, refusing to cooperate, or refusing to follow a doctor's orders. A release of side rails is also a common release form done so to protect the health care facility from liability due to the patient falling out of bed. A release for adoption form is also used in some states, releasing the parents from custody, services and earnings of the child. Another release form is a temporary absence release, giving a patient temporary leave from the hospital.

**release of information**
A consent form which must be signed by the patient before any information may be given out to an insurance company, attorney or any third party.

**relevant**
1. Pertinent. 2. Having to do with the case at hand. 3. Having importance or impact on a issue in a lawsuit.

**reliability**
1. In research, the reproducibility of an experimental result, i.e. how closely a second go-around would yield the same answer as the first go around. 2. As used in testing, a test is reliable if it is repeatable and if it measures accurately and consistently the same things from one time to another. A test that shows predictability over time. See validity, test reliability, test validity.

**Reliance Interest**
One who has depended on the acts or words of another and as a result, has incurred loss. See, Reliance Interest Contract Damages, 46 Yale Law Journal 52-54 (1936).

**relief**
Aid or help provided by a court to a person initiating a claim or a lawsuit. Charitable help given to the poor. rem (Lat.)

**rem**
Radiation-equivalent-man or roentgen-equivalent-man. A unit of radiation dose equivalence.

**rem (Lat.)**
1. Thing or item. 2. Showing that actions are brought against an item rather than a person. See in rem.

**REM (sleep)**
The deep sleep period during which the sleeper exhibits rapid eye movements (REMs); which is one-fifth to one-fourth of total sleep time.

**remand**
1. To return; send back; a higher court may remand a case to a lower court. 2. To commit to custody again. 3. To ask for more information on a particular point.

**remedial**
1. Used as a cure. 2. Able to correct a deficiency; used most often in reference to reading.

**remedial profession**
A professional health care occupation that assists handicapped persons to achieve living and work abilities up to a level that is as near normal as possible. These health care professionals usually include: recreational therapy, occupational therapists, speech therapists, physical therapists, and rehabilitation psychologists.

**remedial statute**
1. A new law created to correct or overcome an inadequacy found in a previously passed law. 2. A law providing a remedy or solution. 3. An intervening law.

**remedy**
1. The process that is used to prevent, redress, or compensate. 2. The result of an action removing or correcting a wrong or misdeed. 3. To make right or provide relief.

**remise**
1. A release of a claim; to give up; surrender. 2. To forgive.

**remission**
Forgiving a penalty or forfeiture.

**remit**
1. To submit or return. 2. To make less severe. 3. To give up. 4. To pay. 5. to forgive or pardon. 6. To refrain from demanding or insisting upon. 7. To send in.

**remittance**
Money sent in or sent forward to another person or to a business, such as a hospital or physician's office.

**remittent fever**
A fever in which there is a wide range of elevated temperatures over a 24-hour period.

**remittitur**
1. The authority of a judge to decrease an award given by a jury. 2. The authority of an appeals court to turn down a new trial if the two parties agree to a smaller award than would be given in court.

**remittitur of record**
A case from an appeals court sent to a lower trial court in order to have the judgment of the higher court carried out.

**remoteness**
1. Far off in time. 2. Lacking cause and effect. 3. Not likely to be related. 4. Lacking proximate cause. 5. Where the relationship between the supposed cause of harm or injury and the actual cause is lacking. 6. So distant that damages cannot be fairly awarded.

**remotivation**
1. A therapy modality used as a means of reaching and motivating long-term, chronic patients residing in nursing homes and mental hospitals, who do not seem to want to move toward better health, improvement or discharge. Remotivation must be followed by therapeutic activities leading toward rehabilitation through programs such as occupational and recreational therapy, vocational and social rehabilitation. Remotivation has been used extensively in nursing homes to stimulate and encourage social participation which is therapeutic. Arts and crafts and group activities such as movies, games or singing are important remotivation factors because they offer social interaction. 2. A group therapy technique

administered by nursing service personnel in a long-term care facility or a mental hospital. Withdrawn patients are put into social situations to stimulate their communication skills and interest in self, others and their environment.

**removable claim**
A claim that may be removed or transferred to another court.

**removal**
The taking away from; the state of being removed. Movement from one place to another.

**removal of a case**
The transferring of a case from one court to another.

**removal of cause**
1. A change of venue. 2. To transfer a lawsuit from one jurisdiction to another.

**renal dialysis (kidney dialysis)**
This service uses an artificial kidney machine to treat patients with chronic kidney problems or kidney failure. Many health care facilities do not have this specialized service. It is the process of cleaning the blood; the blood flows from an artery through an instrument containing an artificial membrane where impurities are removed, and then returns the cleaned blood through a vein.

**render**
1. To declare. 2. To give up. 3. To pay. 4. To perform. 5. To state; pronounce; or utter as a final decision.

**rendering judgment**
The act of giving a decision on a case in court.

**renewal**
1. Retention of a contract; keeping an agreement open. 2. In insurance, this is the continuance of coverage under a policy beyond its original period by the acceptance of a premium for a new policy period.

**renounce**
1. To disown. 2. Failure to accept. 3. To cast off, reject. 4. To give up in an open manner. 5. To abandon. 6. To surrender.

**renunciation**
1. The act of disowning. 2. The giving up of a right; rejecting a right without it going to anyone else. 3. The act of casting off.

**renvoi (French)**
A rule by which a court uses the laws of the accused person's own state to decide a case.

**reparable injury**
Any harm or wrong that can be fixed, repaired, overcome or compensated for with money.

**reparation**
1. The act of paying for an injury; providing redress for a wrong 3. Remedying or overcoming a mistake with the payment of money.

**repeal**
The act of removing a statute by passing a new one to override or take the orginal ones place. To cancel or take away.

**repetitive pattern**
A continual behavior performed mechanically or unconsciously.

**replacement cost**
The inflated current market price of goods or a product and is used to replace a capital purchase of a similar kind.

**replevin**
A court action or a lawsuit used to recover personal property held by another.

**replevy**
The act of returning personal property to the party who owns it and is bringing a lawsuit for the replevin of property.

**replication**
1. A reply. 2. A plantiff's response to a defendant's plea.

**reply**
1. A response provided in the pleading state. 2. The plantiff's returned answer; a response to a counter claim.

**report**
Any formal, written document on proceedings or legal actions. Any written summary or overview.

**reportable diseases**
Those diseases which state and federal laws, regulations, or municipal ordinances require that attending physicians report to the health officer.

**reporter**
1. The pulished decisions of judges. 2. One who compiles or writes reports. 3. Looseleaf binders of current reports and developments in law.

**reports**
The published decisions of cases, usually of certain courts.

**repossession**
1. The legal recovery or taking back of an item that was sold, because payments were not being made. 2 To recover possession.

**represent**
1. To speak or act under one's authority. 2. To do business for. 3. To stand in for or to act for another person.

**representation**
1. The act of representing. 2. A statement of fact. 3. Argument made in behalf of another person. See represent.

**representative**
1. A person authorized to act and speak for others. 2. One who represents another person. 3. A public official elected to the House of Representatives.

**representative action**
The bringing of a lawsuit by a stockholder of a corporation to overcome wrongdoings of other stockholders or claim a right for a company or hospital.

**repression**
A mental or defense mechanism that suppresses or removes unacceptable thoughts, experiences, ideas and emotional impulses from consciousness; to keep out of one's consciousness what is unpleasant or painful.

**reprieve**
Delaying the enforcement of a criminal sentence once it has been handed down.

**reprography**
1. Copying. 2. Photographic copy machine or other copying process. See Xerox.

**repudiate**
1. To refuse to recognize or accept something as due. 2. To disown. 3. To reject. 4. To renounce a responsibility. 5. To refuse an obligation.

**repudiation**
1. The act of repudiating. 2. Rejection. 3. Refusal.

**repudiation of a contract**
Refusing to complete a contract.

**repugnancy**
1. To have high dislike for something. 2. To be contradictory. 3. Inconsistency, as when one part of a document is correct, thus making another part of it false.

**repugnant**
1. To be at variance with or to offer resistance to. 2. Highly distasteful. 3. Opposed to. 4. Contrary and inconsistent.

**required services**
Services which must be offered by a health program in order to meet some external standard. Under Title XIX of the Social Security Act, each state must offer certan basic health services before it can qualify as having a Medicaid program (and thus for eligibility for federal matching funds). The required services are: hospital services; laboratory and x-ray services; skilled nursing facility services for individuals 21 years and over; early and periodic screening, diagnosis and treatment services for individuals under 21; family planning services; physicians' services; and home health care services for all persons eligible for skilled nursing-fare. It is important to note that, within these requirements, states may determine the scope and extent of benefits (limiting hospital care to 30 days a year, etc.). States may offer additional services in their Medicaid

program called optional services because they are offered at the option of the state.

**requirements contract**
1. A contract where a manufacturer agrees to furnish the contractor with as many items as may be required by the contractor. 2. When a health care facility agrees to purchase all of the requirements of a product, i.e., to buy a certain type of syringe and to agree to use only that company's inserts in it.

**requisition**
1. A written request made for something to which you have a right. 2. A claim made by authority. 3. A written demand for items needed.

**res (lat.)**
1. A thing; object or items. 2. The issues or actions that are in rem.

**res adjudicata (Lat.)**
See res judicata.

**rescind**
1. To cancel or terminate. 2. To annul or end a contract. 3. To release a party from obligation.

**research**
Conscious action to acquire deeper knowledge or new facts about scientific or technical subjects. Several different types are distinguished by their concern (such as biomedical and health services) or method.

**resectoscope**
A surgical instrument used in resection of the prostate or tumors from the bladder; an endoscope.

**reserpine**
A drug made from the root of the Rauwolfia serpentina plant. This alkaloid extract is used primarily as a antihypertensive agent. It was once used as an antipsychotic agent because of its sedative effect.

**reserve**
1. An amount of money set aside by an insurance company to guarantee its ability to fulfill its commitments to future claims. 2. To hold back for later use. 3. To keep control of. 4. To keep as your own. 5. Restraint in speech or actions.

**reserves**
Balance sheet accounts set up to report the liabilities faced by an insurance company under outstanding insurance policies. Their purpose is to secure as true a picture as possible of the financial condition of the organization (by permitting conversion of disbursements from a paid to an accrual basis). The company sets the amount of reserves in accord with its own estimates, state laws, and recommendations of supervisory officials and national organizations. Regulatory agencies can accept the reserves or refuse them as inadequate or excessive. For Blue Cross plans, for example, reserves are set aside to cover average monthly claims and operating expenses for some time period. Reserves, while estimated, all

are obligated amounts and have four principal components: reserves for known liabilities not yet paid; reserves for losses incurred but unreported; reserves for future benefits; and other reserves for various special purposes, including contingency reserves for unforeseen circumstances.

**res gestae (Lat.)**
1. Things done or the thing done. 2. The acts and words of an event, which provide a clearer understanding of the event. 3. The transaction. 4. Everything said and done as part of a single incident or deal.

**residency**
A prolonged (usually one or more complete years) period of on the job training which may be a part of a formal educational program or be undertaken separately after completion of a formal program, sometimes in fulfillment of a requirement for credentialing. In medicine, dentistry, podiatry and some other health professions, residencies are the principal part of graduate medical education, beginning either after graduation (increasngly) or internship (traditionally), lasting two to seven years, and providing specialty training. Most physicians now take residencies in one of the 23 specialties in which they are offered, although they are not required for licensure. Residencies are needed for board eligibility.

**resident**

**resident**
1. A graduate of a medical, osteopathic, or dental school serving an A licensed doctor who elects to take further training in a specialty in a hospital. advanced period of graduate training. (This may represent the first year of graduate training or any year thereafter.) 2. Any individual residing within the boundaries of a state regardless of the length of stay.

**residential care**
A house or other domicile-type facility that provides room and board in a protective environment with a program planned to meet the residents' nutritional, social and spiritual needs.

**residential programs**
Accordng to JCAH for psychiatric, alcoholism and drug abuse facilities accreditation purposes, these are programs that provide services to persons who require a less restrictive environment than individuals in an inpatient program and who are capable of self-preservation during an internal disaster. Such programs are usually located in facilities classified as residential occupancies in Chapter 11 of the 1973 edition of the Life Safety Code (NFPA 101).

**residential treatment facility**
A live-in center where a patient receives treatment appropriate for his particular needs while living there. A children's residential treatment facility often will furnish educational training and therapy for the emotionally disturbed child.

**residuary**
1. That which is left over. 2. Pertaining to those parts remaining after other parts have been disposed of or removed.

**residuum (Lat.)**
1. Leftovers. 2. A balance; a residue.

**resile**
1. To withdraw. 2. To recede from an issue, cause or purpose.

**res integra (Lat.)**
1. Whole thing. 2. Yet undecided and without precedent.

**res inter alios acta, alteri nocere non debet (Lat.)**
A transaction between other persons should not prejudice one not a party to it.

**res ipsa loquitur (Lat.)**
1. The thing speaks for itself. 2. The shift of the burden of proof from the defendant. When the obvious becomes evidence in and of itself, such as surgical instrument found inside a patient following an operation. 4. In malpractice, a legal doctrine or presumption that, when an injury occurs to a plaintiff through a situation under the sole and exclusive control of the defendant and where such injury would not normally occur if the one in control had used due care, then it is presumed the defendant is negligent. For example, when a surgeon leaves a sponge or other item in the abdomen.

**resistive behaviors**
Those behaviors which inhibit change, compliance, involvement and cooperation.

**res judicata (Lat.)**
1. A thing decided. 2. A matter once decided by judgment or a competent court cannot thereafter be reconsidered by the same or other court.

**resolution**
1. A decision of the court. 2. An official opinion of a governmental body or legislature. 3. A principle that is created by a vote but doesn't become law.

**resort**
1. To apply to something for help. 2. The gaining of an end. 3. Final end, as in the last resort. 4. A court of last resort is the last court of appeal.

**resource capacity**
The amount, type and distribution of services that can be provided by the usable, available resources in a given geographic area.

**resource requirements**
The identification of the material, money, and manpower necessary in order to reach a goal.

**resources**
Sources of support available to an individual in addition to his regular earned or unearned income. Generally resources refer to an individual's wealth or property (including cash savings, stocks and bonds, a home,

other real estate, the cash value of life insurance, an automobile or jewelry) which could be converted to cash if necessary. Existing programs for the poor generally set a limit on the total amount of resources an individual or family may have and still be eligible. Most existing resource tests exempt a home of reasonable value, on the basis that it would not be reasonable to require selling a home to qualify for benefits. Also used to mean the providers, institutions, health manpower and facilities used for provision of health services in the total health care system.

**resources development**
Activities which focus especially upon the recruitment and education of health care professionals, or the construction and modernization of health care facilities.

**respiration**
The exchange of gases ($O_2$ and $CO_2$) between the lungs and the air in the environment. The respiratory cycle includes inspiration (breathing in) and expiration (breathing out). Rate can be obtained by feeling, seeing, and listening to the patient breathing in and out.

**respiratory care department/service**
According to JCAH for accreditation purposes, this is an organizational unit of the hospital that is designed for the provision of ventilatory support and associated services to patients.

**respiratory therapist**
1. Respiratory therapists work under a physician's supervision and administer prescribed respiratory therapy care and life support to patients with deficiencies and abnormalities of the cardiopulmonary system. They set up, operate, and monitor devices such as respirators, mechanical ventilators, therapeutic gas administration apparatus, environmental control systems, and aerosol generators. They perform bronchopulmonary drainage, assist patients with breathing exercises, and monitor patients' physiological responses to therapy. In many work settings, respiratory therapists are required to exercise a considerable degree of independent clinical judgment in the respiratory care of patients under the direct or indirect supervision of a physician. Further, the respiratory therapist is expected to be capable of serving as a technical resource to the physician regarding current practices in respiratory care, and to the hospital staff regarding safe and effective therapies. In addition, therapists may supervise trainees and technicians. Respiratory therapists are almost always employed by hospitals. They cover intensive care units, newborn nurseries, surgical and medical areas, and emergency rooms. 2. According to JCAH for accreditation purposes, a respiratory is an individual who has successfully completed a training program accredited by the American Medical Association Committee on Allied Health Education and Accreditation in collaboration with the Joint Review Committee for Respiratory Therapy Education, and is eligible to take the registry examination administered by the National Board for Respiratory Therapy, Inc., or has the documented equivalent in training and/or experience. See registered respiratory therapist.

**respiratory therapy services**
Under medical direction, treat, manage, control and perform diagnostic evaluations in the care of patients with deficiencies and abnormalities in the cardio-pulmonary system.

**respiratory therapy technician**
1. Respiratory therapy technicians work under the supervision of a respiratory therapist or a physician and perform clinical duties essentially identical to those of the therapist. Generally, however, they do not engage in teaching, administration, supervision, or evaluation of new equipment and therapeutic modalities. Although duties vary with the employing institution, technicians usually exercise a lesser degree of independent judgment and responsibility, in most cases because their formal training in anatomy, physiology, pharmacology, and clinical practice is less extensive than that of the therapist. Primarily working in hospital settings, technicians provide treatment and maintain patient records. 2. According to JCAH for accreditation purposes, this is an individual who has successfully completed a training program accredited by the American Medical Association Committee on Allied Health Education and Accreditation in collaboration with the Joint Review Committee for Respiratory Therapy Education, and is eligible to take the certification examination administered by the National Board for Respiratory Therapy, Inc., or has the documented equivalent in training and/or experience.

**respite care**
Short-term care provided by non-family members to relieve the family from their 24-hour care and supervision of a mentally retarded child, elderly person, etc.

**respondeat superior (Lat.)**
1. Let the superior answer. 2. A legal principle that an employer is the master and is responsible for the actions of those in his employ, who are carrying out their duties of employment. Liability can exist in situations where wrongful acts are committed by an agent. This principle often applies to the relationship between physicians and allied health care providers. 3. In malpractice, a form of vicarious liability whereby an employer is held liable for the wrongful acts of an employee even though the employer's conduct is without fault. Before liability predicated on respondeat superior may be imposed upon an employer, it is necessary that a master/servant (i.e., controlling) relationship exist between the employer and employee and that the wrongful act of the employee occur within the scope of his employment. The doctrine of respondeat superior does not absolve the original wrongdoer, the employee, of liability for his wrongful act. Not only may the injured party sue the employee directly, but the employer may seek indemnification from him.

**respondent**
1. The one who answers or responds. 2. The party against whom an appeal is made or a motion is filed. 3. An appellee.

**response rate**
That length of time which is generally acceptable as the maximum allowable for a victim to receive medical aid while suffering minimal long term effects from an injury or illness.

**responsibility to duty**
1. An obligation to perform an act or carry out a duty. Often certain circumstances exist between two parties, or a legal duty arises in that one is expected to render reasonable assistance to an injured party, thus a responsibility to duty exists.

**responsive pleading**
A legal document that answers issues presented by the other party's plea.

**rest**
1. A state of repose after exertion. 2. To end; conclude.

**rest a case**
To end the presentation of evidence and to let the other party present their evidence or to let the judge make a final judgment or decision.

**rest homes**
Facilities that provide only custodial care. Some homes offer limited nursing care, but do not have a licensed, well-trained staff such as that found in an intermediate care facility.

**restitution**
1. The act of restoring or giving back. 2. To make things good or keep a promise. 3. The restoration of a right or property to one unjustly deprived of it.

**restrain**
1. To deprive one from liberty. 2. To stop an issue or action. 3. To restrict or limit. 4. To hinder or obstruct. 5. To hold back or interpose on a proceeding.

**restraining order**
A temporary court order given without a trial or hearing which provides for the status quo to remain until a formal action or hearing can be held to determine the necessary action. Also referred to as a TRO (temporary restraining order).

**restraint**
1. An action occasionally used in nursing homes or mental institutions to hold a person down so that he or she will not harm themselves or others. Drugs are now used to calm patients with physical restraints not used as much. Wrongful use of restraints can be legally viewed as a deprivation of liberty or false imprisonment with legal consequences. 2. According to JCAH for psychiatric, alcoholism and drug abuse facilities accreditation purposes, this is a physical or mechanical device used to restrict the movement of the whole or a portion of a patient's body. This does not include mechanisms used to assist a patient in obtaining and maintaining normative body functioning, for example, braces and wheelchairs.

**restrictive indorsement**
Indorsing a check or negotiable instrument so that it ends its negotiability. For example: 'For deposit only to the account of Riverview Hospital."

**resuscitation**
The reviving of a person from lack of breathing or heart activity, which includes cardiac massage and artificial respiration.

**retainer**
An advance fee paid to a professional, used to enlist his services.

**retardation**
The lack of or slowness in the development or progress of a person. There are two types, mental retardation: slowness of intellectual maturation; psychomotor retardation: slow psychic activity or motor activity or both. This form can be observed in pathological depression.

**retention enema**
When an enema (liquid or solution) is introduced into a patient's lower bowel and is not allowed to be expelled. This is one method of applying a local medication or soothing agent. The enema may be retained in the bowel so the body can absorb it to bring about sedation or to help in hydration or provide nourishment. It could also help cool the body or stop local hemorrhage.

**retirement centers**
Usually these facilities are elaborate complexes of homes, apartments, stores, cafeterias, clubs, etc. A retirement center may provide a broad range of apartment-like living arrangements, condominiums, recreational programs and intermediate care facilities. Some short-term skilled nursing care may be provided.

**retirement income credit**
Setting aside income each year for retirement and not paying taxes on it until retirement, when taxes come due but are then lower.

**retract**
1. To take back. 2. To withdraw or disavow a statement, offer or promise.

**retraction**
1. The act of drawing in or taking something back. 2. To admit that a statement was false. See retract.

**retractor**
A surgical instrument used to pull back tissue in order to expose the operation site. This instrument retracts, or pulls the cut edges of skin, muscle and tissue open. It opens up a cavity in which operation procedures are to be conducted. Several types and sizes of retractors are used.

**retro**

**retro-**
1. Before or back; backwards. 2. Behind, previous or past.
Prefix meaning behind.

**retroactive law**
1. Law that changes the legal status of laws already passed or actions previously done. 2. Applying laws to past actions. 3. Laws having the power to affect past acts.

**retroflexion**
The turning of rage onto oneself.

**retrospective reimbursement**
Payment to providers by a third party carrier for costs or charges actually incurred by subscribers in a previous time period. This is the method of payment used under Medicare and Medicaid. See also prospective reimbursement.

**retrospective study**
An inquiry planned to observe events that have already occurred (a case-control study is usually retrospective); compare with a prospective study which is planned to observe events that have not yet occurred.

**return**
1. A report from a court official or peace officer stating that he has carried out an order from the court, or if not, why. 2. An income, yield or profit. 3. To begin or to appear again. 4. To go back to a place. 5. To say in reply.

**return date (day)**
After receiving a summons to appear before a judge or in court This is the date or day by which a party must answer a complaint or pleading.

**return on investment (ROI)**
The monetary gain received for money or resources invested. A measure of a service or production operation's performance; profits divided by assets used in the investment; the profit gain from the product turned over or materials used up.

**rev. (abbrev.)**
1. Revised or a revision. 2. Reviewed.

**revenue**
1. Income. 2. Increase in money, money gained. 3. Money returned on an investment. 4. Money gained through taxation. 5. The gross amount of earnings received by an entity for the operation of a specific activity.

**reversal**
1. To reverse a judgment. 2. The changing or anulling of a decision of a lower court or hearing.

**reverse**
1. To set aside. 2. To annul, vacate or change. 3. Turned backward.

**reversible error**
1. An error made by a lower court or a trial court which has an effect on a appellent's basic rights thus warranting a reversal of the decision by the appellate court.

**revert**
1. To go back to. 2. To return to the former owner.

**reverter**
A reversion

**review**
The process of a court of appeals examining a case.

**revised statutes**
A code or record of statutes in book form with temporary and repealed statutes not included. They are usually placed in the book in the order that they were passed.

**revive**
1. To bring back. 2. To restore to original state or its legal force. 3. To bring back from a state of neglect; to restore life to something.

**revocation**
1. To take back; the retaking of power or authority. 2. To end; make void. 3. The act of annulling a repeal or a reversal.

**revoke**
1. To cancel or rescind. 2. Taking back, cancelling. 3. To reduce or eliminate the legal effect of something.

**rex (Lat.)**
King.

**rider**
1. In insurance, this legal document that modifies the protection provided by an insurance policy which may expand or decrease the payable benefits by adding or excluding certain conditions from policy's coverage. 2. In the process of creating laws, this is an addition to a legislative bill that is added on after it has been through the proper committee. 3. An additional attached to a larger document.

**right**
1. An ethical expectancy. 2. Something that is moral, fair, just, honorable. 3. Right of action; a enforceable claim. 4. To restore to a proper condition; correct. 5. Legal authority to control certain actions of others. Every right has a corresponding duty. Rights as used in law refers to legal rights; those things that are legally just.

**rightful**
Having a just claim according to law.

**right of action**
1. Any legal issue that is enforceable by a court. 2. Any legal claim or fact that is great enough to demand judicial attention. See cause of action.

**right of recovery**
In health insurance, in the event payment is made for any condition for which a third party may be responsible, the insurance company will be entitled to the proceeds of any settlement up to the amount paid. The same applies to payments made in excess of charges.

**Right to privacy**
see Patients/client bill of rights.

**right-to-work law**
State laws prohibiting unions from requiring a person to join a union in order to work at that place of employment or from denying employment because of membership of lack of membership in a labor organization. These laws outlawed closed shops and union shops.

**rigidity**
A psychiatry term meaning a person's resistance to change.

**rigor mortis**
The stiffening of the body after death.

**ripe**
A case that has easily recognizable or obvious and clear legal issues so that a decision is well assured.

**risk**
1. Generally, any chance of loss. 2. In insurance, designates the individual or property insured by an insurance policy against loss from some peril or hazard. 3. Also used to refer to the probability that the loss will occur. See insurable risk and at risk.

**risk charge**
The fraction of a premium which goes to generate or replenish surpluses which a carrier must develop to protect against the possibility of excessive losses under its policies. Profits, if any, on the sale of insurance are also taken from the surpluses developed using risk charges. The risk charge is sometimes referred to as retention or retention rate.

**risk, impaired or substandard**
An insurance applicant whose physical condition does not meet the standards of being healthy.

**risk management**
The assessment and control of the obvious and identifiable risks to which a health care facility has or might be subject to. The management of risk involves analyzing all possibilities of loss and determining how to reduce risk exposures by reducing the risk, eliminating the risk, or transferring the risk, and by obtaining insurance to cover risks that cannot be eliminated.

**rites of passage**
Ceremonial rites marking transition from one social status to another. Used in gerontology and retirement to refer to both explicit and implicit role status that is denoted by some type of occasion or occurrence that allows role change.

**ritual**
1. Automatic activity 2. behavior with a cultural origin.

**ritualistic behavior (ritualism)**
Repetitive acts performed in a compulsive manner to relieve anxiety.

**R.N.**
Registered nurse. See these words.; also nurse

**RNA**
Ribonucleic acid, which is produced by DNA. It is important to memory function. See also DNA.

**robbery**
1. Forcible stealing. 2. The illegal taking of personal property by force or fear.

**roentgen**
The unit of measurement of x-ray or gamma radiation.

**roentgeno-**
Prefix meaning x-rays

**roentgenogram**
A film produced by photography with roentgen rays.

**rogatory letters**
A formal request by a court of one jurisdiction or state to another court asking that a witness be examined by interrogatories and they be returned to the original correct.

**role**
Any pattern of behavior that a person takes on as a part of their own behavior. When a behavior pattern conforms with the expectations of society, it is a complementary role. If it does not conform with the expectation of others, it is a non-complementary role. See also identification, injunction, therapeutic role.

**roleless role**
The ambiguity of no roles caused by retirement, wherein there are few explicit expectations, roles or rules regarding behavior or performance.

**rolfing**
A therapeutic massage used to release emotional stress from the muscles. See structural integration.

**roll**
1. Any official record of a proceeding. 2. A list of names for official purposes.

**room accommodations**
Description of the types of patient care rooms provided in a facility (e.g., private, semi-private, or ward.)

**Rorschach test**
A special type of projective test in which the patient reveals his perceptions, attitudes and emotions by responding to a set of inkblot pictures.

**roster**
A list of patients served by a given health care provider or program (who owns the roster.The roster may be derived from a registry or list of visits but the listing of an individual on a roster does not necessarily imply any ongoing relationship between the program and the individual. See also catchment area.

**rounds**
A physician (or possibly nurse, dietitian, clinic pharmacist, or other health care provider) visiting the bedsides of hospitalized patients to assess treatment and note progress of the patient. See ward rounds, grand rounds.

**routine care**
Care extended to any patient who requires institutionalization as a result of a medical disorder and/or surgery, but whose malady is not severe enough to require special care.

**routine services**
These are the services included by the provider in a daily service charge—sometimes referred to as the "room and board" charge.

**R.R.A.**
Registered Record Administrator. A fully qualified professional in the planning and management of medical information systems and analysis of data generated by those systems, such as quality patient care, medical education, research, epidemic control, drug testing, health planning, and health care evaluation. As manager of the health facility's medical record department, the RRA's duties involve daly contact with the medical staff and administration. As an administrator, the RRA designs health information and medical record management systems. Members of the medical staff are assisted by the RRA via data preparation and reports for patient care evaluation. The RRA's special knowledge of medicolegal decisions in handling subpoenas, working with attorneys and their familiarity with information systems in compiling statistical reports, ensures efficient functioning of the medical record department and the health care facility. See registered record administrators.

**rubber stamp signature**
A physician's signature that is made into a rubber stamp and is used on medical records or prescriptions in health facilities which the physician may not frequent very often, such as a nursing home. The physician may later confirm the rubber stamped signature with his own official signature. See authenticate.

**rubella**

German measles: a mild viral infection marked by a pink mascular rash, fever and lymph node enlargement.

**rubric**

A title or heading for a law.

**rule**

1. A standard. 2. A principle of conduct. 3. An established usage of law. 4. A usual course of action. 5. To govern. 6. To establish by a decision as does a judge in court to settle a legal issue or decide a motion. 7. To settle an objection raised by one side in a legal dispute. 8. In the executive branch of the federal government, an agency statement of general or particular applicability and future effect designed to implement, interpret or prescribe law or policy, or describing the organization, procedure or practice requirements of an agency. Commonly also called a regulation. Rules are published in the Federal Register. The process of writing a rule is called a rule is called a rule-making. A rule, once adopted in accordance with the procedures specified in the Administrative Procedure Act (Title V, U.S.C.), has the force of law.

**rule nisi**

1. Order to show cause. 2. An order that is to take effect unless the person shows cause why it should not.

**rule of discovery**

Statute of limitations does not begin to run until the injured becomes aware of or should have known that the injury or harm has occurred.

**rule of law**

A general guide to conduct in law, government, or health agencies that is applied by government officials, and supported by governmental authority. The highest authority of a government is its laws.

**rules and regulations**

Clear and concise written statements of policy setting forth certain activities allowed or not allowed in a health care facility.

**ruling**

A decision or judgment made on a legal issue.

**run**

1. Having legal effect. 2. To be in effect during a specific time period. 3. To be written or related. 4. To go through successfully. 5. To expose oneself to. 6. To allow or permit. 7. To accrue or mount up. 8. A period of operation. 9. To pursue and catch, as to run down a debt.

**Rx**

Therapy or treatment.

# S

**S.A.**
1. Sociedad Anonima (Spanish). 2. Societe Anonyme (French). Abbreviation for corporation.

**S.A.C.**
Sub Area Advisory Council. A local advisory council to the Health Systems Agency. In some areas these are called Health Advisory Councils (HAC).

**sacrosanct (Lat.)**
Not to be violated, sacred.

**sadism**
1. Deliberate cruelty. 2. Destructive-aggressive attitudes in an individual. 3. A disorder that is often a sexual deviation in which sexual gratification is achieved by inflicting pain and humiliation on the sex partner. This term is also used in a broader , to mean the general inflicting of pain or causing physical harm to others, with no sexual involvement.

**sadist**
One who derives pleasure from inflicting physical or psychological pain on others in both social and sexual encounters.

**sadomasochistic relationship**
Any relationship where enjoyment is achieved due to the suffering by one person and the enjoyment of inflicting pain by the other person. Both are attractions in their relationship. See also masochism, sadism.

**SADR**
Severity adjusted death rate. See case severity.

**safeguard**
1. A person or thing that protects. 2. To provide of security. 3. To protect or defend.

**safe place statutes**
Statutes in some states that require an employer to eliminate all danger from his employees' work place which could reasonably be guarded against.

**safety**
1. The probability that use of a particular drug, device, method or medical procedure will not cause unintended or unanticipated harm, disease, pain or injury. Safety is, in this context, a relative concept which must be balanced against the effectiveness of the drug or procedure in

question. Drugs or procedures known to cause hurt, disease or injury when used are not usually thought of as unsafe if the benefits they give exceed the damage. The Federal Food, Drug and Cosmetic Act requires a demonstration of safety for drugs marketed for human use. No similar requirement exists for most other medical procedures paid for or regulated under federal or state law. 2. Free from hazard or danger. 3. Any device that is protective or keeps an individual from danger, harm or injury.

**said**
1. Already referred to or the one mentioned before. 2. An over-used, unclear term used unnecessarily in legal documents and legal jargon, i.e., 'the said John Doe' or 'said Memorial Hospital.'

**sale**
1. The act of selling. 2. The exchange of a commodity or goods for an agreed upon price. 3. A form of a contract.

**sale-leaseback**
The process of selling a piece of equipment or a machine to an organization or business and then, as part of the same transaction, arranging to lease the equipment back, all of which is agreed upon at the onset of the transaction.

**Salic Law**
A French law that says women cannot inherit land.

**sanatorium**
1. Usually refers to the old tuberculosis hospitals. 2. An older form of institution where patients were treated for chronic physical (such as tuberculosis) or mental illness or where a patient is nursed and treated during a period of recuperation.

**sanction**
1. Formal consent or approval by an official in authority to give it. 2. To condone or approve of another person's actions or behavior. 3. A punishment provided by law to assure that it is obeyed. 4. Power to enforce a law. 5. Consent.

**sane**
1. Mentally sound. 2. Of healthy mind. 3. Relating to good mental health or sanity. 4. Having a competent and stable mental state.

**sanitize**
To reduce the presence of microbiological flora in or on articles or items to levels judged safe by public health authorities.

**sanity**
1. A good mental balance. 2. Soundness of mind. 3. Having a stable emotional and mental state.

**satisfaction**
1. Payment of a debt. 2. Something which satisfies. 3. Reparation for injury or insult. 4. Completion of an obligation.

**satisfaction piece**
A memo from both the plaintiff and defendant which is filed with the court, acknowledging a satisfactory settlement of a lawsuit.

**saturation**
1. In marketing insurance or HMOs, the point at which further penetration is improbable or when costs will be excessive. 2. The state of being filled to capacity; having taken in all that it can. 3. Soaked through.

**satyriasis**
An unhealthy preoccupation with sexual needs or desires in men. This condition may be caused by an organic or psychiatric dysfunction. See also nymphomania.

**save**
1. To spare. 2. To avoid; prevent. 3. To hold until later. 4. To reserve something. 5. To preserve a document.

**save-harmless statutes**
Statutes in some states that permit or require an agency to repay employees for damages lost in civil suits.

**scab**
A nonunion worker; a worker who replaces a union worker out on strike.

**scarcity area**
An area lacking an adequate supply of a particular type of health service (physicians) or all health services; synonymous with medically underserved area.

**schedule**
1. List. 2. A written list of things to be accomplished in a certain order or at a certain time.

**schedule A (Health manpower)**
The list of occupations which the Department of Labor considers to be in short supply throughout the United States for purposes of labor certification. All occupations now listed on schedule A are health occupations, but some health occupations (such as dentists) are not listed.

**scheduled benefit provision**
See allocated benefit provision.

**schedule of controlled substances**
Under the Federal Comprehensive Drug Abuse Prevention and Control Act of 1970 for the purpose of legal control, drugs were classified by schedule. Possession of any controlled substance without a prescription is illegal with no distinction in the penalty language made between drugs or different schedules. For violations concerning the manufacture and sale of controlled substances, a distinction between schedules is made. The schedules of I, II, III, IV, and V are updated and reviewed each year. Briefly each schedule is as follows: *Schedule I,* a drug or substance that has a high potential for abuse and has no current accepted medical use

and lacks accepted safe usage under medical supervision, including drugs such as heroin, LSD, mescaline, psilocybin, DMT, marijuana and hashish. *Schedule II,* a drug or substance that has a high potential for abuse, has currently accepted medical use (even with restrictions) and may lead to severe psychological or physical dependence to include drugs such as (but not limited to) opium, methadone, demerol, codeine and cocaine. *Schedule III,* a drug or substance with a potential for abuse but less potential than those in schedules I and II, has a currently accepted medical use and may lead to moderate or low physical dependence or high psychological dependence to include such drugs as paregoric, barbiturates, doriden and amphetamines. *Schedule IV,* A drug or substance with a low potential for abuse, has current accepted medical use, and abuse may lead to limited physical or psychological dependence to include drugs such as equinol and miltown. *Schedule V,* Drugs with low abuse potential, currently has an accepted medical use and has limited physical and psychological dependence.

**schedule of drugs**
See schedule of controlled substances, drug categories.

**schizocaria**
1. An acute form of schizophrenia, often referred to as 'catastrophic schizophrenia.' 2. A disorder in which the patient's personality deteriorates at a very rapid rate.

**schizoid personality**
A personality disorder characterized by shyness, oversensitivity and sometimes eccentricity. These people are usually detached and apper unemotional in the face of stressful events and experiences.

**schizophrenia**
A serious mental disorder that is in the psychotic area. It is characterized by disturbances in thought processes, mood, disjointed sentences and upset behavior. Thought disturbance is shown through a distortion of reality, manifested by delusions and hallucinations, accompanied by a fragmentation of mental and perceptual associations that results in incoherent speech. Mood disturbance is shown by inappropriate emotional responses. Behavior problems are seen as ambivalence, apathetic withdrawal and bizarre activity. Also known as dementia praecox, the different forms of schizophrenia include simple, hebephrenic, catatonic, paranoid, schizoaffective, childhood, residual, latent, and chronic undifferentiated types and acute schizophrenic episode.

**school health**
The program in schools developed and designed to protect and promote the health and well-being of students and school personnel. Included in the school health program are health education, health promotion, health activation, health services and providing a healthful school environment. Prevention and health promotion are the key concepts in school health.

**school health educator**
Teaches elementary, secondary, and college students principles of personal health sciences, total fitness, family living, consumer and environmental health, and community health trends and resources. See health educator.

**school nurse**
These health care practitioners make up the largest group of health care providers in school health services. It is estimated there are 30-40,000 school nurses practicing in the United States. School nurse responsibilities include activities to promote dental, mental, emotional and physical health; teach about health; serve as a health counselor to students, parents and teachers; and are medical professional liaisons for students, parents, teachers and physicians. School nurses advise schools of unsanitary and environmental conditions; disease control and the spread of communicable disease and provide emergency care for students and school personnel. Also of concern is broken equipment, health hazards, and work with handicapped children and standardizing school facilities. School nurses also participate in a number of preventive programs such as vision and hearing screenings and immunization programs.

**school of nursing**
See collegiate school of nursing.

**school phobia**
A fear of and refusal to go to school; often viewed as a manifestation of separation anxiety.

**scienter (Lat.)**
1. Knowingly; knowledge with guilt. 2. In fraud, knowingly having an intent to deceive.

**Scientology**
A religious movement begun in 1952 which teaches immortality and reincarnation, and claims a sure psychotherapeutic method for freeing the individual from personal problems, increasing human abilities, and speeding recovery from sickness, injury and mental disorder.

**scintilla (Lat.)**
1. A spark; trace; least little bit. 2. Even a little bit is enough; the slightest bit is evidence.

**scire facias (Lat.)**
1. Cause it to be known. 2. A judge's order to a defendant to appear in court and show cause as to why a record should not be used against him.

**scope**

**-scope**
The extent of activities or range of operations that will
Suffix, meaning instrument for visual examination. undertake and/or accomplish.

**scope of employment**
Doing one's duties, i.e., chores, work or professional activities that a person was specifically employed to do, or which may be implied from specific duties.

**scope of services**
The number, type, intensity or complexity of services provided by a hospital or health program. Scope of services is measured, in a number of different ways, so that the capacity and nature of different programs may be compared. A program's scope of services should reflect, and be adequate to meet, the needs of its patient mix.

**scopo-**
Prefix, meaning examination, visual examination.

**scotoma**
A term used in psychology and psychiatry to identify a person's blind spot or unawareness that exists in his or her psychological awareness.

**screening**
1. The use of quick, simple procedures to identify and separate persons who are apparently well, who have, or are having a risk of, a disease from those who probably do not have the disease. It is used to identify suspects for more definitive diagnostic studies. Multiple screening (or multiphasic screening) is the combination of a battery of screening tests for various diseases performed by technicians under medical direction and applied to large groups of apparently well persons. 2. Screening also refers to initial, cursory claims review by insurance companies intended to identify claims which are obviously not covered or deficient in some way. 3. Used in psychology and psychiatry as an initial evaluation of a patient which includes medical and psychiatric history, psychological testing and mental status evaluation to formulate a diagnosis to determine a patient's suitability for a particular treatment modality. See also sensitivity, specificity, preventive medicine, Early Periodic Screening Diagnosis and Treatment program.

**screening clinic**
A clinic where an initial assessment of patients seeking care is done to determine what services they need, with what priority, and sometimes, where treatment of minor problems is done. See also triage.

**screening panels**
In malpractice, screening panels are fact finding bodies and are used during the early stages of a malpractice dispute. There are two basic types of screening panels in use: physicians' defense panels, which seek to develop the best possible defense for the physician who faces a real or potential malpractice claim and joint physician and lawyer panels whose purpose is to look at the facts of the case for both the physician and the plaintiff and decide on its merits.

**screen memory**
A memory that one could cause and use to serve as a cover-up or repression of a painful memory.

**scurrilous**
1. Using abusive language. 2. Vulgar; indecent. 3. Having abuse.

**scut work**
A term used by housestaff and others in hospitals to describe work they dislike, usually dirty or trivial in nature, paperwork or work which could be done by anybody else.

**S.E.**
South Eastern Reporter of the National Reporter System.

**seal**
An authenticating mark on a document, such as a Notary or corporate seal.

**sealed verdict**
A verdict decided while a court is not in session, thus the verdict is placed in an envelope and sealed, and the jury separates. The verdict is pronounced later in court.

**search warrant**
A court order issued by a magistrate upon a showing of probable cause so that a police officer, is allowed him to search real or personal property for evidence, stolen goods, or illicit materials.

**seasonable**
Within a reasonable period of time.

**S.E.C.**
Securities and Exchange Commission.

**seclusion**
According to JCAH for psychiatric, alcoholism and drug abuse facilities accreditation purposes, this is a procedure that isolates the patient to a specific environmental area removed from the patient community.

**second aid**
The performance of assistance after the time of any immediate or temporary need; continuous health care. See secondary care.

**secondary authority**
Any indirect authority, opinions or sources other than actual decisions by an appellate court in the governing jurisdiction.

**secondary boycott**
Indirect pressure or indirectly withholding of services.

**secondary care**
Services provided by medical specialists who generally do not have first contact with patients (e.g., cardiologists, urologists, dermatologists). In the United States, however, there has been a trend toward self-referral for these services, rather than referral by primary care providers. This route is quite different from the path usually followed in England, for example, where all patients first seek care from primary care providers and are

then referred to secondary and/or tertiary providers, as needed. See also tertiary care. See care, secondary.

**secondary care facilities**
Facilities that render care which requires a degree of sophistication and skills and which are usually associated with the confinement of the care seeker for a defininte period of time. Refers to that health care which is usually associated with the care rendered in general acute hospitals or specialized outpatient facilities, such as ambulatory surgical centers.

**secondary evidence**
Evidence that is not from primary or forthright sources, as oral testimony of the contents of a lost document.

**secondary gain**
The recognition, attention and advantage that a person gains from being ill, such as gifts, pampering and the release from responsibility. See also primary gain.

**secondary psychological prevention**
Those measures needed to prevent an emotional or mental disease process through prevention based on early findings, therapy and treatment.

**section 1122**
A section of the Social Security Act added by P.L. 92-603. The section provides that payments will not be made under Medicare or Medicaid for certain disapproved capital expenditures determined to be inconsistent with state or local health plans. P.L. 93-641, the National Health Planning and Resources Development Act of 1974, requires states to participate in the section 1122 program to have the new state health planning and development agency serve as the section 1122 agency for purposes of the required review. See also capital expenditure review and certificate-of-need.

**section 222**
A section of the Social Security Amendments of 1972, P.L. 92-603, which authorized the former Secretary of HEW (now HHS), to undertake, with respect to Medicare, studies, experiments or demonstration projects on: prospective reimbursement of facilities, ambulatory surgical centers (surgicenters), intermediate care and homemaker services (with respect to the extended care benefit under Medicare); elimination or reduction of the three-day prior hospitalization requirement for admission to a skilled nursing facility; determination of the most appropriate methods of reimbursing the services of physicians' assistants and nurse practitioners; provision for day care services to older persons that are eligible under Medicare and Medicaid; and possible means of making the services of clinical psychologists more generally available under Medicare and Medicaid.

**section 223**
A section of the Social Security Amendments of 1972, P.L. 92-603, which requires the Secretary to establish limits on overall direct or indirect costs which will be recognized as reasonable under Medicare for

comparable services in comparable facilities in an area. The Secretary is also permitted to establish maximum acceptable costs in such facilities with respect to items or services (for example, food or standby costs). The beneficiary is liable (except in the case of emergency care) for any amounts determined as excessive (except that he may not be charged for excessive amounts in a facility in which his admitting physician has a direct or indirect ownership interest). Under rules issued for this section, reimbursement for hospital inpatient routine service costs is limited to a figure derived from the 80th percentile (plus 10 percent of the median) for each class of hospitals. Classification of hospitals is based on whether the hospital is located in a Standard Metropolitan Statistical Area (SMSA) or not, percapita income in the area, and hospital bed capacity.

**section 224**

A section of the Social Security Amendments of 1972, P.L. 92-603, which places a limit on Medicare and Medicaid reimbursement of charges recognized as reasonable. The law recognizes as reasonable those charges which fall within the 75th percentile of all charges for a similar service in a locality. Increases in physicians' fees allowable for Medicare purposes are indexed to a factor which takes into account increased costs of practice and the increase in general earnings levels in an area. Section 224 further provides that, with respect to reasonable charges for medical supplies and equipment, only the lowest charges at which supplies and equipment of similar quality are widely and consistently available in a locality may be recognized.

**section 314 (d)**

A section of the PHS Act which authorized formula grants by the federal government to the states for their unrestricted use in funding state and local health programs and activities. Therefore sometimes called a health revenue sharing program.

**secure**

1. Free from fear, care, or worry. 2. Confident. 3. To provide confidence in the payment of an obligation. 4. To guarantee repayment. 5. To gain possession of.

**secured creditor**

One to whom money is owed and is protected by a mortgage or security interest in the property of the debtor.

**securities**

Stocks, bonds, or other documents or notes that show a share or exists in a company.

**security**

1. The quality or state of being safe; certain. 2. In insurance, a policy offers protection or security. 3. Something given as a guarantee of performance, protection or payment. 4. A quasi-police program or officer in a health care facility.

**sedative**
1. Tending to calm or soothe. 2. A drug used to reduce anxiety and calm a person. 3. Any drug that produces a calming or relaxing effect through central nervous system depression. Some sedative drugs are barbiturates, chloral hydrate, paraldehyde, and bromide.

**sedition**
The promotion of public disorder against the government.

**seductive**
1. To lead astray. 2. To entice from duty. 3. To tempt to do wrong.

**seemly**
Fit or becoming; decent; proper. To have seemly behavior.

**seize**
To take property legally. To legally possess; to put into possession.

**seizure**
A public official taking property into custody as a direct result of a person violating the law.

**selectman**
A person chosen to sit on a board of officials. Mostly used in New England towns to serve in the capacity as a mayor to carry on the business of a town.

**self-actualization**
The term used by Abraham Maslow to describe the highest level of mental and emotional development and personality adjustment.

**self-care**
Individuals are taught and encouraged to go beyond participating in health decision making and learn minor medical procedures including the observation and reporting of symptoms, vital signs, and to do health record keeping and self-treatment of 70% of one's illnesses *not* requiring a physician. Many training programs and books are available such as self-care at the family level, and helping the diabetic care for oneself.

**self-dealing**
A person who is working in a place of trust. One who acts for himself rather than helping his agent or the person for whom he works.

**self-defense**
The right to employ aggression or physical force against a person who is threatening one's own person, property or name. Force is acceptable only when the threat was not provoked, and if there is no reasonable escape, and the force is not disproportionate to the threat.

**self-executing**
1. A law or court action that requires no further official action in order for it to be enforced or put into effect. 2. A will executed by the testator and witnesses and verified by a notary public, which needs no other proof to be admitted into probate.

**self-help**
1. Taking a legal action without authority and planning to suffer the consequences. 2. Giving first aid or primary health care to oneself or family; called medical self-help, or self-care. See self-care, medical self-help.

**self-insure**
The practice of an individual, group of individuals, employer or organization assuming complete responsibility for losses which might be insured against, such as malpractice losses, medical expenses and/or other losses due to illness. In such cases, medical expenses would most likely be financed out of current income, personal savings, a fund developed for the purpose, and/or some other combination of personal assets. Self-insurance is contrasted to the practice of purchasing insurance, by the payment of a premium, from some third party (an insurance company or government agency).

**self-pay**
Patients who pay their own hospital bill out of their own pockets without insurance benefits.

**self-pity**
A mental or defense mechanism that shifts the responsibility of lifes disappointments from one's self to others or to the environment. The conscious mind shares the feeling of thwarted desire of the unconscious mind, thus creating inner harmony. As one feels sorry for himself, self-pity is a form of projection. Self-pity is destructive to the personality as it is a negative cognitive set and promotes a defeatist attitude.

**semen**
Seminal fluid combined with sperm prior to ejaculation.

**semi-**
Prefix, meaning half.

**semi-private**
Hospital room with two beds.

**Senate**
One group or body of a state legislature of the U.S. Congress.

**senescence**
A part of the aging process, usually the second half of life, which could increase vulnerability to any life occurrence possible to be experienced,

**senile dementia**
A mental disorder associated with aging. An organic brain syndrome marked by some degree of mental deterioration, accompanied by childish behavior, self-centeredness, sometimes hostility, and difficulty in dealing with life's experiences.

**senile psychosis**
One form of mental illness predominantly found in the aged. It may be marked by the physiological involution of the brain itself. See chronic brain syndrome.

**senility**
A vague term that is loosely used to describe emotional and mental degeneration that occurs in old age.

**senior citizen policies**
Contracts insuring persons 65 years or over with policies that are supplemental to the coverage afforded by the Medicare program.

**senior citizens' residences**
Apartment complexes usually limited to the elderly who can manage fairly well for themselves, but need daily supervision. A clinic is provided and a nurse may be available to visit residents in need of assistance. Some facilities have "resident clubs" or an association which plans activities and provides services for residents. Most of these residences have a manager, special services and grounds are well maintained and kept safe and comfortable for the elderly residents.

**senior interest**
Any right that takes precedent over or ahead of others.

**seniority**
Longevity on a job or in a position.

**sensation**
The feeling experiences when sensory nerve endings of any of the six senses (sight, sound, taste, touch, smell, kinesthesia) are stimulated.

**sensitivity**
1. A measure of the ability of a diagnostic or screening test, or other predictor to correctly identify the positive (or sick) people, the proportion of true positive cases (sick people) correctly identified as positive. Sensitivity = true positives ÷ (true positives + false negatives). A test may be quite sensitive without being very specific. 2. Capable of responding to a stimulus, such as bacteria responding to an antibiotic. 3. A high level of understanding and awareness of a person's emotional, mental and social needs.

**sensoristasis**
The need for sensory stimulation.

**sensory deficit**
Partial or complete impairment of any stimulus to one's sensory organs.

**sensory deprivation**
A lack of sensory stimulation or the impulses that are conveyed from the sensory organs to the brain.

**sensory overload**
Excessive amounts of sound or visual sensory stimulation.

**sentence**
The punishment handed down by a court and given to a person convicted of a crime.

**separate maintenance**
Support money paid by one married person to the other while separated and not living together as husband and wife.

**separation**
1. A husband and wife no longer living together by mutual agreement. 2. A legal separation. 3. A separation agreement is a document designed to distinguish who gets what and who pays what. This is usually temporary, but in some cases can be permanent.

**separation of powers**
The balancing of power of each branch of the government, i.e., the executive, legislative and the judicial; by having different jobs and roles so each can keep the other from becoming too powerful.

**sepso-**
Prefix, meaning infection.

**septic**
Putrefaction or decomposition.

**septic (hectic) fever**
Intermittent fever with wide fluctuations and periods when it falls to normal or below normal levels.

**sequester**
1. To isolate. 2. To hold aside. 3. To deposit. 4. To set apart. 5. To seclude, as to sequester witnesses during a trial.

**seriatim (Lat.)**
One by one; in order of occurrence or priority.

**serum**
The clear substance of a fluid; the liquid portion of blood as opposed to the solid particles.

**servant**
1. A person employed by and subject to another person's control as to what and how work is to be done. 2. In agency law it is the agent; a person serving as a servant or agent is responsible to carry out the orders given by the master or principal. The master or principal is also responsible for the acts of the servant (see respondent superior). Legally speaking a physician is a master, the nurse or other allied health care provider is the servant in this working relationship. See master, agent.

**service**
1. The act of delivering or issuing a legal document such as a summons, a court order, an injunction, or a writ to the person named in it and done so in the prescribed legal manner as to comply with due process of law. 2. Professional functions and duties. 3. To receive a special benefit or advantage. 4. Continual and regular payments on a debt. 5. To provide help or aid to those in need of such help. 6. A unit of health care. There is no standard term for a single unit of health care, whatever that unit may be. Both service and procedure are often used to refer to units of health care, i.e., a health service or a medical procedure. Service

is sometimes used synonymously with encounter, but they should be differentiated, since an encounter may include several services. It is used synonymously with department.

**service area**
See medical trade and catchment area.

**service benefits**
Those received as a result of prepayment or insurance, whereby payment is made directly to the provider of services or the hospital or other medical care programs for covered services provided by them to eligible persons. Service benefits may be full service benefits, meaning that the plan fully reimburses the hospital, for example, for all services provided during a period so that the patient has no out-of-pocket expenses. Full service benefits may also be available when the program itself provides the service as in a prepaid group practice. Partial service benefits cover only part of the expenses, the remainder to be paid by the beneficiary through some form of cost-sharing. See also indemnity benefits and vendor payment.

**service-connected disability**
In the Veterans Administration health care program, a disability incurred or aggravated in the line of duty in active military service. In this context disability includes disease. These disabilities are the primary concern of the program. See also nonservice-connected and adjunct disability.

**service of process**
Official notification that in some way a person is involved in a legal action or court proceeding. Notification may be done in person or, under certain situations, by mail or by publication of the notice in a newspaper.

**service patient**
A patient whose care is the responsibility of a health program or institution (usually a hospital). Service patients are often cared for by an individual practitioner paid by the program (typically a member of a hospital's housestaff), but the program, not the individual, is paid for the care. Sometimes called a public or ward patient. See also private patient.

**services**
1. Refers to groupings of patients, departments, treatments, personnel and physicians. For example, pediatric, surgical, medical, obstetrical or outpatient services. Most groupings of services and personnel are called departments for example; x-ray and nursing. 2. Care or services as provided by health care providers at different levels are defined below. For health insurance purposes, each of these levels are given a code number from the procedure coding manual for each type of care provided.

—minimal services. In health insurance a level of service including injections, dressings, minimal care, etc., not necessarily requiring the presence of the physician.

—brief services. In health insurance a level of service requiring a brief period of time, with minimal effort of the physician.

—limited services. In health insurance, a level of service requiring limited effort or judgment, such as abbreviated or interval history, limited examination or discussion of findings and/or treatment.
—intermediate services. In health insurance a level of service such as a complete history and examination or one or more organ systems, or an in-depth counseling or discussion of the findings, but not requiring a comprehensive examination of the patient as a whole.
—extended services. In health insurance a level of service requiring an unusual amount of time, effort or judgment but not a complete examination of the patient as a whole.
—comprehensive services. In health insurance a level of service providing an in-depth evaluation of the patient.
—unusually complex services. In health insurance an unusually complex medical problem necessitating a comprehensive history and complete examination, extensive review of prior medical records, compilation and assessment of data.
3. According to JCAH for accreditation purposes this is used to indicate a functional division of the hospital or of the medical staff. Also used to indicate the delivery of care. See level of service, care.

**services, critical care**
See critical care services.

**servient**
1. Serving. 2. Being a slave to something.

**servitude**
1. Slavery; bondage. 2. To place restrictions and burdens upon something.

**session**
1. The meeting together of an assembly of people such as a court, hearing or legislature. 2. A day or a period of time in which a court or legislature meets. 3. Continuous periodic gatherings or meetings.

**session laws**
The publication of laws and statutes in the order, or by session, in which they were ruled upon and passed.

**set aside**
1. To cancel. 2. To void or annul. 3. To revoke a judgment or a court ruling. 4. Declaring a verdict void.

**set down**
To schedule a case or lawsuit for trial or hearing.

**set-off**
1. A counter claim which is unrelated to the lawsuit at hand. 2. To try to extinguish or mitigate the claim brought against the defendant by payment of money.

**settle**
1. To reach an agreement about an issue, disagreement, damage, debt, or the disposition of a lawsuit. 2. To finish or end completely. 3. To put into a fixed state or position. 4. To agree on or adjust to. 5. To make

final, firm and solid. 6. To dispose of. 7. To become fixed and assume a lasting form. 8. To determine. 9. To create a trust.

**settlement**
1. The payment of a debt or obligation. 2. The adjustment made on a dispute. 3. In insurance, to pay up to the policy holder claims made against the insurance.

**sever**
1. To end or cut off. 2. To pull apart. 3. To be torn apart. 4. To hear a person's case in a separate place and a different time removed from a current trial.

**severable**
1. Divided; disunited. 2. Separable. For instance, one cause of action may be disunited from earlier action of which it was previously a part. 3. Capable of a separate existence.

**several**
1. Having many or more than one. 2. To be distinct and separate. 3. Individual. 4. Independent.

**severally**
Each its own way; separate, distinct.

**severalty ownership**
1. Having single or sole ownership. 2. A health facility or nursing home with ownership by one person.

**sewer service**
Reporting to the court that a summons or court order was properly served, when it was actually thrown away or flushed down a toilet.

**sex-typed behavior**
The behavior which elicits positive responses for one's sex.

**sexual dimorphism**
The physical, emotional and psychological differences between males and females.

**shall**
According to JCAH for psychiatric, alcoholism and drug abuse facilities accreditation purposes, this is used to indicate a mandatory standard.

**shall or must**
According to JCAH, this term is used to indicate a mandatory statement, the only acceptable method under the current standards. See should and may.

**sham**
1. False; fake. 2. Deceiving. 3. A pretense or fraud.

**sham pleading**
A pleading that appears fair on the surface but is founded on an error or mistakes in the facts or has a fraudulent pretense.

**share**
1. A stock in a corporation. 2. An equitable part given. 3. To have a common possession.

**shared services**
The coordinated, or otherwise explicitly agreed upon, sharing of responsibility for provision of medical or non-medical services on the part of two or more otherwise independent hospitals or other health programs. The sharing of medical services might include, for example, an agreement that one hospital provide all pediatric care needed in a community and no obstetrical services while another undertook the reverse. Examples of shared non-medical services would include joint laundry or dietary services for two or more nursing homes. Common laundry services purchased by two or more health programs from one independent retailer of laundry services are not usually thought of as shared services unless the health programs own or otherwise control the retailer.

**shared support services**
Those services shared by health care institutions such as laundry, purchasing, data processing, etc. See shared services.

**S.H.C.C.**
State Health Coordinating Council. Serves as an advisory body to the Health Planning Agencies in a state or region.

**S.H.C.C. activities**
The functions of the State Health Coordinating Council listed in Section 1524 of the Act pertaining to the establishment of the HSP. Identifies the actions the S.H.C.C. is to undertake in the development and implementation of the HSP.

**shelter**
1. Having a title to property that is sound. 2. Investing money to minimize taxes.

**Shepard's Citations**
A legal publication for use in reference to cases and statutes, which reflects all subsequent cases which cite or refer to a principal case.

**sheriff**
The head police officer of a county.

**sheriff's deed**
A legal document giving ownership to a buyer of property at a police auction or sale.

**Sherman Act**
A federal anti-trust law used to stop combinations in restraint of trade or monopolies.

**shielding**
High density protective materials placed over or between a radioactive source and its surroundings to reduce the radiation exposure.

**shifting**
1. Changing. 2. Transferring or changing position. 3. To change testimony or an account of what happened. 4. Also used in interest on money, called shifting interest.

**shock**
Primarily, the rapid fall in circulation and blood pressure following injury, operation, or the administration of anesthesia.

**shop book rule**
If books are kept in the usual course of business they may be entered into court as evidence so long as they are proper and held in proper custody.

**shop steward**
One who is elected by a labor union to represent the workers in dealings with the employer and to help enforce union policy and rules.

**short cause**
Also referred to as short calendar. That part of a lawsuit or a case that must be heard by a judge, but will not take up much time, thus the waiting period is shortened.

**shorting**
Dispensing a quantity of a drug which is less than the quantity prescribed for the purpose of increasing profit by charging for the prescribed amount. See also kiting and fraud.

**short-range actions**
Well defined changes that must be made in the next year if long-range actions are to be implemented and objectives achieved by the time specified. Short-range actions are more explicit than long-range actions in that they usually specify individuals or agencies who should take primary responsibility for the implementation of a short-range action.

**short sale**
A contract made for the quick sale of stock by a seller who does not own it. Used to profit from an expected fall in price of the stock in question.

**short-stay (acute inpatient) setting**
Providing health care services to patients who stay overnight in the institution but fifty percent or more of whom return to their normal place of residence within thirty days of entering the institution. See short-term hospital.

**short-stay hospital**
See hospital, acute care hospital.

**short-term capital gain**
In tax law, this refers to the amount of profit from the sale of a capital asset held less than one year. Thus, it qualifies as a long term capital gain, therefore is taxed as ordinary income.

**short-term disability income insurance**
A provision in insurance to pay benefits to a disabled person as long as he remains disabled. Coverage is usually up to a specified period of time not to exceed 2 years.

**short-term hospital**
Also refered to as an acute care facility these are determined by the average length of stay of the inpatients. According to the American Hospital Association, a short-term hospital has over 50 percent of all inpatients admitted staying less than 30 days. See hospital, general hospital, short-stay setting.

**short title**
In Congress, the shorter, less formal common title given an Act of Congress by its authors. Health Maintenance Organization Act of 1973 (P.L. 93-222), and National Health Planning and Resources Development Act of 1975 (P.L. 93-641) are short titles.

**should**
According to JCAH, this term is used in the interpretation of a standard to reflect the commonly accepted method, yet allowing for the use of effective alternates. See shall or must and may.

**show cause**
A court order issued to require someone to appear in court in order for him to explain why the court should not carry out a decision or a proposed act. If he fails to appear or to give good enough reasons why the court should not act on the issue, then the court will go ahead with the decision on the action.

**S.H.P.D.A.**
State Health Planning Development Agency. The state government's planning agency which cooperates and coordinates plans and activities with Health Systems Agencies.

**shyster**
A dishonest or unscrupulous person.

**si (Lat.)**
If.

**sic (Lat.)**
Thus; so; in such a way. Same in context, meaning this error in the writing was made in the original document and copied correctly by the last writer. Not an error in the reproduction.

**sickness**
Used synonymously with disease and illness, generally not clearly defined. Common in the insurance field.

**sick role**
To assume a role of wanting to be pampered and freed from life's responsibilities because of illness.

**sic utere tuo ut alienum non laedas (Lat.)**
Use your own so as not to injure another.

**side effect**
The effects or outcomes that are not wanted or intended, such as physical, emotional or mental disorders which are complications of a drug.

**sight (or at sight)**
Payable when presented or requested. Also referred to as sight bill, sight draft, or at sight.

**sigmoidoscope**
A specialized instrument that is used to visually examine the sigmoid colon.

**sigmoidoscopy**
Examination of the interior of the sigmoid colon by the use of an endoscope or sigmoidoscope.

**signatory**
One who signs.

**signature**
1. One's name signed by hand. 2. The name of a person in his own handwriting.

**simple**
1. Plain; uncomplicated. 2. Not aggravated or complicated. 3. Not involved or elaborate.

**simple contract**
An orally expressed contract. A contract that is not sealed.

**simple treatment**
Used in health insurance to refer to radiation therapy and oncology treatment of benign or malignant diseases requiring simple field localization or simple beam shaping devices, single field treatment, or surface or intracavitary therapy applied without general anesthesia.

**simpliciter (Lat.)**
Plainly, purely, simply, naturally, summarily. See simple.

**Sim's position**
A semi-prone examination position, in which a patient lies on his left side with his right knee and thigh drawn up above his left leg. The left arm is placed back of the patient and hanging over the edge of the examining table. The patient's chest is forward so that the patient rests on it.

**simulate**
1. To make a pretense. 2. To take on the appearance of. 3. To imitate or to be fake. 4. Pretend.

**sine (Lat.)**
Without.

**sine die (Lat.)**
1. Without day. 2. Adjournment, without setting a date for another appearance or meeting.

**sine prole (Lat.)**
1. Without issue. 2. Without child.

**sine qua non (Lat.)**
1. Without. 2. A condition or situation that cannot be done away with. 3. An indispensable element.

**single-name paper**
A negotiable instrument with only one original signer or originator.

**single proprietorship**
1. A one owner business. 2. A business owned by one individual person.

**single specialty group**
A group or clinic that provides medical and health care services in one area of medical specialization. Common specialty groups include anesthesiologists, orthopedic surgeons, family practice, pathologists and radiologists.

**sings**
A spiritual healing ceremony ritual conducted by a native American medicine man for healing purposes.

**sit**
1. To officially occupy a seat. 2. To meet or hold a session of court. 3. To formally carry on official business.

**sit-down strike**
Once on the job, employees strike by stopping work and refusing to leave the work site.

**situs (Lat.)**
1. Place. 2. A fixed locale. 3. A location.

**size of group**
The size of a group practice is determined by the full-time equivalent (FTE) numbers of physicians practicing in a group.

**skill**
A learned psychomotor ability to do a function or activity or to apply something in order to carry out an activity.

**skilled nursing facility (SNF)**
Under Medicare and Medicaid, an institution which as a transfer agreement with participating hospitals and which:
is primarily engaged in providing skilled nursing care and related services for patients who require medical or nursing care, or rehabilitation services for the rehabilitation of injured, disabled or sick persons;
has formal policies, which are developed with the advice of a group of professional personnel, including one or more physicians and one or more registered nurses, to govern the skilled nursing care and related medical

or other services it provides; has a physician, a registered professional nurse or a medical staff responsible for the execution of such policies; has a requirement that the health care of every patient be under the supervision of a physician, and has a physician available to furnish necessary medical care in case of an emergency; maintains medical records on all patients; provides 24-hour nursing service and has at least one registered professional nurse employed full time (40 hours/week); provides appropriate methods and procedures for the dispensing and administering of drugs and biologicals; has in effect a utilization review plan which meets the requirements of the law; in the case of an institution in any state in which state or applicable local law provides for the licensing of institutions, as meeting the standards established for such licensing; has in effect an overall plan and budget, including an annual operating budget and a three-year capital expenditures plan; provides for a regular program of independent medical review of the patients in the facility to the extent required by the programs in which the facility participates (including medical evaluation of each patient's need for skilled nursing facility care); meets life safety code; meets any other conditions relating to the health and safety of individuals who are furnished services in such institution or relating to the physical facilities.

**skilled nursing services**

Under Medicare for home health care, means patient care services pertaining to the curative, restorative and preventive aspects of nursing performed by or under the supervision of a registered nurse pursuant to the plan of treatment established in consultation with the care team. Skilled nursing services is nursing care emphasizing a high level of nursing direction, observation and skill.

**skimming**

The practice in health programs paid on a prepayment or capitation basis, and in health insurance, of seeking to enroll only the healthiest people as a way of controlling program costs (since income is constant whether or not services are actually used). Contrast with adverse selection. Sometimes known as creaming. See also skimping.

**skimping**

The practice in health programs paid on a prepayment or capitation basis of denying or delaying the provision of services needed or demanded by enrolled members as a way of controlling costs (since income is constant whether or not services are actually used). The classic example is the denial or delay of a cataract extraction. See also skimming and adverse selection.

**slander**

Oral defamation. Malicious speaking of untrue, false, and defamatory remarks that injure a person's profession, reputation, business, rights, etc.

**slating**

To carry out booking; as booking someone into jail.

**sliding scale deductible**
A deductible which is not set at a fixed amount but rather varies according to income. A family is usually required to spend all (a spend-down) or a set percentage of their income over some base amount (for example, all or 25 percent of any income over $5,000) as deductible before a member can receive medical care benefits. There may be a maximum amount on the deductible. The sliding scale concept can also be applied to coinsurance and copayments.

**slight negligence**
The absence of the level of care which persons of extraordinary prudence and foreseeability are accustomed to.

**sling**
A support used to rest an injured limb, usually an arm, so that pain is reduced and healing in correct position is enhanced.

**slip**
1. Decisions printed on a sheet. 2. U.S. Supreme Court decisions (or other court decisions) that are printed and made readily available soon after the decisions are handed down. Also referred to as a slip sheet, slip decision or slip opinion.

**slip law**
In Congress, the final version of an Act of Congress and its first official publication. Each public law is printed in the form of a slip law which also lists, but does not include, the legislative history of the Act, whatever earlier Act may be amended by the new law, as it is amended, or any explanation or interpretation of the law. See also Public Health Service Act.

**slipper pan**
A specialized bedpan that has one end flattened in order to easily place it under the patient.

**slit lamp**
An instrument with a narrow beam of light, usually used with a special microscope.

**slot**
Position in a work, education program such as medical school, nursing school, physical therapy, etc.

**sludge**
1. Any muddy or slushy mess. 2. Precipitated solid matter arising from sewage treatment processes.

**small business**
A company or business that has a limited number of employees and has less sales volume, or smaller amounts of money to deal with. A group, clinic, or private nursing home may be considered a small business.

**small claims**
A special court that handles small cases concerning a limited amount of money.

**smart money**
Money paid in the form of punitive damages.

**smog**
Irritating smoke or particulate matter in the air that can be turned to haze from the sun's effect on pollutants in the air, notably those from automobile and industrial exhaust.

**smoke**
Any suspension of particles in the air, often originating from combustion. Carbon or soot particles result from the incomplete combustion of carbonaceous materials such as coal or oil. Smoke generally contains water or other droplets as well as dry particles. Tobacco smoke, for example, is a wet smoke composed of minute tarry droplets.

**smoke compartment**
For JCAH long term care facilities this is a subdivision of a floor that is protected by smoke partitions and that provides an area of refuge should another part of the floor become filled with smoke from a fire.

**smoke door**
For JCAH long term care facilities accreditation this is a door installed in a smoke partition and constructed to resist the passage of smoke. Wood doors serving this function must have at least a $1\frac{3}{4}$-inch solid wood core.

**smoke partition/wall**
For JCAH long term care facilities accreditation, this is a wall or barrier that is constructed to resist the passage of smoke and that has a minimum fire resistance rating of one-half hour. Smoke partitions are required to subdivide any floor providing sleeping accommodations for 30 or more patients/residents in existing facilities and to limit the maximum smoke compartment length to 150 feet.

**S.M.S.A.**
1. Standard Metropolitan Statistical Area. 2. The geographic area designated by population by the U.S. Bureau of the Census for statistical reporting purposes.

**smuggling**
1. To bring, carry or handle something in secret. 2. Secretly bringing illegal, prohibited or taxable items into a country.

**Snellen chart**
A special chart used to roughly check a person's vision. It is rows of capital letters placed in random order and graduated in size, which is correlated with the ability to read them at a certain distance.

**So.**
Southern Reporter of the National Reporter System.

**S.O.A.P.**
A term describing an approach to the recording of information in a patient's medical record, based on the problem oriented medical method.

S — Subjective (what the patient or other information source has told you.) If S is other than the patient, state who.
O — Objective (what you have observed).
A — Assessment (affirmative statement of the situation.)
P — Plan of action (future plans).

Not all the letters need to be used with each recording of the narrative. Soaping is needed for an explanation in documentation. There is no necessity for one to be redundant if the flow sheet in the medical record says what you want it to.

**social adaptation**

1. Adjustment to society. 2. Acceptable interpersonal relationships and transactions. 3. The ability to live in society and express oneself. 4. To live in accordance with society's restrictions and demands. See also adaptational approach.

**Social and Rehabilitation Service (SRS)**

The administration within HHS which manages welfare and related programs including Medicaid, which is the responsibility of SRS's Medical Services Administration. Since SRS is not under the direction of HHS's Assistant Secretary for Health, this means that Medicaid is administered separately from the Department's other health programs.

**social assessment**

According to JCAH for psychiatric, alcoholism and drug abuse facilities accreditation purposes, this is the process of evaluating each patient's environment, religious background, childhood history, military service history, financial status, reasons for seeking treatment, and other pertinent information that may contribute to the development of the individualized treatment plan.

**social breakdown syndrome**

The construct that a part of a mental patient's symptomatology is a direct result of treatment and living conditions in facilities and not a part of the primary illness. Factors related to this condition are labeling, learning the chronic sick role, dysfunctional or lost work and social skills and role identification with the maladjusted and ill.

**social characteristics**

The social aspects of the population of the state and their presumed impact on health and health care.

**social diagnosis**

The assessment of the major factors having a negative effect on the quality of life found in a population by clarifying concerns in economics, housing, nutrition, work, unemployment, illegitimacy, civic disturbance, etc.

**social indicator**

A numerical value given to a social situation which reflects a change in the quality of life.

**social insurance**

A device for the pooling of risks by their transfer to an organization, usually governmental, that is required by law to provide indemnity (cash) or service benefits to or on behalf of covered persons upon the occurrence of certain pre-designated losses. This is characterized by the following conditions: coverage is compulsory by law; except during a transition period following its introduction, eligibility for benefits is derived, in fact or in effect, from contributions having been made to the program by or in respect of the claimant or the person as to whom the claimant is a dependent; there is no requirement that the individual demonstrate inadequate financial resources, although a qualified status may need to be established; the methods for determining the benefits are prescribed by law; the benefits for any individual are not usually directly related to contributions made by or in respect of him but instead usually redistribute income so as to favor certain groups such as those with low former wages or a large number of dependents; the cost is borne primarily by contributions which are usually made by covered persons, their employers, or both; the plan is administered or at least supervised by the government; and the plan is not established by the government solely for its present or former employees. Examples in this country include social security, railroad retirement, and workman's and unemployment compensation. In other countries, health insurance is often a government sponsored social insurance program.

**socialization**

The learning of adequate interpersonal skills and proper interaction with other members of a group according to and in conformity with one's society.

**socialized medicine**

A medical care system where the organization and provision of medical care services are under direct government control, and providers are employed by or contract for the provision of services directly with the government; also a term used more generally, without recognized or constant definition, referring to any existing or proposed medical care system believed to be subject to excessive government control.

**social problem**

A set of circumstances or a situation that has an effect on a significant number of people that are the victims of difficulty based on the local situation, one's perception including an objective view of the situation as well as a social interpretation.

**social psychiatry**

A branch of psychiatry that deals with the ecological, sociological, and cultural variables that cause maladaptive behavior and the treatment of the related problems.

**Social Security Administration (SSA)**

The agency within the Department of HHS which manages the social security program including Medicare, which is the responsibility of the SSA's Bureau of Health Insurance. Since SSA is not under the direction of HHS's Assistant Secretary for Health, this means that Medicare is administered separately from the Department's other health programs.

**social service aide/assistant**

A person who assists social workers. They may interview applicants for services, refer people to available community resources, and do simple follow-up studies under supervision of a social worker. There are no specific educational requirements beyond a high school diploma. A 2 year associate degree may be preferred by some employers.

**social service department**

The social services of health care facilities are carried out by medical and psychiatric social workers who focus on the social, economic, mental and community factors that influence the patient's condition. Community resources are used to reduce the social, environmental and emotional barriers to recovery, such as financial problems, post-hospital care, discharge planning and assistance to the patient's family. Social service programs often work very closely with psychiatry and psychiatric social work services.

**social services designee**

A person identified in an extended care, or long-term care facility to provide social services, under the direction of a social work consultant. A designee should have at least two years of college education and, preferably, a B.A. degree. State licensure is not required in any state because the function of social service designee is not itself an occupation, but a role specified in Medicare regulations and assigned to an otherwise employed member of the facility staff.

**social work assistant**

According to JCAH for accreditation purposes, this is an individual with the baccalaureate, preferably with a social welfare sequence, who is given training on the job for specific assignments and responsibilities in the provision of social work services; or who has the documented equivalent in education, training, and/or experience.

**social worker**

A professionally trained person providing social services, either as a member of a health team, a social service section of a health facility, or on a consultant basis. Social services are provided to enable a patient, family members, or others to deal with problems of social functioning affecting the health or well-being of the patient. Most trained social workers now hold a master's degree in social work (MSW). The B.A. in social work (BSW) is a beginning professional degree. The National Association of Social Workers (NASW) requires that social workers engaging in independent practice have at least an MSW and two years of professionally supervised practice in the methods to be employed in independent practice.

**social worker, psychiatric**

A professional, trained in social work, who works with psychologists and psychiatrists in a clinic or institutional setting. This professional's role is to assess family, environmental and social factors that contribute to the patient's illness, intake and work with new patients and may follow up after discharge are also activities that are incorporated in their skills in case work. Psychiatric social workers also do individual, family, and group psychotherapy.

**social worker, qualified**

1. According to JCAH for psychiatric, alcoholism and drug abuse facilities accreditation purposes, this is an individual who has a master's degree from an institution accredited by the Council on Social Work Education, or who has been certified by the Academy of Certified Social Workers, or who has the documented equivalent in education, training, and/or experience. 2. A person who is licensed, if applicable, by the state in which practicing, is a graduate of a school of social work accredited or approved by the Council on Social Work Education, and has 1 year of social work experience in a health care setting. (social worker, qualified consultant-Medicare.)

**Society of Prospective Medicine**

Provides an opportunity for individuals to keep up with the rapid changes in the practice of health maintenance and health enhancement. Through identifying the actual and potential health risks for a person, followed by a personalized plan of risk reduction, is the ultimate in comprehensive and continuing high level wellness care. Large industrial corporations, life insurance companies, labor unions, community action groups, colleges and universities, religious organizations and individuals utilize wellness programs based on the principles of the Society of Prospective Medicine. The goals include: 1) assist in the development of appropriate risk factors for identified causes of disability and death, such as overweight, sedentary lifestyles, smoking, and excessive stress, to name only a few. 2) seek to identify additional causes of disability and death. 3) provide for quality evaluation and availability of risk factor data. 4) advance the teaching of prospective medicine and personal health in medical schools, residency programs, community hospitals, other educational institutions, and in all appropriate forms. 5) serve as a clearing house for professional and lay information about procedures that will enable individuals to adopt healthful life styles. 6) promote research to evaluate the effectiveness of these changes and mechanisms to motivate individuals to decrease risks and practice positive wellness.

**sociogram**

Pictoral or diagrammatic presentation of the occurrence of choices, rejections, and indifferences in a number of persons involved in a life situation.

**sociology**

The study of groups and social organization.

**sociometric distance**

A method used to measure degree of perception that one person has for another. It is suggested that the greater the sociometric distance between persons, the more inaccurate is one's evaluation of social relationships.

**sociometrist**
An investigator or researcher who measures interpersonal relations and social structures and vital statistics of a community.

**sociopath**
A person who does not adhere to societies' moral and ethical standards at the expense of others, sometimes this type of person will commit bizarre crimes.

**sodomy**
1. Unnatural sexual intercourse such as anal intercourse, or placing the penis in the mouth between humans. 2. Anal intercourse; a crime in most states.

**soft money**
Money that is given to a program or organization on a short-term basis and in limited amounts. When the specific amount is gone, the program or job ends. Sources of soft money are usually grants in specific amounts from federal or state governments, philanthropic organizations, or businesses. See hard money.

**software**
1. The collection of programs and routines such as application programs, operating system, programming languages and translators, used with a computer. 2. Films, audio tapes, videotapes, slides, etc. used on projectors and media equipment.

**sole proprietorship**
A single, one-owner business. A one-physician, one-dentist, one-psychologist solo practice approach to ownership of an unincorporated business entity. One of the simplest forms of practicing one's profession, where the physician or psychologist hires an associate on a salary while retaining responsibility for legal matters, management, policy development and budgetary and financial matters. The advantage of sole proprietorship are sole ownership, self determination, a simple decision making, simple financial arrangement, finding compatible employees, with the disadvantages being: sole legal and financial responsibility, limited information in decision making, limited consultations and professional interactions.

**solicitation**
1. To ask for. 2. Something urgently needed. 3. Something that is enticing. 4. To seek or strongly request.

**solicitor**
Used to refer to an English lawyer.

**solicitor general**
A lawyer or officer for the Department of Justice who represents the United States government in actions which it is involved.

**solid waste**
Waste material that requires oxidation or enzyme action to break down into its elements, e.g., paper; tin cans.

**solo practice**
Lawful practice of a health occupation as a self-employed individual. Solo practice is thus by definition private practice but is not necessarily general practice or fee-for-service practice (solo practitioners may be paid by capitation, although fee for service is far more common). Solo practice is common among physicians, dentists, psychologists, podiatrists, optometrists and pharmacists; less common and sometimes illegal in other professions.

**solvency**
1. Being able to pay debts. 2. Having enough money to pay one's debts, possessing more assets than liabilities.

**solvent**
1. Having the authority to end or dissolve something. 2. Being capable of paying off a debt. 3. A substance or agent which could be water, but often an organic compound which dissolves another substance.

**somatic**
Referring to the physical body.

**somnambulism**
Sleepwalking movement or motor activity during sleep. It is commonly seen in children. In adults it is seen in the schizoid personality disorder and certain types of schizophrenia.

**somno-**
Prefix, meaning sleep.

**somo- or somato-**
Prefix, meaning body.

**sono-**
Prefix, meaning sound.

**sonoplacentography**
A technique utilizing ultrasound waves to ascertain the exact position of the placenta during pregnancy.

**sonotopography**
A technique utilizing ultrasound to determine the position of a structure within the body.

**sound**
1. Together; whole. 2. Not deteriorating or decaying. 3. In good condition. 4. Healthy. 5. Founded on what is believed to be true. 6. Free from error. 7. Carefully thought out. 8. Dependable. 9. Valid.

**sound mind**
1. Having a sane, competent, healthy mental state. 2. Competent to make reasonable and thought out decisions.

**source document**
A paper on which data are originated, this may be handwritten or machine written. A medical chart or doctor's order or a medical insurance form can be a source document.

**sovereign immunity**
1. The government's ability to allow or not allow claims to be brought against it. 2. Immunity from laws or claims due to its state of being, i.e., the source of power and laws. 3. Designed for a particular purpose.

**special**
1. Uncommon. 2. Extraordinary. 3. Differing or distinctive from others. 4. Limited. 5. Unusual.

**special appearance**
Appearing in court for a special reason, such as to contest the jurisdiction of a court to hear a case.

**special care**
That care which is limited to a particular branch of medicine or surgery. Delivered by staff who by virtue of their advanced training are qualified to deliver such care in a specialized setting.

**special care unit**
According to JCAH for accreditation purposes, this is an appropriately equipped area of the hospital where there is a concentration of physicians, nurses, and others who have special skills and experience to provide optimal medical care for critically ill patients.

**special class insurance**
Health insurance coverage for applicants who cannot qualify for a standard policy for reason of poor health.

**special damages**
Those damages which are the actual, but not the necessary result of the injury.

**special hospital**
Unique health care facilities for mentally ill patients who are a danger to themselves and must be kept separate and under security.

**special injunction**
A court order or writ that prohibits acts of a party such as dumping of pollutants indiscriminately.

**specialist**
A physician, dentist or other health professional who limits his practice to a certain branch of medicine or dentistry related to: specific services or procedures, e.g., surgery, radiology, pathology; certain age categories of patients, e.g., pediatrics, geriatrics; certain body systems, e.g., dermatology, orthopedics, cardiology; or certain types of diseases, e.g., allergy, psychiatry, periodontics. Specialists usually have special education and training related to their practice and may or may not be certified as specialists by the related specialty board. See also board eligible and certified, general practice, secondary care and RVS.

**special master**
An official of the court who represents the state to determine the validity of certain facts or the real circumstances surrounding a case.

**special pleading**
Presentation of new facts that offset the matter presented by the opposing party.

**special risk insurance**
Insurance coverage for risks or hazards of a special or unusual nature.

**special services**
In health insurance, this is a service which is generally not part of basic services, but which involve additional services of physicians. They generally are adjunctive to common services. See services.

**specialty**
A completed contract. An agreement in final form and delivered to the parties involved.

**specialty boards**
Organizations that certify physicians and dentists as specialists or subspecialists in various fields of medical and dental practice. The standards for certification relate to length and type of training and experience and include written and oral examination of applicants for specialty certification. The boards are not educational institutions and the certificate of a board is not considered a degree. Specialties and their boards are recognized and approved by the American Board of Medical Specialties in conjunction with the AMA Council on Medical Education. See also board certified and board eligible.

**special verdict**
A decision in which the jury states bare facts as they are determined, upon which a verdict is based.

**specific gravity**
The weight of an agent or substance, compared to the weight of an equal volume of some other substance that is a known standard, such as water; the specific gravity of water is 1.

**specificity**
A measure of the ability of a diagnostic or screening test or other predictor to correctly identify the negative (or healthy) people; the proportion of true negative cases (healthy people) correctly identified as negative. Specificity = true negatives ÷ (true negatives + false positives). A test may be quite specific without being very sensitive.

**specific performance**
To be compelled to perform in a contract, when money damages for breach of the contract would not be satisfactory.

**specified disease insurance**
Insurance which provides benefits, usually in large amounts or with high maximums, toward the expense of the treatment of the specific disease or diseases named in the policy. Such policies are rarely written these days,

being more common in the past for such diseases as polio and spinal meningitis, but coverage of end-stage renal disease under Medicare can be thought of as an example.

**specified professional personnel**
According to JCAH for accreditation purposes this is individuals who are duly licensed practitioners, members of the house staff, and other personnel qualified to render direct medical care under the supervision of a practitioner who has clinical privileges in the hospital, and who are capable of effectively communicating with patients, the medical staff, and hospital personnel.

**speculum**
A specialized instrument used to open a body orifice in order to view an internal cavity.

**speech disturbance**
A general term for a variety of verbal or nonverbal communication disorders not due to an organic problem. See aphasia, alexia.

**speech/hearing therapy aide**
Assists in testing, evaluating, and treating the problems of people with speech and hearing difficulties.

**speech pathologists**
1. These health care providers are prepared to diagnose and evaluate individual speech and language competencies, including assessment of speech and language skills as related to educational, medical, social and psychological factors. They plan, direct, and conduct habilitative and rehabilitative treatment programs to establish and promote communicative efficiency in individuals with communication problems arising from neurological disturbances or defective articulation. They provide counseling and guidance to speech and language handicapped individuals and their families. Speech pathologists frequently work closely with the health care team, as in the care of the aphasic stroke patient, and may provide consultant services to educational, medical, and other professional groups. They may teach scientific principles of human communication in educational institutions, direct scientific projects, or conduct research in the areas of voice, speech, and language. 2. Speech pathologist or audiologist (qualified consultant) (Medicare) A person who is licensed, if applicable by the state in which practicing and is eligible for a certificate of clinical competence in the appropriate area granted by the American Speech and Hearing Association under its requirements in effect on the publication of this provision; or meets the educational requirements for certification, and is in the process of accumulating hours of supervised experience required for certification. See qualified speech-language pathologist.

**speech screening**
According to JCAH for psychiatric, alcoholism and drug abuse facilities accreditation purposes, this is a process that may include such tests as articulation in connected speech and formal testing situations; voice in terms of judgments of pitch, intensity, and quality and determinations of

appropriate vocal hygiene; and fluency, usually measured in terms of frequency and severity of stuttering or dysfluency (based upon evaluation of speech flow-sequence, duration, rhythm, rate, and fluency).

**speech therapy**
The study, examination, appreciation and treatment of defects and diseases of the voice, of speech and of spoken and written language, as well as the use of appropriate substitutional devices and treatment. See also speech pathologist.

**spell of illness**
In Medicare, the benefit period during which Part A hospital insurance benefits are available. A benefit period begins the first time an insured person enters a hospital after his hospital insurance begins. It ends after he has not been an inpatient in a hospital or skilled nursing facility for 60 days in a row. During each benefit period the insured individual is entitled to up to 90 days of hospital care, 100 days in a skilled nursing facility, and 100 home health visits. An additional lifetime reserve of 60 hospital days may be drawn upon when more than 90 days of hospital care is needed in a benefit period. There is no limit to the number of benefit periods an insured person may have. The spell of illness concept means that the program may pay for more than 90 days in a hospital in a given year, because with a new spell of illness, the benefit becomes available again. Where a spell of illness continues for a long period of time, as over a several year period, the program pays less than 90 days of care per year, because it does not pay in the second or third year if there has not been a break in the spell of illness. Additionally, under Medicare, the deductible is tied to each spell of illness. Thus an individual who is hospitalized three times in a year, each in a separate spell of illness, has to pay the deductible of the cost of an inpatient hospital day three times.

**spendable income**
Income after taxes and expenses, which can be used or spent.

**spend down**
A method by which an individual establishes eligibility for a medical care program by reducing gross income through incurring medical expenses until net income (after medical expenses) becomes low enough to make him eligible for the program. The individual, in effect, spends income down to a specified eligibility standard by paying for medical care until his bills become high enough in relation to income to allow him to qualify under the program's standard of need, at which point the program benefits begin. The spend-down is the same as a sliding scale deductible related to the over-all income level of the individual. For example, persons are eligible for program benefits if their income is $200/month or less, a person with a $300/month income would be covered after spending $100 out-of-pocket on medical care; a person with an income of $350 would not be eligible until he incurred medical expenses of $150. The term spend-down originated in the Medicaid program. An individual whose income makes him ineligible for welfare but is insufficient to pay for medical care, can become Medicaid-eligible

as a medically needy individual by spending some income on medical care. Medicaid only covers an individual if aged, blind, disabled, or a member of a family where one parent is absent, incapacitated, or unemployed—that is, fitting one of the categories of individuals who are covered under the welfare cash payment programs.

**sperm**
The male reproductive cell.

**spermacide**
Foams, jellies, or creams inserted into the vagina before intercourse to stop or destroy the sperm.

**sphygmocardiograph**
A device used to record a continuous heartbeat via a person's pulse, which is recorded on a moving graph or oscilloscope.

**sphygmograph**
A device used to record a continuous pulse of an artery with the strength and rate displayed.

**sphygmomanometer**
The blood pressure cuff; the instrument used to measure blood pressure.

**sphygmophone**
An instrument used to record activity of the heart using amplified sound waves played through a set of earphones or a speaker.

**sphygmoscope**
An instrument used for showing the activity of the heart as displayed on an oscilloscope.

**spiral bandage**
A method of applying a bandage to parts of the body extremities, usually to joints, and holds a dressing or splint in place.

**spiral reverse bandage**
A bandage applied to extremities of the body to hold dressings in place. Because the limbs are tapered, the bandage is given one turn with each wrap to keep it tight.

**spirogram**
The record made by a spirograph.

**spirograph**
A device used to record respiration/breathing movements on a graph.

**spirometer**
A device for measuring the volume of air inhaled and exhaled.

**spirometry**
Measurement of pulmonary capacities.

**spite fence**
A fence erected to irritate a neighbor which affects his access or view.

**splint**
A special rigid support to maintain or immobilize a body part or limb.

**spoliation**
1. Intentional destruction or mutilation by a third party or an outsider, i.e., the failure of one side of a dispute to come forward with evidence which it has. 2. Intentional change or mutilation by an unauthorized party.

**sponge**
1. Any absorbent pad used in hospitals or surgical operations. 2. A porous, absorbent mass, such as a pad of gauze or cotton surrounded by gauze.

**sponge, gelatin absorbable**
A sterile, absorbable, water-insoluble, gelatin-base material used in the control of bleeding.

**sponging, cold**
See cold sponging.

**sponsor**
A subscriber to a prepaid health care plan who has dependent beneficiaries.

**sponsored malpractice insurance**
A malpractice insurance plan which involves an agreement by a professional society (such as a state medical society) to sponsor a particular insurer's medical malpractice insurance coverage, and to cooperate with the insurer in the administration of the coverage. The cooperation may include participation in marketing, claims review, and review of ratemaking. They have been replaced by professional society operated plans, joint underwriting associations, state insurance funds and other arrangements.

**sporadic disease**
A disease that occurs in occasional scattered cases.

**spore**
A destruction-resistant body formed by certain microorganisms; resistant cells.

**spot zoning**
Where zoning is applied to a certain area or property, while surrounding land has a different zoning. Sometimes special changes or spot zoning is allowed for special purposes, such as allowing a nursing home to be built in a residential area.

**sprain**
Accidental pulling, wrenching or twisting of a joint, causing a partial rupture of the ligaments. There may be damage to the associated blood vessels, muscles, tendons, and nerves.

**sputum**
The mucus secreted from the lungs, bronchi, and trachea.

**S.R.S.**
Social and Rehabilitative Service. (see these words) A branch of the U.S. Department of Health and Human Services.

**S.S.A.**
Social Security Administration. (see these words). A branch of the U.S. Department of Health and Human Services that is responsible for old age and disability insurance.

**S.S.I.**
Supplemental Security Income. See these words.

**stab wound**
A puncture wound caused by a sharp instrument such as a knife.

**staff development (Medicare)**
An ongoing educational program is planned and conducted for the development and improvement of skills of all the facility's personnel, including training related to problems and needs of the aged, ill, and disabled. Each employee receives appropriate orientation to the facility and its policies, and to his position and duties. Insevice training includes at least prevention and control of infections, fire prevention and safety, accident prevention, confidentiality of patient information, and preservation of patient dignity, including protection of his privacy and personal and property rights. Records of training are to be maintained which indicate the content of, and attendance at, such staff development programs.

**staffing patterns (Medicare)**
The facility furnishes to the state survey agency information from payroll records setting forth the average numbers and types of personnel (in full-time equivalents) on each tour of duty during at least 1 week of each quarter. Such week will be selected by the survey agency.

**staffing ratio**
The total number of employees in a health care facility if it is to be an overall facility staffing ratio or total numbers of employees on a unit within the facility that are full time employees (FTE - full time equivalents) divided by the average daily census of the facility or by the census of the unit if it is to be a unit staffing ratio.

**staff privilege**
The privilege, granted by a hospital, or other inpatient health program, to a physician, or other independent practitioner, to join the hospital's medical staff and hospitalize private patients in the hospital. A practitioner is usually granted staff privileges after meeting certain standards, being accepted by the medical staff and board of trustees of the hospital, and committing himself to carry out certain duties for the hospital such as teaching without pay, or providing emergency or clinic services. It is common for a physician to have staff privileges at more than one hospital. On the other hand, since hospitals accept a limited number of physicians, some practitioners are excluded and end up with no access to hospital facilites, having no staff privileges. The standards used to determine staff privileges sometimes include evaluation by the

county medical society, which may give preference to or require membership in that society, which in turn may require membership in the American Medical Association. This practice is formally opposed by the AMA. Some hospitals limit privileges for certain services to board eligible or certified physicians. Full time, or hospital-based physicians, and physicians working in a system such as a prepaid group practice with its own hospital are not usually thought of as having staff privileges; Many hospitals have several different levels of staff privileges with names like active, associate, courtesy or limited. Sometimes staff privileges are called admitting, hospital, practice or clinical privilege.

**stakeholder**
A noninvolved party who is selected to hold funds or property which are in dispute, with the understanding that he will turn the goods over once the matter is settled.

**stale check**
A check or negotiable instrument that has been held beyond its time limit before cashing it. The time period to cash a check is set by law or is written on the check.

**stamina**
Endurance, strength.

**stamp tax**
A tax that requires revenue stamps to be bought and placed on a legal document in order to make it them valid.

**stand**
1. The location where a witness sits to testify. 2. To remain. 3. To refuse to change or reconsider.

**standard**
1. A professionally developed expression of the range of acceptable variation of performance from a norm or criterion. 2. The value assigned to a particular criterion when measuring health service characteristics. 3. A measure of quantity, quality, weight, extent or value that is set up as a rule by authority.

**standard deviation**
In statistics, it is a measure of variation and is derived by squaring each deviation in a set of scores, taking the average of these squares, and taking the square root of the result. The standard deviation, represented byς, the Greek letter sigma, is one of the most useful measures of variation in statistical computations.

**standard error**
In statistics, it is a measure used to determine how much variation exists in test results and how much is due to chance and error. It shows how much is due to experimental influences. The standard error of the mean is arrived at by dividing the standard deviation by the square root of the numbers of measures, or, when the number of measures is less than 30, by the square root minus 1.

**standard of care**
1. Skill and learning commonly possessed by members of their chosen profession that are needed to deliver an expected level of care. 2. Reasonable and ordinary care, skill and diligence that ordinary and prudent health care providers and professionals in good standing should exercise in like or similar cases or situations. This definition is used to include locality or community rules, that is, the health care provider would be expected to deliver the usual level of care given in that locality or community, however, the locality rule has mostly been done away with. The reasonable man concept and the principle of foreseeability are closely aligned with the standard of care.

**standard of reasonableness**
The expected level at which prudent individuals are to act under certain circumstances. See reasonable man.

**standard rates**
See rates.

**standards**
Generally, a measure set by competent authority as the rule for measuring quantity or quality. Conformity with standards is usually a condition of licensure, accreditation, or payment for services. Standards may be defined in relation to: the actual or predicted effects of care; the performance or credentials of professional personnel; and the physical plant, governance and administration of facilities and programs. In the PSRO program, standards are professionally developed expressions of the range of acceptable variation from a norm or criterion. Thus, the criteria for care of a urinary tract infection might be a urinalysis and urine culture and the standard might require a urinalysis in 100 percent of cases and a urine culture only in previously untreated cases.

**standby commitment**
In finances, this is a commitment to issue a loan, usually for a period of one of five years once construction is completed in the event a regular permanent loan cannot be obtained. This type of loan is usually at a higher interest rate than a permanent loan and a standby fee is charged.

**standing**
The right to bring a lawsuit as the party involved is directly affected by the issues being disputed in the case.

**standing to sue**
Where a party has enough cause or enough personal interest in a matter to cause him to seek relief.

**stand mute**
A refusal to plead "guilty" or "not guilty." Such a stand is often treated as a "not guilty" plea.

**Stanford-Binet intelligence test (scale)**
A verbal psychological test administered individually to children and adults to test levels of intelligence. See also I.Q., mental age.

**stare decisis (Lat.)**
1. Let the decision stand. 2. To stand by previous decisions; judge made law. 3. A doctrine involved with precedent in deciding cases. A court should stick to a legal principle created by a previous decision and apply it to all future cases with similar facts unless there is a strong reason not to. 4. To stick to a precedent.

**stat**
Used in a hospital crisis or emergency, meaning at once; immediately.

**state**
1. To say. 2. To set forth. 3. To declare. 4. A condition or situation.

**State Comprehensive Health Planning Agency (state CHP or 314(a) agency).**
A former health planning agency assisted under section 314(a) of the PHS Act, added by P.L. 89-749, the Comprehensive Health Planning and Public Health Service Amendments of 1966. The agencies were to develop state comprehensive health planning programs, with the assistance of a health planning council which was broadly representative of the general public and private health organizations in the state with a majority of consumers among its members. P.L. 89-749 has been superceded by P.L. 93-641, the National Health Planning and Resources Development Act of 1974, which authorizes assistance for state health planning and development agencies to replace 314(a) agencies. These new agencies prepare annual state health plans and medical facilities plans. The state agency also serves as the designated section 1122 review agency and administer a certificate-of-need program.

**state cost commissions**
State agencies assigned various health services cost and charge regulation or review responsibilities. The duties of a commission may include assuring that: total hospital costs are reasonably related to total services offered; aggregate rates bear a reasonable relationship to aggregate costs; and rates are applied equitably to preclude any possibility of discriminatory pricing among various services and patients of a hospital.

**state health manpower plan**
That plan developed by the SHPDA that concerns itself with health manpower in the state. See SHPDA, State Health planning and Development Agency.

**state health manpower priorities**
The ranking of the state's health manpower needs and concerns in order of importance.

**State Health Plan (SHP)**
A combination of the Health Systems Plans in a state, as modified by the State Health Coordinating Council to represent its decisions as to broad strategic actions and health resource changes recommended over the next five years or more, plus recommendations for their implementation, to alter the future health system in order to attain explicitly stated goals.

**state health planning and development agency (SHPDA)**
Section 1521 of the PHS Act, added by P.L. 93-641, requires the establishment of state health planning and development agencies in each state. As a replacement for existing state CHP agencies, SHPDAs prepare an annual preliminary state health plan and the state medical facilities plan (Hill-Burton). The agency will also serve as the designated review agency for purposes of section 1122 of the Social Security Act and administer a certificate-of-need program. Many SHPDAs have been closed down or have assumed a planning role for state owned and controlled agencies such as public health departments.

**state health priorities**
Health needs and concerns of the population of the state ranked according to importance, and amenable to intervention by the State Health Planning and Development Agency and the Health Systems Agency. See priorities.

**State Medical Facilities Plan (SMFP)**
A document presenting the decisions reached by the State Health Planning and Development Agency and approved by the State Health Coordinating Council specifying the State requirements for medical facilities, the Title XVI (P.L. 93-641) financial assistance which should be provided for medical facility construction, modernization and conversion and the priorities for such assistance.

**statement of affairs**
A financial summary form which is used when filing bankruptcy.

**Statement of Construction**
A JCAH document that must be completed by each long term care facility prior to survey. A properly completed Statement of Construction describes and verifies the basic structural and fire protection characteristics of each building in which patients/residents are housed. In addition, a plan of correction for all physical plant deficiencies identified by either authorized inspection agencies or indicated in the JCAH Statement of Construction and Fire Protection must be submitted.

**statement of managers**
See conference.

**state's evidence**
Evidence given by an accomplice to a crime, by testifying against his partners in the crime.

**statewide health coordinating council (SHCC)**
A state council of providers and consumers (who shall be in the majority) required by section 1524 of the PHS Act, added by P.L. 93-641. Each SHCC generally will supervise the work of the state health planning and development agency, and review and coordinate the plans and budgets of the state's health systems agencies (HSA). It will also annually prepare a state health plan from HSA plans and the preliminary plans of the state agency. The SHCC will also review applications for HSA planning and resource development assistance.

**statewide issues/needs**
Concerns identified by entities of state government which are considered as being of statewide importance.

**statim (Lat.)**
Immediate.

**statistical significance.**
A statistical measure of the reliability that shows something occurs other than by chance.

**status**
1. A condition. 2. The position, state or basic standing of a person or situation. 3. The condition of affairs. 4. The legal state of affairs.

**status health**
The state of or level of a person or group's well being.

**status of the health delivery system**
A description of the existing health delivery system and the structures utilized in the provision of health services to the residents of the state.

**status value**
The total worth of a person as measured by criteria such as income, social prestige, intelligence, professional status and education; used as an assessment of one's position in the society.

**statute**
Any law passed by a legislative body, i.e., an ordinance or law passed by a lawmaking body. A written law, such as criminal law.

**statute of frauds**
Requiring long-term contracts to be written and signed in order for them to be valid. A concept based on old English law. See fraud.

**statute of limitations**
A law that establishes and fixes the period of time during which an action may be started. Time limitation often depends on the type of legal action, or circumstances of the issue or dispute.

**statutes at large**
Statutes that were passed by a legislature. They are collected and printed in the order of their passage.

**statutory**
1. Established or declared by law or statute. 2. Having to do with a statute. 3. Created by or conforming to statute. 4. Defined, or required by a statute.

**statutory law**
A law passed by a legislature that is a city, county, state, provincial or federal law making body.

**statutory rape**
An adult or grown man having sexual intercourse with a female under a certain age.

**stay**
1. To stop or halt. 2. To stop a proceeding. 3. A temporary act by a court order.

**stenographic recording**
The writing or recording of testimony or court proceedings by a court reporter who uses a paper-punching recording machine, a tape recorder or a notebook.

**step-rate plan**
Health insurance coverage in which premiums increase with the age of the enrolled member.

**stereotaxy**
A specialized surgical procedure used in brain surgery. Deep areas of the brain are operated on once a pinpointed position has been determined utilizing 3 point measurements. The actual procedure is done with electricity, heat, cold or mechanical means.

**stereotype**
1. Beliefs and values held in common by the members of a group that conforms to a fixed belief system or cultural pattern. 2. Oversimplified evaluation, judgment or bias about a person or group.

**stereotypy**
Unusual or excessive continuous repetition of speech or physical activities. A characteristic of catatonic schizophrenia.

**sterile**
Free from microorganisms; aseptic.

**sterile technique**
See surgical asepsis.

**sterility**
Inability (either temporary or permanent) to reproduce.

**sterilization**
1. The process of making sterile; the destruction of all forms of life by heat and/or chemical means. 2. The surgical procedure that renders an individual incapable of reproduction, such as vasectomy or tubal ligation.

**stertor**
Snoring or sonorous respiration.

**stethoscope**
An auditory instrument used to hear and listen to the sounds produced within the body.

**stillbirth**
The delivery of a fetus that died before or during delivery. The term is used to refer to either such a delivery or such a fetus. Some definitions are limited to fetuses of an age or weight that are potentially or usually viable (e.g., 1,000 grams). A fetal death is sometimes synonymous,

sometimes limited to those which occur before delivery. See also perinatal mortality.

**stimulant**
Any drug that produces an exciting or arousing effect, increases physical activity and promotes an unusually high sense of well-being. There are different types of stimulants, such as central nervous system stimulants, cardiac stimulants, and respiratory stimulants.

**stimulus**
Anything from the environment, internal or external, that arouses or incites action or a response.

**stipulation**
A written agreement about legal procedures or matters between lawyers of different parties.

**stock**
1. Items or goods for sale by a business. 2. The supply of goods on hand. 3. Shares in a corporation.

**stockholder's derivative suit**
The bringing of a lawsuit by a stockholder of a corporation for the corporation while the company itself is not suing.

**stockinette**
A soft cloth material that is placed next to the skin under a cast to protect the skin.

**stock insurance company**
A company owned and controlled by stockholders and operated for the purpose of making a profit, and contrasted with a mutual insurance company. In the former the profits go to the owners, in the latter they go to the insured.

**stool**
Waste products from the large intestine; feces. See feces.

**stopcock**
A valve that controls the flow of fluid through a tube.

**stop order**
To give notice to a bank to refuse payment on a check.

**stoppage in transit**
A merchant's right to stop the delivery of an item or goods even after it has been sent.

**stores**
See materials management.

**strabismus**
Crossed eyes or squint.

**straight-line depreciation**
Dividing the cost of an item by the number of years it will be useful and deducting that amount each year from income tax.

**strain**
1. Overstretching of a muscle or part of a muscle. 2. Sometimes used synonymously with stress.

**stranger**
One who is not part of a business transaction; a third party. A person not known to the first party.

**strategy**
A methodological approach or plan of action that takes into account any problem or barriers and limited resources necessary to achieve specific objectives.

**straw man**
1. A person who is present or involved only on a superficial level. 2. One who takes part in a business transaction in name only.

**stress**
A physical, chemical, psychological or emotional factor that causes bodily or mental tension, anxiety, upset and which may be a factor in disease causation or fatigue, which stems from a deviation of optimal conditions that an individual cannot easily cope with, adapt or adjust to. See stressor, distress, benestressor, eustruess, dystressor.

**stress immunity**
The failure to react to stress.

**stressor**
Any changes, occurrences, events, or experiences that upset or threaten the physical, mental, spiritual, emotional, social values, belief system, relationship or economic status of the human organism, which cannot be effectively coped with or adapted to. If poor adaptation to stress occurs and if coping skills are lacking, this tends to diminish one's natural resistance to disease and proper functioning at the emotional, social and physiological levels. When an upset in the normal balance of the body occurs, then stress causes a mental and physiological breakdown of the person. See stress, dystressor, benestressor.

**strict**
1. Exacting. 2. Severe. 3. Precise. 4. Rigid; governed by rigid or exact rules.

**strict foreclosure**
1. The right of a creditor to regain property, but only in a special situation. 2. To cancel a debt with the creditor without the debtor being able to sue.

**strict liability**
1. To be legally responsible for harm done or injury caused even if not at fault. 2. Liability without the identification of any fault, negligence,

malpractice knowledge, or acts of omission. 3. Liability by being involved in an act that results in harm or injury.

**strike**
1. Employees purposely stopping work or not showing up for work in order to gain benefits or win concessions from an employer. 2. To hit or dash against; to deal a blow.

**stroke**
A cerebrovascular accident, apoplexy, or any hemorrhage or softening of the brain that results in damage to the cerebral arteries. Paralysis, aphasia, and coma are among the neurological symptoms that accompany this condition. This is caused by a sudden rupture or blockage of a blood vessel in the brain, depriving the brain of its blood supply, resulting in loss of consciousness, paralysis, or other disorders depending on the site and extent of brain damage. A stroke is referred to as a CVA. See cerebral vascular accident.

**struck jury**
The most qualified, or at least unobjectionable, group of persons selected as a jury to try a case.

**structural inteqration**
A deep-massage technique, developed by Ida P. Rolf, Ph.D., which is designed to help a person realign the body by altering the length and tone of myofaxcial tissues. Practitioners of "Rolfing", as the technique is commonly known, believe that misalignment of body structure, resulting from inaccurate learning about posture, as well as emotional and physical trauma, may have a detrimental effect on an individual's health, energy, self-image, perceptions, and muscular efficiency.

**structural measure**
See input measure.

**Stryker frame (Foster frame)**
A canvas-covered frame on which the patient lies. It is attached to a metal frame on wheels. The canvas-covered frame is connected at a pivot joint, so that the entire frame turns when the patient is turned from his back to his abdomen and vice versa. When turning the patient, a second canvas-covered frame is placed on top of the patient and the two frames are secured with the patient between them like a sandwich. Safety belts are used to hold the frames together.

**Stryker saw**
A hand-held electrical saw with a half-blade that oscillates rather than rotates. It has no guards, as the manufacturer claims they are not needed. It is used to remove casts from patients' limbs or is used in autopsy work, or in medical education in the dissection of cadavers. Stryker is a brand name. Similar saws are manufactured by other companies.

**stupor**
A disorder or reaction that causes a disturbance of one's consciousness where the patient is nonreactive and unaware of his surroundings.

Organically, it is the same as unconsciousness. In psychiatry, it is a form of mutism and is found in catatonia disorders and psychotic depression.

**sua sponte (Lat.)**
1. Voluntarily; on his own; of his own will. 2. On a judge's own motion. 3. Lack of a formal request from the parties of a dispute.

**sub (Lat.)**
Under.

**subacute**
An illness, disease, disorder or condition that is not quite as serious as an acute disorder, but may become so if not properly cared for.

**sub-area**
Subdivisions of a Health Service area which are used for localizing input, involvement and advice by HSAs.

**Sub-area Advisory Councils (SAC)**
Organizations established by Health Systems Agencies (HSA.) under P.L. 93-641 to advise them on the performance of their functions and to provide an advisory link between the HSA and local communities. Also referred to as (HACs) Health Advisory Councils (HACs).

**subchapter "S" corporation**
A business or organization that receives protection of a corporation but is being taxed as a partnership.

**subcoma insulin treatment**
A form of shock treatment in which insulin is used to produce sleepiness and cause a sense of well-being instead of a shock or coma.

**subconscious**
The preconscious or unconscious mind. A term now obsolete in psychiatry.

**subcutaneous**
Beneath the layers of skin; hypodermic.

**subjective data**
1. Signs and symptoms of dysfunction or disease perceived by the person, which are real to them, such as pain or nausea. 2. Information based on personal opinion rather than facts.

**subjectivity**
An appraisal, evaluation and interpretation of something influenced by one's own feelings, perceptions and thinking as to a quality of the object or experience.

**sub judice (Lat.)**
To be considered by the court; before the court; for the court's consideration.

**sublimation**
The channeling of unacceptable behavior into socially acceptable behavior; a mental mechanism.

**subluxation of the spine**
An incomplete or partial dislocation of two adjacent vertebrae. Normally the vertebral bodies are squarely situated atop one another; however, when such things as trauma or certain forms of arthritis intervene, one vertebral body may shift with respect to its neighbor. When the shift does not completely abolish contact between the two normally adjacent surfaces but does alter their position with respect to one another, the abnormally positioned vertebra is said to be subluxed or partially dislocated. Services of chiropractors are covered under Medicare only when such subluxation is demonstrated on an x-ray.

**submission**
The act of referring of issues to the arbitration process or other legal processes.

**submit**
1. To refer to the judgment of another. 2. To present for. 3. To refer to. 4. To yield or surrender. 5. To allow to. 6. To introduce evidence.

**sub nomine (Lat.)**
1. Under the name; in the name of. 2. Indicating that the name of a case has been changed.

**subordinate**
1. Lower in rank. 2. To have less power or authority. 3. Of less value or importance.

**subordination**
The signing of an official document in a manner that indicates that your interest or position is weaker than another, or that your claim is secondary to another.

**subordination agreement**
A special agreement whereby an encumbrance is made based on or subject to another encumbrance. A loan for land purchase is made once a subsequent construction loan is finalized.

**suborn**
1. To induce. 2. To give false testimony. 3. To bribe or entice another to commit perjury.

**subornation of perjury**
Forcing or enticing a person to lie under oath; which is a crime.

**subpoena**
An order of a court commanding a person to appear in court to testify. A penalty may be imposed in the event of failure to appear.

**subpoena duces tecum (Lat.)**
A subpoena which directs a person to bring certain documents to court. For example, a nurse or physician would bring medical records to court.

**subrogation**
1. To substitute one party for another in order to claim a right or debt. 2. A provision of an insurance policy which requires an insured

individual to turn over any rights he may have to recover damage from another party to the insurer, to the extent to which he has been reimbursed by the insurer. Some experts have argued that private health insurance (including Blue Cross or group insurance) should have subrogation rights similar to those in most property insurance policies, e.g., auto, fire. Having paid the hospital bill of a policyholder, the health insurance company could assume its right to sue the party whose negligence might have caused the hospitalization, and be reimbursed for its outlay to the policyholder. Subrogation rights could help insure prompt payment of medical expenses without duplication of benefits. (Refer to Michigan Hospital Service v. Sharpe, 339 Mich. 357, 63 N.W. 2d., 638, 1954 for ruling on subrogation by Michigan Supreme Court.) Others respond that subrogation is time consuming, expensive and may not offer companies adequate protection against loss. Few insurers use it voluntaily and some insurance commissioners forbid its use.

**sub rosa (Lat.)**
1. Secretly or privately. 2. Literally means under the rose, or hidden.

**subscribe**
1. To write or sign one's name to a document, such as a contract. 2. To sign.

**subscriber**
1. One who pays into or belongs to a group health insurance plan, also called enrollee, certificate holder, insured, policyholder, client, member, patient, or beneficiary but in a strict sense means only the individual (family head or employee) who has elected to contract for, or participate in (subscribe to) an insurance or HMO plan for either himself or himself and his eligible dependents.

**subsequent negligence**
When a defendent sees or is aware of a possible danger or a situation where harm could be done to the plaintiff and fails to exercise due care and precaution to prevent the injury to the plaintiff from occurring.

**sub silentio (Lat.)**
1. Under silence; with silence. 2. Without giving notice or any indication.

**substance**
The real or essential part of anything. The essence of or the main point of a document.

**substance abuse plan (alcoholism and drug abuse)**
Plan of an entity of the state that addresses the provision of services to those individuals known to be abusers of intoxicants and controlled substances.

**substandard health insurance**
An individual health insurance policy issued to a person who cannot meet the minimal health requirements of a standard health insurance policy. Protection is provided but with an increase in the premium and by a waiver of medical condition, or under special qualified impairment clause.

**substantial**
1. Having a real existence; actual. 2. Valuable. 3. Not imaginary. 4. Real, worthwhile or of real worth. 5. Complete enough; considerable. 6. Real and true for the most part.

**substantial performance**
In contract law where there has been performance on the substantial part of the contract but not necessarily on other less important details or parts.

**substantiate**
1. To establish the existence of a fact or evidence. 2. To prove true; to verify.

**substantive law**
1. The legal principles that determine rights and duties, as opposed to procedural or adjective law which determines procedure and process in legal concerns. See procedural law.

**substituted service**
A substituted legal procedure as in the service or process by other than the usual in person delivery; such as by mail, or publication in a newspaper.

**substitution**
1. The filling of a prescription by a pharmacist with a drug product therapeutically and chemically equivalent to, but not, the one prescribed. Many states have anti-substitution laws which prohibit the pharmacist from filling a prescription with any product other than the specific product of the manufacturer whose brand name is used on the prescription. See also maximum allowable cost and generic name. 2. A mental or defense mechanism that replaces one thing by another; unattainable or unacceptable goals are replaced by ones that are attainable or acceptable.

**succession**
The act of transferring a dead person's property to his or her heirs.

**succinylcholine**
A drug used as a powerful muscle relaxant. It is used in anesthesia and in electroconvulsive treatment.

**suctioning**
The drawing of secretions from out of the body by a tube connected to a suction machine.

**sue**
1. To initiate a civil legal proceeding. 2. To start a lawsuit.

**suffer**
1. To allow or to permit something to happen. 2. To sustain injury, harm, loss or damage.

**sufficient**
1. Adequate, solvent or responsible. 2. Equal to the proposed goal.

**suggestibility**
Open to the power of suggestion or influence. A common observation in persons with hysterical symptoms.

**sui generis (Lat.)**
1. Of its own class. 2. One of a kind.

**sui juris (Lat.)**
1. Of his own right; competent. 2. Having full legal rights.

**suit**
1. A lawsuit. 2. A civil action taken to court. 3. To seek favor. 4. An action, court procedure or process at law other than in criminal law.

**summary**
1. A short abridged statement. 2. To be brief and concise; an abstract or shortend form., 3. Immediate; without a full trial; i.e., summary judgment is when one side of a lawsuit is successful in proving the case before the conclusion of the trial.

**summary judgment**
A judgment given on an issue or motion in a lawsuit where pleadings, depositions, testimony, interrogatories, admissions, and all other evidence show that there are no controverted material facts; thus, the party who initiated the motion is entitled to a decision from the court or a judgment as a matter of law.

**summons**
A document that has been certified by the clerk of the court which is a brief summary of a complaint and states the number of days within which the defendant has to answer or appear.

**sumptuary law**
Statutes created to control the sale or use of socially undesirable, harmful, or wasteful products or substances.

**superbill**
An itemized statement furnished to the patient, giving all pertinent information so that the patient may bill the insurance company directly. See super ticket.

**superego**
An unconscious part of the psyche that monitors the id and the ego; concerned primarily with morality, ethics and social standards. A term of psychoanalytic theory created by Sigmond Freud.

**superior**
1. High in place, rank or position. 2. To have power and control over. 3. Preferable or higher in quality. 4. Above.

**superior court**
Court of general and extensive jurisdiction.

**supersede**
1. To have something set aside. 2. To wipe out. 3. To take the place of. 4. To make old laws or policies unnecessary; to replace a law or document with another one.

**supersedeas (Lat.)**
In practice; a court order that temporarily stops or delays a hearing or court from proceeding.

**supersedeas bond**
A bond used to gain a suspension of judgment resulting in a delay in the execution of a pending appeal.

**superticket**
A medical bill and related insurance claims are combined onto a single sheet in order to avoid duplication and to keep costs down. Commonly referred to as a fee ticket and is utilized in outpatient, emergency care or ambulatory services. See superbill.

**supervening**
1. Newly effective. 2. Interposing. 3. A new policy or procedure.

**supervision (Medicare)**
Authoritative procedural guidance by a qualified person for the accomplishment of a function or activity within his sphere of competence, with initial direction and periodic inspection of the actual act of accomplishing the function or activity. Unless otherwise stated in regulations, the supervisor must be on the premises if the person does not meet assistant-level qualifications specified in these definitions.

**supination**
Turning the palm upwards, or lying on the back.

**supine**
The position of lying on one's back, facing upward.

**supplemental health insurance**
Health insurance which covers medical expenses not covered by separate health insurance already held by the insured; which supplements another insurance policy. For example, many insurance companies sell insurance to people covered under Medicare which covers either the costs of cost-sharing required by Medicare, or services not covered, or both. Where cost-sharing is intended to control utilization, the availability of supplemental health insurance covering cost-sharing limits its effectiveness.

**supplemental health services**
The optional services which HMOs may provide in addition to basic health services and still qualify for federal assistance. They are defined in section 1302(2) of the PHS Act.

**supplemental security income (SSI)**
A program of income support for low-income aged, blind and disabled persons, established by title XVI of the Social Security Act. SSI replaced state welfare programs for the aged, blind and disabled. A federally-administered program now paying a monthly basic benefit; states may

supplement this basic benefit amount. Receipt of a federal SSI benefit or a state supplement under the program is often used to establish Medicaid eligibility.

**Supplementary Medical Insurance Program (Part B, SMI)**
The voluntary portion of Medicare in which all persons entitled to the hospital insurance program (Part A) may enroll. The program is financed on a current basis from monthly premiums paid by persons insured under the program and a matching amount from federal general revenues. During any calendar year, the program will pay (with certain exceptions) 80 percent of the reasonable charge (as determined by the program) for all covered services after the insured pays a deductible on the costs of such services. Covered services include: physician services, home health care, medical and other health services, outpatient hospital services, and laboratory, pathology and radiologic services. Any individual over 65 may elect to enroll in Part B. However, indivduals not eligible for Part A who elect to buy into Part A must also buy into Part B. State welfare agencies may buy Part B coverage for elderly and disabled public assistance recipients and pay the premiums on their behalf. The program contracts with carriers to process claims under the program. The carriers determine amounts to be paid for claims based on reasonable charges. The name, Part B, refers to part B of title XVIII of the Social Security Act, the legislative authority for the program. See medical eligibility.

**supplementation**
Partial payment for a portion of the cost of nursing home care by the patient or his family. Supplementation was, prior to 1972, a common requirement in state Medicaid programs in several of the southern states; the practice was stopped in response to a directive of the Senate Finance Committee set forth in the report on the 1967 Social Security Amendments. Supplementation should not be confused with the practice of requiring an individual to contribute his excess income to assist in payment for his nursing home care. Generally, under Medicaid, a nursing home must agree to accept reimbursement from the state as the full amount of its payment for service. Under a system of supplementation, a state pays a rate but the nursing home does not agree to accept that amount as full payment; accepting supplementation of the state rate by the individual or his family. The amount the homes collect in supplement is not under the control of the state. Supplementation generally was used where the state rate was admittedly not sufficient to pay for the cost of the care.

**supplier**
Generally, any institution, individual or agency that furnishes a medical item or service. In Medicare, suppliers are distinguished from providers, including hospitals, and skilled nursing facilities. Institutons classified as providers are reimbursed by intermediaries on a reasonable cost basis while suppliers, including physicians, nonhospital laboratories and ambulance companies, are paid by carriers on the basis of reasonable charges.

**supplies**
Inexpensive medical items, usually of a disposable nature, such as bandages, tongue depressors, rubbing alcohol, etc. Supplies should be distinguished from permanent and durable capital goods (those whose use lasts over a year).

**supply**
In health economics, the quantity of services supplied as the price of the service varies, income and other factors being held constant. For most services, increases in price induce increases in supply. Increases in demand (but not necessarily, in need) normally induce an increase in price.

**support**
1. The financial, moral, and social obligation to provide food, clothing, and shelter for your immediate family. To bear the weight of; to endure; to bear or put up with. 3. To verify or prove.

**supportive services**
Social, nutritional and related health care services that are provided to individuals in their homes in order to avoid institutionalization. Such services include home health care, meals-on-wheels, etc.

**support services**
See ancillary services.

**support staff**
According to JCAH for psychiatric, alcoholism and drug abuse facilities accreditation purposes, these are employees or volunteers whose primary work activities involve clerical, housekeeping, security, laboratory, record keeping, and other functions necessary for the overall clinical and administrative operation of the facility.

**support system**
Those activities and people who can support or assist a person in an emergency or crisis.

**suppress**
1. To subdue. 2. To prevent or disallow. 3. To conceal or keep in. 4. To restrain.

**suppress evidence**
To subdue or conceal evidence from being used in a criminal trial by trying to show that it was obtained illegally or that it is irrelevant.

**suppression**
1. The controlling, hindering or inhibiting an impulse, emotion, experience or idea. Suppression is different from repression in that the latter is an unconscious process. 2. Sudden stoppage. 3. A mental or defense mechanism whereby unpleasant feelings and experiences are kept from conscious awareness.

**Supremacy Clause**
Article VI, Section 2, U.S. Constitution—All legal documents or laws made, under the authority of the United States, shall be the supreme law

of the land; and the Judges in every State shall be bound by them and anything in the Constitution or laws of any State.

**supremacy of law**
In any government the highest authority is the law, not the citizen's wants. See supremacy clause.

**surcharge**
1. Additional money added onto something already paid for. 2. An excessive or added charge above the regular price. 3. Any additional word or mark. 4. To overload or overburden.

**surety**
1. Certainty; that which makes security; assurance that something will happen. 2. A guarantee; security; insurance. 3. One who guarantees or gives assurance.

**surgery**
Any operative or manual procedure undertaken for the diagnosis or treatment of a disease or other disorder; the branch of medicine concerned with diseases which require or are responsive to such treatment; or the work done by a surgeon (one who practices surgery). See also operation, psychosurgery, and major, minor, elective and cosmetic surgery.

**surgical asepsis**
Those methods or measures taken that render items or objects free from all pathogenic microorganisms as well as non-pathogens, and maintain them in this state of sterility.

**surgical expense insurance**
A type of health insurance policy that provides benefits toward the doctor's operating fees. Benefits usually consist of scheduled amounts for each surgical procedure.

**surgical insurance benefits**
A type of medical or health insurance used to insure against loss due to surgical expenses.

**surgical schedule**
A list of cash allowances which are payable for various types of surgery, with the maximum amounts based upon the severity of the operations.

**surgical scrub**
A thorough cleansing procedure of the hands, wrists, and forearms prior to surgery or entering a sterile situation, in which the hands are held higher than the elbows in order to maintain sterility.

**surgical services**
The diagnosis and treatment of physical diseases and conditions or their symptoms by means of operative techniques, in conjunction with the administration of anesthesia when appropriate. In insurance these services mean the work performed by a surgeon in treating diseases, injuries and deformities by manual or operative means.

**surgical team**
In health insurance, under some circumstances highly complex procedures requiring the concomitant services of several physicians, often of different specialties, plus other highly skilled, specially trained personnel and various types of complex equipment are carried out under a surgical team concept with a single, global fee for the total service. The services included in the global charge vary widely.

**surgical technologist**
Works as a general technical assistant on the surgical team by arranging supplies and instruments in the operating room, maintaining antiseptic conditions, preparing patients for surgery and assisting the surgeon during the operation. (formerly operating room technician)

**surplus**
In insurance, the excess of a company's assets (including any capital) over liabilities. Surpluses may be used for future dividends, expansion of business, or to meet possible unfavorable future developments. Surpluses may be developed and increased intentionally by including an amount in the premium in excess of the pure premium needed to meet anticipated liabilities known as a risk charge. Surpluses are sometimes earmarked in part as contingency reserves and in part as unassigned surplus.

**surplussage**
1. Excess; surplus. 2. Something over and above the required amount. 3. Something superfluous or unnecessary.

**surprise**
When one party is brought to trial with no intent or purpose on the part of the opposite party and is presented with something or an issue that was completely unexpected and unanticipated, resulting in difficulty in presenting his side of the case. This situation could cause a new trial or a delay in the present trial.

**surrebutter**
A form of pleading no longer used. Current practice in court usually allows two or three pleadings, whereas five or more were formerly allowed.

**surrejoinder**
See surrebutter.

**surrender**
1. To give back or give up. 2. To return.

**surrogate**
1. A person appointed to act for another. 2. A substitute. 3. A judge presiding over matters of probate and intestate succession. 4. A court officer who deals with proving of wills and estates. 5. A substitute person or object.

**surrogate parent**
Any parental or authority figure who acts as a parent for a child and is reactive and sensitive to emotions, feelings and responses in the child.

**surtax**
1. Any tax imposed on an item or service that is above the normal or expected tax. 2. A tax placed on a tax.

**survive**
To outlive; to live longer than another; to live beyond or through an event.

**survivorship, right of**
The legal right of a person to property of another due to outliving or surviving that person.

**suspect**
1. To believe in the possible guilt of an illegal act without having proof. 2. To conjecture; to consider as questionable. 3. One who is believed to be involved with the committing of a crime.

**suspect class**
Any class of persons identified by a statute for special (discrimatory) treatment; classes identifiable by monetary worth, nationality, race, age or sex. Having to do with violation of the 14th Amendment.

**suspended sentence**
A sentence that is formally handed down for a crime committed, but is not actually served. A sentence that is removed.

**suspicion**
1. To be held temporarily by the police, as they believe you are involved in something harmful or illegal which has occurred. 2. To be held without specific charges stated or brought against you.

**sustain**
1. To maintain or uphold. 2. To suffer or undergo loss. 3. To confirm or grant. 4. To bear out.

**susto (Spanish)**
Shock; frieght. A mental and emotional disorder common to the Mexican-American culture characterized by shock, fright or sudden terror. It is founded on emotional and supernatural powers.

**suture**
Surgical sewing or stitches used to close accidental or surgical openings in the organs or tissues of the body.

**S.W.**
South Western Reporter of the National Reporter System.

**swap maternity**
A provision in group health insurance plans providing immediate maternity benefits to a newly covered woman but terminating coverage on pregnancies in progress upon termination of a woman's coverage. See also switch and flat maternity.

**switch maternity**
A provision in group health insurance plans providing maternity benefits to female employees only when their husbands are covered in the plan as their dependents. Has the effect of denying maternity benefits to single women. See also flat and swap maternity.

**syllabus**
1. A summary , or abstract of a case. 2. An outline or overview.

**sym-**
Prefix, meaning together; with.

**symbiosis**
A dependent relationship that is created between two mentally ill persons. This relationship helps to reinforce each other's pathological condition.

**symbolic delivery**
The giving of an item of value to be used as a legal symbol of ownership, i.e., giving a key to an automobile is a symbolic delivery of the actual gift.

**sympathetic nervous system**
The part of the autonomic nervous system that is reactionary rather than voluntary and is helpful in dealing with threatening situations by preparing one's body for fight or flight.

**sympathomimetic drug**
Any drug that can reproduce or cause the same reactions that are produced by the sympathetic nervous system. Examples are amphetamine and epinephrine.

**sympathy**
Showing pity or some concern of another's fears by sharing another person's feelings, ideas and experiences. This is opposed to empathy, and is not objective.

**symptom**
Any abnormal manifestation or reaction that departs from the normal function, appearance, or sensation experienced by a patient. Any sign indicative of disease.

**symptom formation**
See symptom substitution.

**symptom substitution**
A psychological process where repressed desire shows itself and is indirectly released through psychological or behavioral symptoms. Such symptoms can include obsession, compulsion, phobia, dissociation, anxiety, depression, hallucination and delusion. The reaction is also known as a symptom formation.

**syn-**
Prefix meaning together, with.

**syncope**
Being faint; having temporary loss of consciousness.

**syncretic-thought**
Concrete and specific thought processes. (A term introduced by Jean Piaget.)

**syndicate**
1. Any group of persons organized for a special undertaking. 2. A joint adventure.

**syndrome**
A group of effects, signs and symptoms of a condition, disorder or disease that constitute a typical clinical picture.

**synergistic effect**
An agent or substance that affects the action of another agent or substance so that their combined effect is greater than both.

**synopsis**
A summary, abstract or overview of a document or case.

**syntaxic thought**
A term used to describe logical, goal-directed and reality-oriented thought processes. (A term of psychologist Harry Stack Sullivan.)

**synthesis**
The combining of the elements or parts of a whole.

**syntropy**
Healthy or wholesome relationships.

**syphilis**
A venereal disease that is treatable, but if left untreated can cause organic psychosis.

**systemic**
Pertains to the systems of the body; something like infection throught an entire system.

**systems planning**
Also referred to as systems approach. This is the continuous planning methodology which addresses the segments of a continuum as they relate to the whole.

**systolic pressure**
The greatest amount of pressure exerted by the blood being forced against the arterial wall during contraction of ventricles of the heart.

# T

**T.A.**
Transactional Analysis. A form of psychotherapy and self-counseling. See transactional analysis.

**tablet**
A drug, medicine, or medication in solid pill form.

**tachycardia**
An accellerated heart rate of over normal.

**tachypnea**
An abnormally high respiratory rate.

**tacit**
1. Saying nothing or making no sound. 2. Unspoken, still or silent. 3. Implied. 4. Understood without being spoken.

**tactic**
A method, technique or approach used as a part of a strategy.

**tactile**
Pertaining to the sense of touch.

**Taft-Hartley Act**
A 1947 federal law, that created rights for the employer, related to or counter to union rights created by the Wagner Act. It helped control unfair union and labor practices such as forcing an employee to join a union.

**tail**
1. Curtailed. 2. Limited in a specific way as to inheritance limited to only children or grandchildren. 3. To cut. 4. To set down a tally. 5. To limit; as by an entail.

**talc**
A silicate powder used in ceramics, cosmetics, paint and pharmaceuticals as a powder and a filler in soap, putty and plaster.

**talesman**
1. A person called in to serve as a juror. 2. A person summoned as a spokesman.

**tamper**
1. To make changes by meddling or interfering. 2. To plot or scheme. 3. To make secret illegal arrangements. 4. To make corrupt or illegal.

**tampon**
A cotton sponge used to plug a cavity subject to bleeding, such as the nose or vagina.

**tamponade**
A plug, usually of cotton, used to stop hemorrhage.

**tangible**
Something real that can be held or touched.

**tariff**
1. A list of items. 2. That which has a form or substance to it. 3. An explanation or information given especially about fees to be paid. 4. To set a price or tax on an item, goods, or service; an import tax.

**T.A.T.**
Thematic Apperception Test. A psychological test using projective techniques in which the subject supplies interpretations of a series of pictures, revealing his own feelings, perceptions and attitudes.

**tautology**
Needless repeating the same idea using different words; redundancy, repetition.

**tax**
1. A compulsory payment of money to a government. 2. To assess or determine judicially the amount of levy for the support of certain government functions for public purposes. A charge or burden, usually pecuniary, laid upon persons or property for public purposes; a forced contribution of wealth to meet the public needs of a government. See also tax credit and deduction, and regressive, proportional and progressive tax.

**taxable income**
1. Money or profit gained that is legally taxable or filed under the tax laws. 2. The income against which taxes are paid.

**tax, ad valorem**
1. A tax according to value. 2. A portion or percentage of the value on an article that is taxable.

**tax avoidance**
Taking advantage of all legal tax breaks, deductions, exemptions, etc.

**tax credit**
A reduction of tax liability for federal income tax purposes. Several national health insurance proposals allow businesses and/or individuals to reduce their taxes dollar for dollar for certain defined medical expenses. The effect of using a tax credit approach rather than a tax deduction is to give persons and businesses an equal benefit for each dollar expended on health care. A tax credit favors lower over higher income people while a tax deduction is worth more the higher the marginal tax rate. See also Medicredit.

**tax deduction**

A reduction in one's income base upon which federal income tax is calculated. Health insurance expenditures are deductible by businesses as a business expense. Since the tax rate for most large businesses is 48 percent, this means there is a reduction of tax liability of nearly $1 for each $2 the business spends on health insurance. Individuals may take a medical deduction on their personal income tax of one-half the cost of health insurance premiums up to $150 plus all medical expenses and premiums that exceed 3 percent of income. Since the marginal tax rate is related to income and is higher for higher income persons and businesses, the value of a tax deduction for income spent on medical care increases as income increases; thus, the subsidy is effectively greater for the higher income person or more profitable corporation. See also tax credit.

**tax evasion**

1. Not paying any taxes or paying less taxes than required by law. 2. Committing tax fraud by paying taxes in less amounts than is true or can be accounted for.

**tax expenditure budget**

In the federal budget, an enumeration of revenue losses resulting from tax expenditures. Section 301 of the Congressional Budget and Impoundment Control Act of 1974 requires that estimated levels of tax expenditures be presented by major functions in the Congressional and Presidential budgets.

**tax expenditures**

Revenues lost to government because of any form of legal tax reduction or tax forgiveness, including tax credits and deductions. The term emphasizes that such revenues foregone for specific purposes (such as subsidizing private purchase of health insurance through the federal income tax deduction for health insurance) are budgetarily equivalent to actual federal expenditures. See also tax expenditure budget.

**taxing cost**

Legally causing one party in a lawsuit to pay the other party's legal fees.

**T-binder**

A binder used in dressing wounds or surgical areas or bandage-type cloth shaped in a T and used to retain dressings in the genital areas.

**teaching facilities**

Areas dedicated for use by students, faculty, or administrative or maintenance personnel for clinical purposes, research activities, libraries, classrooms, offices, auditoriums, dining areas, student activities, or other related purposes necessary for, and appropriate to, the conduct of comprehensive programs of education. Such term includes interim facilities but usually does not include off-site improvements or living quarters.

**teaching hospital**

A hospital which provides undergraduate and/or graduate medical education, usually with one or more medical, dental or osteopathic (AMA, ADA or AOA approved) internship and residency programs and affiliation with a medical school. Hospitals which educate nurses and other health personnel without training physicians are not generally thought of as teaching hospitals. Nor are those which have only programs of continuing education for practicing professionals. See also housestaff and affiliated hospital.

**teaching hospital, graduate associated**
Teaching hospitals that have one or more training programs directed by medical school clinical departments, and may also have training programs independent of the medical school.

**teaching hospital, principal**
Teaching hospitals in which medical school clinical departments direct all aspects of graduate training programs.

**teaching hospitals, independent**
Teaching hospitals that conduct only their own graduate and undergraduate medical education programs.

**teaching hospital, undergraduate associated**
Teaching hospitals that have a tie to a school for undergraduate clinical training, and conduct their own independent graduate medical education program.

**teaching physician**
A physician who has responsibilities for the training and supervision of medical students, interns, and residents. Teaching physicians are often, but not necessarily salaried by the institution in which they teach. A common arrangement is that a physician in private practive must donate a certain amount of time for teaching and supervision in return for being granted staff privileges. Appropriate reimbursement of the activities of these physicians has been a subject of condiderable controversy. Under Medicare, hospitals are reimbursed under the hospital insurance program for the costs they incur in compensating physicians for teaching and supervisory activities and in paying the salaries of residents and interns in approved teaching programs; in addition, reasonable charges are paid under the supplementary medical insurance program for teaching physicians' services to patients. See physician.

**teaching rounds**
See ward rounds.

**technical**
1. Having to do with unique or special aspects, skills, knowledge or teminology of a profession, i.e., x-ray technicians or medical technicians have special unique knowledge and skills. 2. In law it is specific steps or procedures to have a case dismissed for technical reasons, usually a failure to follow specific step-by-step procedures or rules.

**technical assault**
Assault without the intent to injure, such as giving an injection with a hypodermic needle.

**technical component**
When filing an insurance claim, the health care provider, under certain circumstances, may make a charge for a technical procedure component alone. Under those circumstances the technical component charge is identified by adding this modifier number to the usual procedure number as provided by the procedure coding manual.

**technician**
1. A person with highly specialized training in a focused area of expertise. 2. A person knowledgeable and skillful in some field or subject.

**technicist**
A technician; a person skilled in technics or having special skill or knowledge.

**Technicon Medical Information System (TMIS)**
A comprehensive computerized medical information system first used at El Camino Hospital of Mountain View, California. It uses a computer to accept, store and send data to physicians, nurses, technologists, clerks, etc. A broad range of medical data, physicians' orders, test results, etc. as well as administrative data such as charges, insurance coverage, etc. is all processed by the computer system.

**technic, technique**
Rarely used words for technical.

**technique**
1. A specialized procedure, skill or method. 2. A degree of expertise or expertness.

**technologist**
A technician; one versed, skilled and knowledgeable in technology. One with specialized training and skills in a specialized and focused area or field.

**technology**
Applied science using specialized instruments, electronics, tools, devices, equipment with the accompanying terminology to perform specialized techniques, tasks or skills not possible without the specialized equipment; advanced skills, techniques and knowledge gained through electronics and instrumentation.

**tele-**
Prefix meaning distant; far.

**temperament**
Inborn predisposition to act or react in a specific way to experiences. Temperament can and does vary from person to person.

**temperature**
1. The level of heat of a living body as expressed in degrees. 2. The balance between the heat produced and the heat lost in the body.

**temporary disability**
An illness or injury of such a kind or nature that temporarily prevents an insured person from performing the functions of his regular job.

**temporary restraining order**
A court order causing one party or the other to take or to refrain from taking certain actions prior to a hearing being held on an issue or dispute.

**tenacious**
Holding firmly or strongly; cohesive, stubborn.

**tenancy**
1. The act of or condition of being a tenant. 2. Interests of a tenant. 3. The duration of occupancy.

**tenancy in common**
Property that is common to two or more persons with each having a right to the property or of occupying it. The right of survivorship to the property is often excluded.

**tenancy, joint**
An undivided interest in property held by two or more parties, which is established by one document with a right of survivorship included.

**tenant**
A person who occupies property, real estate, or rents.

**tenant at will**
A tenant who is allowed to remain in possession of a property, but whose right to remain can be withdrawn at any time.

**tender**
1. To offer money or something of value to pay for goods or services; money offered to end or pay on a debt. 2. To present for acceptance. 3. To offer an official or former offer. 4. An item, such as money, used to complete an agreement, deal or to satisfy an obligation. Tender is money but also can be any item or goods used to complete a deal. Two sacks of wheat could tender a deal as well as money.

**tender offer**
1. The offering of payment to satisfy a debt or claim; a willingness to pay; the show of a willingness. 2. To complete an offer or deal. 3. In corporate law, a tender offer is an offer made to the public to buy a specific number of stocks at a specific price, which enable the offeror to take over the corporation.

**tenement**
1. Any house, apartment, building, or place in which one could live. 2. A dwelling place. 3. Any type of permanent housing or property that is held by tenure.

**tenement house.**
A house divided into a number of living places or apartments. A word often used to refer to poorer, run-down, overcrowded, deteriorating apartments which present public health problems in central city areas.

**tenor**
1. A mode of continuation. 2. A general direction. 3. Of a general nature. 4. Train of thought or idea that is basic to or runs through an issue. 5. The exact wording of a legal document. 6. An exact legal copy. 7. The tone or implication of a statement or act.

**tension**
Unpleasurable emotions and anxiety characterized by a strenuous increase in mental and physical activity. Another word for stress.

**tergiversate**
1. To turn one's back on an issue. 2. To use subterfuge. 3. To desert a cause. 4. To equivocate.

**term**
1. A fixed or definite period of time; a time period set for something to happen; a set time or date. 2. A point of time to determine the beginning or ending of a period or agreement. 3. A word or words with a certain meaning. 4. In insurance, it is the period of time for which an insurance policy is issued.

**terminal decline**
A decline in one's ability to think and reason, thought by some to occur shortly prior to death. Perhaps a result of disruptions within the central nervous system; a marked drop in intellectual functioning as death draws near.

**terminal digit filing**
One approach used in filing medical records. This method uses consecutively issued record numbers, divided into groups of two digits each and filed first by the last two or terminal digits. This method effects a near perfect distribution of the most recent records among other records in the file. For example, record 21-44-65 would be filed by the terminal digits (65), next by the middle digits (44) and finally, by the first two digits (21).

**termination**
1. The end of something. 2. The ending of an agreement or dispute. 3. The ending of a contract legally, without it being breached or broken by either party.

**term of court**
The established time for a court to hold sessions or to hear cases.

**territorial**
Having to do with limited, specific areas or jurisdictions.

**territorial courts**
Federal courts used in each U.S. territory to serve as federal and state courts.

**territorial jurisdiction**
The authority of a court to hear cases from within a designated or limited geographical area or region.

**territory**
1. An assigned or designated area. 2. A province of action or existence.

**terror**
1. Intense fear. 2. An unmanageable person.

**terrorize**
1. To frighten or to appall. 2. To alarm, shock or terrify.

**tertiary care**
Services provided by highly specialized providers (e.g., neurologists, neurosurgeons, thoracic surgeons, intensive care units). Such services frequently require highly sophisticated technological and support facilities. The development of these services has largely been a function of diagnostic and therapeutic advances attained through basic and clinical biomedical research. See also care, primary and secondary care.

**tertiary care facility**
Facilities which render highly specialized services requiring highly technical resources. This type of care is usually associated with those services rendered in university medical centers or specialty hospitals (e.g., burn centers).

**tertiary case, see tertiary care.**

**tertiary psychological prevention**
Those measures taken to reduce emotional and mental impairment or disability following a physical or emotional condition; rehabilitation programs.

**testacy**
To create and leave a valid will. See testate.

**testament**
1. A will. 2. A legal document with instructions concerning the disposition of a person's personal property upon death of the person writing it.

**testamentary capacity**
Having the mental ability and competence necessary to make a valid will.

**testate**
Having died and left a will.

**testator**
One who has made a will.

**test case**
A lawsuit that is considered highly important as it may establish a new or important legal issue, principle or right. Test cases are usually filed to establish the constitutionality of a new statute.

**testes**
The male gonads.

**testify**
To give verbal evidence while under oath in a hearing, a court, or to an official of the court.

**testimony**
The evidence given by a witness while testifying under oath. See testify.

**test, patient liability**
Proposed guidelines which describe the obligations and extent of financial participation of patients in paying for physician services in a teaching setting.

**test, physician role**
Guidelines which establish criteria for the payment of physicians on a fee-for-service basis in a teaching setting.

**test reliability**
See reliability.

**test validity**
See validity.

**tetanus**
An infectious disease caused by the toxic byproducts of the bacteria Clostridium tetani. It is characterized by muscle spasms. Also called "lockjaw."

**T-group (training group)**
A method of group therapy that emphasizes self-awareness and group dynamics. It is now used more in management than in psychotherapy. A sensitivity training group therapy program used to increase one's sensitivity to others while improving skills in humaa relations by disclosing and discussing feelings about and behaviors with one another. This encounter group technique is rarely used any more.

**thanatoid**
1. Apparently dead. 2. Being close to or having a condition similar to death.

**thanatologist**
A person who studies or is a specialist or expert on the dying process or death.

**thanatology**
1. The study of death. 2. An account of the death process.

**thanatophobia**
The fear of death.

**thanatopsis**
Meditation on death.

**thanatos**
A Greek mythical figure in which death is personified. 2. A death wish.

**theft**
Stealing, or the act of taking something that does not belong to you, which can be either a misdemeanor or a felony, depending on the value of the property.

**therapeutic activity services**
According to JCAH for psychiatric, alcoholism and drug abuse facilities accreditation purposes, these are goal-oriented activities designed to help an individual develop expressive and/or performance skills through participation in art, crafts, dance, drama, movement, music, prevocational, recreational, self-care, and social activities.

**therapeutic agent**
Any substance or person that promotes healing in a maladaptive person. In group therapy, it refers mainly to people who help others.

**therapeutic community**
Any treatment setting that provides a curative or helpful environment for behavioral change through resocialization and rehabilitation.

**therapeutic environment**
Any social environment which is supportive of health or the restoration of physical or mental health.

**therapeutic equivalents**
Drug products with essentially identical effects in treatment of some disease or condition. Such products are sometimes, but not necessarily always, chemically equivalent or bioequivalent. Therapeutic equivalents are sometimes defined as chemically equivalent, and drugs with the same treatment effect, which are not chemically equivalent, called clinically equivalent. This is a useful distinction but inconsistently used.

**therapeutic group**
Group of patients together in one room under the leadership of a therapist for the purpose of working together for the treatment of each patient's emotional disorders or maladaptive behaviors.

**therapeutic radiology services**
The department, people and instruments used to treat physical diseases, usually cancerous tumors, through the use of radiant energy.

**therapeutic recreation**
See recreational therapy.

**therapeutic recreation specialist (qualified consultant) (Medicare)**
A person who if required by state law is licensed or registered, to practice, and is eligible for registration as a therapeutic recreation specialist by the National Therapeutic Recreation Society (Branch of National Recreation and Park Association) under its requirements in effect. See recreation therapist.

**therapy**

**-therapy**
A suffix meaning treatment.
The treatment of physical, mental or emotional disease.

**therapy services**
The therapeutic techniques used in implementing a program of habilitation or rehabilitation designed to meet the needs of an ill or disabled individual.

**thermal trauma**
Injury caused from excessive heat or cold.

**thermo-**
Prefix meaning heat.

**thermogram**
The picture produced by thermography. Hot spots are shown on the picture as they produce infrared radiation.

**thermography**
A method of assessing the heat produced by different parts of the body using film which is photosensitive to infrared radiation.

**thing**
1. Any item, matter, issue, circumstance, object, affair or concern. 2. A process or step by step procedure. 3. That which is an object of concern, discussion, spoken of or conceived. 4. A tangible object, not a concept or idea. 5. An act, transaction, event, matter or that which is done. 6. That which is mentioned but unnamed and nonspecific. 7. That which can be owned or possessed such as property. 8. That which is not a person.

**third degree**
Using illegal or physical means to force a person to confess to an illicit action or crime.

**third party**
An individual or party who is uninvolved or not associated directly with a deal, claim, dispute, or lawsuit, but who may be a part to it or be affected by it or subject to it.

**third party beneficiary**
In contract law a person who is not a party to a contract, but who has a legal interest in the contract and for whose benefit it was drawn up.

**third-party billing**
Bills and statements prepared by a health care practitioner, group, hospital, nursing home or other provider and then sent to a third-party payor on behalf of the patient.

**third party paid**
Paid patients have part or all of their health care paid for by someone else, like an insurance company or the government. This third party pays to the patient and/or the health care provider.

**third party payer**

An insurance carrier who steps in to pay hospital or medical bills instead of the patient. Also known as third party carrier. 2. Any organization, public or private, that pays or insures health or medical expenses on behalf of beneficiaries or recipients (e.g. Blue Cross and Shield, commercial insurance companies, Medicare, and Medicaid). The individual generally pays a premium for coverage in all private and some public programs. The organization then pays bills on the patients behalf; such payments are called third party payments and are distinguished by the separation between the individual receiving the service (the first party), the individual or institution providing it (the second party) and the organization paying for it (the third party). See also service and indemnity benefits.

**thought process disorder**

A symptom of schizophrenia that involves problems with intellectual functions. It is shown by incoherence of the patient's verbal processes.

**threshold**

1. The level at which first effects occur. 2. The point at which a person just begins to notice a sound is becoming audible.

**threshold limit value**

In occupational health it is an exposure level under which most people can work consistently for 8 hours a day, day after day, with no harmful effects

**tic**

Involuntary, repetitive behavior in a small segment of the body. Mainly psychogenic, it may be seen in certain cases of chronic encephalitis.

**tidal irrigation**

This is also referred to as "thru and thru irrigation" which is an automatic continuous process of introducing a solution and then emptying it out (usually in the bladder) through a closed catheter system.

**time draft (time bill or loan)**

A draft bill or loan that is payable at a specified time.

**time is of the essence**

1. This phrase is used in a contract to mean that if what is specified in the contract is not done by a specified time, a breach of the contract can occur. 2. A phrase used in contracts to insure certain acts are completed when time is a factor in the situation.

**time is of the essence contract**

1. A contract that places emphasis on a time limitation and upon expiration of the contract if not completed by a stated time. 2. One limitation is that no one can demand an extension of time for performance.

**time limit**

The period of time in which a notice of an insurance claim or proof of loss must be filed.

**timeliness**
1. The timing was to one's advantage. 2. Happening at a good or proper time. 3. Being timely. 4. Completed or happening at a suitable time. 5. Being of good time. 6. Having good timing.

**timely**
1. Well timed; being in good time; early. 2. Completed on time. 3. Opportune timing. 4. Done at a suitable time.

**time-price doctrine**
The allowing of a higher price to be charged for items bought on credit. This is a way to get around state usury doctrines.

**time-sharing**
Arrangement that permits two or more health care facilities or enterprises to be users and to share the same computer.

**tinnitus**
Noises or sounds in one's ears, such as ringing and whistling, which is occasionally a side effect of some anti-depressant drugs.

**tissue**
A large group of similar cells, bound together and dedicated to the performance of a particular function.

**tissue committee**
A committee, which usually functions in a hospital setting, and reviews and evaluates all surgery performed in the hospital on the basis of the extent of agreement among the preoperative, postoperative, and pathological diagnoses; and on the relevance and acceptability of the procedures undertaken for the diagnosis. The committee derives information from the use of pathologic findings from tissue removed at surgery as a key element in the review.

**title**
1. The official document that shows the right to ownership of property.
2. Certificate of ownership.

**titled patient**
One whose health care services are reimbursed under Titles V, XVIII, or XIX of the Social Security Act.

**Title XIX(19)**
The title of the Social Security Act which contains the principal legislative authority for the Medicaid program, and therefore a common name for the program.

**Title XVIII(18)**
The title of the Social Security Act which contains the principal legislative authority for the Medicaid program, and therefore a common name for the program.

**titometer**
An instrument used to measure the depth of color in a liquid.

**TLV**
Threshold limit value.

**TMIS**
Technicon Medical Information System. A computerized information system used in hospitals.

**to have and to hold**
A phrase formerly required in a deed to make the transfer of land official.

**toilet training**
Teaching a child or elderly person to control his bladder and bowel functions.

**tolerance**
1. Sympathy for beliefs or behaviors differing from one's own beliefs. 2. Capacity for endurance or adapting. 3. Putting up with a deviation from normal or expected behavior. 4. In drug use/abuse this means that if the same dose of a drug is taken day after day the effects gradually disappear.

**toll**
1. To remove. 2. To defeat. 3. To take away. 4. To entice or allure. 5. A tax or duty paid. 6. To draw attention to. 7. A loss of a large number of items, money or property.

**tolling statute**
A law passed that allows the statute of limitations to be delayed, put off, or to put off its future effects.

**-tome**
Suffix meaning instrument to cut.

**tomography**
An image gathering technique using either x-ray or ultrasound to produce an image of structures of the body at a specified depth. See CT scanner, computerized axial tomography.

**-tomy**
Suffix meaning cutting; incision; section.

**tonometer**
An instrument used to measure pressures within a body part such as the eye, which uses an ophthalmotonometer.

**tonsillectomy**
The surgical procedure involving the removal of a tonsil or tonsils.

**tontine**
A type of life insurance in which persons pay into an insurance fund and only those still alive by a certain time receive benefits or payments. This type of insurance approach has been outlawed in most states.

**topectomy**
A psychosurgical procedure performed on chronic psychotic patients in cases that do not respond to other treatment methods such as psychotherapy or drug therapy.

**topical**
The application of heat, ointment, drugs, etc. to the external surfaces of the body.

**topo-**
Prefix meaning place; position; location.

**topography**
The geography, structure or configuration of a surface, including its relief and the natural and man-made features.

**tort**
1. A wrongful or negligent act done to another person or property that results in harm, injury or damage. 2. A civil wrong that does not involve a contract and usually is not a crime. 3. When a health care person violates a duty owed to another person and damages occur. 4. When wrongful conduct on the part of one party has caused harm to a second party and those who suffer the harm then seek compensation for the loss and suffering through some form of legal process or lawsuit. 5. When a duty owed is breached. Some torts include negligence, malpractice, battery, slander and libel.

**tortfeasor**
1. One who does harm or damage or commits a tort. 2. A wrongdoer.

**tortious**
A wrongful occurance; the act of committing a tort.

**total disability**
An illness or injury that completely prevents an insured person from performing every duty pertaining to his job or occupation, or from engaging in any other type of work to earn his livelihood.

**total loss constructive**
Any loss or damage that is of sufficient magnitude to make the cost of repairing a damaged property more than it is worth.

**total maternity care**
Includes antepartum care, delivery and postpartum care. The services normally provided in uncomplicated maternity care.

**totten trust**
Placing money into an account in one's own name as a trustee for another person. It can be returned or reclaimed, or if you die, it then becomes the property of the other person.

**tourniquet**
A device that is wrapped around a limb to compress the blood vessels and completely stop the flow of blood.

**to wit**
That is to say; namely. It can be replaced by "to know". The punctuation mark of a colon as it is used to introduce lists.

**Towne's projection**
A posteroanterior x-ray film used to produce an image of the entire skull and mandible.

**township**
A division of state land having a certain mile limit on each side, creating the boundaries of a city.

**toxemia**
Poisoning by way of the blood stream.

**toxic dust**
Any dust that may enter the body through the respiratory tract into the blood and may be harmful to the respiratory system or to other parts of the body.

**toxicity**
A chemical agent that produces harmful effects on some biologic function including the condition under which this poisonous effect occurs.

**toxico-**
Prefix meaning poison.

**toxicologist**
Concerned with the nature and extent of the injurious response to the ingestion of chemical compounds and the determination of safe levels of exposure or ingestion in may and other species.

**toxicology**
The study of toxic substances or poisons.

**toxic psychosis**
A form of mental illness produced by toxic substances produced by the body itself, or introduced into it, such as chemicals or drugs.

**toxin**
A poisonous substance that is the byproduct of the metabolism of a living organism.

**toxo-**
A prefix meaning poison.

**TPR**
Temperature, pulse and respiration rates.

**tracers**
Selected conditions or diseases chosen for appraisal in programs which seek to assess the quality of medical care because it is believed that the quality of care given for the tracers is typical or representative of the quality of care given generally or to all diseases.

**tracheostomy**

A surgically created vertical slit in the windpipe in the front portion of the neck; a single or double cannula or tube airway is inserted into the opening to facilitate breathing and the adequate exchange of oxygen and carbon dioxide in the lungs. The main tube is held in place by ties around the neck.

**tracheostomy care**

To assist in the aspiration of secretions from a patient's tracheostomy opening through use of a sterile catheter connected to a suction machine. The cleansing of the inner cannula or tube of the tracheostomy tube and the anterior part of the neck is also a part of this care procedure.

**traction**

1. The process of placing a pulling force on injured parts of the body by means of pulleys and/or weights. 2. To support a bone by means of a strut or a pulling force on the neck or a limb as a part of the treatment process.

**trade**

1. To buy and sell. 2. Commerce. 3. A job, occupation or profession. 4. To barter; to swap or exchange for money. 5. The collective aspects of a profession. 6. Merchandise or traffic.

**trademark**

A distinguishing symbol, design, mark, motto or sign that a company can claim and reserve by law for its exclusive use in identifying its products or its organization.

**trade name**

See brand name.

**training center for allied health professions**

A junior college, college or university A) which provides programs of education leading to a baccalaureate or associate degree (or to the equivalent of either) or to a higher degree in medical technology, optometric technology, dental hygiene, or in any of such other of the allied health professions curricula as are specified by regulation, for full credit toward a baccalaureate or equivalent degree in the allied health professions or designed to prepare the student to work as a technician in a health occupation; B) which provides training for not less than a total of twenty persons in such curricula; C) which, if in a college or university which does not include a teaching hospital or in a junior college, is affiliated with a hospital, and D) which is in a college or university which is accredited by a recognized body or bodies approved for such purpose by the Commissioner of Education, or which is in a junior college which is accredited by the regional accrediting agency for the region in which it is located or there is satisfactory assurance afforded by such accrediting agency that reasonable progress is being made toward accreditation by such junior college.

**training program, approved**
Any graduate physician training program for interns and/or residents which is approved by the Liaison Committee on Graduate Medical Education, the Committee of Post Doctoral Education of the American Osteopathic Association, or the Council on Dental Education of the American Dental Association.

**training program, non-approved**
A graduate physician training program that has not received or has not sought approval from the Liaison Committee of Post Doctoral Education of the American Osteopathic Association, or the Council on Dental Education of the American Dental Association.

**trance**
A sleep-like state. A state or condition of reduced consciousness; not as deep or serious as a coma.

**tranquilizer**
A psychotropic drug that produces a calming, soothing, quieting or pacifying effect without clouding one's thought processes. Major tranquilizers include antipsychotic drugs, and the minor tranquilizers are antianxiety drugs.

**trans-**
A prefix meaning across.

**transaction**
1. A deal. 2. Something that takes place. 3. An interaction. 4. The making of a contract. 5. Any event that causes action; an affair. 6. A business agreement. 7. In psychology, it is an interpersonal interaction between two or more persons.

**transactional analysis**
A system of psychotherapy introduced by Eric Berne that focuses on interactions in the treatment sessions. The system includes 1) analysis of intrapsychic occurance, 2) the determination of the dominant ego states (parent, child, or adult) of each participant, 3) identification of the games played in their interactions and 4) uncovering the causes of the patient's emotional problems. Transactional analysis is used in individual and group psychotherapy.

**transcript**
1. An official copy of a record or a court proceeding. 2. An official record or copy of a document.

**transfer**
1. The passing or changing of a right, a title, or of property from one person to another or to the rightful owner. 2. Movement of a patient from one treatment service or location to another.

**transfer agreement**
As used in JCAH long term care facilities accreditation, this is a written arrangement that provides for the reciprocal transfer of patients/residents between health care facilities.

**transference**
The displacement of emotions or feelings during therapy (or otherwise) toward a psychotherapist, counselor, psychologist, or psychiatrist, stemming from life's earlier experiences with one's father or other authority figures.

**transfer tax**
A tax placed on large transactions or the transfer of property or money. Often these transactions are made without something of value given in return. Also called a "gift tax."

**transient**
1. Passing away with time. 2. Passing through; transitory. 3. Not permanent. 4. One who is temporary, passing through or staying only for a short time.

**transient situational disturbance**
A disorder that represents an acute reaction to overwhelming stress such as the severe crying spells, loss of appetite, sexual dysfunction, reaction to an unwanted situation manifested by suicidal gestures and hostility. The disturbance generally recedes as the stress diminishes.

**transillumination**
An information gathering or diagnostic technique that uses a bright light shown through part of the body to allow for its examination, i.e., the sinuses of the skull.

**transitory action**
1. A lawsuit that is possible to be heard in many of several places. 2. An action which may be brought in any state or county as opposed to a local action.

**transsexualism**
1. A belief that a person of one sex is trapped in the body of another sex. 2. The desire to change one's sex.

**transvestite**
An individual who wears clothing of the opposite sex and/or desires to be accepted as a member of the opposite sex.

**transvestitism (transvestism)**
The act of dressing in the clothing of the opposite sex.

**T ratio**
A statistical method used to test significance if fewer than 30 subjects are involved. The ratio is used to determine whether the found differences could occur just from chance. See also critical ratio.

**trauma**
1. In psychiatry, a stressful and upsetting experience or event that precipitates a mental crisis. 2. A blow or injury to one's physical body. 3. Sudden stressful or psychological upset. 4. Damage.

**traumatology**
The branch of medicine that deals with accidents and emergency surgery of wounds and disabilities as a result of traumatic injury.

**travel accident policy**
A limited contract covering only those accidents that occur while an insured person is traveling.

**traverse**
1. The denial of facts of a pleading by denying all, or denying only certain facts. 2. To cross horizontally.

**treason**
1. Violating an allegiance, betraying one's country, or levying war against one's government. 2. Helping the enemy by aiding and comforting them. 3. Betrayal of trust.

**treasure trove**
Found treasure.

**treatise**
A comprehensive written work on a subject of concern. It provides a special discussion of facts, evidence, principles and their conclusions.

**treatment**
The management and care of a patient for the purpose of combating disease or disorder.

**Treatment Authorization Request**
A special insurance form used in gaining authorization to render a specific service to a patient on the Medi-Cal program.

**treatment week**
Usually in health insurance this is, four or more treatment days in a calendar week. If three treatments or less in a week are given, a "treatment day" charge is used. Used mostly in radiation therapy and oncology.

**treble damages**
A triple amount awarded for damages provided to the plaintiff in some lawsuit in order to strongly discourage certain wrongful or harmful acts.

**trench mouth**
Inflammation of the mouth and gums with ulcerations.

**trend analysis/population projections**
A description of the population trends and the statistical measurements of the movement (growth) of the population of the state.

**Trendelenburg position**
Used in operating on a patient. The feet are lowered, and the head and shoulders are slightly lowered, with the abdominal area sightly elevated.

**trespass**
The illegal, unlawful or wrongful entry onto or into another person's property. An unlawful and harmful incursion on another's property, for which money damages may be awarded.

**trespass on a case**
In common law, it was a form of action used to collect damages for injury or harm as an indirect result of a wrongful act of another party.

**triad**
1. Three; a group of three items, objects or structures that are similar or alike. 3. Three symptoms or effects that occur together. 3. Three persons in a group, such as in psychotherapy.

**triage**
1. Commonly used to describe the sorting out or screening of patients seeking care, to determine which service is initially required and with what priority. A patient coming to a facility for care may be seen in a triage, screening or walk-in clinic. Here it will be determined, possibly by a triage nurse, whether, for example, the patient has a medical or surgical problem, or requires some non-physician service such as social work consultation. A screening or rapid assessment unit merely refers patients to the most appropriate treatment service, or may also give treatment for minor problems. Originally used to describe the sorting of battle casualties into groups who could wait for care, would benefit from immediate care, and were beyond care. 2. According to JCAH this is the sorting or classification of patients in accordance with the nature or degree of injury or illness.

**trial**
1. The process of presenting facts and/or an issue to proof; to try. 2. Testing; the testing of qualifications. 3. The process, procedures and proceedings used for the formal examination of facts of a dispute or case by a court to decide the validity of a claim or charge.

**trial court**
The court in which facts and evidence related to a dispute or crime is presented to a judge or jury for a decision.

**trial per pais**
Trial by jury.

**tribunal**
1. A court. 2. A seat of judgment. 3. The stand of a judge; the judge's bench.

**tribune**
1. The benches and witness stand of a court. 2. An elevated place to speak from.

**trichology**
The study of hair.

**trichotillomania**
Morbid compulsion to pull out one's hair.

**tricyclic drug**
An antidepressant drug that is presently the most popular drug in the treatment of pathological depression.

**trimester**
A three month period.

**T.R.O.**
Temporary restraining order.

**trocar**
A sharp pointed instrument used to withdraw fluids out of the body, used mostly in embalming procedures.

**troche**
Lozenge.

**troika**
A Russian term referring to a carriage drawn by three horses abreast; a team consisting of three horses. In health care administration this term is often used to refer to the three components of health care administration, which usually are administration, medical staff and nursing. The governing body, The administration and the medical staff have also been referred to as the hospital management troika.

**trolley car policy**
A facetious name for an insurance policy wich is so hard to collect benefits upon that it is as though it provided benefits only for injuries resulting from being hit by a trolley car. Typically used in mail order insurance.

**trover**
1. An action used to recover property or goods from someone who supposedly found them. 2. A writ against the wrongful holding of personal property. 3. All that is needed is to prove that the goods belong to you and that they are held by another person. A dated principle.

**true bill**
An indictment made by a grand jury.

**trust**
1. A fiduciary relationship. 2. An agreement where one party holds a title but controls and administers the property for the benefit of another. 3. The transfer of money or property to a second person for the benefit of another. 4. A combination of corporations in a similar industry. 5. Confidence, integrity, honesty in a deal or relationship. 6. Depending on aother person's integrity, honesty and rightness. 7. The confidence reposed in a person by giving ownership of property which is to be kept, used, or administered for another's benefit.

**trustee**
1. One who holds, executes, or administers a trust. 2. A group, committee or governing board appointed to manage the affairs of a hospital or other health care facility or health service. 3. A person who

has a fiduciary relationship with another person, such as a physician or psychologist.

**trust funds**

Funds collected and used by the Federal government for carrying out specific purposes and programs according to terms of a trust agreement or statute, such as the social security and unemployment trust funds. Trust funds are administered by the government in a fiduciary capacity for those benefitted and are not available for the general purposes of the government. Trust fund receipts whose use is not anticipated in the immediate future are generally invested in interest bearing government securities and earn interest for the trust fund. The Medicare program is financed through two trust funds--the Federal Hospital Insurance Fund which finances Part A, and the Federal Supplementary Medical Insurance Trust Fund which finances Part B. See also social insurance, funded, and Congressional and Presidential budgets.

**try**

1. To separate or pick out. 2. To sift through or sort out facts. 3. To examine, test or prove; to put to the test or to the proof. 4. To settle, test, or contest; to examine, argue and decide in court or law. 5. To determine the guilt or innocence of a person within the scope of the law.

**turkey**

Deprecating housestaff term for an inpatient who they feel does not need hospital admission. Such patients are not usually malingerers.

**turnaround time**

In health insurance, the time it takes from receipt of claim or inquiry, until an answer is provided or the bill is paid. This applies to inquiries from both providers and subscribers (enrolled members).

**turnkey system**

As used in major equipment purchases or in computers. As used in computer installation in which the computer sales agency assumes all responsibilities for installing a computer, which includes analysis, selection, installation, maintenance, training, and documentation. When completed, the user, figuratively, has only to turn the key to have it an operational system. This term was derived from a real estate construction term where a new facility would be totally completed so the new owner would only have to turn the key and open the door to have it a functioning facility.

**turnover**

In financial terms it is the number of times that assets, such as accounts receivable, are paid up during a certain time period. Accounts receivable turnover is figured by total billings on account for a period divided by average accounts receivable balance for the period.

**turpitude**

1. Depravity; shameful, unjust, dishonest or immoral activity. 2. Wickedness.

**two headed**
Ruled or arranged by two different heads or directors.

**two surgeons**
A term used by health insurance companies, where under certain circumstances the skills of two surgeons (usually with different skills) may be required in the management of a specific surgical problem (e.g., a urologist and a general surgeon in the creation of an ileal conduit, etc.)

**type of patient**
See new patient, established patient, ward patient, private patient.

**tyrant**
A cruel dictator and oppressive ruler. One who exercises absolute power and authority in his management of others. A hospital or health administrator who is cruel, rigid and insensitive to needs of employees. An administrator who rules without concerns with policy, the governing board, or the employees.

# U

**uberrima fides (Lat.)**
In the utmost good faith.

**ubi (Lat.)**
Where.

**ubi jus ibi remedium (Lat.)**
There is no wrong without a remedy.

**U.C.C.**
Uniform Commercial Code.

**U.C.C.C.**
Uniform Consumer Credit Code.

**U.C.M.J.**
Uniform Code of Military Justice.

**ulcer**
A localized destruction of skin tissue or mucous membrane commonly associated with varicosities or hyperactivity of the gastrointestinal tract, with or without pain. See pressure sore.

**ultima (Lat.)**
1. The most remote. 2. The final or last answer or response; the farthest possible or ultimate response, act or possibility.

**ultima ratio (Lat.)**
1. The final and last argument. 2. The last resort; final try.

**ultimate fact**
1. A fact, the truth of which is decided by the jury and which is essential to a case or the cause of action. 2. Basic fact based on evidence and reason.

**ultra-**
Prefix meaning beyond; excess.

**ultra (Lat.)**
1. Beyond the expected limit. 2. Outside of or in excess of; extreme. 2. One who proposes extreme measures or holds extreme opinions. 3. An ultraist.

**Ultradian rhythm**
A rhythm which cycles over minutes or hours.

**ultrasonics**
The production of sound at frequencies above the audio range.

**ultrasonogram**
The record produced by the process of ultrasonography.

**ultrasonography**
A radiologic diagnostic technique through which deep body structures are visualized by recording the reflection or echoes of ultrasonic waves.

**ultrasound**
High-frequency sound which causes radiant energy.

**ultraviolet**
A type of radiation with powerful properties, between the violet rays and the roentgen rays.

**ultra vires (Lat.)**
1. Beyond authority delegated to a person; beyond powers. 2. Acts performed by a corporation that are beyond the scope of its corporate power. 3. Acts that are beyond the authority of a public official or public organization, such as the Environmental Protection Agency or Occupational Safety and Health Administration.

**ululation**
The constant sobbing of a psychotic or hysterical person.

**unallocated benefit**
A policy provision in an insurance policy providing reimbursement up to a maximum amount for the costs of all extra miscellaneous hospital services, but not specifying how much will be paid for each type of service.

**unauthorized practice**
1. Unqualified persons doing the practices and skills that only specific health care providers are trained, licensed, and permitted to do. 2. Practicing acts or providing services that may be prohibited by law unless licensed, registered or certified.

**una voce (Lat.)**
With one voice; unanimous.

**unclean hands principle**
1. A person seeking equitable relief must not have acted with bad faith, malice or illegally, or he will not be entitled to relief. 2. Transactions must have been in good faith and with probity.

**unconditioned reflex**
Any automatic response to a stimulus, such as pulling a hand away from a hot stove.

**unconscionability**
1. Sales practices that are extremely unfair. 2. Merchandising practices that a court will not permit.

**unconscionable**
1. Exceeding the limit of any reasonable claim or expectation. 2. Unreasonable; unscrupulous; not influenced by conscience.

**unconscionable bargain**
1. A bargain that is unreasonable and offends public policy. 2. To enter into a deal that exceeds the limits of a reasonable bargain.

**unconscious**
1. Parts of the mind in which psychic material such as repressed desires, wishes and memories exist but are not directly accessible to one's awareness. 2. A mental state of unawareness with the absense of sensation and perception. See also conscious.

**unconstitutional**
Laws, penalties, or actions that are against or not permitted by the U.S. Constitution.

**underachievement**
Failure to reach an adequate level of achievement in school due to biological or psychological underdevelopment.

**underachiever**
A person who does not perform or function to his ability or capacity. Usually a bright child whose school test grades fall below expected levels of capability.

**undergraduate medical education**
Medical education given before receipt of the M.D. or equivalent degree, which is usually the four years of study in medical, osteopathic, dental or podiatric school leading to a degree. This use contrasts with that in general education where undergraduate education refers to college education leading to the bachelor degree.

**undernutrition**
Inadequate intake of vitamins, minerals, calories, etc.

**undersigning**
Not designing or crafty; straightforward.

**undertaking**
A promise, guarantee, or assumption of responsibility.

**underwrite**
1. To sign one's name to. 2. To agree to pay or give of certain things by signing a document. 3. To insure. 4. To assume liability to the amount specified.

**underwriter**
One who underwrites insurance.

**underwriting**
In insurance, the process of selecting, classifying, evaluating and assuming risks according to their insurability. Its fundamental purpose is to make sure that the group insured has the same probability of loss and probable amount of loss, within reasonable limits, as the universe on which premium rates were based. Since premium rates are based on an expectation of loss, the underwriting process must classify risks into classes with about the same expectation of loss.

**underwriting profit**
That portion of the earnings of an insurance company that comes from the function of underwriting. It excludes earnings from investments (other than interest earnings required by law or regulation to be assumed to have been earned for purposes of determining the reserves held) either in the form of income from securities or sale of securities at a profit. The remainder is found by deducting incurred losses and expenses from earned premium.

**undetermined**
1. Not limited. 2. Not defined; not determined.

**undo**
1. To put an end to. 2. To bring to ruin. 3. To put distress upon. 4. To find an answer or explanation. 5. To reverse, annul or cancel.

**undoing**
A mental or defense mechanism in which something unacceptable and already done is symbolically acted out repetitiously in reverse, in the hope of relieving anxiety.

**undue**
1. Not just, legal or lawful. 2. Improper; not suitable or appropriate. 3. Excessive or unreasonable. 4. More than needed.

**undue influence**
Controlling another to the point that he or she is no longer capable of being a free agent or is prevented from being one.

**unemployemnt insurance**
A form of social insurance that operates by means of a payroll tax, the revenues from which are used to pay calculated benefits for defined periods to people who qualify (usually by virtue of accumulated amounts of covered employment) as being unemployed, as defined in the law. Of interest because people receiving unemployment insurance do not usually continue to receive group health insurance coverage obtained through their most recent place of employment.

**unemployment compensation disability**
Insurance which covers off-the-job injury or sickness and is paid for by deductions from a person's paycheck. This program is administered by a state agency and is sometimes also known as State Disability Insurance.

**unethical conduct**
Acts that violate a profession's standards.

**unfair labor practice**
Acts by a union or by an employer that are prohibited by law.

**uniform**
1. Always the same; applying generally; regular; equally. 2. Having a consistent form, manner or procedure.

**uniform acts**
Laws on various subjects proposed by the Commissioners on Uniform State Laws, so that most codes are adopted by most states.

**Uniform Commercial Code**
1. A code that regulates commercial transactions. 2. A comprehensive set of laws on business law. 3. Statutory codes used to control business transactions and are uniformly accepted from state to state.

**Uniform Consumer Credit Code**
Laws developed to protect the consumer against unscrupulous and unfair business practices.

**uniform cost accounting**
The use of a common set of accounting definitions, procedures, terms, and methods for the accumulation and communication of quantitative data relating to the financial activities of several enterprises. The American Hospital Association, for example, encourages the use of its Chart of Accounts as a system which can be employed by hospitals in the United States.

**Uniform Hospital Discharge Data Set (UHDDS)**
A defined set of data which give a minimum description of a hospital episode or admission. Collection of a UHDDS is required upon discharge for all hospital stays reimbursed under Medicare and Medicaid. The UHDDS was defined in a policy statement of the Secretary of the old HEW and includes data on the age, sex, race and residence of the patient, length of stay, diagnosis, responsible physicians, procedures performed, disposition of the patient and sources of payment. The PSRO program uses a slightly larger data set called the PSRO Hospital Discharge Data Set (PHDDS). The Uniform Hospital Discharge Abstract (UDHA) used to collect the UHDDS is one example of a discharge abstract.

**Uniform Individual Policy Provisions**
A set of provisions regarding the nature and content of individual health insurance policies, developed in a recommended model law by the NAIC and adopted (with minor variations) by almost all jurisdictions and permitted in all.

**unilateral**
One-sided, such as a unilateral contract.

**unilateral contract**
1. A contract in which only one side promises performance with no promise of return payment or performance by the other side. 2. A contract wherein one side performs and the other side merely promises to perform.

**unincorporated association**
A business or organization created without any legal process, charter or incorporation procedures. This is often the business approach used in solo practice or a partnership. This form of association has many similarities to a corporation, such as a manager, transferability of interests, continuity

of organization with each person involved being personally legally responsible for all professional and business transactions of the association.

**unions**
An organized group of workers united for a purpose, usually for improving benefits, economic status and working conditions through collective bargaining with their employers. Public Law 93-360 (July 1974) extended the Labor Management Relations Act of 1947 to all private health care institutions. Passage of this law means that every health care facility, regardless of its size, may be subject to unions organizing its employees.

**union shop**
A business, hospital or shop where all employees must eventually join a union.

**union shop contract**
A labor agreement with an employer for continued employment being contingent upon joining a union.

**unit**
According to JCAH for accreditation purposes this is used to indicate a functional division or facility of the hospital.

**unit clerk**
Serves in a support capacity in a nursing unit. Handles routine clerical and reception work: receiving patients and visitors, scheduling appointments, monitoring the location of all ward staff, and where hospital policy permits, transcribing doctor's orders, ordering supplies, and updating information on patients' charts. (ward clerk)

**United States Court of Appeals**
Federal courts that take appeals from U.S. District Courts.

**United States Government Organization Manual**
The official legal handbook of the United States Government containing descriptions of the agencies of the legislative, judicial and executive branches.

**United States Pharmacopeia (USP)**
A legally recognized compendium of standards for drugs, published by the United States Pharmacopeial Convention, Inc., and revised periodically. It includes also assays and tests for the determination of strength, quality and purity. See also National Formulary.

**unit manager**
Supervises and coordinates administrative management functions for one or more patient care units: oversees unit clerks, initiates clerical procedures and serves as a liaison for the unit with other hospital departments. Also refered to as ward service manager, ward supervisor, charge nurse, supervisor nurse.

**unit of employees**
Two or more employees who share common employment and conditions.

**unitrust**
A trust in which a percentage is paid each year to its beneficiaries.

**universal donor**
A person with type O blood.

**unjust enrichment**
To return money or property gained unfairly, even though it was gained legally. The object is not to give so much restitution to a plaintiff as to prevent the defendant from profiting without payment. A doctrine where a defendant may sue in equity to regain that which is rightfully his, if it was lost by misrepresentation, unfair practice or without complete disclosure.

**unlawful**
1. Against or contrary to law. 2. Illegal or illicit. 3. Unauthorized by law. 4. An illegal act. Any action that violates a federal, state or municipal ordinance, statute or law.

**unlawful detainer**
A court order to leave property when holding onto buildings or property beyond the legal time one has a right to occupy them.

**unliquidated**
1. Not settled; not cleared up. 2. Undetermined; not ascertained.

**unpalatable**
Distasteful, unpleasant to the taste.

**unstable**
1. In reference to emotional or mental well-being, this refers to a person's lack of emotional and behavioral control. 2. In health care, this refers to the unpredictable health status of an ill patient as to his or her ability to recover and regan one's health. 3. Concerning radiation, this refers to all radioactive elements since they emit particles and decay to form other elements.

**untoward**
Adverse.

**unusually complex services**
See services, also levels of service.

**unusual services**
In health insurance, when services are provided that are greater than those usually required for usual procedure listed in the procedure coding manual.

**unwritten law**
1. Common or customary law; the usual acts people do that are considered right, just, expected or usual. Lex non scripta (Lat.).

**urban**
Relating to city dwelling.

**urinalysis**
The analysis of urine by physical, chemical or microscopic means for diagnostic purposes.

**usage**
1. Well-established or continued usual practice; customary use. 2. The way a custom, act, or practice is done. 3. The known way a business of a specific kind is carried out.

**usage of trade**
The regular, usual, or customary method of dealing in a vocation or trade as to justify an expectation with respect to the transaction at hand or in question.

**U.S.C.**
United States Code.

**U.S.C.A.**
United States Code Annotated; United States Court of Appeals.

**U.S.D.A.**
United States Department of Agriculture.

**U.S.D.C.**
United States District Court.

**use of outside resources (Medicare)**
If the facility does not employ a qualified professional person to render a specific service to be provided by the facility, there are arrangements for such a service through a written agreement with an outside resource—a person or agency that will render direct service to patients or act as a consultant. The responsibilities, functions, and objectives, and the terms of agreement, including financial arrangements and charges, of each such outside resource are delineated in writing and signed by an authorized representative of the facility and the person or the agency providing the service. The agreement specifies that the facility retains professional and administrative responsibility for the services rendered. The financial arrangements provide that the outside resource bill the facility for covered services (either Part A or B for Medicare beneficiaries) rendered directly to the patient, and that receipt of payment from the program(s) to the facility for the services discharges the liability of the beneficiary or any other person to pay for the services. The outside resource, when acting as a consultant, apprises the administrator of recommendations, plans for implementation, and continuing assessment through dated, signed reports, which are retained by the administrator for follow-up action and evaluation of performance.

**usual and customary charge**
Variation of UCR utilized by insurance carriers which do not have contracts with physicians (such as Blue Cross) and cannot guarantee acceptance of payment by physician as "in full".

**usual charge**
See customary charge.

**usual, customary and reasonable (UCR)**
Refers to the charges (fees) of a physician.

**usual, customary and reasonable (UCR)charge**
A benefit description implying paid-in-full physicians' bills so long as the charge is the usual one for the specified service and that it is withing the range of fees for that service customarily charged by other physicians in the community. The term "reasonable" has come to mean a fee which meets the criteria of usual and customary or, is justified in the special circumstances of the case in question.

**usual customary and reasonable plans (UCR)**
Health insurance plans that pay a physician's full charge if: it does not exceed his usual charge; it does not exceed the amount customarily charged for the service by other physicians in the area (often defined as the 90 or 95 percentile of all charges in the community), or it is otherwise reasonable. In this context, usual and customary charges are similar, but not identical to customary and prevailing charges, respectively, under Medicare. Most private health insurance plans, except for a few Blue Shield plans, use the UCR approach.

**usufruct**
1. The right to use an item just so it is not changed or used up. 2. In civil law, it is the right to use, and make profits from property owned by another party.

**usufructuary**
The agent or party having the usufruct of property.

**usurious**
Pertaining to usury. See usury.

**usury**
Lending money at higher rates of interest than are allowed by law.

**utilization**
Use. Utilization is commonly examined in terms of patterns of use or rates of use of a single service or type of service, e.g., hospital care, physician visits, prescription drugs. Measurement of utilization of all medical services in combination is usually done in terms of dollar expenditures. Use is expressed in rates per unit of population at risk for a given period, e.g., number of admissions to hospital per 1,000 persons over 65 per year, or number of visits to a physician per person per year for family planning services.

**utilization review (UR)**
1. Evaulation of the necessity, appropriateness and efficiency of the use of medical services, procedures and facilities. In a hospital this includes review of the appropriateness of admissions, services ordered and provided, length of stay, and discharge practices, both on a concurrent and retrospective basis. Utilization review can be done by a utilization review committee, PSRO, peer review group, or public agency. 2. According to JCAH for psychiatric, alcoholism and drug abuse facilities accreditation purposes, this is the process of using predefined criteria to

evaluate the necessity and appropriateness of allocated services and resources to assure that the facility's services are necessary, cost efficient and effectively utilized. See also medical review.

**utilization review committee**

1. A group of physicians, nurses, administrators, allied health and other personnel from outside of the hospital or nursing home who review patient records to review length of stay, medical and nursing procedures and insure that it is necessary for patients to be in the health care facility. This committee is a requirement for participation in Medicare. The committee studies the medical course and care plan of every patient in the facility to ensure that services received are within skilled nursing care. Any care that is more or less than skilled care would qualify a patient to be transferred to another facility to receive the level of care for which he or she is eligible. The utilization review committee not only review level of care and duration of stay, but also must conduct medical care evaluation studies to ensure the quality of care. The findings of these studies may be used to improve services, treatment and programs in hospitals or skilled nursing facilities. The utilization review committee cannot be employed by or have an interest in the facility. A minimum of two physicians is required and other allied health professionals or nurses may participate. A certified social worker or professional nurse is desirable to help clarify matters that are not medical determinations but effect a need for a continued stay. Facility personnel that could attend include the medical director, the director of nursing, social workers, administrative director, the records coordinator and the physical therapist. 2. In long term care facilities accreditation by JCAH this is a committee that reviews a facility's resources in striving to provide high-quality patient/resident care in the most cost-effective manner. Based on this review, the committee makes recommendations, including plans for follow-up action, to the governing body of the facility.

**utter**

1. Unconditional; completely unqualified. 2. To put into circulation. 3. To give out or put forth (not used much anymore except for counterfeit money). 4. To pronounce, say, or speak; to express in any way. 5. To make known; to divulge or reveal.

**ux (Lat. abbrev.)**

Abbreviation for uxor.

**uxor (Lat.)**

Wife.

# V

**v.**
Abbreviation for versus or against. Used in the title of a case, i.e., John Doe v. Jane Roe.

**V.A.**
Veterans Administration. See hospital, veterans.

**vacate**
1. To annul. 2. To leave; move out. 3. To empty. 4. To take back. 5. To set aside.

**vacate a judgment**
To annul, set aside or completely remove a previous decision or judgment.

**vaccine**
A suspension of disease-producing microorganisms modified by killing or attenuation so that it will not cause disease and can stimulate the formation of antibodies upon inoculation.

**vagrancy**
1. A wandering in talk or thought. 2. Wandering through or from place to place. 3. Shiftless; unpredictable or idle, hanging around without money or work.

**vagrant**
1. A beggar, tramp, vagabond, prostitute, or roaming person. 2. Having no direction, plan or course.

**vague**
1. Indefinite, unclear, not certain. 2. Not precise in thought or explanation.

**valid**
1. Good; binding; in force; legal; sound. 2. Properly completed, executed and binding by law. 3. Well founded in evidence.

**validate**
To make valid.

**validity**
1. The extent to which results of a study are correct. 2. The extent to which something like a test does what it is professed or believed to do. 3. The extent to which a situation reflects the true situation. See also reliability.

**validity, (test)**
Validity of a test is how well the test measures whatever it is that the test was constructed to measure. A test is only valid to the extent that it measures what it claims to measure. A test may be reliable, even though it is not valid. A valid test is always reliable. See reliability.

**valuable consideration**
1. The real reason, usually for money or other items of value that a contracting party enters into an agreement. 2. The valuable material, cause, or reason for a contract. 3. The important motive of a stipulation.

**value**
1. To think highly of; to esteem, prize or hold with much respect or worth. 2. Having worth. 3. For value means consideration. See valuable consideration, consideration.

**vaporization (evaporation)**
To cause a solid or liquid to turn into a gas.

**vapors**
The gaseous form of substances under normal conditions which are in the solid or liquid state.

**variance**
1. In pleading a case, variance occurs when an inconsistency between allegations and proof exists. 2. A lack of agreement between the testimonies of the parties of a legal proceeding and evidence presented. 3. Not in agreement with each other. 4. In statistics, it is a measure. Variance is arrived at by squaring all the deviations in a set of measures, summing them, and then dividing them by the number of measures. Variance is helpful in analyzing how much variation in the data is due to chance or to intervening variables or experimental treatment. 5. In environmental health law it is license, granted by government, to pollute beyond acceptable limits in return for promises and plans on curbing pollution.

**variation**
A statistical measure used to determine the different results obtained in measuring the same phenomenon. See variance

**vasectomy**
A form of male birth control through sterilization, in which the seminal ducts are tied off. Potency, sexual performance and sexuality are not affected.

**vaso-**
Prefix meaning vessel, or duct.

**vector**
A carrier, especially the animal (usually an arthropod) which transfers an infective agent from one host to another; animals or insects that transfer pathogens from one host to another.

**vector analysis**
Used to determine the magnitude, nature and direction of a moving force. For example, the electrocardiogram is used as a vector analysis to measure movement, magnitude, nature and force of the cycles of the heartbeat.

**vehicle**
A transporting agent or medium.

**vehicles of infection**
The mechanism or means by which infectious agents are transported. Water, food, insects, and inanimate objects are usual vehicles of infection. Insect or rodent vehicles are also called vectors. See this word.

**vel non (Lat.)**
Or not.

**vendee**
Buyer, one who purchases.

**vendor**
1. Seller. 2. A provider; an institution, agency, organization or individual practitioner who provides health or medical services. Vendor payments are those payments which go directly to institutions or providers from a third party program like Medicaid.

**vendor payment**
Used in public assistance programs to distinquish those payments made directly to vendors of service from those cash income payments made directly to assistance recipients. The vendors, or providers of health services, are reimbursed directly by the public assistance programs for services they provide to eligible recipients. Vendor payments are essentially the same as service benefits provided under health insurance and prepayment plans.

**venire facias (Lat.)**
1. Make to come; used in common law. 2. A writ to the sheriff to have him assemble a jury.

**venire facias de novo (Lat.)**
1. Make to come again. 2. A writ for a second trial, due to some irregularity in the original trial. It is also called "venire de novo."

**venireman**
A juror.

**veno-**
Prefix meaning vein.

**ventilation**
Causing fresh air to circulate in order to simultaneously replace foul air.

**ventilation of the lungs**
The act of breathing; the filling of lungs with air.

**ventriculography**
An X-ray or other radiological examination of the ventricles of the brain by the insertion of air or other radiopaque medium.

**venue**
1. Locality; region; area. 2. Jurisdiction over a geographical area. 3. The locality in which a cause of action occurs or a crime is committed. 4. The judicial district or area in which a case is tried and the jury is

selected. 5. A writ that designates the county or geographical area a trial is to be held or where an affidavit is sworn.

**verba (Lat.)**
Words.

**verbigeration**
Meaningless use of words or the repetition of words or phrases. Also known as cataphasia, a serious disorder seen in catatonic schizophrenia.

**verdict**
The declaration of a jury's findngs, signed by the jury foreman and presented to the court. 2. The final judgment of a jury. 3. Deciding which side wins a case. 4. A decision or judgment pronounced; the decision of a jury on any dispute or matter being tried in court.

**verdict of acquittal**
A defense used in court to show that the evidence is not sufficient enough to proceed, thus the case should be dismissed.

**verdict, special**
The results and facts of a case with a judge or court comparing the evidence and facts to the law and how it applies.

**verify**
1. To establish the truth of a document. 2. To prove to be true. 3. To establish proof through facts, evidence, and testimony. 4. The truthfulness or conformity of a statement. 5. The quality of being real or actual.

**vermin**
External animal parasites such as ticks, lice and fleas.

**vertical opening**
According to JCAH for long term care facilities accreditation, a penetration in a floor slab and assembly which creates an opening between floors of a building. Examples include stairwells, elevators, chutes, and shafts.

**vertigo**
Dizziness; the sensation that the environment is revolving around you.

**vesicant**
Anything that produces blisters.

**vesicle**
A small blister on the skin.

**vest**
1. Fixed. 2. To place in the control of a group or organization, i.e., as giving authority as power to such a party. 3. To give full rights and power. 4. To take effect.

**vested**
1. Settled; absolute or complete. 2. Established; fixed. 3. Not contingent upon an act or event.

**vested interest**
Personal interest in a deal; personal gain or property, whether present or future.

**vested remainder**
See remainder.

**Veterans' Administration hospital**
A health care facility where medical, mental health and dental services are rendered to a veteran who has a service-related disability.

**veterinarian**
An individual dedicated to protecting the health and welfare of both animals and people. Veterinarians are primarily animal doctors, highly educated and skilled in preventing, diagnosing and treating animal health problems. However, because their special knowledge and training extend into a number of closely related areas, veterinarians are involved in much more than animal medicine. Today's veterinarian is a member of a major health profession with its own system of education, licensure, organization and ethics. In taking the veterinarian's oath, the doctor solemnly swears to use his or her scientific knowledge and skills for the benefit of society, through the protection of animal health, the relief of animal suffering, the conservation of livestock resources, the promotion of public health, and the advancement of medical knowledge.

**veterinary services**
Work with the care, use, production, and husbandry of animals in medical settings.

**veto**
1. When the president or a governor fails to sign a bill into law or refuses to sign a bill into law. 2. To turn down; to refuse to consent to.

**vexatious**
1. Troublesome; harassing; annoying. 2. Instituted without real grounds. 3. For the main purpose of causing annoyance to the defendant.

**vexatious litigation**
A lawsuit brought or charges made against a person without a good reason or a just cause shown.

**viability**
Capability of living; ability to function.

**viable**
Capable of living; the power of a fetus to live outside the uterus.

**vial**
A small glass bottle with a rubber stopper.

**vicar**
1. A term often used in a church or governmental context, indicating a person who acts in the place of another. 2. One with delegated authority; a deputy.

**vicarious**
Substitute.

**vicarious liability**
Indirect legal responsibility; liability suffered by one person because of another; as an employer being responsible for his employee's on-the-job mistakes or negligence

**vice**
1. A serious fault in character. 2. Evil and illegal conduct. 3. Immoral or depraved habits. 4. A character fault or defect such as obsessive gambling or prostitution.

**vide (Lat.)**
See.

**vide ante (Lat.)**
Look at the words that come before this one.

**videlicet**
To wit; namely. See viz.

**vi et armis (Lat.)**
1. With force and arms. 2. With direct force or violence.

**viro-**
Prefix meaning virus; poison.

**virtue**
1. Goodness, moral uprightness. 2. Chastity, especially in women. 3. By the power of; because. 4. Excellence; good quality. 5. On the grounds of.

**virulence**
The capacity of a microorganism to produce disease.

**virulent**
Extremely poisonous or venomous; capable of overcoming bodily defensive mechanisms.

**virus**
A class or very small germs of infecting agents which cause many diseases. They are capable of multiplying on or in the living cells of some organism.

**vis (Lat.)**
With force or violence.

**vis a vis**
One who is opposite to.

**viscosity**
The quality of being gummy or sticky.

**vision, abnormal**
See astigmatism, cataract, hyperopia, myopia or presbyopia.

**vision, normal**
The normal lens of the eye is such that an object 20 feet away will be in focus without any accommodation reflex activities. If you have no difficulty reading a standard-sized letter at this distance, you are said to have normal 20/20 vision. If, however, you can see a standard-sized letter at 20 feet, which a normal person can see at 40 feet, you are said to have 20/40 vision. Thus, the higher the second number, the greater your vision problem.

**visit**
1. An encounter between a patient and a health professional which requires either the patient to travel from his home to the professional's usual place of practice (an office visit), or vice versa (a housecall or home visit). 2. In health insurance, a visit is an office call, and is considered a personal interview between the enrolled member and the physician and shall not include telephone calls or any other situations where the enrolled member is not personally examined by the physician. This definition is used to determine benefits for office calls.

**Visiting Nurse Association (VNA)**
See visiting nurse services.

**visiting staff**
Physician, physical therapists, physician assistants, nurse practitioners and other allied health care providers who have a private practice, yet utilize the hospital for the care of their patients.

**vis major (Lat.)**
Force majeur. An act of nature or other superior force which occurs without intervention of man and could not have been prevented through reasonable action.

**VISTA**
Volunteers in Service to America.

**Visting Nurse Services (VNS).**
A voluntary health agency which provides nursing services in the home, including health supervision, education and counseling; bedside care; and the carrying out of physicians' orders using nurses and other personnel such as home health aides who are specifically trained for specific tasks of personal bedside care. These agencies had their origin in the visiting nursing program provided to the sick and poor in their homes by voluntary agencies in the 1870s, such as the New York City Mission. The first visiting nurse associations were established in Buffalo, Boston and Philadelphia in 1886-87. See also home health agency.

**visual hallucination**
A false visual occurrence or perception; seeing something that is not there.

**vita-**
Prefix meaning life.

**vital signs**
The various signs produced by normal body functions that reflect the physiological state, which govern the body's vital organs (brain, heart, lungs) that are necessary to sustain life. The vital signs are: temperature, pulse, respiration and blood pressure.

**vital statistics**
Statistics relating to births (natality), deaths (mortality), marriages, health and disease (morbidity). Vital statistics for the United States are published annually by the National Center for Health Statistics of the Health Resources Administration, the Department of Health and Human Services. Each state also publishes its own vital statistics.

**vitamins**
Organic chemical substances found in food which are essential for nutrition, normal metabolism and life.

**vitiate**
1. To make imperfect. 2. To destroy the legal effect. 3. To cause to fail; to corrupt; to weaken morally. 4. To make a document legally ineffective to take away the legal force or make invalid.

**vito-**
Prefix meaning life.

**viva voce (Lat.)**
1. Expressed orally; with living voice. 2. By word of mouth. 3. Oral testimony or other than written expression.

**viz**
Short for videlicet, meaning: to wit; that is to say. Used to introduce a list.

**vocational assessment**
According to JCAH for psychiatric, alcoholism and drug abuse facilities accreditation purposes, this is the process of evaluating each patient's past experiences and attitudes toward work; current motivations or areas of interest; and possibilities of future education, training, and/or employment.

**void**
1. Null; having no binding force. 2. Having no legal effect. 3. To wipe out or destroy its validity.

**voidable**
That which can be legally made void or declared invalid.

**voidable contract**
A contract that may not be legally binding on either party, if one party seeks to avoid it.

**void contract**
Any legal obligation or agreement that is no longer in force, as it lacks some legal element.

**voir dire (French)**
"Look-speak." To speak truthfully. The act of selecting potential jurors by lawyers and a judge to decide whether or not a person is worthy, unprejudiced and competent to sit on the jury of a case.

**volatile**
Substances that evaporate rapidly.

**volens (Lat.)**
Willing.

**volenti non fit injuria (Lat.)**
1. To the consenting, no wrong is done. 2. To not allow a lawsuit to be brought against another if the person originally consented to allow the act to be done that caused the harm, injury, or damage.

**voluble.**
1. Speaking up or out with clarity, ease and fluency. 2. Talkative.

**voluntary health agency**
Any non-profit non-governmental agency, governed by lay and/or professional individuals, organized on a national, state or local basis, whose primary purpose is health-related. The term usually designates agencies supported primarily by voluntary contributions from the public at large, and engaged in a program of service, education, and research related to a particular disease, disability, or group of diseases and disabilities; for example, the American Heart Association, American Cancer Society, National Tuberculosis Association, and their state and local affiliates. The term can also be applied to such agencies as non-profit hospitals, visiting nurse associations, and other local service organizations which have both lay and professional governing boards, and are supported by both voluntary contributions, and fees for services provided.

**voluntary hospital**
Any hospital that is owned and/or operated by any fraternal, religious or not-for-profit community organization. See hospital

**voluntary manslaughter**
The act of committing a homicide in the heat of passion or when provoked.

**voluntary nonsuit**
When a plaintiff abandons the required legal procedure of his case and allows a judgment and costs to be brought against him because of failure to respond to the litigation process.

**volunteer services**
Also referred to as auxiliaries. People from the community donate their time and service to provide non-medical assistance and aid in the efficient running of the health care facility. They assist in a variety of tasks such as delivering flowers, manning desks and reception counters, escorting families or patients, preparing bandages, operating a gift shop or snack bar, etc. Teenage volunteers are called Candy Stripers.

**voodoo**

Practice of witchcraft or magic.

**vouch**

1. To attest or give evidence. 2. To testify, affirm or guarantee. 3. To call as a witness; to call into court to give warranty of title.

**voucher**

1. A document or paper attesting to facts and which can be used as evidence. 2. A receipt or evidence of payment or accuracy of the status of an account. 3. One who vouches, attests, assures or warrants something is true or factual through testimony.

**voyeurism**

The unhealthy behavior or desire to look at sexual organs or sexual acts.

**vs**

Abbreviation; versus; against. See "v."

# W

**wage assignment**
An agreement allowing a person to pay his wages directly to a creditor.

**Wagner Act**
The first federal act (1935) that established rights of unions. It prohibited any attempts at keeping employees out of a union. It derived the concept of unfair labor practices and created the National Labor Relations Board to enforce the newly created labor laws.

**Wagner-Murray-Dingell Bill**
One of the original national health insurance proposals, first introduced by Congressmen, Wagner, Murray and Dingell in the 1940s.

**WAIS**
Wechsler Adult Intelligence Scale. An intelligence test created specifically for adults.

**waiting list**
A list of patients awaiting admission to a hospital or nursing home. The number of patients on a list to be admitted for special treatments or surgery.

**waiting period**
1. Also known as excepted period. 2. The time which must elapse before an indemnity is paid on health insurance. 3. A period of time an individual must wait either to become eligible for insurance coverage, or to become eligible for a given benefit after overall coverage has commenced (see exclusions). This does not generally refer to the amount of time it takes to process an application for insurance, but rather is a defined period before benefits become payable. Some policies will not pay maternity benefits, for example, until nine months after the policy has been in force. Another common waiting period occurs in group insurance offered through a place of employment where coverage may not start until an employee has been with a firm for over 30 days. For disabled persons to be covered under Medicare, there is a waiting period of two years; a person must be entitled to social security disability benefits for two years before medical benefits start.

**waive**
1. To voluntarily give up a right; to relinquish a privilege. 2. To abandon or relinquish. 3. To renounce; to disclaim a right.

**waived**
To have voluntarily renounced or given up a privilege.

**waiver**

1. The giving up of a privilege or right. 2. The voluntary surrender of a claim. 3. To allow a policy or procedure to not be in effect or to not apply. 4. In insurance, this is an agreement attached to an insurance policy which exempts certain disabilities or injuries from coverage that are normally covered by the policy.

**waiver of premium**

A provision included in some health insurance policies that exempts the insured person from paying premiums if he is disabled during the period of the insurance contract.

**waiving time**

To allow more time than usual to try a case or answer a charge.

**want**

1. To desire; to wish. 2. To suffer from the lack of or the need of something.

**wanton**

1. In need. 2. Reckless; without giving heed or caution. 3. Negligent; malicious; undisciplined; immoral. 4. Lacking in foreseeability.

**wanton negligence**

When a party acts or fails to act and is conscious and aware that this could cause injury and he or she has a reckless indifference to the consequences of the act or the omission of an act, yet has no actual intent to cause harm. See negligence.

**ward**

1. To fend off or turn aside. 2. One under the care of a guardian. 3. To put into custody. 4. The guardianship of a child or person unable or not capable of caring for himself. 5. The court seizing custody and taking over the guardianship of a person (usually a child) to care for that person when the legal guardian seems incompetent to care for him or her. 6. A floor or geographical location housing patients in a hospital. 7. A section or division; subsection of a larger area or organization.

**ward accommodation**

A hospital room with three or more beds.

**ward clerk**

See unit clerk.

**ward patients**

Indigent or medically indigent patients who are kept in a special hospital ward and are usually are treated in city or county hospitals or a medical school teaching hospital. In the past, these patients were kept and treated on open wards instead of in semi-private or 3 to 6 patients per room arrangements.

**ward rounds**

Teaching rounds. When the teaching physician takes his or her medical students, interns or residents to the bedside of patients in a teaching hospital or teaching unit to review the patients' diseases, disorders or disabilities for the purpose of instructing and providing clinical training.

**warrant**
1. To promise, by contract or deed. 2. To assure; to promise. 3. The legal authority by a writ to arrest a person. 4. Permission given by a judge or court to arrest a person, seize property, search a house, etc. 5. To promise that the facts of a situation are true.

**warranty**
1. In malpractice, actions against physicians are normally based on negligence, but in certain circumstances the plaintiff can bring his action on the basis of a warranty. A warranty arises if the physician promises or seems to promise that the medical procedure to be used is safe or will be effective. One of the advantages to bringing an action on warranty grounds, rather than for negligence, is that the statute of limitations is usually longer. A warranty action may be brought and maintained if there is an express warranty offered by the physician to the patient. 2. In insurance; a promise, made as part of an insurance contract, upon which the transaction depends. An insurance company could refuse to pay a claim if a statement is misleading, invalid, false or if the promise is not kept. 3. In business; any representation made by a seller to a buyer on a sale of goods that they are fit for use. 4. A promise that facts are true.

**warranty of fitness**
A promise that an item is fit for the purposes for which it is sold.

**waste**
The destroying or abuse of someone else's property in your possession.

**Waters projection**
A posteroanterior x-ray showing parts of the face.

**weekend hospital**
A type of health care facility used for partial hospitalization in which the patient spends only weekends in the health care facility and functions in the outside world during the week.

**weight of evidence**
1. The relative importance of the facts or evidence; the greater influence. 2. The consequence of the evidence given. 3. The most firm and believable evidence; the quality of evidence given.

**welfare**
1. The state of doing or being well. 2. Public assistance to the poor. 3. To be "on welfare" is to receive governmental aid due to poverty, sickness, unemployment, or other justifiable deprivation.

**wheal**
1. A pustule; a pimple. 2. A raised area of skin; a ridge or strip of skin that is elevated, such as in an insect bite.

**whereas**
Because.

**whereby**
1. By means of. 2. How.

**whole law**
The actual laws of a state as well as other laws regarding choice-of-laws.

**wholistic**
An integrated whole system of healing and well-being embracing the qualities of holism; the taking into account in the healing or health processes more than disease and physiology, and including the mental, emotional and spiritual, value system, social and cultural dimensions as well. This also includes being in contact with one's own healing process and health maintenance.

**WIC**
Women's, Infant's and Children's nutrition program. See these words.

**wildcat strike**
A strike initiated without permission, support or authorization of the union.

**will**
1. To decree or to ordain. 2. To wish, desire, or long for. 3. A legal document stating the wishes of a person concerning the disposition of his or her belongings, personal property, and estate upon his death. 4. A command or decree.

**willful**
1. Intentionally done. An act deliberately and purposely done. 2. Willing and ready. 3. Following one's desires or wishes without reason or rationality; to be stubborn.

**willful negligence**
Often rejected by the courts, as it could be viewed as a criminal charge of battery rather than an act of negligence, the term is used to show a higher and more aggravated form of negligence than gross negligence. When a person has a willful determination to not perform an expected and known duty. A conscious and intentional omission of duty or acts of proper care so to disregard the health, life, rights and/or safety of another person.

**windfall**
Excessive and unexpected gain.

**withdrawal**
The retreating or going away. One symptom seen in the schizophrenic or depressed person. It is characterized by an unhealthy retreat from interpersonal relations, contacts and social involvement, resulting in self-preoccupation.

**withdrawal symptoms**
Vomiting, shaking, profuse sweating, hallucinations and other physical and emotional symptoms resulting from withdrawal from addictive or habituating drugs.

**withholding tax**
The withholding of money by an employer from an employee's pay check and paying it to the government as a prepaid income tax for the employee.

**without day**
1. An indefinite time. 2. Not final. 3. A date not given or set.

**without recourse**
A conditional endorsement of a negotiable instrument meaning that if payment is refused, the signer will not be responsible for the outcome or the end results.

**witness**
1. One who sees or is present at an event, act, situation, or occurrence. 2. One who attests to the signing of a document. 3. A person who provides testimony or statements under oath.

**witnessing**
Testifying, providing verbal evidence, one telling what he has seen, heard or otherwise observed.

**Women's, Infant's and Children's nutrition program (WIC)**
Recognizing the important role of nutrition during pregnancy and early childhood growth and development, Congress enacted legislation in 1972 creating the Supplemental Food Program for Women, Infants and Children (WIC), as a major nutritional intervention program for this target population. WIC serves as an adjunct to health care by providing nutritious foods to supplement a participant's diet as well as nutrition education services. As a result, it has facilitated health improvements by reducing rates of anemia, overweight, underweight, short stature, prematurity and low birth weight infants. Pregnant, breastfeeding and postpartum women are eligible for services if they demonstrate signs of anemia, overweight, underweight; are younger than age 20 or over 35, have a poor obstetrical history (miscarriages, still births, previous low-birth weight infants, multiple births, etc.) or have nutritionally related medical conditions such as toxemia, diabetes and other conditions which predispose them to inadequate nutritional patterns or nutritionally related medical conditions.

**word processing**
Computer information system that utilizes recording and retrieval of data at high speeds.

**word salad**
A mixture of words and phrases. This is a speech problem resulting from a disturbance in thought processes. A common symptom in advanced states of schizophrenia.

**Words and Phrases**
A set of lawbooks that provide definitions of legal words, phrases and the actual quotes from the cases from which they were taken.

**working capital**
The sum of an institution's investment in short-term or current assets including cash, marketable (short-term) securities, accounts receivable, and inventories. Net working capital is defined as the excess of total current assets over total current liabilities.

**working through**
Process of obtaining insight into emotional or personal problems and personality changes through examination of a conflict or problem.

**workman's compensation**
State based insurance programs that make cash benefits available to workers or their dependents who are injured, disabled or die in the course of and as a result of work. The injured employee is entitled to benefits for some or all of the medical services necessary for his or her treatment and restoration to a useful life and a productive job. These insurance programs are mandatory under state laws in all states.

**Workman's Compensation Insurance**
An insurance contract which insures a person against on-the-job injury or illness. The employer pays the premium for his employees.

**workmen's compensation programs**
State social insurance programs which provide cash benefits to workers or their dependents injured, disabled, or deceased in the course, and as a result, of employment. The employee is also entitled to benefits for some or all of the medical services necessary for treatment and restoration to a useful life and possibly a productive job. These programs are mandatory under state laws in all states.

**work-product rule**
A legal rule in that one party need not show any facts discovered by the party's attorney to the other party unless the other side can show that it would be unfair or unjust for such information not to be shared.

**writ**
1. A court or judge's order; a written order issued by the authority of a court. 2. The order by a judge or court to have something done outside the actual courtroom.

**write-off**
A debt that cannot be collected, thus is considered a bad debt and is deducted or written off the gross income.

**write-off method**
Accepting that an uncollectible account is a loss as determined by a specific time account receivables are identified as no longer collectible.

**writ of course**
A court order granting that which one has right or is entitled to.

**writ of entry**
See entry, writ of.

**writ of prohibition**
1. An order from a higher court to a lower court to stop operating out of its jurisdiction. 2. Also used to direct a person from doing an act which the court has precedence over.

**writ of right**
A legal order protecting the rights in freehold real estate.

**written authorization**
Consent, permission or authority given in writing, specifically empowering someone to do something.

**written law**
Lex scripta (Lat.). Statutes, codes and regulations.

**written premium**
A total amount of insurance premiums obtained in a year from all policies issued by an insurance company.

**wrong**
1. Not morally right. 2. Not in accordance with expected or established principles and standards; not suitable. 3. Contrary to fact and truth. 4. Incorrect acts or judgments. 5. Incorrectly done. 6. A violation of a legal right. 7. Malice actions. 8. A tort.

**wrongful**
Injurious, unjust and unfair. Illegal; unlawful, illicit.

**wrongful death**
1. Death due to wrongful acts. 2. A lawsuit filed by the living family members of a dead person against the one causing the death. Monetary damages are sought if the act that caused the death was wanton, wrongful, negligent, or willful.

**wry**
1. Turned; bent; twisted. 2. One-sided. 3. Having a distorted meaning.

# X

**X**

A symbol used in statistics meaning mean or average.
1. Roman numeral for 10. 2. A person or thing unknown or unrevealed; an unknown.

**xanthine**

A group of substances containing, caffeine, such as coffee, cola drinks and chocolate.

**xantho-**

Prefix meaning yellow.

**xeno-**

Prefix meaning foreign; alien.

**xenophobia**

Fear of strangers.

**xero-**

Prefix meaning dry.

**xerography**

A printing process used for copying printed material or other images or pictures by the machine transferring and reproducing the exact or similar image on another sheet of paper.

**Xerox**

A brand of photocopying that reproduces exact images on a new sheet of paper. See xerography, reprography.

**x-ray**

1. To examine or treat with x-rays. 2. A widely used technique in medicine to study, diagnose and treat.

# Y

**yang**
A positive force in Chinese folk medicine that regulates health; represents the male, warmth, light and fullness.

**yea**
An affirmative vote or statement.

**yellow dog contract**
An illicit contract for employment forcing an employee to promise that he will not join a union.

**yellow journalism**
The use of cheap, sensational and unscrupulous means to attract readers or to sway public opinion.

**yield**
1. To give in return. 2. To submit to. 3. To give up or to surrender. 4. To give place. 5. To lose precedence. 6. To admit the truth of. 7. To admit the justice and force of. 8. To grant or to allow. 9. The amount or profits gained.

**yin**
A negative force in Chinese folk medicine that regulates health; represents the female, coldness, darkness, and emptiness.

**yttrium-90**
An artificial radioactive isotope of the element yttrium. An element which emits beta rays, which is used in radiation therapy.

**Z**
A mark or sign used to fill blank spaces left in a legal document to insure that they will not be filled later.

# Z

**Z (Regulation Z)**
A set of principles laid down by the Federal Reserve Board governing truth in lending laws.

**za (Greek)**
1. Argumentative. 2. Intensive. 3. Used to express a high degree of quality in a scientific way.

**Zen**
A Buddhist sect that seeks enlightenment through introspection and intuition, rather than from scripture.

**zero**
1. A cipher or naught. 2. The lowest point. 3. The point halfway between positive and negative quantities. 4. A crucial or decisive moment (zero hour).

**zero population growth (ZPG)**
An attempt to control the birth rate of a population where births are only to replace in numbers the persons who die to keep population at a constant level.

**Zionism**
A movement to reestablish the state of Israel; a Jewish movement.

**zip**
To move with speed or energy.

**zip code**
A several-digit code number representing a regional location or place with the intent of helping the mail to move in a more efficient and speedy manner.

**zone**
1. A region or area that is distinct and different in its use from other areas. 2. Any special area or district in a city or county that is restricted by law for certain and specified use, i.e., business, factories, apartment complexes, health facilities, etc.

**zoning**
When a community sets certain sections of land aside for different purposes by ordinances; regulation of land and its use; community planning of land use. See zone.

**zoo-**
Prefix meaning animal life.

**zoonoses (plural), zoonosis (singular)**
Those diseases and infections which are naturally transmitted between vertebrate animals and man. Also called zoonotic disorders or diseases.

**zoophobia**
Fear of animals.

**zoopsia**
A hallucination of animals.

**ZPG**
Zero Population Growth. See these words.

**zygote**
The fertilized reproductive egg.

**zymology**
The science and study of yeasts and fermentation.

# APPENDICES

**Appendix I**

## FORMULAS FOR CALCULATION OF VITAL STATISTICS RATES

1. CRUDE BIRTH RATE:

$$\frac{\text{Number of live births reported during a given year}}{\text{Estimated population as of July 1 of the same year}} \times 1000$$

2. SPECIFIC BIRTH RATE:

$$\frac{\text{Number of live births to women of a specific age reported during a given year}}{\text{Estimated female population of the same age as of July 1 of the same year}} \times 1000$$

3. CRUDE DEATH RATE:

$$\frac{\text{Number of deaths reported during a given year}}{\text{Estimated population as of July 1 of the same year}} \times 1000$$

4. MORTALITY RATE FOR A SPECIFIC DISEASE:

$$\frac{\text{Deaths assigned to the specific cause during a given year}}{\text{Estimated population as of July 1 of the given year}} \times 1000$$

5. INFANT MORTALITY RATE:

$$\frac{\text{Number of deaths under 1 year of age reported during a given year}}{\text{Number of live births reported during the same year}} \times 1000$$

6. NEONATAL MORTALITY RATE:

$$\frac{\text{Number of deaths under 28 days of age reported during a given year}}{\text{Number of live births reported during the same year}} \times 1000$$

7. MATERNAL MORTALITY RATE:

$$\frac{\text{Number of deaths assigned to causes related to pregnancy during a given year}}{\text{Number of live births reported during the same year}} \times 1000$$

8. CASE-FATALITY RATE:

$$\frac{\text{Number of deaths assigned to a specific disease during a given year}}{\text{Number of cases reported of the same disease during the same year}} \times 1000$$

9. PROPORTIONAL MORTALITY RATE:

$$\frac{\text{Number of deaths assigned to a specific cause during a given year}}{\text{Number of deaths reported from all causes during the same year}} \times 1000$$

10. MORBIDITY RATES FOR A SPECIAL DISEASE:

a. Incidence:

$$\frac{\text{Number of new cases of a specific disease reported during a given year}}{\text{Estimated population as of July 1 of the same year}} \times 100{,}000$$

b. Prevalence:

$$\frac{\text{Number of cases present at a given time}}{\text{Estimated population at the same time}} \times 100{,}000$$

**Appendix II**

## ABBREVIATIONS OF MEDICAL DIPLOMATE SPECIALTIES AND FELLOWS OF COLLEGES

### Diplomates in Specialties

| | Abbreviations |
|---|---|
| Diplomate American Board of Anesthesiology | D-A |
| Diplomate American Board of Dermatology | D-D |
| Diplomate American Board of Internal Medicine | D-IM |
| Diplomate American Board of Neurological Surgery | D-NS |
| Diplomate American Board of Opthalmology | D-O |
| Diplomate American Board of Obstetrics and Gynecology | D-OG |
| Diplomate American Board of Orthopedic Surgery | D-OS |
| Diplomate American Board of Pathology | D-PA |
| Diplomate American Board of Preventive Medicine, Inc. | D-PM |
| Diplomate American Board of Physical Medicine and Rehabilitation | D-PMR |
| Diplomate American Board of Psychiatry and Neurology | D-PN |
| Diplomate American Board of Proctology | D-PR |
| Diplomate American Board of Plastic Surgery | D-PS |
| Diplomate American Board of Radiology | D-R |
| Diplomate American Board of Surgery | D-S |
| Diplomate American Board of Urology | D-U |
| Licentiate American Board of Pediatrics | L-P |
| Diplomates certified by National Board of Medical Examiners | N-B |

### Fellows of Specialty Colleges

| | |
|---|---|
| Associate Fellow of American College of Allergists | AFACAL |
| Fellow of American College of Allergists | FACAL |
| Fellow of American College of Angiology | FACA |
| Fellow of American College of Anesthesiologists | FACAn |
| Fellow of American College of Cardiology | FACC |
| Fellow of American College of Chest Physicians | FCCP |
| Fellow of American College of Gastroenterology | FACG |
| Fellow of American College of Hospital Administrators | FACHA |
| Fellow of American College of Nursing Home Administrators | FACNHA |
| Fellow of American College of Obstetricians and Gynecologists | FACOG |
| Fellow of College of American Pathologists | FCAP |
| Fellow of American College of Physicians | FACP |
| Fellow of American College of Preventive Medicine | FACPM |
| Fellow of American College of Radiology | FACR |
| Fellow of American College of Surgeons | FACS |
| Fellow of International College of Surgeons | FICS |

**Appendix III**

## Medical Specialties And Their Abbreviations

| | |
|---|---|
| A | Allergy |
| ANES | Anesthesiology |
| C | Cardiology |
| CD | Cardiovascular Disease |
| CHP | Child Psychiatry |
| CS | Cardiovascular Surgery |
| D | Dermatology |
| DIA-R | Diagnostic Radiology |
| EM | Emergency Medicine |
| END | Endocrinology |
| EP | Emergency Physician |
| FP | Family Practice |
| GE | Gastroenterology |
| GER | Geriatrics |
| GP | General Practice |
| GYN | Gynecology |
| HAd | Hospital Administration |
| HEM | Hematology |
| HS | Hand Surgery |
| I | Internal Medicine |
| IND | Industrial Medicine |
| N | Neurology |
| NEPH | Nephrology |
| NS | Neurological Surgery |
| NM | Nuclear Medicine |
| ObG | Obstetrics |
| OB-GYN | Obstetrics & Gynecology |
| OM | Occupational Medicine |
| Onc | Oncology |
| Oph | Opthalmology |
| Or | Orthopedic Surgery |
| OS | Oral Surgery |
| OTO | Otology, Laryngology, Rhinology |
| P | Psychiatry |
| Path | Pathology |
| Pd | Pediatrics |
| PDS | Pediatric Surgery |
| PH | Public Health |
| Pharm | Pharmacology |
| PL | Plastic surgery |
| PM | Preventive Medicine |
| PMR | Physical Medicine & Rehabilitation |
| PN | Psychiatry & Neurology |
| Pr | Proctology |
| Pul | Pulmonary Diseases |

| | |
|---|---|
| R | Radiology & Roentgenology |
| RHEUM | Rheumatology |
| S | Surgery |
| TR | Therapeutic Radiology |
| TS | Thoracic Surgery |
| U | Urology |
| VS | Vascular Surgery |

Appendix IV

# STATEMENT

## AMERICAN HOSPITAL ASSOCIATION

## A PATIENT'S BILL OF RIGHTS

*The American Hospital Association Board of Trustees' Committee on Health Care for the Disadvantaged, which has been a consistent advocate on behalf of consumers of health care services, developed the* Statement on a Patient's Bill of Rights, *which was approved by the AHA House of Delegates February 6, 1973. The statement was published in several forms, one of which was the S74 leaflet in the Association's S series. The S74 leaflet is now superseded by this reprinting of the statement.*

The American Hospital Association presents a Patient's Bill of Rights with the expectation that observance of these rights will contribute to more effective patient care and greater satisfaction for the patient, his physician, and the hospital organization. Further, the Association presents these rights in the expectation that they will be supported by the hospital on behalf of its patients, as an integral part of the healing process. It is recognized that a personal relationship between the physician and the patient is essential for the provision of proper medical care. The traditional physician-patient relationship takes on a new dimension when care is rendered within an organizational structure. Legal precedent has established that the institution itself also has a responsibility to the patient. It is in recognition of these factors that these rights are affirmed.

1. The patient has the right to considerate and respectful care.

2. The patient has the right to obtain from his physician complete current information concerning his diagnosis, treatment, and prognosis in terms the patient can be reasonably expected to understand. When it is not medically advisable to give such information to the patient, the information should be made available to an appropriate person in his behalf. He has the right to know, by name, the physician responsible for coordinating his care.

3. The patient has the right to receive from his physician information necessary to give informed consent prior to the start of any procedure and/or treatment. Except in emergencies, such information for informed consent should include but not necessarily be limited to the specific procedure and/or treatment, the medically significant risks involved, and the probable duration of incapacitation. Where medically significant alternatives for care or treatment exist, or when the patient requests information concerning medical alternatives, the patient has the right to such information. The patient also has the right to know the name of the person responsible for the procedures and/or treatment.

4. The patient has the right to refuse treatment to the extent permitted by law and to be informed of the medical consequences of his action.

5. The patient has the right to every consideration of his privacy concerning his own medical care program. Case discussion, consultation, examination, and treatment are confidential and should be conducted discreetly. Those not directly involved in his care must have the permission of the patient to be present.

6. The patient has the right to expect that all communications and records pertaining to his care should be treated as confidential.

7. The patient has the right to expect that within its capacity a hospital must make reasonable response to the request of a patient for services. The hospital must provide evaluation, service, and/or referral as indicated by the urgency of the case. When medically permissible, a patient may be transferred to another facility only after he has received complete information and explanation concerning the needs for and alternatives to such a transfer. The institution to which the patient is to be transferred must first have accepted the patient for transfer.

8. The patient has the right to obtain information as to any relationship of his hospital to other health care and educational institutions insofar as his care is concerned. The patient has the right to obtain information as to the existence of any professional relationships among individuals, by name, who are treating him.

9. The patient has the right to be advised if the hospital proposes to engage in or perform human experimentation affecting his care or treatment. The patient has the right to refuse to participate in any such research projects.

10. The patient has the right to expect reasonable continuity of care. He has the right to know in advance what appointment times and physicians are available and where. The patient has the right to expect that the hospital will provide a mechanism whereby he is informed by his physician or a delegate of the physician of the patient's continuing health care requirements following discharge.

11. The patient has the right to examine and receive an explanation of his bill regardless of source of payment.

12. The patient has the right to know what hospital rules and regulations apply to his conduct as a patient.

No catalog of rights can guarantee for the patient the kind of treatment he has a right to expect. A hospital has many functions to perform, including the prevention and treatment of disease, the education of both health professionals and patients, and the conduct of clinical research. All these activities must be conducted with an overriding concern for the patient, and, above all, the recognition of his dignity as a human being. Success in achieving this recognition assures success in the defense of the rights of the patient.

## Appendix V

### Department of Health, Education, and Welfare
### Skilled Nursing Facilities Standards for Certification and Participation in Medicare and Medicaid Programs
### Section 405.1121 — Standard (k) — Patients' Rights
### Effective October 3, 1974

The governing body of the facility establishes written policies regarding the rights and responsibilities of patients and, through the administrator, is responsible for development of, and adherence to, procedures implementing such policies. These policies and procedures are made available to patients, to any guardians, next of kin, sponsoring agency(ies), or representative payees selected pursuant to section 205(j) of the Social Security Act, and Subpart Q of Part 404 of this chapter, and to the public. The staff of the facility is trained and involved in the implementation of these policies and procedures. These patients' rights policies and procedures ensure that, at least, each patient admitted to the facility:

1) Is fully informed, as evidenced by the patient's written acknowledgement, prior to or at the time of admission and during stay, of these rights and of all rules and regulations governing patient conduct and responsibilities;
2) Is fully informed, prior to or at the time of admission and during stay, of services available in the facility, and of related charges including any charges for services not covered under titles XVIII or XIX of the Social Security Act, or not covered by the facility's basic per diem rate;
3) Is fully informed, by a physician, of his medical condition unless medically contraindicated (as documented, by a physician, in his medical record) and is afforded the opportunity to participate in the planning of his medical treatment and to refuse to participate in experimental research;
4) Is transferred or discharged only for medical reasons, or for his welfare or that of other patients, or for non-payment for his stay (except as prohibited by titles XVIII or XIX of the Social Security Act), and is given reasonable advance notice to ensure orderly transfer or discharge, and such actions are documented in his medical record;
5) Is encouraged and assisted, throughout his period of stay, to exercise his rights as a patient and as a citizen, and to this end may voice grievances and recommend changes in policies and services to facility staff and/or to outside representatives of his choice, free from restraint, interference, coercion, discrimination, or reprisal;
6) May manage his personal financial affairs, or is given at least a quarterly accounting of financial transactions made on his behalf

should the facility accept his written delegation of this responsibility to the facility for any period of time in conformance with state law;

7) Is free from mental and physical abuse, and free from chemical and (except in emergencies) physical restraints except as authorized in writing by a physician for a specified and limited period of time, or when necessary to protect the patient from injury to himself or to others;

8) Is assured confidential treatment of is personal and medical records, and may approve or refuse their release to any individual outside the facility, except, in case of his transfer to another health care institution, or as required by law or third-party payment contract;

9) Is treated with consideration, respect, and full recognition of his dignity and individuality, including privacy in treatment and in care for his personal needs;

10) Is not required to perform services for the facility that are not included for therapeutic purposes in his plan of care;

11) May associate and communicate privately with persons of his choice, and send and receive his personal mail unopened, unless medically contraindicated (as documented by his physician in his medical record);

12) May meet with, and participate in activities of social, religious, and community groups at his discretion, unless medically contraindicated (as documented by his medical record);

13) May retain and use his personal clothing and possessions as space permits, unless to do so would infringe upon rights of other patients, and unless medically contraindicated (as documented by his physician in his medical record); and

14) If married, is assured privacy for visits by his/her spouse; if both are inpatients in the facility, they are permitted to share a room, unless medically contraindicated (as documented by the attending physician in the medical record).

All rights and responsibilities specified in paragraphs (k) (1) through (4) of this section—as they pertain to (a) a patient adjudicated incompetent in accordance with state law, (b) a patient who is found, by his physician, to be medically incapable of understanding these rights, or (c) a patient who exhibits a communication barrier—devolve to such patient's guardian, next of kin, sponsoring agency(ies), or representative payee (except when the facility itself is representative payee) selected pursuant to section 205(j) of the Social Security Act and Subpart Q of Part 404 of this chapter.

**Appendix VI**

## VITAL SIGNS OF THE BODY

TEMPERATURE

Normal Body Temperature

Children: 99° F.
Adults: 98.6° F.

Rectal thermometer readings tend to be one-half degree higher than those recorded by mouth thermometers, with temperatures lowest upon rising in the morning. One's temperature may rise as much as one degree toward the end of the day.

### Centigrade and Fahrenheit Comparisons

| | Centrigrade | Fahrenheit |
|---|---|---|
| Normal Body Temperature | 37.0° | 98.6° |

To convert Fahrenheit to Centigrade: subtract 32 and multiply by 5/9.
To convert Centigrade to Fahrenheit: multiply by 9/5 and add 32.

### THE RELATIONSHIP OF TEMPERATURE TO PULSE

An increase of one degree of temperature above 98° F. is approximately equivalent to a rise of 10 beats in pulse rate.

| | | | | | | | | |
|---|---|---|---|---|---|---|---|---|
| Temperature. | 98 F. | corresponds | with | pulse | of | 70 | per | minute. |
| | 99 F. | ,, | ,, | ,, | ,, | 80 | ,, | ,, |
| | 100 F. | ,, | ,, | ,, | ,, | 90 | ,, | ,, |
| | 101 F. | ,, | ,, | ,, | ,, | 100 | ,, | ,, |
| | 102 F. | ,, | ,, | ,, | ,, | 110 | ,, | ,, |
| | 103 F. | ,, | ,, | ,, | ,, | 120 | ,, | ,, |
| | 104 F. | ,, | ,, | ,, | ,, | 130 | ,, | ,, |
| | 105 F. | ,, | ,, | ,, | ,, | 140 | ,, | ,, |

### RESPIRATION: NORMAL BREATHING RATES

| Age | Number of respirations/minute |
|---|---|
| Up to one year | 25 to 35 |
| 12th to 17th year | 20 to 25 |
| Adult | 16 to 18 |

Breathing rates tend to rise with the rate of the pulse.

**Appendix VI (cont.)**

## PULSE RATES

| | Average Beats per Minute |
|---|---|
| The Unborn Child | 140 to 150 |
| Newborn Infants | 130 to 140 |
| During first year | 110 to 130 |
| During second year | 96 to 105 |
| During third year | 86 to 105 |
| 7th to 14th year | 76 to 90 |
| 14th to 21st year | 76 to 85 |
| 21st to 60th year | 70 to 75 |
| After 60th year | 67 to 80 |

Pulse rates normally rise during emotional excitement, following physical exertion or exercise and during digestion.
The pulse rate is generally more rapid in females.
The pulse rate is influenced by the rate of breathing.

## BLOOD PRESSURE

Average Normal Blood Pressure

| Age | Systolic Pressure | Diastolic Pressure |
|---|---|---|
| 10 years | 103 | 70 |
| 15 years | 113 | 75 |
| 20 years | 120 | 80 |
| 25 years | 122 | 81 |
| 30 years | 123 | 82 |
| 35 years | 124 | 83 |
| 40 years | 126 | 84 |
| 45 years | 128 | 85 |
| 50 years | 130 | 86 |
| 55 years | 132 | 87 |
| 60 years | 136 | 89 |

Systolic pressure is the pressure or force with which blood is pumped during the heart's contraction; diastolic pressure is the pressure or force with which blood is pumped during relaxation of the heart.

**Appendix VII**

## GREEK ALPHABET

| | | | | | | | | |
|---|---|---|---|---|---|---|---|---|
| Alpha | Α | α | Iota | Ι | ι | Rho | Ρ | ρ |
| Beta | Β | β | Kappa | Κ | κ | Sigma | Σ | σ |
| Gamma | Γ | γ | Lambda | Λ | λ | Tau | Τ | τ |
| Delta | Δ | δ | Mu | Μ | μ | Upsilon | Υ | υ |
| Epsilon | Ε | ϵ | Nu | Ν | ν | Phi | Φ | ϕ |
| Zeta | Ζ | ζ | Xi | Ξ | ξ | Chi | Χ | χ |
| Eta | Η | η | Omicron | Ο | ο | Psi | ψ | ψ |
| Theta | Θ | θ | Pi | Π | π | Omega | Ω | ω |

**Appendix VIII**

# NUMBERS AND SYMBOLS COMMONLY USED IN CHARTING MEDICAL RECORDS

The following are standard numbers and symbols that are most frequently used.

One $\overline{\text{i}}$

Two $\overline{\text{ii}}$

Three $\overline{\text{iii}}$

Four $\overline{\text{iv}}$

Nine $\overline{\text{ix}}$

Ten $\overline{\text{x}}$

Eleven $\overline{\text{xi}}$

Twelve, etc. $\overline{\text{xii}}$

and et, +, &

greater than >

less than <

dram ʒ

ounce ℥

Five $\overline{\text{v}}$

Six $\overline{\text{vi}}$

Seven $\overline{\text{vii}}$

Eight $\overline{\text{viii}}$

grain gr

one-half $\overline{\text{ss}}$

one and one-half $\overline{\text{iss}}$

three ounces ℥ $\overline{\text{iii}}$

two drams ʒ $\overline{\text{ii}}$

number #, no.

with $\overline{\text{c}}$

without $\overline{\text{s}}$

## Appendix IX

# ABBREVIATIONS USED IN MEDICAL RECORDS

Guidelines for Medical Record Charting Using Abbreviations

Abbreviations used in medical records should be used in a consistent manner. Made-up or personally developed abbreviations have no place in the medical record.

Abbreviations are used in the portions of the medical record least likely to be utilized for legal purposes.

Abbreviations are used to save time and space; however, if a question might arise, the word should be written out.

| | |
|---|---|
| $\bar{a}\bar{a}$ | of each |
| abd | abdomen |
| a.c. | before meals |
| accom | accomodation |
| ACTH | adrenocorticotropic hormone |
| ad | to, up to |
| ad. lib. | as desired |
| adm | admission |
| alb | albumin |
| alk | alkaline |
| A.M. | morning |
| amb | ambulate, ambulatory, walking |
| amp | ampule |
| amt | amount |
| ant | anterior |
| A-P | anterior-posterior |
| APC | aspirin, phenacetin, caffeine |
| approx | approximately, about |
| ASA | acetasalicylic acid (aspirin) |
| ASHD | arteriosclerotic heart disease |
| A.V. node | atrioventricular node |
| ax | axillary, armpit |
| BCG | bacillus Calmette-Guerin (tuberculosis vaccine) |
| b.i.d. | twice a day |
| bisp | bispinous or interspinous diameter (pelvic measure) |
| B.M. | bowel movement |
| BMR | basal metabolic rate |
| B.P. | blood pressure |
| BPH | benign prostatic hyperplasia |
| BRP | bathroom privileges |
| $\underline{C}$ | centrigrade |
| $\bar{c}$ | with |
| $C_1$, $C_2$ (etc) | first cervical vertebra, second cervical vertebra (etc) |

APPENDIX IX

| | |
|---|---|
| Ca | calcium |
| CA | cancer; carcinoma |
| cap | capsule |
| cath | catheter; catheterized |
| C.C. | chief complaint |
| cc | cubic centimeter |
| CCU | coronary care unit |
| CD | communicable disease |
| CHF | congestive heart failure |
| CHO or carbo | carbohydrate |
| Cl | chloride |
| cm | centimeter |
| cmp | compound |
| CNS | central nervous system |
| $CO_2$ | carbon dioxide |
| c/o | complains of |
| COLD | chronic obstructive lung disease |
| comp | compound |
| cont | continued; continuous |
| CPR | cardiopulmonary resuscitation |
| C.S. | central service; cesarean section |
| CSF | cerebrospinal fluid |
| CVA | cerebrovascular accident |
| CVP | central venous pressure |
| clysis | hypodermoclysis (fluid under the skin) |
| cysto | cystoscope; cystoscopy |
| | |
| DC | discontinue |
| D.C. | diagonal conjugate (pelvic measurement) |
| D&C | dilatation and curettage |
| diab | diabetic |
| diag | diagnosis |
| diam | diameter |
| disc | discontinue |
| dist. | distilled |
| DNP | do no publish |
| DNS | do now show |
| DOA | dead on arrival |
| Dr | doctor |
| dr | dram |
| D.T.s | delirium tremens |
| D/W | distilled water |
| Dx | diagnosis |
| | |
| ECG | electrocardiogram |
| EDC | expected date of confinement |
| EEG | electrocardiogram |
| EENT | eye, ear, nose and throat |
| EKG | electrocardiogram |

| | |
|---|---|
| elix | elixir |
| EOM | extraocular movement |
| epith | epithelial |
| ER | emergency room |
| et | and |
| etc | and so on |
| exam | examination |
| exp. lap. | exploratory laparotomy |
| expir | expiration or expiratory |
| ext | extract or external |
| | |
| F | Fahrenheit |
| F. cath. | Foley catheter |
| Fe | iron |
| F.H. | family history |
| FHS | fatal heart sound |
| fl, fld | fluid |
| fract | fracture |
| ft | feet |
| | |
| G in W or glyc. in W | glycerin in water |
| gal | gallon |
| G.B. | gallbaldder |
| G.C. | gonorrhea |
| G.I. | gastrointestinal |
| Gm, gm | gram |
| gr | grain |
| Grav.I, Grav.II, (etc) | primigravida, secundigravida (etc) |
| gt | drop |
| gtt | drops |
| G.U. | genitourinary |
| gyn | gynecology |
| | |
| H or (H) | hypodermic |
| h | hour |
| H et H or H&H | hemoglobin and hematocrit |
| H&P | history and physical |
| Hb or Hgb | hemoglobin |
| HCl | hydrochloric acid |
| Hct | hematocrit |
| Hg | mercury |
| Hgb | hemoglobin |
| hi-cal | high calorie |
| hi-vit | high vitamin |
| $H_2O$ | water |
| $H_2O_2$ | hydrogen peroxide |
| HOB | head of bed |
| hosp | hospital |
| hr | hour |

| | |
|---|---|
| h.s. | hour of sleep; bedtime |
| ht | height |
| | |
| I | iodine |
| ICU | intensive care unit |
| I&D | incision and drainage |
| IICU | infant intensive care unit |
| I.M. | intramuscular |
| inspir | inspiration or inspiratory |
| inter | between |
| invol | involuntary, without knowledge |
| I&O | intake and output |
| IPPB | intermittent positive pressure breathing |
| irrig | irrigate |
| iss | one and one-half |
| I.T. | inhalation therapy or intertubenous (pelvic measurement) |
| I.V. | intravenous (within the vein) |
| | |
| K | potassium |
| Kg | kilogram |
| $KMnO_4$ | potassium permanganate |
| | |
| L | liter |
| L or lt | left |
| $L_1$, $L_2$, $L_3$ (etc) | first lumbar vertebra, second lumbar vertebra, third lumbar vertebra (etc) |
| lab | laboratory |
| lap | laparotomy |
| lat | lateral |
| lb | pound |
| lg | large |
| liq | liquid |
| LLL | left lower lobe (lung) |
| LLQ | left lower quadrant (left lower section of abdomen) |
| LMP | last menstrual period |
| L.P. | lumbar puncture |
| L.R. | lactated Ringer's (I.V. solution) |
| LUL | left upper lobe (lung) |
| LUQ | left upper quadrant (left upper section of abdomen) |
| L&W | living and well |
| | |
| M | male, meter, minum |
| max | maximum |
| mcg | microgram |
| med | medicine, medical |
| mEq | milliequivalent |
| mg | magnesium |
| mid | middle |
| mg, mgm | milligram |

| | |
|---|---|
| M.I. | myocardial infarction |
| min | minute or minimum |
| ml | milliliter |
| mm | millimeter |
| Mn | manganese |
| mo | month |
| M.S. | morphine sulphate; multiple sclerosis |
| N | normal; nitrogen |
| Na | sodium |
| N.B. | newborn |
| neg | negative |
| neuro | neurology, neurological |
| no. | number |
| noc., noct | nocturnal (night) |
| non. rep. | do not repeat |
| NPN | non protein nitrogen |
| NPO | nothing by mouth |
| N.S. | neurosurgery |
| N/S | normal saline |
| N&V | nausea and vomiting |
| ‘o’ | orally |
| $O_2$ | oxygen |
| $O_2$ cap | oxygen capacity |
| $O_2$ sat | oxygen saturation |
| obs or OB | obstetrics |
| O.C. | obstetrical conjugate (pelvic measurement) |
| occ | occasional |
| occ. th. | occupational therapy |
| o.d. | daily |
| O.D. | right eye |
| oint | ointment |
| op | operation |
| ophth | ophthalmology |
| o.pt. | outpatient |
| opt | optimal |
| O.R. | operating room |
| ortho | orthopedic |
| O.S. | left eye |
| O.T. | occupational therapy |
| oto | otology |
| O.U. | both eyes |
| oz | ounce |
| P | pulse; potassium |
| $\bar{p}$ | after or post |
| P-A | posterior-anterior |
| palp | palpable |
| PAR | post anesthesia recovery |

| | |
|---|---|
| Para I, Para II (etc) | primipara, secundipara (etc) |
| paracent | paracentesis |
| path | pathology |
| p.c. | after meals |
| P.E. | physical education |
| pedi, peds | pediatrics |
| per | by or through |
| percuss. & ausc. | percussion and ausculation |
| PKU | phenylketonuria |
| P.H. | past history |
| pH | hydrogen concentration |
| P.I. | present illness |
| PID | pelvic inflammatory disease |
| P.M. | afternoon |
| PMP | previous menstrual period |
| PNP | pediatric nurse practitioner |
| P.O. | phone order |
| p.o. | per os (by mouth) |
| poplit | popliteal |
| pos | positive |
| post-op | postoperative |
| prep | preparation |
| pre-op | preoperative |
| PRN | whenever necessary |
| prog | prognosis |
| prot | protein |
| psych | psychology; psychiatric |
| pt | patient; pint |
| P.T. | physical therapy |
| pulv | powder |
| PZI | protamine zinc insulin |
| | |
| q | every |
| qd | every day |
| q.i.d. | four times a day |
| qh | every hour |
| q2H, q3H, (etc) | every 2 hours, every 3 hours (etc) |
| q.o.d. | every other day |
| q.n. | every night |
| q.n.s. | quantity not sufficient |
| q.s. | quantity or quantitative |
| qt | quart |
| quant | quantity or quantitative |
| | |
| R or resp | respiratory or respiration |
| RBC | red blood count |
| req | request or requisition |
| RHF | right heart failure |
| RLL | right lower lobe (lung) |
| RLQ | right lower quadrant (right lower section of abdomen) |

| | |
|---|---|
| RML | right middle lobe (lung) |
| ROM | range of motion |
| rt | right |
| rt'd | returned |
| RUL | right upper lobe (lung) |
| RUQ | right upper quadrant (right upper section of abdomen) |
| Rx | therapy or treatment |
| $\bar{s}$ | without |
| SAD | sugar and acetone determination |
| S.A. node | sinus atrial node |
| S.C. | subcutaneous |
| SCIV | subclavian intravenous |
| scop | scopolamine |
| S.H. | social history |
| sig | wirte or label |
| sm | small |
| SMR | submucous resection |
| sod. bicarb | sodium bicarbonate |
| sol | solution |
| SOS | may be repeated once if urgently required |
| spec | specimen |
| sp. fl. | spinal fluid |
| sp. gr. | specific gravity |
| SS | soap suds |
| ss enema | soap suds enema |
| ss | one half |
| Staph | Staphylococcus |
| stat | immediately, once only, at once |
| stillb | stillbirth |
| Strep | Streptococcus |
| subcu | subcutaneous |
| subling | sublingual (under the tongue) |
| surg | surgery; surgical |
| sympt | symptom |
| syr | syrup |
| T | temperature |
| T&A | tonsillectomy and adenoidectomy |
| tab | tablet |
| TAT | tetanus antitoxin |
| Tb | tubercle bacillus |
| Tbc | tuberculosis |
| tbsp | tablespoon |
| temp | temperature |
| t.i.d. | three times a day |
| tinct | tincture |
| T.L. | tubal ligation; team leader |
| TLC | tender loving care; total lung capacity |
| TLV | total lung volume |

| | |
|---|---|
| TPR | temperature, pulse, respiration |
| tr | tincture |
| trach | tracheostomy |
| tsp | teaspoon |
| TUR | transurethral resection |
| | |
| U | unit |
| U.A. | urinalysis |
| ung | ointment |
| URI | upper respiratory infection |
| urol | urology; urological |
| | |
| vag | vaginal |
| V.C. | vital capacity |
| V.D. | venereal disease |
| V.I. | volume index |
| via | by the way of |
| vit | vitamin |
| vit. cap. | vital capacity |
| V.O. | verbal orders |
| vol | volume |
| V.S. | vital signs |
| | |
| WBC | white blood cells, white blood count |
| wd | well-developed |
| wn | well-nourished |
| wt | weight |

## Appendix X

### Abbreviations Used in Charting in Medical Laboratories

| | |
|---|---|
| acid p'tase | acid phosphatase |
| AFB | acid fast bacillus |
| A-G | albumin-globulin ratio |
| alk | alkaline |
| alk p'tase | alkaline phosphatase |
| ANA | antinuclear antibody (test for Lupus erythematosus) |
| ASO or ASTO | antistreptolysin |
| baso | basophile |
| bili | bilirubin |
| bl. cult. | blood culture |
| Bl. time | bleeding time |
| Br | bromide |
| BSP | bromosulphalein |
| BUN | blood urea nitrogen |
| C | carbon |
| Ca | calcium |
| CBC | complete blood count |
| ceph. floc. | cephalin flocculation test |
| chol | cholesterol |
| chol. est. | cholesterol ester |
| CI | color index |
| Cl | chloride |
| CPK | creative phosphokinase |
| $CO_2$ | carbon dioxide |
| coag. time | coagulation time |
| creat | creatinine |
| CRPA | C-reactive protein antiserum |
| diff | differential count |
| eos | eosinophils |
| FBS | fasting blood sugar |
| Fe | iron |
| fib | fibrinogen |
| glob | globulin |
| gluc | glucose |
| Gm O/O | grams per hundred milliliters of serum or blood |
| Hct. | hematocrit |
| Hgb or Hb | hemoglobin |
| h.p.f. | per high powered field (used only in describing urine sediments) |

## APPENDIX X

| | |
|---|---|
| I | iodine |
| ict. ind. | icterus index |
| LDH | lactic dehydrogenase |
| L.E. cell | lupus erythematosus cell |
| lymph | lymphocytes |
| MCH | mean corpuscular hemoglobin |
| MCV | mean corpuscular volume |
| mg O/O | milligrams per hundred milliliters of serum or blood |
| mono | monocytes |
| $NH_3N$ | ammonia nitrogen |
| NPN | non protein nitrogen |
| PBI | protein bound iodine |
| $pCO_2$ | partial pressure of carbon dioxide |
| pH | hydrogen concentration |
| PKU | phenylketonuria |
| $PO_4$ | inorganic phosphorus |
| polys | polymorphonuclear leukocytes |
| pro. time | prothrombin time |
| PSP | phenolsulfonphthalein |
| RBC | red blood count |
| sed. rate | sedimentation rate |
| SGOT | serum glutamic oxaloacetic transaminase |
| SGPT | serum glutamic pyruvic transaminase |
| SMA-12 | sequential multiple analysis of 12 chemistry constituents |
| STS | serologic test for syphilis |
| $T_3$ test | triiodothyronine test |
| TGT | thromboplastin generation time |
| TPI | treponema pallidum immobilization test |
| U.A. | urinalysis |
| VDRL | flocculation test |
| WBC | white blood count |
| Zn | zinc |

## Appendix XI

### Abbreviations Used in Charting in Radiography

| | |
|---|---|
| ABD | ABDOMEN |
| AC JOINTS | Acromioclavicular joints |
| AP | Anterior posterior |
| BE | Barium enema |
| BA. BE. | Barium enema |
| BA. SWALLOW | Barium swallow (esophagram) |
| BI LAT | Bilateral |
| BPD | Biparietal diameter |
| CA | Cancer (carcinoma) |
| CHF | Congestive heart failure |
| CLAV | Clavicle |
| COPD | Chronic obstructive pulmonary disease |
| C/S | With and without contrast |
| CS | Central supply |
| C SPINE | Cervical spine |
| CXR | Chest x-ray |
| DIP | Distal interphalangeal |
| ER | Emergency room |
| FU | Follow up |
| GB | Gall bladder series |
| GI | Gastro-intestinal |
| HYSTERO | Hysterosalpingogram |
| IV | Intravenous |
| IVA | Ivac intravenous monitor |
| IVP | Intravenous pyelogram |
| KUB | Kidney, ureter, bladder (one view ABD) |
| LAT | Lateral |
| L SPINE | Lumbar spine |
| LS SPINE | Lumbar sacral spine |
| LSP | Lumbar spine |
| LUQ | Left upper quadrant |
| LUQ | Lower upper quadrant |
| MIF | Myocardial infarction |
| MISC | Miscellaneous |
| MP JOINTS | Metacarpal joints |

APPENDIX XI

| | |
|---|---|
| MVA | Motor vehicle accident |
| | |
| NB | Newborn |
| NMI | No middle initial |
| | |
| OP | Out patient |
| OR | Operating room |
| O2 | Oxygen |
| | |
| PEDS | Pediatrics |
| PORT | Portable |
| PP | Post partum |
| PREOP | Preoperative |
| POST OP | Post operative |
| PROM | Premature rupture of membrane |
| PULM | Pulmonary |
| | |
| R/O | Rule out |
| RUQ | Right upper quadrant |
| RLQ | Right lower quadrant |
| | |
| SI JOINTS | Sacral iliac joints |
| SOB | Short of breath |
| SM BOWEL | Small bowel |
| SONO | Sonogram |
| | |
| T SPINE | Thoracic spine |
| | |
| UGI | Upper gastrointestinal series |
| UNI LAT | Unilateral |
| US | Ultrasound |
| | |
| X-TABLE | Cross table |

## Appendix XII

# MEDICATIONS AND TREATMENTS: ABBREVIATIONS AND LATIN DERIVATIONS

| Abbreviation | Explanation | Latin word |
|---|---|---|
| a.c. | before meals | ante cibum |
| ad lib. | freely, as desired | ad libitum |
| agit. | shake, stir | agita |
| aq. | water | aqua |
| aq. dest. | distilled water | aqua destillata |
| b.i.d. | twice a day | bis in die |
| c̄ | with | cum |
| cap. | capsule | capsula |
| comp. | compound | compositus |
| dil. | dissolve, dilute | dilatus |
| elix. | elixir | elixir |
| h. | an hour | hora |
| h.s. | at bedtime | hora somni |
| M. or m. | mix | misce |
| no. | number | numerus |
| non rep. | do not repeat | non repatatur |
| OS or o.l. | left eye | oculus sinister or laevus |
| OD | right eye | oculus dexter |
| o.u. | each eye | oculus uterque |
| p.c. | after meals | post cibum |
| p.o. | by mouth | per os |
| p.r.n. | when needed | pro re nata |
| q. | every | quaque |
| q.d. | every day | quaque die |
| q.a.m. (o.m.) | every morning | quaque ante meridiem |
| q.h. (qlh.oh) | every hour | quaque omni hora (omni hora) |
| q.2h. | every 2 hours | quaque 2 hora |
| q.3h | every 3 hours | quaque 3 hora |
| q.4h | every 4 hours | quaque 4 hora |
| q.6h | every 6 hours | quaque 6 hora |
| q.h.s. (.n.) | every night | quaque hora somni (omni nocte) |
| q.i.d. | four times a day | quater in die |

| | | |
|---|---|---|
| q.o.d. | every other day | |
| q.s. | sufficient quantity | quantum satis |
| rept. | may be repeated | repetatur |
| Rx | take | recipe |
| s̄ | without | sine |
| Sig. or S. | label | signa |
| s.o.s. | if it is needed | si opus sit |
| ss | a half | semis |
| stat. | at once | statim |
| sup. or supp. | suppository | |
| susp. | suspension | |
| t.i.d. | three times a day | ter in die |
| tr. or tinct. | tincture | tinctura |

## Appendix XIII

# WEIGHT EQUIVALENTS: METRIC AND APOTHECARIES'

| Metric | Apothecaries' |
|---|---|
| 0.1 mg | 1/600 grain |
| 1.12 mg | 1/500 grain |
| 0.15 mg | 1/400 grain |
| 0.2 mg | 1/300 grain |
| 0.25 mg | 1/250 grain |
| 0.3 mg | 1/200 grain |
| 0.4 mg | 1/150 grain |
| 0.5 mg | 1/120 grain |
| 0.6 mg | 1/100 grain |
| 0.8 mg | 1/80 grain |
| 1 mg | 1/60 grain |
| 1.2 mg | 1/50 grain |
| 1.5 mg | 1/40 grain |
| 2 mg | 1/30 grain |
| 3 mg | 1/20 grain |
| 4 mg | 1/15 grain |
| 5 mg | 1/12 grain |
| 6 mg | 1/10 grain |
| 8 mg | 1/8 grain |
| 10 mg | 1/6 grain |
| 12 mg | 1/5 grain |
| 15 mg | 1/4 grain |
| 20 mg | 1/3 grain |
| 25 mg | 3/8 grain |
| 30 mg | 1/2 grain |
| 40 mg | 2/3 grain |
| 50 mg | 3/4 grain |
| 60 mg | 1 grain |
| 100 mg (0.1 gm) | 1½ grains |
| 150 mg (0.15 gm) | 2½ grains |
| 200 mg (0.2 gm) | 3 grains |
| 300 mg (0.3 gm) | 5 grains |
| 400 mg (0.4 gm) | 6 grains |
| 500 mg (0.5 gm) | 7½ grains |
| 600 mg (0.6 gm) | 10 grains |
| 1 gram | 15 grains |
| 1.5 gm | 22 grains |
| 2 gm | 30 grains |
| 3 gm | 45 grains |
| 4 gm | 60 grains (1 dram) |
| 5 gm | 75 grains |
| 6 gm | 90 grains |
| 7.5 gm | 120 grains (2 drams) |

APPENDIX XIII

| | |
|---|---|
| 10 gm | 2½ drams |
| 30 gm | 1 ounce (8 drams) |
| 500 gm | 1.1 pounds |
| 1000 gm | 2.2 pounds (1 kilogram) |